Radiologic Science for Technologists

PHYSICS, BIOLOGY, AND PROTECTION

Radiologic Science for Technologists

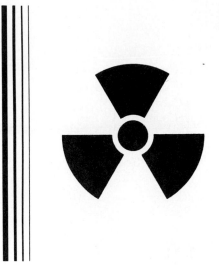

PHYSICS, BIOLOGY, AND PROTECTION

FOURTH EDITION   with 712 illustrations

Stewart C. Bushong, Sc.D.

Professor, Department of Radiology,
Baylor College of Medicine,
Houston, Texas

The C. V. Mosby Company

ST LOUIS • WASHINGTON, D.C. • TORONTO   1988

MOSBY

A TRADITION OF PUBLISHING EXCELLENCE

Editor: David Culverwell
Project manager: Kathleen L. Teal
Production editor: Teresa Breckwoldt
Manuscript editor: Roger McWilliams
Designer: Gail Morey Hudson

Fourth Edition

The C.V. Mosby Company
11830 Westline Industrial Drive, St. Louis, Missouri 63146

Library of Congress Cataloging in Publication Data

Bushong, Stewart C.
  Radiologic science for technologists.

  Includes index.
    1. Diagnosis, Radioscopic.   2.   Radiology, Medical.
3.   Radiation—Safety measures.   4.   Radiobiology.
I.   Title.
RC78.B86   1988
ISBN 0-8016-1532-1   616.07′572   87-34782

GW/D/D/ 9 8 7 6 5 4 3

To

BETTIE,

LESLIE,

STEPHEN,

ANDREW,

BUTTERSCOTCH,†

JEMIMAH,†

GERALDINE,†

CASPER,†

GINGER,†

SEBASTIAN,†

BUFFY,†

BRIE,†

and EBONEY

†R.I.P.

Preface

This textbook is the outgrowth of a series of annual lectures incorporated into radiologic science courses for students and technologists in the programs of the University of Houston and the Houston Community College. These students receive their clinical training in one of several hospitals and assemble together for much of the didactic instruction. This textbook therefore is designed to meet the needs of students who may be receiving clinical training in a wide spectrum of environments and whose classwork may be presented on several levels of difficulty.

This is not simply a physics textbook but rather a text in radiologic science. Its purpose is to guide the student technologist through material that need not be as difficult as some portray it and to prepare the student as painlessly as possible for ultimate certification as a Registered Technologist. Throughout the book emphasis is placed on the radiation protection aspects of medical x-ray use.

The fundamentals of radiologic science cannot be totally divorced from mathematics, but for the purposes of this textbook little prior mathematic background is required of the student. Mathematic equations are presented in selected segments, but they are always followed by sample problems, which usually have a direct clinical application. Additional problems presented at the end of each chapter are intended for either homework assignments or review sessions. Answers to numeric problems can be found at the end of the book in Appendix F.

The practice and the equipment of diagnostic radiology have remained relatively stable over the past 70 years. Truly great changes during this time can be counted on the fingers of one hand: the Crookes tube, the Potter-Bucky diaphragm, and image intensification, for example.

However, since the publication of the first edition of this textbook in 1975, several truly great and innovative developments have come into routine use in diagnostic radiology: computed tomography, diagnostic ultrasound, digital subtraction angiography, and, most recently, magnetic resonance imaging. These developments have transformed radiology into an imaging science. Several of the newest imaging techniques employ nonionizing radiation, and this also is changing the knowledge requirements of radiologic technologists. Each of these newer imaging modalities is given special treatment in this edition.

A revised edition of the accompanying workbook is also available. It contains worksheets that are complementary to the newly added material in this text. Both the student and the instructor will find the revised edition of the workbook helpful in providing a fuller understanding of the content of the textbook.

In the spring of 1978 Great Britain became the last of the western nations, except the United States, to adopt the International System of Units (SI). This system is essentially what some of us have learned as the MKS system (meters, kilograms, seconds). Although the United States has not formally adopted SI, we are committed to its introduction into our technology. With this system come corresponding units of radiation and radioactivity. The roentgen, the rad, and the rem are being replaced by the coulomb/kilogram (C/kg), the gray (Gy), and the seivert (Sv), respectively. Radioactivity is to be expressed in the unit bequerel (Bq). Consequently, throughout this fourth edition, where there has been reference to units other than SI, the SI equivalent will follow in parentheses. A summary of SI units and the factors necessary to convert from conventional to SI units is given in Table 1-4 of the text.

Additional nomenclature is continually being introduced into diagnostic radiology, and, where appropriate, newer forms are employed in this text. SID (source–to–image receptor distance), PBL (positive beam limitation), linearity, reproducibility, and HU (Hounsfield unit) are examples of some of the new vocabulary. In many instances, when conversion from English to metric is made, the result is rounded off. For example, 40 inches target-to-film distance (TFD) is actually 101.6 cm, but it is identified throughout as being equivalent to 100 cm SID.

For the preparation of this fourth edition, I am indebted to the many readers and users of the earlier editions who submitted suggestions, criticisms, corrections, and compliments. For this edition I enlisted the help of many clinical technologists and educators in hopes of making the text and workbook more consistent with one another and more helpful as educational tools. I believe we succeeded, and for that I am grateful to Pedro D. Balanag, Mount Sinai Medical Center, Miami Beach, Florida; J. Edward Barnes, General Electric Medical Systems, Milwaukee, Wisconsin; Judith Baron, College of Lake County, Grayslake, Illinois; Ronald J. Bohland, St. Charles Hospital, Oregon, Ohio; Gary S. Brink, Mallinckrodt Institute of Radiology, St. Louis, Missouri; Evelyn Burns, Houston Community College, Houston, Texas; Priscilla F. Butler, George Washington University Medical Center, Washington, D.C.; Janet Carey, St. Joseph Hospital, Lorain, Ohio; Quinn B. Carroll, Midland College, Midland, Texas; Victor Ciaravino, University of Texas Health Science Center, San Antonio, Texas; Charles Collins, San Diego Mesa College, San Diego, California; John E. Cullinan, Eastman Kodak, Rochester, New York; Terry R. Eastman, Agfa-Gevaert, Irving, Texas; Dan Finley, Santa Fe, New Mexico; Michele Gable, The Methodist Hospital, Houston, Texas; Mary M. Gerald, Del Mar College, Corpus Christi, Texas; Buhrmann D. Gilbert, El Paso Community College, El Paso, Texas; Daniel Hagan, El Paso Community College, El Paso, Texas; Steven Hayes, Midwestern State University, Wichita Falls, Texas; Jim Heck, Angelina College, Lufkin, Texas; Joleen A. Herrmann, St. Joseph

Medical Center, Wichita, Kansas; Trudi James-Parks, Lorain Community College, Elyria, Ohio; Manfred Kratzat, Phillips Medical Systems, Shelton, Connecticut; Robert A. Luke, Boise State University, Boise, Idaho; Margaret Matczynski, Mount Sinai Medical Center, Miami, Florida; Mary Moore, Cooper Hospital/University, Camden, New Jersey; C. William Mulkey, Midlands Technical College, Columbia, South Carolina; Carolyn Nicholas, Baptist Hospital, Beaumont, Texas; Don Nichols, University of Oklahoma Health Science Center, Oklahoma City, Oklahoma; Virginia L. Olsen, Lakewood Community College, White Bear Lake, Minnesota; Patricia R. Paris, Del Mar College, Corpus Christi, Texas; Linda Parsell, Phillips Medical Systems, Houston, Texas; Ruth Reinhart, Parkview Memorial Hospital, Fort Wayne, Indiana; Alan M. Rosich, Lorain Community College, Elyria, Ohio; Cheryl Ross, Hazel Hawkins Hospital, Hollister, California; Bette A. Schans, Swedish Medical Center, Denver, Colorado; Diana L. Shatraw, Aims Community College, Greeley, Colorado; Linda Shields, El Paso Community College, El Paso, Texas; Michele Smith, Northern Ohio Imaging Center, Elyria, Ohio; Gary D. Stevens, Kaskaskia College, Centralia, Illinois; Dwayne J. TerMaat, St. Louis Community College, St. Louis, Missouri; Christi Thompson, El Paso Community College, El Paso, Texas; James A. Wasseen, Medical College of Virginia, Richmond, Virginia; Allen West, University of Alabama at Birmingham, Birmingham, Alabama; Ezell Westbrook, University of District of Columbia, Washington, D.C.; and Randy Whitmore, San Jacinto Junior College, Pasadena, Texas.

I am also deeply indebted to my associates Sharon Glaze, Benjamin Archer, and Nicholas Schneider, who have assisted me with this revision. The illustrations are the product of Kraig Emmert, Spencer Phippen, Ann Sparks, and Angela Dinnean. Their caricatures and cartoons help considerably in easing any pain associated with physics. I am also particularly indebted to Jo Ann Dinnean, Bettie McCoy, and Elaine Casey for the many times they had to struggle through my handwritten notes, my slurred dictation, and the unfamiliar symbols and equations. I appreciate their conscientious approach in preparing the final manuscript.

Finally, I would invite users of this fourth edition to let me know if you have additional changes or comments. Our common goal, of course, is to enhance the level of professionalism within the radiologic community by elevating the educational standards as painlessly as possible.

"Physics Is Fun" is the motto of my radiologic science courses, and I believe this text will help make it enjoyable for the student technologist. Then we can all join together to **legalize physics.**

Stewart C. Bushong

Contents

1

Concepts
of
radiation

NATURE OF OUR SURROUNDINGS

In a physical analysis, all things visible and invisible can be classified as matter or energy.

Matter is anything that occupies space and has form or shape. It is the material substance of which physical objects are composed. All matter, basically, is composed of fundamental building blocks called atoms, arranged in various complex ways. These atomic arrangements will be considered at greater length in Chapter 3.

A primary, distinguishing characteristic of matter is **mass,** the quantity of matter contained in any physical object. We generally use the term "weight" when describing the mass of an object, and for our purposes we may consider mass and weight to be the same, although they are not in the strictest sense. Mass is actually described by its energy equivalence, whereas weight is the force exerted by a body under the influence of gravity.

For example, we know that a 200 lb (91 kg) man will "tip the scales" more easily than a 120 lb (55 kg) woman. This occurs because of the mutual attraction, called the force of gravity, between the earth's mass and the mass of people. On the moon these same people would weigh only about one sixth what they weigh on earth because the mass of the moon is much less than that of the earth. The masses of the people remain unchanged at 91 kg and 55 kg, respectively. The kilogram is the scientific unit of mass and is unrelated to gravitational effects. The prefix **kilo** stands for 1000; a kilogram (kg) is equal to 1000 g.

Although mass, the quantity of matter, remains unchanged regardless of its surroundings, it can be transformed from one size, shape, and form to another. Consider a 1 kg block of ice. Its shape changes as the block of ice melts into a puddle of water. If the puddle is allowed to dry, the water apparently disappears entirely. We know, however, that the ice is transformed

1

from a solid state to a liquid state, and that liquid water becomes water vapor suspended in the air. If we could gather all the molecules making up the ice, the water, and the water vapor and measure their masses, we would find that each form has the same mass.

Energy is the ability to do work. Like matter, energy can exist in several forms:

Potential energy is the ability to do work by virtue of position. A heavy guillotine blade held 20 ft (6.1 m) in the air by a rope and pulley is an example of an object that possesses potential energy (Fig. 1-1). If the rope is cut, the blade will descend and do its ghastly task. Work was required to get the blade to its high position, and because of this position, the blade is said to possess

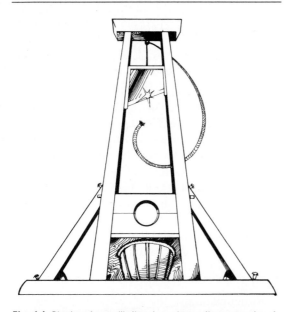

Fig. 1-1. Blade of a guillotine is a dramatic example of both potential and kinetic energy. When the blade has been pulled to its maximum height and locked in place, its position gives it the potential, or ability, to do work when the blade lock is removed. This situation represents potential energy. During the short time that the blade falls, energy is released in the form of kinetic energy.

potential energy. Other examples of objects that possess potential energy include a roller coaster on top of a hill and the stretched spring of an open screen door.

Kinetic energy is the energy of motion. It is possessed by all matter in motion—a moving automobile, a turning windmill wheel, a falling guillotine blade. These systems can all do work because of their motion.

Chemical energy is the energy released by way of a chemical reaction. An important example of this type of energy is the energy provided to our bodies through chemical reactions involving the food we eat. At the molecular level this area of science is called **biochemistry.** The energy released when a stick of dynamite explodes is a more dramatic example of chemical energy.

Electrical energy represents the work that can be done when an electron or an electronic charge moves through an electric potential. The most familiar form of electrical energy is normal household electricity, which involves the movement of electrons through a copper wire under an electric potential of about 110 volts (V). All electric apparatus, such as motors, heaters, and blowers, function through the use of electrical energy.

Thermal (heat) energy is the energy of motion at the atomic or molecular level and in this regard may be viewed as the kinetic energy of atoms. Thermal energy is measured by temperature. The faster the atoms and molecules of a substance are moving, the more heat energy the substance contains, and the higher its temperature.

Nuclear energy is the energy contained in the nucleus of an atom. We control the release and use of this type of energy in nuclear electric-power–generating plants. An example of the uncontrolled release of nuclear energy is the atomic bomb.

Electromagnetic energy, perhaps the least familiar of these forms, is the most important for our purposes because it is the type of energy in an x ray. For the time being electromagnetic energy will be described as an electric and magnetic (electromagnetic) disturbance traveling through space at the speed of light. In addition to x rays, electromagnetic energy includes radio waves, microwaves, and visible light.

Just as matter can be transformed from one size, shape, and form to another, so energy can be transformed from one type to another. In radiology, for example, electrical energy in the x-ray machine is used to produce electromagnetic energy (the x ray), which then is converted to chemical energy in the radiographic film.

Reconsider now the statement that all things can be classified as matter or energy. Look around you and think of absolutely anything, and you should be convinced of this statement. You should be able to classify anything as matter, energy, or both. Frequently matter and energy exist side by side. A moving automobile has mass and kinetic energy. Boiling water has mass and thermal energy. The Leaning Tower of Pisa has mass and potential energy.

Perhaps the strangest property associated with matter and energy is their interchangeability of form, a characteristic first predicted by Albert Einstein in his famous theory of relativity. Einstein's **mass-energy equivalence** equation is a cornerstone of that theory.

(1-1)

$$E = mc^2$$

where E is energy; m, mass; and c, the speed of light.

This mass-energy equivalence is the basis for the atomic bomb, nuclear power plants, and nuclear medicine. As we shall see later, it also has some relevance to radiology.

Energy emitted and transferred through matter is called **radiation.** When a piano string vibrates, it is said to radiate sound; the sound is a form of radiation. Ripples, or waves, radiate from the point where a pebble is dropped into a still pond. Visible light, a form of electromagnetic energy, is radiated by the sun and often is called **electromagnetic radiation.** In fact, electromagnetic energy usually is referred to as electromagnetic radiation, or simply, **radiation.**

Matter that intercepts radiation and absorbs part or all of it is said to be **exposed** or **irradiated.** When one spends a day at the beach, one is exposed to ultraviolet light, and that exposure may result in a sunburn. During a radiographic examination, the patient is exposed to x rays, or, as some would say, the patient is irradiated.

Ionizing radiation is a special type of radiation that includes x rays. Ionizing radiation is any kind of radiation capable of removing an orbital electron from an atom with which it interacts. Fig. 1-2 depicts this type of interaction between radiation and matter, called **ionization.** Ionization occurs when incident ionizing radiation, on passing through matter, passes close enough to an orbital electron of a target atom to transfer sufficient energy to the electron to remove it from the atom. The ionizing radiation may interact with and ionize additional atoms. The orbital electron and the atom from which it was

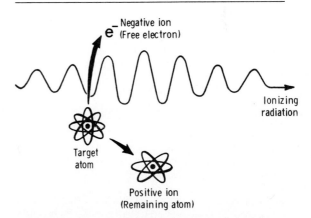

Fig. 1-2. Ionization is the process whereby an electron is removed from a target atom. Ionizing radiation interacts with the orbital electrons of the target atom, ejecting one from the atom. The ejected electron and the resulting positively charged atom are called an ion pair.

separated are called an **ion pair;** the electron is a negative ion, and the remaining atom is a positive ion.

Thus any type of energy or matter-energy combination capable of ionizing matter is known as ionizing radiation. X rays and gamma rays are the only electromagnetic radiation with sufficient energy to ionize matter. Some fast-moving particles (particles with high kinetic energy) are also capable of ionization. Examples of particle-type ionizing radiation are alpha and beta particles. Although alpha and beta radiations are sometimes called rays, such designation is a misnomer because they are particles.

SOURCES OF IONIZING RADIATION

Many types of radiation are harmless, but ionizing radiation can severely injure humans. We are exposed to many sources of ionizing radiation (Table 1-1). One source is **natural environmental radiation,** which results in an annual dose of approximately 100 mrad (1 mGy). An mrad (millirad) is ¹⁄₁₀₀₀ of a **rad.** The rad is the unit of radiation absorbed dose; it is used to express the quantity of radiation absorbed by humans. The approximate annual dose resulting from medical

applications of ionizing radiation is 90 mrad (0.90 mGy). Unlike the natural radiation dose, this level takes into account those persons not receiving an x-ray examination and those receiving several within the period of a year. The medical radiation exposure for some segments of our population will be zero, but for others it may be quite high. Although this average level is comparable to natural radiation levels, it is actually a rather small amount of radiation. One could question, therefore, why it is necessary to be concerned with radiation control and radiation safety in radiology.

Remember, however, that humans have existed on the earth for approximately 100,000 years in the presence of this natural background radiation level. Human evolution and the development of the environment undoubtedly have been influenced by this natural radiation. Some geneticists contend that evolution is influenced primarily by ionizing radiation. If this is so, then we must indeed be concerned with control of unnecessary radiation exposure because over the last 90 years, with the increasing medical applications of radiation, the average annual exposure of our population to radiation has nearly doubled. It is necessary to institute proper radiation-control measures now, since later it may be too late.

Medically employed x rays constitute the largest source of man-made ionizing radiation. The benefits derived from the application of x rays in medicine are indisputable; however, such applications must be made with prudence and with regard to reducing unnecessary exposure of patients and personnel. This responsibility falls primarily on the radiologic technologist, since the technologist usually controls the operation of the x-ray machine during radiologic examination.

Other sources of man-made radiation include nuclear power generation, nuclear weapons testing, industrial sources, and consumer items. At the height of atmospheric nuclear weapons testing in the early 1960s, fallout contributed approximately 5 mrad/yr to our radiation dose.

Table 1-1. Estimated average annual whole-body radiation doses (mrad) in the United States from natural and man-made sources

Radiation source	Annual dose
Natural	
Cosmic rays	39
External terrestrial, principally from ^{226,228}Ra, ^{220,222}Rn, ^{14}C	35
Internal radionuclides, principally ^{40}K	26
Subtotal	100
Man-made	
Fallout	1
Diagnostic x rays	80
Radiopharmaceuticals	10
Miscellaneous	4
Subtotal	95
TOTAL	195

Now it is less than 1 mrad. Nuclear power stations and other industrial applications contribute insignificantly to our radiation exposure. Consumer products such as watch dials, exit signs, smoke detectors, television receivers, camping lantern mantles, and airport surveillance systems contribute a few mrad to our annual radiation dose.

DISCOVERY OF X RAYS

X rays were not developed; they were discovered, quite by accident. During the 1870s and 1880s, many university physics laboratories were involved in the investigation of the conduction of **cathode rays,** or electrons, through a large, partially evacuated glass tube known as a **Crookes tube.** Sr. William Crookes was an Englishman from a rather humble background who was a self-taught genius. The tube that bears his name was the forerunner of modern fluorescent lamps and neon sign–type lamps. Fig. 1-3 is a rendering of the type of Crookes tube with which Wilhelm Roentgen was experimenting when he discovered x rays. There were many different types of Crookes tubes; the majority of them were capable of producing x rays.

On November 8, 1895, Roentgen was working in his laboratory at Würzburg University in Germany. He had darkened his laboratory and completely enclosed his Crookes tube with black photographic paper so that he could better visualize the effects of the cathode rays in the tube. A plate coated with barium platinocyanide, a fluorescent material, happened to be lying on a bench top several feet from the Crookes tube. No visible light escaped from the Crookes tube because of the black paper enclosing it, but Roentgen noted that the barium platinocyanide fluoresced regardless of its distance from the Crookes tube. The intensity of fluorescence increased as the plate was brought closer to the tube; consequently, there was little doubt about the origin of the stimulus for fluorescence. Roentgen's immediate approach to investigating this "X-light," as he called it, was to interpose various materials—wood, aluminum, his hand—between the Crookes tube and the fluorescing plate. He feverishly continued these investigations for several weeks.

There are several amazing features about the discovery of x rays that cause it to rank high in the events of human history. First, the discovery was quite by accident. Second, probably no fewer than a dozen contemporaries of Roentgen had

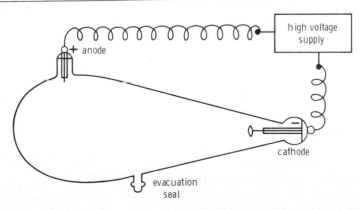

Fig. 1-3. Schematic representation of type of Crookes tube Roentgen was using when he discovered x rays. Cathode rays (electrons) leaving the cathode are attracted to the anode by the high voltage. Many of the cathode rays travel directly to the opposite end of the tube, however, and there x rays and fluorescent light are produced.

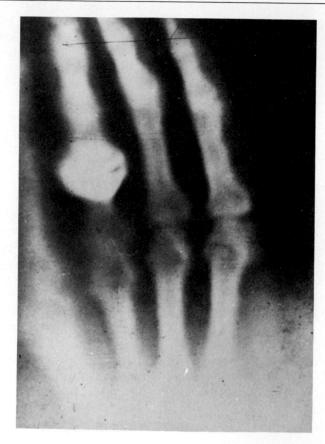

Fig. 1-4. Hand shown in this x-ray film is Mrs. Roentgen's. This was the first indication of the possible future medical applications of x rays and was made within a few days of their discovery. (Courtesy Deutsches Roentgen-Museum.)

previously observed x-radiation, but none of these other physicists had recognized its significance or investigated it. Third, Roentgen followed his discovery with such scientific vigor that within little more than a month he had ascribed to x-radiation nearly all the properties recognized today. His initial investigation was extremely thorough, and he was able to report his experimental results to the scientific community before the end of 1895. For this work he received in 1901 the first Nobel prize in physics. Finally, Roentgen recognized the value of his discovery to medicine. He produced and published the first medical x-ray, one of his wife's hand (Fig. 1-4).

Fig. 1-5 is a reproduction of a photograph of what is reported to be the first x-ray examination in the United States, conducted in early February, 1896, in the physics laboratory at Dartmouth College.

DEVELOPMENT OF MODERN RADIOLOGY

There are two general types of x-ray procedures: **radiographic** examinations and **fluoroscopic** examinations. Radiographic examinations employ x-ray film and usually an x-ray tube mounted from the ceiling on a track that allows the tube to be moved in any direction. Such

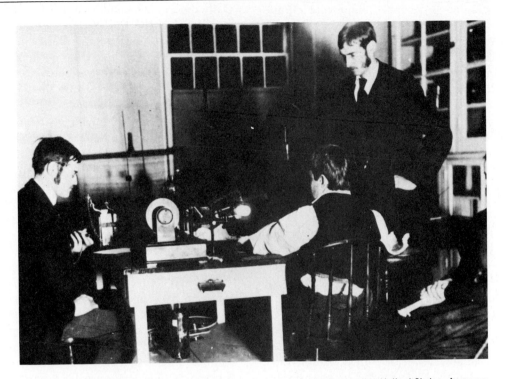

Fig. 1-5. This photograph records the first medical x-ray examination in the United States. A young patient, Eddie McCarthy of Hanover, New Hampshire, broke his wrist while skating on the Connecticut River and submitted to having it photographed by the "X-light." With him are (left to right) Professor E.B. Frost, Dartmouth College; his brother, Dr. G.D. Frost, Medical Director, Mary Hitchcock Hospital; and Mrs. G.D. Frost, the hospital's first head nurse. The apparatus was assembled by Professor F.G. Austin in his physics laboratory in Reed Hall, Dartmouth College, February 3, 1896. (Courtesy Mary Hitchcock Hospital.)

examinations provide the radiologist with fixed photographic images. Fluoroscopic procedures are usually conducted with an x-ray tube located under the examining table. The radiologist is provided with moving, or dynamic, images portrayed on a fluoroscopic screen or television monitor. There are many variations of these two basic types of examinations, but in general the x-ray equipment is similar. Although the x-ray equipment used today is quite sophisticated, there have not been many basic changes since Roentgen's time.

To produce a satisfactory x ray, one must supply the x-ray tube with a high voltage and a sufficient electric current. X-ray voltages are measured in kilovolts peak (**kVp**). One kilovolt (**kV**) is equal to 1000 V of electric potential. X-ray currents are measured in milliamperes (**mA**), where the ampere (**A**) is a measure of electric current. Normal household current is a few amperes. The prefix **kilo** stands for 1000; the prefix **milli**, for 1/1000, or 0.001. Today voltage and current are supplied to an x-ray tube through rather complicated electric circuits, but in Roentgen's time simple static generators were all that were available. These units could only provide currents of a few milliamperes and voltages to perhaps 50 kVp.

Radiographic procedures employing equipment with these limitations of electric current and potential often required exposure times of 30 or more minutes for a satisfactory examination. One development that helped reduce this exposure time was the use of a fluorescent **intensifying screen** in conjunction with the glass photographic plates. Michael Pupin is said to have demonstrated this technique in 1896, but only several years later did it receive adequate recognition and use. Radiographs during Roentgen's time were made by exposing a glass plate with a layer of photographic emulsion coated on one side. Charles L. Leonard found that by exposing two glass x-ray plates with the emulsion surfaces together, exposure time was reduced and the image was considerably enhanced. This demonstration of double emulsion radiography was conducted in 1904, but double emulsion film did not become commercially available until 1918.

During World War I, radiologists began to make use of film rather than glass plates. Much of the high-quality glass used in radiography came from Belgium and other European countries. This supply was interrupted during World War I. The demands of the army for increased radiologic services made a substitute for the glass plate necessary. The substitute base for the photographic emulsion was **cellulose nitrate.** It quickly became apparent that the substitute was better than the original.

The **fluoroscope** was developed in 1898 by the American inventor Thomas A. Edison. Edison's original fluorescent material was barium platinocyanide, a widely used laboratory material. He investigated the fluorescent properties of over 1800 other materials, including zinc cadmium sulfide and calcium tungstate, two materials in use today. There is no telling what further inventions Edison might have developed had he continued his x-ray research, but he abandoned it when his assistant and long-time friend, Clarence Dally, suffered a severe x-ray burn that eventually required amputation of both arms.

Dally died in 1904 and is counted as the first x-ray fatality in the United States.

Two devices designed to reduce the exposure of patients to x rays and thereby minimize the possibility of x-ray burn were introduced before the turn of the century by a Boston dentist, Dr. William Rollins. Dr. Rollins used x rays to visualize teeth and found that restricting the x-ray beam by a diaphragm and inserting a leather or aluminum filter improved the diagnostic quality of his radiographs. This first application of **collimation** and **filtration** was followed very slowly by general adoption of these techniques. It was later recognized that these devices reduce the hazard associated with the application of x rays.

Two developments that occurred at approximately the same time transformed the use of x rays from a novelty in the hands of a few physicians and physicists into a valuable, large-scale medical specialty. In 1907 H.C. Snook introduced a substitute high-voltage power supply, an interrupterless transformer, for the static machine and induction coils then in use. Although the Snook transformer was far superior to these other devices, its capability greatly exceeded the capacity of the Crookes tube. It was not until the introduction of the Coolidge tube that the Snook transformer was widely adopted.

The type of Crookes tube that Roentgen used in 1895 had existed for a number of years. Although some modifications were made by x-ray workers, it remained essentially unchanged into the second decade of the twentieth century. After considerable clinical testing, William D. Coolidge unveiled his hot-cathode x-ray tube to the medical community in 1913. It was immediately recognized as far superior to the Crookes tube. It was a vacuum tube and allowed x-ray intensity and energy to be selected separately and with great accuracy. This had not been possible with gas-filled tubes, which made standards for techniques difficult to obtain. X-ray tubes in use today are refinements of the **Coolidge tube.**

The era of modern radiography is dated from

the matching of the Coolidge tube with the Snook transformer; only then did acceptable levels of kVp and mA become possible. Few developments since that time have had major influence on diagnostic radiology. In 1921 the Potter-Bucky grid, which greatly increased image contrast, was developed. In 1946 the light amplifier tube was demonstrated at the Bell Telephone Laboratories. This device was adapted for fluoroscopy by 1950. Today image-intensified fluoroscopy is commonplace. Table 1-2 chronologically summarizes some of the more important developments.

REPORTS OF RADIATION INJURY

The first x-ray fatality in the United States occurred in 1904. Unfortunately, radiation injuries occurred fairly frequently in the early years. These injuries usually took the form of skin damage (sometimes severe), loss of hair, and anemia. Physicians and, more commonly, patients were afflicted, primarily because of the long exposure time required for an acceptable radiograph and the low energy of radiation that was available at the time.

By about 1910 these acute injuries began to be controlled as the biologic effects of x-radiation

Table 1-2. Some important dates in the development of modern radiology

Date	Event
1895	Roentgen discovers x rays
1896	First medical applications of x rays in diagnosis and therapy are made.
1900	The American Roentgen Society, the first American radiology organization, is founded.
1901	Roentgen receives the first Nobel Prize in physics.
1905	Einstein introduces his theory of relativity and the famous equation $E = mc^2$.
1907	The Snook interrupterless transformer is introduced.
1913	Bohr theorizes his model of the atom, featuring a nucleus and planetary electrons.
1913	The Coolidge hot-filament x-ray tube is developed.
1916-1918	Cellulose nitrate film base is widely adopted.
1919-1921	Several investigators demonstrate the use of soluble iodine compounds as contrast media.
1920	The American Society of Radiologic Technology is founded.
1921	The Potter-Bucky grid is introduced.
1922	Compton describes the scattering of x rays.
1925	The First International Congress of Radiology is convened in London.
1929	Forssmann demonstrates cardiac catherization . . . on himself!
1929	The rotating anode tube is introduced.
1930	Tomographic devices are shown by several independent investigators.
1937	The International Committee on X-ray and Radium Protection offically defines the roentgen.
1942	Morgan exhibits an electronic phototiming device.
1948	Coltman develops the first fluoroscopic image intensifier.
1951	Multidirectional tomography (Poly Tome) is introduced.
1953	The rad is officially adopted as the unit of absorbed dose.
1956	Xeroradiography is demonstrated.
1957	Automatic film processing is introduced by Eastman Kodak.
1966	Diagnostic ultrasound enters routine use.
1972	Rare-earth radiographic intensifying screens are introduced.
1973	Hounsfield completes development of first computed tomographic (CT) scanner (EMI, Ltd.)
1973	Damadion and Lauterbur produce first magnetic resonance images (MRI).
1979	Mistretta demonstrates digital fluoroscopy.
1982	Picture archiving and communications systems (PACS) become available.
1984	Laser-stimulable phosphors for direct digital radiographs appear.

were scientifically investigated and reported. With the introduction of the Coolidge tube and the Snook transformer, the frequency of reports of injuries to superficial tissues decreased. Years later it was discovered that radiologists were developing blood disorders such as aplastic anemia and leukemia at a much higher rate than other physicians. Because of these observations, protective devices and apparel, such as lead gloves and aprons, were developed for use by radiologists. X-ray workers were routinely observed for any effects of their occupational exposure and were routinely provided with personnel radiation-monitoring devices. This attention to radiation safety in radiology has resulted in the disappearance of reports of any type of radiation effect on x-ray workers. Radiology is now considered a completely safe occupation.

Today the emphasis on radiation control in diagnostic radiology has shifted back to protection of the patient. Current studies suggest that even the low doses of x-radiation employed in routine diagnostic procedures may result in a small incidence of latent harmful effects. It is also well established that the human fetus is highly sensitive to x-radiation early in pregnancy. This sensitivity decreases as the age of the fetus increases. There is growing concern that even low levels of radiation exposure may produce harmful genetic results.

It is hoped that this introduction has emphasized the importance of providing adequate protection for both technologist and patient. As you progress through your training in radiologic technology, you will quickly learn how to operate your x-ray equipment safely, with minimal radiation exposure, by adhering to certain standard techniques and procedures. One caution is in order early in your training. After having worked with x-ray machines for a period of time, you will become so familiar with your work environment that you may become complacent about radiation control. Do not allow yourself to develop this attitude. It can lead to an accidental overexposure.

BASIC RADIATION PROTECTION

Minimizing radiation exposure to technologist and patient is easy if the radiographic and fluoroscopic devices designed for this purpose are recognized and understood. Fig. 1-6 identifies the primary devices of this kind. A brief description of some follows:

Filtration. Metal filters, usually aluminum, are inserted into the x-ray tube housing so that the low-energy x rays emitted by the tube are absorbed before they can reach the patient. These x rays have little diagnostic value.

Collimation. Collimators take many different forms. Blade-type diaphragms, adjustable light-localizing collimators, and cones are the most frequently employed collimating devices. Collimation restricts the useful x-ray beam to that part of the body requiring examination and thereby spares adjacent tissue from unnecessary exposure. Collimation also reduces scatter radiation and thus enhances image contrast.

Intensifying screens. Today most x-ray films are exposed in a cassette with intensifying screens on either side of the film. Examinations conducted with intensifying screens reduce the exposure of the patient to x rays by more than 95% compared with examinations conducted without intensifying screens.

Protective apparel. Lead-impregnated leather or vinyl is used to make aprons and gloves worn by radiologists and technologists during fluoroscopy and some radiographic procedures.

Gonadal shielding. The same lead-impregnated material used in aprons and gloves is used to fabricate gonadal shields. Gonadal shields should be employed with all persons of childbearing age when their gonads are in or near the useful x-ray beam and when use of such shielding will not interfere with the diagnostic value of the examination.

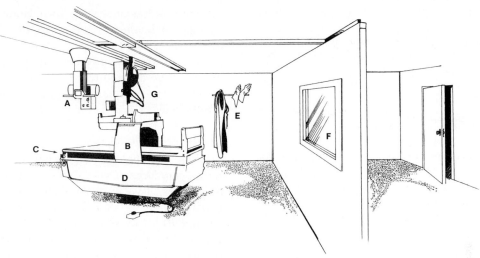

Fig. 1-6. General purpose x-ray room usually includes *(A)* an overhead radiographic tube and *(D)* a fluoroscopic examining table with an x-ray tube under the table. Some of the more common radiation protection devices are *(B)* leaded curtain, *(C)* Bucky slot cover, *(E)* leaded apron and gloves, and *(F)* protective viewing window. The location of the image intensifier *(G)* and associated imaging equipment is also shown.

Protective barriers. The radiographic control console is always located behind a protective barrier. Often the barrier is lead lined and equipped with a leaded glass window. Under normal circumstances personnel remain behind the barrier during radiographic examination.

There are also certain procedures that should be followed. Abdominal films of expectant mothers should never be taken during the first trimester unless absolutely necessary. Every effort should be taken to ensure that an examination will not have to be repeated because of technical error. Repeat examinations subject the patient to twice as much radiation as necessary. When selecting patients for x-ray examination, one should consider the medical management of the patient. In general, examination of asymptomatic patients is not indicated. Patients who require assistance during examination should never be held by x-ray personnel. Usually it is best for a member of the patient's family to pro-

vide the necessary assistance. This person should be given protective apparel and should be carefully instructed before each exposure.

Many aspects of radiation protection will be considered in more detail later. For the time being, the following list should serve as a summary and ready reference of the more important aspects of radiation protection in diagnostic radiology. Chapters 30 and 32 contain a more complete discussion of apparatus, techniques, and legislative guides for the control of unnecessary x-ray exposure.

Ten basic radiation-control principles in diagnostic radiology

1. Understand and apply the cardinal principles of radiation control: time, distance, and shielding.
2. Do not allow familiarity to result in false security.
3. Never stand in the primary beam.
4. Always wear protective apparel when not behind a protective barrier.

5. Always wear a personnel monitoring device and position it outside the protective lead apron on the collar.
6. Never hold a patient during radiographic examination. Use mechanical restraining devices when possible. Otherwise, use parents or friends of the patient or other hospital employees. No other hospital employee should be *routinely* used for this purpose.
7. The person holding the patient must always wear a lead apron and, if possible, lead gloves.
8. Use gonadal shields on all persons within childbearing age when such use will not interfere with the examination.
9. Examination of the pelvis and lower abdomen of women of reproductive capacity should be limited to the 10-day interval following the onset of menstruation. During known pregnancy, these examinations, when appropriate, should be postponed until the conclusion of the pregnancy or at least until its latter half.
10. Always collimate to the smallest field sizes appropriate for the examination.

Table 1-3. Standard scientific and engineering prefixes

Multiple	Prefix	Symbol
10^{18}	exa-	E
10^{15}	peta-	P
10^{12}	tera-	T
10^{9}	giga-	G
10^{6}	*mega-	M
10^{3}	*kilo-	k
10^{2}	hecto-	h
10	deka-	da
10^{-1}	deci-	d
10^{-2}	*centi-	c
10^{-3}	*milli-	m
10^{-6}	*micro-	μ
10^{-9}	nano-	n
10^{-12}	pico-	p
10^{-15}	femto-	f
10^{-18}	atto-	a

*Prefixes frequently used in radiologic science.

DEFINITIONS

Every profession has its own language. Radiologic technology is no exception. Several words and phrases characteristic of radiologic technology already have been identified; many more will be defined and used throughout this book. For the time being, an introduction to this terminology should be sufficient.

Numeric prefixes

Often in radiologic technology we must describe very large or very small multiples of standard units. Two units, milliamperes and kilovolts peak, have already been dealt with. By writing 70 kVp instead of a 70,000 volts peak, we can understandably express the same quantity with fewer characters. For such economy of expression, scientists have devised a system of prefixes and symbols (Table 1-3).

EXAMPLE: How many kilovolts are 37,000 V?
ANSWER: $37,000 \text{ V} = 37 \times 10^3 \text{ V}$
$$= 37 \text{ kV}$$

EXAMPLE: The diameter of a blood cell is about 10 μm (micrometers). How many meters is that?
ANSWER: $10 \ \mu\text{m} = 10 \times 10^{-6} \text{ m}$
$$= 10^{-5} \text{ m}$$
$$= 0.00001 \text{ m}$$

Radiologic units

Five units are used to measure radiation. They should become a familiar part of your vocabulary. Fig. 1-7 relates four of them to a hypothetical situation in which they would be used. Table 1-4 shows the relationship of the customary radiologic units to their SI equivalents.

Roentgen (R) (C/kg). The roentgen is the unit of radiation exposure or intensity. It is equal to the radiation intensity that will create 2.08×10^9 ion pairs in a cubic centimeter of air; that is, $1 \text{ R} = 2.08 \times 10^9$ ion pairs/cm³. The official definition, however, is in terms of electric

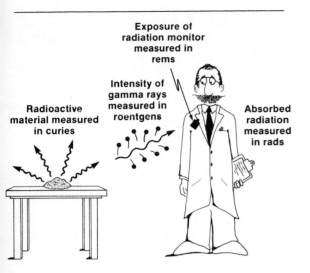

Fig. 1-7. Radiation is emitted by radioactive material. The quantity of radioactive material is measured in curies. Radiation quantity is specified in roentgens, rads, or rems, depending on the conditions under which it is measured and the use of the measurement. In diagnostic radiology we may consider 1 roentgen equal to 1 rad equal to 1 rem.

charge per unit mass of air (1 R $= 2.58 \times 10^{-4}$ C/kg). The charge refers to the electrons liberated by ionization. The roentgen was first defined as a unit of radiation quantity in 1928. Since then, the definition has been revised many times. Radiation measuring instruments usually are calibrated in roentgens. The output of x-ray machines is specified in roentgens or sometimes milliroentgens (mR). The roentgen applies only for x rays and gamma rays and their interactions with air.

Rad (Gy). The rad is the unit of radiation absorbed dose. Biologic effects usually are related to the radiation absorbed dose, and therefore the rad is the unit most often used when describing the radiation quantity received by a patient or an experimental animal. Use of the rad allows quantitation of the amount of ionizing radiation energy transferred by any type of radiation to any target material, not just air. One rad is equal to 100 ergs/g (10^{-2} Gy), where the **erg (joule)** is a unit of energy, and the **gram (kilogram)** is a unit of mass.

Table 1-4. The special quantities of radiologic science and their associated special units

| Quantity | Customary unit | | SI unit | |
	Name	Symbol	Name	Symbol
Exposure	roentgen	R	coulomb per kilogram	C/kg
Absorbed dose	rad	rad	gray	Gy
Dose equivalent	rem	rem	seivert	Sv
Activity	curie	Ci	becquerel	Bq

Multiply number of ____"A"____ by ____"B"____ to obtain number of ____"C"____

Divide number of ____"C"____ by ____"B"____ to obtain number of ____"A"____

A	B	C
R	2.58×10^{-4}	C/kg
rad	0.01	Gy
rem	0.01	Sv
Ci	3.7×10^{10}	Bq

Rem (Sv). Personnel monitoring devices, such as film badges, are analyzed in terms of rems (**rad e**quivalent **man**). The rem is the unit of dose equivalent (**DE**) or occupational exposure. It is used to express the quantity of radiation received by radiation workers. Some types of radiation produce more damage than x rays. The rem accounts for these differences in biologic effectiveness. This is particularly important to persons working near nuclear reactors or particle accelerators.

Curie (Ci) (Bq). The curie is a unit of radioactivity related to the three preceding units of radiation. It is a unit of the quantity of radioactive material and not the radiation emitted by that material. One curie is that quantity of material in which 3.7×10^{10} atoms disintegrate every second (3.7×10^{10} Bq). The millicurie (mCi) and microcurie (μCi) are common quantities of radioactive material.

Electron volt (eV). The energy of an x ray is measured in electron volts or, more often, thousands of electron volts (keV). An electron that is accelerated by an electric potential of one volt will acquire energy equal to eV. One eV is equivalent to 1.6×10^{-19} J. Most x rays used in diagnostic radiology have energy up to 150 keV, whereas those in radiotherapy are measured in MeV. Other radiologically important energies, such as electron and nuclear binding energies and mass-energy equivalence, are also expressed in eV.

• • •

Because diagnostic radiology is concerned primarily with x rays, for our purposes we may consider 1 R equal to 1 rad equal to 1 rem (2.58×10^{-4} C/kg = 0.01 Gy = 0.01 Sv). With other types of ionizing radiation this generalization is not true. Your facility with and understanding of these terms will increase as they are considered individually in various applications.

REVIEW QUESTIONS

1. Define or otherwise identify the following:
   a. Energy
   b. Einstein's mass-energy equivalence equation
   c. Ionizing radiation
   d. The mrad
   e. The average level of background radiation
   f. The Coolidge tube
   g. Fluoroscopy
   h. Collimation
   i. The unit of radioactivity
2. Match the following dates with the appropriate event:

1901	Roentgen discovers x rays
1907	Roentgen wins first Nobel Prize in physics
1913	The Snook transformer is developed
1895	The Coolidge hot-cathode x-ray tube is introduced

3. An x-ray machine is operated at 86 kVp and 200 mA. What is the maximum number of volts across the tube? What is the current through the tube when expressed in amperes?
4. An x-ray photon has 36 keV of energy. What is the photon energy in electron volts?
5. A normal chest x-ray examination exposes the patient to approximately 15 mR (3.87 μC/kg). How many roentgens is that?
6. What is the purpose of filtration?

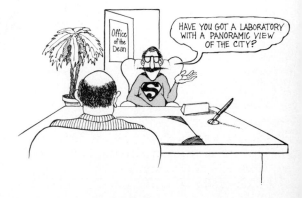

2

Fundamentals
of
physics

REVIEW OF MATHEMATICS
UNITS OF MEASUREMENT
MECHANICS
HEAT

Physics is basically the study of the interactions of matter and energy in all their diverse forms. Like all scientists, physicists strive for exactness or certainty in describing these interactions. Consider, for example, the act of a man kicking a football. If several observers were asked to describe this event, each would give a description based on his or her perception of it. One might describe the stature of the man and his kicking stance. Another might simply conclude that "a man kicked a football about 30 yards." There could be as many different descriptions as observers.

Physicists, however, try to remove uncertainties by eliminating subjective descriptions such as these. A physicist describing this event might determine quantities such as the mass of the football, the initial velocity of the ball, the wind velocity, and the exact distance the football travels. Each of these requires a measurement and ultimately can be represented by a number. As-

suming that all measurements are correctly made, each observer using the methods of physics will obtain exactly the same results.

REVIEW OF MATHEMATICS

Physics owes a great deal of its certainty to the use of mathematics, and accordingly most of the concepts of physics can be expressed mathematically. It is therefore important in the study of radiologic physics to have a solid foundation in the basic concepts of mathematics. The following sections will review fundamental mathematics. You should become proficient at working each type of problem presented in this review.

Fractions

1. Addition and subtraction (require a common denominator)

$$\frac{2}{3} + \frac{4}{5} = \frac{10}{15} + \frac{12}{15} = \frac{22}{15} = 1\frac{7}{15}$$

2. Multiplication

$$\frac{2}{5} \times \frac{7}{4} = \frac{14}{20} = \frac{7}{10}$$

3. Division (invert second term and multiply)

$$\frac{7}{9} \div \frac{3}{5} = \frac{7}{9} \times \frac{5}{3} = \frac{35}{27} = 1\,{}^{8}\!/_{27}$$

$$\frac{1}{2} \div 2 = \frac{1}{2} \times \frac{1}{2} = \frac{1}{4}$$

Decimals

Fractions in which the denominator is a power of ten may easily be converted to decimals.

$$\frac{3}{10} = 0.3 \qquad\qquad \frac{3}{10,000} = 0.0003$$

$$\frac{3}{100} = 0.03 \qquad\qquad \frac{161}{10,000} = 0.0161$$

$$\frac{3}{1000} = 0.003 \qquad\qquad \frac{1527}{10,000} = 0.1527$$

If the denominator is not a power of ten, the decimal equivalent can be found by division.

$$\frac{5}{12} = 12\overline{)5.000} \;\; .41\overline{6}$$

$$
\begin{array}{r}
.41\overline{6} \\
12\overline{)5.000} \\
4\,8 \\
\hline
20 \\
12 \\
\hline
80 \\
72 \\
\hline
80 \\
72 \\
\end{array}
$$

The bar above the 6 indicates that this digit is repeating. When one divides 5.000000 by 12, the answer is $0.41666\overline{6}$.

Significant figures

Most beginning physics students wonder how many decimal places to report in an answer. For example, suppose you were asked to find the area of a circle with a radius of 1.25 cm. Recalling the formula for the area of a circle and substituting yields the following:

$$
\begin{aligned}
A &= \pi r^2 \\
&= (3.14)(1.25 \text{ cm})^2 \\
&= (3.14)(1.5625 \text{ cm}^2) \\
&= 4.90625 \text{ cm}^2
\end{aligned}
$$

However, this answer is unsuitable, since it implies much greater precision in the measurement of the radius than we actually have. This result must be rounded off according to specific rules. **In addition and substraction, round to the same number of decimal places as the entry with the least number of decimal places.**

EXAMPLE:
$$
\begin{array}{r}
5.0631 \\
117.2 \\
21.42 \\
\hline
143.6831
\end{array}
$$
ANSWER: Since 117.2 has one digit, 2, to the right of the decimal point, the answer is 143.7.

In multiplication and division, round to the same number of digits as the entry with the least number of significant figures.

EXAMPLE:
$$
\begin{array}{r}
17.24 \\
\times\ 0.382 \\
\hline
6.58568
\end{array}
$$
ANSWER: Since 0.382 has three significant figures (the zero is not significant) and 17.24 has four, the answer must have three digits. The answer is 6.59.

EXAMPLE: How would you report the area of the circle discussed previously?
ANSWER: 4.91 cm^2

Algebra

Algebraic rules provide definite ways to manipulate equations to solve for unknown quantities. Usually the unknowns are designated by an alphabetic symbol such as **x** or **y.** The following examples illustrate the three principal algebraic rules used in the solutions of problems of diagnostic radiology.

Rule 1: *When an unknown is multiplied by a number, divide both sides of the equation by the number.*

EXAMPLE: Solve the equation $5x = 10$ for x.
ANSWER: $5x = 10$

$$\frac{5x}{5} = \frac{10}{5} \qquad \text{(by \textit{Rule 1})}$$

$$x = 2$$

Rule 2: *When numbers are added to an unknown, subtract that number from both sides of the equation.*

EXAMPLE: Solve the equation $y + 7 = 10$.

ANSWER: $y + 7 - 7 = 10 - 7$ (by *Rule 2*)

$$y = 3$$

Rule 3: *When an equation is presented in fractional form, cross multiply and then solve for the unknown.*

EXAMPLE: Solve the equation $\dfrac{b}{5} = \dfrac{3}{8}$ for b.

ANSWER: The crossed arrows show the direction of cross multiplication:

$$\frac{b}{5} \bowtie \frac{3}{8} \qquad \text{(by Rule 3)}$$

This gives: $8b = 3 \times 5$

$$8b = 15$$

$$\frac{8b}{8} = \frac{15}{8} \qquad \text{(by Rule 1)}$$

$$b = 1\tfrac{7}{8}$$

EXAMPLE: Solve the following for x:

a. $6x + 3 = 15$

b. $\dfrac{4}{x} = \left(\dfrac{3}{4}\right)^2$

c. $ABx + C = D$

ANSWERS:

a.

$$6x + 3 = 15$$
$$6x + 3 - 3 = 15 - 3$$
$$6x = 12$$
$$\frac{6x}{6} = \frac{12}{6}$$
$$x = 2$$

b.

$$\frac{4}{x} = \left(\frac{3}{4}\right)^2$$
$$\frac{4}{x} = \frac{9}{16}$$
$$9x = 64$$
$$\frac{9x}{9} = \frac{64}{9}$$
$$x = 7\tfrac{1}{9}$$

c.

$$ABx + C = D$$
$$ABx + C - C = D - C$$
$$ABx = D - C$$
$$\frac{ABx}{AB} = \frac{D - C}{AB}$$
$$x = \frac{D - C}{AB}$$

Note that examples a and c are nearly identical in form. As we shall see, symbols are often used in physics equations instead of numbers.

Number systems

We use a system of numbers fundamentally composed of multiples of 10, called the number system to the **base 10.** Numbers in this system can be represented in various ways, four of which are shown in Table 2-1. The logarithmic form, although particularly useful in some areas of physics and mathematics, has little application in radiology except in the description of some characteristics of radiographic film.

The superscript on 10 in the exponential form column of Table 2-1 is called the **exponent.** The **exponential form,** often referred to as **power-of-ten notation** or **scientific notation,** is particularly useful in diagnostic radiology. Note that very large and very small numbers are difficult to write in decimal and fractional form. In radiology many numeric quantities are either very large or very small. Scientific notation allows these numbers to be written and manipulated with relative ease.

To express a number in scientific notation, first write the number in decimal form, accurately locating the decimal point. If there are

Table 2-1. Various ways to represent numbers in a number system to the base 10

Fractional form	Decimal form	Exponential form	Logarithmic form
10,000	10,000	10^4	4.000
1000	1000	10^3	3.000
100	100	10^2	2.000
10	10	10^1	1.000
1	1	10^0	0.000
$\frac{1}{10}$	0.1	10^{-1}	-1.000
$\frac{1}{100}$	0.01	10^{-2}	-2.000
$\frac{1}{1000}$	0.001	10^{-3}	-3.000
$\frac{1}{10,000}$	0.0001	10^{-4}	-4.000

digits to the left of the decimal point, the exponent will be positive. To determine the value of this positive exponent, position the decimal point after the first digit and count the number of digits the decimal point was moved. For example, the national debt of the United States is approximately 2100 billion dollars ($2,100,000,000,000.00). To express this in scientific notation, we must position the decimal point after the 1 and count the number of digits it was moved. This indicates that the exponent will be +12.

$$\$2,100,000,000,000.00 = \$2.1 \times 10^{12}$$

If there are no nonzero digits to the left of the decimal point, the exponent will be negative. The value of this negative exponent is found by positioning the decimal point to the right of the first nonzero digit and counting the number of digits the decimal point was moved. For example, a string on Waylon Jennings' guitar has a diameter of 0.00075 m. What is its diameter in scientific notation? First position the decimal point between the 7 and the 5. Next count the number of digits the decimal point has moved, and express this quantity as the negative exponent.

$$0.00075 \text{ m} = 7.5 \times 10^{-4} \text{ m}$$

One common quantity used in physics is a number called **Planck's constant,** symbolized by

h. Planck's constant is related to the energy of an x ray. Its decimal form follows:

h = 0.000000000000000000000000000663 erg-s
h =
0.0000000000000000000000000000000000663
joule-s

Obviously this form is too cumbersome to write each time. Thus Planck's constant is always written in scientific notation:

$$h = 6.63 \times 10^{-27} \text{ erg-s}$$
$$h = 6.63 \times 10^{-34} \text{ joule-s}$$

EXAMPLE: Write the following in scientific notation: 4050, 125, 0.035, ½₀₀₀.

ANSWER: $4050 = 4.05 \times 10^3$
$125 = 1.25 \times 10^2$
$0.035 = 3.5 \times 10^{-2}$
$\frac{1}{2000} = 0.0005 = 5.0 \times 10^{-4}$

Rules for exponents

The primary advantage of handling numbers in exponential form is evident in operations other than addition and subtraction. The general rules for these types of numerical operations are shown in Table 2-2.

The following examples should sufficiently emphasize the principles involved.

EXAMPLE: Simplify the following:
a. $2^3/2^5$
b. $(3 \times 10^{10})^2$
c. $(2.718 \times 10^{-4})^3$
d. $2^3/3^2$

Table 2-2. Rules for handling numbers in exponential form

Operation	Rule	Example
Multiplication	$10^X \times 10^Y = 10^{X+Y}$	$10^2 \times 10^3 = 10^{2+3} = 10^5$
Division	$10^X \div 10^Y = 10^{X-Y}$	$10^6 \div 10^4 = 10^{6-4} = 10^2$
Raising to a power	$(10^X)^Y = 10^{XY}$	$(10^5)^3 = 10^{5 \times 3} = 10^{15}$
Inverse	$10^{-X} = 1/10^X$	$10^{-3} = 1/10^3 = 1/1000$
Unity	$10^0 = 1$	$3.7 \times 10^0 = 3.7$

ANSWER:

a. $2^3/2^5 = 2^{3-5} = 2^{-2} = \frac{1}{2}^2 = \frac{1}{4}$

b. $(3 \times 10^{10})^2 = 3^2 \times (10^{10})^2$
$= 9 \times 10^{20}$

c. $(2.718 \times 10^{-4})^3 = (2.718)^3 \times (10^{-4})^3$
$= 20.08 \times 10^{-12}$
$= 2.008 \times 10^{-11}$

d. $2^3/3^2 = \dfrac{2 \times 2 \times 2}{3 \times 3} = \dfrac{8}{9}$

Note, as the last example indicates, that the rules for exponents apply only when the bases are the same.

EXAMPLE: Given a $= 6.62 \times 10^{-27}$, b $= 3.766 \times 10^{12}$, what is

a. a $\times$ b?

b. a $\div$ b?

ANSWER:

a. a $\times$ b $= 6.62 \times 10^{-27} \times 3.766 \times 10^{12}$
$= (6.62 \times 3.766) \times (10^{-27} \times 10^{12})$
$= 24.931 \times 10^{-27 + 12}$
$= 24.93 \times 10^{-15}$
$= 2.49 \times 10^{-14}$

b. a $\div$ b $= \dfrac{6.62 \times 10^{-27}}{3.766 \times 10^{12}}$

$= \left(\dfrac{6.62}{3.766}\right) \times \left(\dfrac{10^{-27}}{10^{12}}\right)$

$= 1.758 \times 10^{-27 - 12}$
$= 1.76 \times 10^{-39}$

Graphing

Knowledge of graphing is essential to the study of radiologic science. It is important not only to be able to read information from graphs but also to graph data obtained in the laboratory.

Most graphs consist basically of two **axes:** a horizontal, or **x axis,** and a vertical, or **y axis.** The point where the two axes meet is called the **origin** (labeled 0 in Fig. 2-1). Coordinates have the form of **ordered pairs** (x,y), where the first number of the pair represents a distance along the x axis and the second number indicates displacement in the y direction. For example, the ordered pair (3,2) represents a point three units over on the x axis and up two units on the y axis.

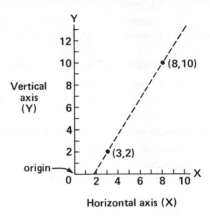

Fig. 2-1. Principal features of any graph are x and y axes that intersect at the origin. Points of data are entered in ordered pairs.

This point is plotted in Fig. 2-1. How does it differ from the point (2,3)? If the value of one additional ordered pair is known, a graph can be constructed.

In physics the axes of graphs are not usually labeled x and y. Generally, the relationship between two specific quantities is desired. Suppose, for example, that you were asked to graphically determine the effect of radiographic milliampere-seconds (mAs) on film density (darkening) given the following data:

mAs	Density
0	0.20
10	0.25
20	0.46
30	0.70
40	0.91
60	1.24
80	1.45
100	1.60

The first step would be to draw the axes on graph paper. In this example the data are recorded in ordered pairs, where mAs represents the x value and density represents the y value. Next, note the range of each quantity and choose a convenient scale that allows the graph to adequately fill the page. Very small graphs should generally be avoided. Then label the axes and carefully plot each point. Finally, draw the best *smooth* curve through the points. The curve need not touch each of the plotted points. A completed graph of the data on p. 19 is shown in Fig. 2-2.

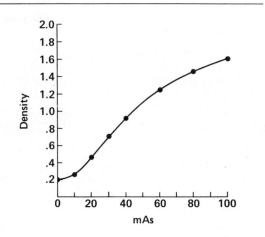

Fig. 2-2. Relationship of film density and mAs from the data presented in the text.

UNITS OF MEASUREMENT

In addition to seeking certainty, physicists strive for simplicity. Thus only three measurable quantities are set aside as the basis or building blocks of all others. These **base quantities** are **mass, length,** and **time.** Fig. 2-3 indicates the role these base quantities play in supporting some of the other quantities used in physics. The secondary quantities are called **derived quantities,** since they are derived from a combination of one or more of the three base quantities. For example, volume is length cubed (1^3), density is mass divided by volume (m/l^3), and velocity is length divided by time (l/t). There are additional quantities designed to support measurement in specialized areas of science and technology. These are called **special quantities;** in radiology the special quantities are those of **exposure, dose, dose equivalent,** and **activity.**

Whether a physicist is studying something large, such as the universe, or a small object, such as an atom, meaningful measurements must be reproducible. Therefore once the fundamental quantities are established, it is essential that they be related to a well-defined and invariable **standard.** Standards are normally defined by international organizations and usually

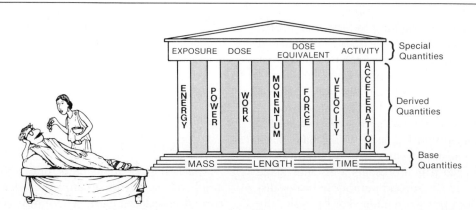

Fig. 2-3. Base quantities support derived quantities, which in turn support the special quantities of radiologic science.

redefined when the progress of science requires greater precision.

Standard of length

For many years the standard unit of length was accepted to be the distance between two lines engraved on a platinum-iridium bar kept at the International Bureau of Weights and Measures in Paris, France. This distance was *defined* to be exactly one **meter (m)**.

The English-speaking countries also base their standards of length on the meter.

$$1 \text{ yd} = 0.9144 \text{ m}$$
$$1 \text{ in} = 2.54 \text{ cm}$$

In 1960 the need for a more accurate standard of length led to the redefinition of the meter in terms of the wavelength of orange light emitted from an isotope of krypton (^{86}Kr). One meter is now defined as $1,650,763.73$ wavelengths of this light.

Standard of mass

In the same vault in Paris where the standard meter is kept, there is a cylinder of platinum-iridium that represents the standard of mass—the **kilogram (kg).** The kilogram was defined to represent the mass of 1000 cm^3 of water at 0° Celsius (C). As discussed in Chapter 1, mass is not the same quantity as weight. The kilogram is a unit of mass, whereas the **newton** or the **pound,** a British unit, is a unit of weight. The differences will be discussed later in this chapter.

Standard of time

The standard unit of time is the **second (s)**. Originally the second was defined in terms of the rotation of the earth on its axis—the mean solar day. In 1956 is was redefined to be a certain fraction of the tropical year 1900. In 1964 the need for a better standard of time led to another redefinition. Now time is measured by an atomic clock and is based on the vibrations of cesium atoms. The atomic clock is capable of keeping time correctly to about 1 second in 5000 years. The accuracy of future hydrogen maser clocks promises to be even greater—perhaps to 1 second in several million years!

Systems of units

Every measurement has two parts: a dimension or magnitude and a unit. For example, this book is 23 cm long. The magnitude, 23, is not meaningful unless a unit is also designated. Here the unit of measurement is the centimeter.

Table 2-3 shows that there are four **systems of units** to represent the base quantities. The MKS (meters, kilograms, seconds) and the CGS (centimeters, grams, and seconds) systems are more widely used in science and in most countries of the world than is the British system. Le Systeme International d'Unités (The International System, SI) is an extension of the MKS system and represents the present state of the art for units. SI includes the three base units of the MKS system plus an additional four. There

---

Table 2-3. Systems of units

	SI*	MKS	CGS	British
Length	Meter (m)	Meter (m)	Centimeter (cm)	Foot (ft)
Mass	Kilogram (kg)	Kilogram (kg)	Gram (g)	Pound (lb)†
Time	Second (s)	Second (s)	Second (s)	Second (s)

*The SI includes four additional base units.
†The pound is actually a unit of force but is related to mass.

are **derived units** and **special units** of SI to represent derived quantities and special quantities. The SI units for the special radiologic quantities (exposure, dose, dose equivalent, and activity) are C/kg, J/kg, J/kg, and s^{-1}, respectively. The latter three special units have special names in SI: the **gray (Gy)**, the **seivert (Sv)**, and the **becquerel (Bq)**.

Rule: *The same system of units must always be used when working problems or reporting answers.*

EXAMPLE: The following answers would be unacceptable because of improper units:

Density $= 8.1$ g/m^3
Pressure $= 700$ lb/cm^2

Density should be reported with units of either grams per cubic centimeter or kilograms per cubic meter, whereas the pressure could be given in terms of pounds per square inch or newtons per square meter.

EXAMPLE: The dimensions of a rectangular box are found to be 30 cm × 86 cm × 4.2 m. Find the volume.
ANSWER: The formula for the volume of a rectangle is given by

$$V = length \times width \times height$$

or

$$V = lwh$$

However, since the dimensions are given in different systems of units, we must choose only one system. Therefore

$$V = (0.30 \text{ m})(0.86 \text{ m})(4.2 \text{ m})$$
$$= 1.1 \text{ m}^3$$

Note that the units are multiplied also: m × m × m = m^3.

EXAMPLE: Find the density of a ball with a volume of 200 cm^3 and a mass of 0.4 kg.

ANSWER: $D = mass/volume$ (change 0.4 kg to
     $= 400$ g/200 cm^3 400 g)
     $= 2$ g/cm^3

MECHANICS

Mechanics is a segment of physics that deals with the motion of objects. Many of the quantities studied in mechanics depend on the direction of motion and are known as vectors. A **vector** is a quantity that has both **magnitude** and **direction.** Quantities that have magnitude only are called **scalars.** A vector description of a distance might be 30 m, North. This distance reported as a scalar would be 30 m.

Velocity

The motion of an object can be described by the use of two terms: **velocity** and **acceleration.** Velocity, sometimes called **speed,** is a measure of how fast something is going or, more precisely, the rate of change of its position with time. You know that the velocity of a car is measured in miles per hour (kilometers per hour). Units of velocity in the metric system are usually meters per second. A defining equation for velocity is

(2-1)

$$v = \frac{d}{t}$$

where d represents the distance traveled in time t.

EXAMPLE: What is the velocity of a ball that travels 60 m in 4 s?
ANSWER: $v = d/t$
     $= 60$ m/4 s
     $= 15$ m/s

Often the velocity of an object changes as its position changes. For example, a dragster running a race starts from rest and finishes with a velocity of 80 m/s. As shown in Fig. 2-4, the **initial velocity** designated by v_o is 0. The **final velocity** represented by v_f is 80 m/s. The **average velocity** can be calculated from the expression

(2-2)

$$\bar{v} = \frac{v_o + v_f}{2}$$

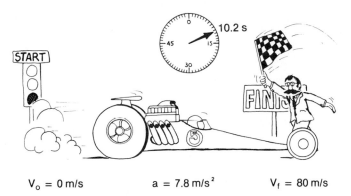

Fig. 2-4. Drag racing provides a familiar example of the relationships between initial velocity, final velocity, acceleration, and time.

where the bar over the v represents average velocity. Substitution gives

$$\bar{v} = \frac{0 \text{ m/s} + 80 \text{ m/s}}{2}$$

$$= 40 \text{ m/s}$$

Acceleration

Acceleration is the rate of change of velocity with time, that is, how "fast" the velocity is changing. Since acceleration is velocity divided by time or a distance divided twice by time, the unit is meters per second squared.

If velocity is constant, the acceleration is zero. On the other hand, constant acceleration of 2 m/s² means that the velocity of an object increases by 2 m/s each second. The defining equation for acceleration is given by

(2-3)

$$a = \frac{v_f - v_o}{t}$$

From the example in Fig. 2-4, the acceleration could be determined.

$$a = \frac{80 \text{ m/s} - 0 \text{ m/s}}{10.2 \text{ s}}$$

$$= 7.8 \text{ m/s}^2$$

Newton's laws of motion

In the year 1686 English mathematician Sir Isaac Newton presented three principles that, even today, are recognized as **fundamental laws of motion.**

Newton's first law states that **a body will remain at rest or continue moving with a constant velocity in a straight line unless acted on by an external force.** This law says in effect that if no force acts on an object, there will be no acceleration. The property of matter that acts to resist a change in its state of motion is called **inertia.** Newton's first law is thus often referred to as the **law of inertia.** Fig. 2-5 illustrates this principle. A portable x-ray machine obviously will not move until forced by a push or motion. However, once in motion it will continue to move forever, even when the pushing force is removed, unless an opposing force is present—friction!

Newton's second law is a definition of the concept of **force.** Force can be thought of as a push or a pull on an object. If a body of mass m has an acceleration a, then **the force on it is given by the mass times the acceleration.** Newton's second law is illustrated in Fig. 2-6. In equation form this law can be expressed as

Newton's 1st Law

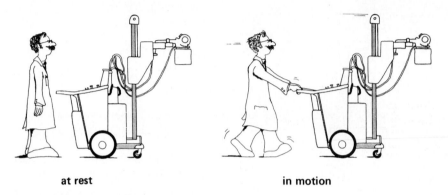

at rest   **in motion**

Fig. 2-5. Newton's first law states that a body at rest will remain at rest and a body in motion will continue in motion until acted on by an outside force.

Newton's 2nd Law

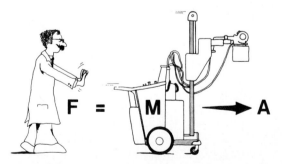

Fig. 2-6. Newton's second law states that the force applied to move an object is equal to the mass of the object times the accelerated movement.

$$(2\text{-}4)$$

$$F = ma$$

The SI unit of force is the **newton (N).** In the CGS system the unit is the **dyne** $(1 \text{ N} = 10^5$ dyne).

EXAMPLE: Find the force on a 55 kg mass accelerated at 14 m/s².

ANSWER: $F = ma$
$$= (55 \text{ kg}) (14 \text{ m/s}^2)$$
$$= 770 \text{ N}$$

Newton's third law of motion states that **to every action there is an equal and opposite reaction.** According to this law, if you push on a heavy block, the block will push back on you with the same force that you apply. If you exert a very large force, the block will begin to accelerate away, continuing to equalize the interaction. On the other hand, if you were the physics professor illustrated in Fig. 2-7, whose crazed students had tricked him into the clamp room, no matter how hard you pushed, the walls would continue to close.

Weight

Weight (Wt) is a **force** on a body caused by the downward pull of gravity on it. Experiments have shown that objects falling to earth accelerate at a constant rate. This rate, termed the acceleration **of gravity** and represented by the symbol **g,** has the following values on earth:

SI g = 9.8 m/s²
CGS g = 980 cm/s²
British g = 32 ft/s²

The value of gravity on the moon is only about one sixth that on the earth. "Weightlessness" observed in outer space is due to the absence of gravity. Thus the value of gravity in space is zero. The weight of an object can be determined from the product of its mass and the acceleration of gravity.

$$(2\text{-}5)$$

$$Wt = mg$$

The units of weight are the same as those for force: newtons and dynes. In the British system, weight is measured in pounds.

EXAMPLE: A student has a mass of 75 kg. What is his weight on earth? In space?

ANSWER:
Earth: $g = 9.8 \text{ m/s}^2$

$$Wt = mg$$
$$= 75 \text{ kg} (9.8 \text{ m/s}^2)$$
$$= 735 \text{ N}$$

Space: $g = 0 \text{ m/s}^2$

$$Wt = mg$$
$$= 75 \text{ kg} (0 \text{ m/s}^2)$$
$$= 0 \text{ N}$$

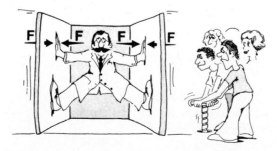

Fig. 2-7. Crazed student technologists performing a routine physics experiment.

This example displays an important concept. The weight of an object can vary according to the value of gravity acting on it. Note, however, that the mass of an object does not change, regardless of its location. The student's 75 kg mass remains the same on the earth, in space, or on other planets.

Momentum

The product of the mass of an object and its velocity is called **momentum,** represented by **p.**

(2-6)

$$p = mv$$

The greater the velocity of an object, the more momentum the object possesses. A truck accelerating down a hill, for example, gains momentum at an ever-increasing rate as its velocity increases.

The **conservation of momentum** is a law stating that **the total momentum before any interaction is equal to the total momentum after the interaction.** To illustrate this principle, imagine a billiard ball colliding with two other balls at rest. The total momentum before the collision is the mass times the velocity of the moving ball. After the collision this momentum is shared by the three balls. Thus the original momentum of the moving ball is conserved after the interaction.

Work

Work, as used in physics, has a specific meaning. The work done on an object is the force applied times the distance over which it is applied. In mathematic terms:

(2-7)

$$Work = Fd$$

The units of work are the joule (J) in SI and the erg in CGS. When you lift a heavy suitcase, you are doing work. However, when the suitcase is merely held motionless, no work (in the physics sense) is being performed, even though considerable effort is being expended.

EXAMPLE: Find the work done in lifting a suitcase weighing 90 N to a height of 3 m.
ANSWER: $Work = Fd$
$$= (90 \text{ N})(3 \text{ m})$$
$$= 270 \text{ J}$$

Power

Power is the rate of doing work. Recall that the same amount of work is required to lift a suitcase to a given height, whether it takes 1 second or 1 year to do so. Power gives us a way to include the time required to perform the work. The defining equation for power is

(2-8)

$$P = Work/t$$

The SI unit of power is the joule/second (J/s), which is called the **watt (W).** The British unit of power is the **horsepower (hp).**

$$1 \text{ hp} = 746 \text{ W}$$
$$1000 \text{ W} = 1 \text{ kilowatt (kW)}$$

EXAMPLE: A technologist lifts a 0.8 kg x-ray film cassette from the floor to the top of a 2 m table with an acceleration of 3 m/s². What is the power exerted if it takes 1.2 s?
ANSWER: This is a multistep problem. We know that $P = work/t$; however, the value of work is not given in the problem. Recall that $work = Fd$, and $F = ma$. First find F:

$$F = ma$$
$$= (0.8 \text{ kg}) (3 \text{ m/s}^2)$$
$$= 2.4 \text{ N}$$

Next find $work$:

$$Work = Fd$$
$$= (2.4 \text{ N}) (2 \text{ m})$$
$$= 4.8 \text{ J}$$

Now P can be determined:

$$P = Work/t$$
$$= 4.8 \text{ J}/1.2 \text{ s}$$
$$= 4 \text{ W}$$

Energy

Energy is the ability to do work. There are many forms of energy, as discussed in Chapter

1. The law of conservation of energy states that **energy may be transformed from one form to another, but it cannot be created or destroyed;** the total energy is constant. For example, electrical energy is converted into light and heat energy in an electric light bulb. The units of energy and work are the same.

There are two forms of **mechanical energy** that are often used in radiologic science.

Kinetic energy (KE) is the energy associated with the motion of an object. From the defining equation

(2-9)

$$KE = \tfrac{1}{2}\, mv^2$$

it is apparent that kinetic energy depends on the mass of the object and on the **square** of its velocity.

EXAMPLE: Consider two cars, A and B, with the same mass. If B has twice the velocity of A, verify that the KE of car B is **four** times that of car A.

ANSWER:

Car A: $KE_A = \tfrac{1}{2}\, m_A v_A^2$
Car B: $KE_B = \tfrac{1}{2}\, m_B v_B^2$
However, $m_A = m_B$, $v_B = 2\, v_A$
therefore $KE_B = \tfrac{1}{2}\, m_A\, (2\, v_A)^2$
$= \tfrac{1}{2}\, m_A\, (4\, v_A^2)$
$KE_B = 2\, m_A v_A^2 = 4\,(\tfrac{1}{2}\, m_A v_A^2) = 4\, KE_A$

Potential energy (PE) is the stored energy of position or configuration. A book on a table has PE because of its height above the earth. It has the ability to do work by falling back to the ground. Gravitational potential energy can be calculated from the equation

(2-10)

$$PE = mgh$$

where h is the distance above the earth's surface.

A coiled spring and a stretched rubber band are examples of other systems that have PE because of their unstable configurations.

If a scientist held a ball in the air atop the Leaning Tower of Pisa, as shown in Fig. 2-8, the ball would have only PE, no KE. When it is

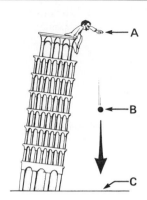

Fig. 2-8. Potential energy results from the position of an object. Kinetic energy is the energy of motion. *A,* Maximum potential energy; no kinetic energy. *B,* Potential energy and kinetic energy. *C,* Maximum kinetic energy; no potential energy.

released and begins to fall, the PE decreases as the height decreases. At the same time the KE is increasing as the velocity increases. Just before impact, the KE of the ball becomes maximum as its velocity reaches maximum. Since it now has no height, the PE becomes zero. All the initial PE of the ball has been converted into KE during the fall.

Table 2-4 presents a summary of the quantities, units, and equations used in mechanics.

HEAT

Heat is a form of energy that is highly important to the radiologic technologist. Excessive heat is a deadly enemy of an x-ray tube and can cause permanent damage. For this reason the student technologist should be aware of properties of heat.

The standard definition of **heat is the random disordered motion of molecules.** The more rapid and disordered the motion, the more heat the body contains. The unit of heat, the **calorie,** is defined as the heat necessary to raise the temperature of 1 g of water 1° C. The same amount of heat will have different effects on different

Table 2-4. Summary of terms used in mechanics

Quantity	Symbol	Defining equation	Units		
			SI	CGS	British
Velocity	v	$v = d/t$	m/s	cm/s	ft/s
Average velocity	$\bar{v}$	$\bar{v} = \dfrac{v_o + v_f}{2}$	m/s	cm/s	ft/s
Acceleration	a	$a = \dfrac{v_f - v_o}{t}$	m/s²	cm/s²	ft/s²
Force	F	$F = ma$	N	dyne	lb
Weight	Wt	$Wt = mg$	N	dyne	lb
Momentum	p	$p = mv$	kg-m/s	g-cm/s	ft-lb/s
Work		$Work = Fd$	J	erg	ft-lb
Power	P	$P = Work/t$	W	erg/s	hp
Kinetic energy	KE	$KE = \frac{1}{2}\,mv^2$	J	erg	ft-lb
Potential energy	PE	$PE = mgh$	J	erg	ft-lb

materials. For example, the heat required to change the temperature of 1 g of silver by 1° C is approximately 0.05 calorie, or only one twentieth that required for a similar temperature change in water.

Heat is transferred from one place to another in three ways:

1. **Conduction** is the transfer of heat by molecular motion from a high temperature. Conduction is easily observed when a hot object and cold object are placed on contact. After a short time heat conducted to the cooler object will result in equalization of temperatures.

2. **Convection** is the mechanical transfer of "hot" molecules in a gas or liquid from one place to another. A steam radiator or a forced-air furnace warms a room by convection. The air around the radiator is heated, causing it to rise, while cooler air circulates in and takes its place. A forced-air furnace blows heated air into the room, providing forced circulation to complement the natural convection.

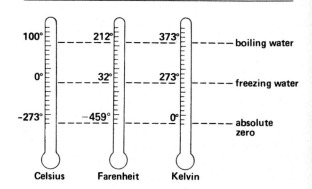

Fig. 2-9. Three principal scales used to represent temperature. Celsius is the universally adopted scale for reporting purposes.

3. **Thermal radiation** is a method of heat transfer that depends on the temperature of the object. The reddish glow emitted by hot objects is evidence of heat transfer by thermal radiation. **An x-ray tube relies primarily on thermal radiation for cooling.**

Temperature is normally measured with a reproducible scale called a **thermometer.** A thermometer is usually calibrated at two reference points: the freezing and boiling points of water. Fig. 2-9 shows the relationship of three scales that have been developed to measure temperature: Fahrenheit (F), Celsius (C), and Kelvin (K).

These scales are interrelated by the following equations, where the subscripts c, f, and k refer to Celsius, Fahrenheit, and Kelvin, respectively.

(2-11)

$$T_c = \tfrac{5}{9}\,(T_f - 32)$$

(2-12)

$$T_f = \tfrac{9}{5}\,T_c + 32$$

(2-13)

$$T_k = T_c + 273$$

EXAMPLE: Convert 77° F to degrees Celsius.

ANSWER: $T_c = \tfrac{5}{9}\,(T_f - 32)$
$= \tfrac{5}{9}\,(77 - 32) = \tfrac{5}{9}\,(45) = 25°\ C$

Magnetic resonance imaging (MRI) with a superconducting magnet requires extremely cold liquids called **cryogens.** Liquid nitrogen, which boils at 77 K, and liquid helium, which boils at 4 K, are the two cryogens most often used.

REVIEW QUESTIONS

1. Define or otherwise identify the following:
   a. Base quantity
   b. Derived quantity
   c. Special quantity
   d. Unit
   e. Inertia
   f. Acceleration
2. Determine your height in the SI system; the CGS system.
3. Discuss the difference between mass and weight.
4. Solve the following:
   a. $\dfrac{7}{8} + \dfrac{5}{32} =$
   b. $1^4/_9 \times {}^3/_8 =$
   c. $\dfrac{16}{2} \div {}^4/_9 =$
5. Write the following as decimals:
   a. $\dfrac{7}{10} =$
   b. ${}^{81}/_{1000} =$
   c. $\dfrac{7}{15} =$
6. Write the following in scientific notation:
   a. 1,480,000
   b. 0.0040
   c. 711,000
7. Solve the following:
   a. $(2 \times 10^6) \times (4 \times 10^4)$
   b. $(8 \times 10^{15}) \div (2 \times 10^5)$
   c. $3x - 9 = 12$
   d. $\dfrac{x}{3} = \dfrac{5}{7}$
8. The mass of an x-ray tube is 12 kg. What is its weight on earth in newtons? How much does it weigh on the moon (g = 1.63 m/s²)?
9. Find the KE of a 4380 N portable x-ray unit moving with a velocity of 6 m/s.
10. Superman weighs 667 N (192 lb) on earth.
    a. What is his mass?
    b. Assume he returned to Krypton, where his weight is 944 N. Find the acceleration of gravity on Krypton.

3

The atom

CENTURIES OF DISCOVERY
Greek atom

One of civilization's most pronounced, continuing scientific investigations has been precisely determining the structure of matter. The earliest recorded reference to this investigation comes from the Greeks, several hundred years before the time of Christ. They thought all matter was composed of four substances: earth, water, air, and fire. According to them, all matter could be described in terms of combinations of various proportions of these four basic substances, modified by four basic essences: wet, dry, hot, and cold. Fig. 3-1 depicts the manner in which this theory of matter was represented at that time.

The Greeks employed the term **atom,** meaning indivisible, to describe the smallest part of the four substances of matter. Each type of atom was represented by a symbol, as shown in Fig. 3-2, A. Today over one hundred substances, or

elements, have been identified; ninety-two are naturally occurring, and an additional fifteen have been artificially produced in high-energy particle accelerators. We have a reasonably clear understanding of the atom, the smallest particle of matter that has the properties of an element and can react chemically. There are many particles much smaller than the atom, called subatomic particles.

Dalton atom

The Greek description of the structure of matter persisted for many hundreds of years. It was the theoretical basis for the vain efforts by medieval alchemists to transform lead into gold. It was not until the nineteenth century that the foundation for modern atomic theory was laid. In 1808 John Dalton, an English schoolteacher, published a book summarizing his experiments, which showed that the elements could be classified according to integral values of atomic

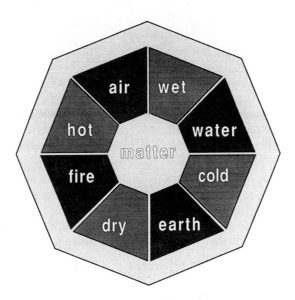

Fig. 3-1. Symbolic representation of the substances and essences of matter as viewed by the ancient Greeks.

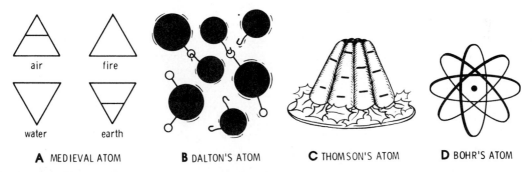

A MEDIEVAL ATOM   **B** DALTON'S ATOM   **C** THOMSON'S ATOM   **D** BOHR'S ATOM

Fig. 3-2. Through the years the atom has been represented by many symbols. Shown here are four symbols of the more significant developments in our knowledge of the atom. **A,** The Greeks envisioned four different atoms, representing air, fire, earth, and water. These symbols were adopted by medieval alchemists. **B,** Dalton's atoms had hooks and eyes to account for chemical combination. **C,** Thomson's model of the atom has been described as a plum pudding, with the plums representing electrons. **D,** The Bohr atom has a small, dense, positively charged nucleus surrounded by electrons in precise energy levels.

Group →

Period	I	II							Transitional Elements							III	IV	V	VI	VII	VIII
	Alkali metals	Alkaline-earth metals																		Halogens	Noble gases
1	1 **H** 1.00797																				2 **He** 4.0026
2	3 **Li** 6.939	4 **Be** 9.0122														5 **B** 10.811	6 **C** 12.01115	7 **N** 14.0067	8 **O** 15.9994	9 **F** 18.9984	10 **Ne** 20.183
3	11 **Na** 22.9898	12 **Mg** 24.312														13 **Al** 26.9815	14 **Si** 28.086	15 **P** 30.9738	16 **S** 32.064	17 **Cl** 35.453	18 **A** 39.948
4	19 **K** 39.102	20 **Ca** 40.08	21 **Sc** 44.956	22 **Ti** 47.90	23 **V** 50.942	24 **Cr** 51.996	25 **Mn** 54.9380	26 **Fe** 55.847	27 **Co** 58.9332	28 **Ni** 58.71	29 **Cu** 63.54	30 **Zn** 65.37				31 **Ga** 69.72	32 **Ge** 72.59	33 **As** 74.9216	34 **Se** 78.96	35 **Br** 79.909	36 **Kr** 83.80
5	37 **Rb** 85.47	38 **Sr** 87.62	39 **Y** 88.905	40 **Zr** 91.22	41 **Nb** 92.906	42 **Mo** 95.94	43 **Tc** [99]*	44 **Ru** 101.07	45 **Rh** 102.905	46 **Pd** 106.4	47 **Ag** 107.870	48 **Cd** 112.40				49 **In** 114.82	50 **Sn** 118.69	51 **Sb** 121.75	52 **Te** 127.60	53 **I** 126.9044	54 **Xe** 131.30
6	55 **Cs** 132.905	56 **Ba** 137.34	★ 57–71	72 **Hf** 178.49	73 **Ta** 180.948	74 **W** 183.85	75 **Re** 186.2	76 **Os** 190.2	77 **Ir** 192.2	78 **Pt** 195.09	79 **Au** 196.967	80 **Hg** 200.59				81 **Tl** 204.37	82 **Pb** 207.19	83 **Bi** 208.980	84 **Po** [210]*	85 **At** [210]*	86 **Rn** [222]*
7	87 **Fr** [223]*	88 **Ra** [226]*	+ 89–103																		

*A value given in brackets denotes the mass number of the most stable known isotope.

★ Rare-earth metals

+ Actinide metals

Fig. 3-3. Periodic table of the elements.

mass. According to Dalton, an element was composed of identical atoms that behaved identically in a chemical reaction. For example, all oxygen atoms were alike. They looked alike; they were constructed alike; and they reacted alike. However, they were very different from atoms of any other element. The physical combination of one type of atom with another was visualized as being an eye-and-hook affair. The size and number of the eyes and hooks were different for each element. Fig. 3-2, *B*, is a schematic view of Dalton's model of the atom.

Some 50 years following Dalton's work a Russian scholar, Dmitri Mendeleev, was credited with showing that if the elements were arranged in order of increasing atomic mass, a periodic repetition of similar chemical properties occurred. At that time about sixty-five elements had been identified. Mendeleev's work resulted in the first periodic table of the elements. Although there were many holes in Mendeleev's table, it showed that all the then-known elements could be placed in one of eight groups.

Fig. 3-3 is a rendering of the modern periodic table of the elements. Each block represents an element. The superscript is the atomic number, and the subscript is the elemental mass. All elements in the same group react chemically in a similar fashion and have similar physical properties. For example, except for hydrogen, the elements of group I, called the alkali metals, are all soft metals that combine readily with oxygen and react violently with water. The elements of group VII, called halogens, are gaseous or easily vaporized and combine with metals to form water-soluble salts. Group VIII elements, called the noble gases, are highly resistant to reaction with other elements. These elemental groupings are determined by electronic configurations, which will be considered more fully later.

Thomson atom

Following the publication of Mendeleev's original periodic table, additional elements were separated and identified, and the periodic table slowly became filled. Our knowledge of the structure of atoms, however, remained scanty. Around the turn of the century, atoms were considered indivisible, the only difference between the atoms of one element and the atoms of another being their mass. Through the efforts of many researchers, it slowly became apparent that there was an electrical nature to the atomic structure of matter. In the late 1890s, while investigating the physical properties of **cathode rays** (electrons), J.J. Thomson concluded that electrons were an integral part of all atoms. He described the atom as looking something like a plum pudding, where the plum represented negative electric charges (electrons), and the pudding was a shapeless mass of uniform positive electrification (Fig. 3-2, *C*). The number of electrons was thought to equal the quantity of positive electrification because the atom was known to be electrically neutral.

Through a series of ingenious experiments, Ernest Rutherford in 1911 disproved Thomson's model of the atom. Rutherford introduced the nuclear model, which described the atom as containing a small, dense, positively charged center surrounded by a negative cloud of randomly located electrons. He called the center of the atom the **nucleus.**

Bohr atom

In 1913 Niels Bohr extended Rutherford's description of the atom. Bohr's model was a miniature solar system in which the orbital electrons revolved about the nucleus in prescribed shells or **energy levels.** Today the Bohr atom (Fig. 3-2, *D*) is accepted as the atomic model most representative of the true nature of matter. Simply put, the Bohr atom contains a small, dense, positively charged nucleus surrounded by negatively charged electrons that revolve in fixed, well-defined orbits about the nucleus. In the normal atom the number of electrons is equal to the number of positive charges in the nucleus.

COMBINATIONS OF ATOMS

Atoms of various elements may combine to form rigid structures called **molecules;** molecules in turn may combine to form even larger structures. For example, two atoms of hydrogen (H_2) and two atoms of oxygen (O_2) can combine to form two molecules of water ($2\ H_2O$). The following chemical equation represents this atomic combination:

$$2H_2 + O_2 \rightarrow 2H_2O$$

An atom of sodium (Na) can combine with an atom of chlorine (Cl) to form a molecule of sodium chloride (NaCl), which is common table salt:

$$Na + Cl \rightarrow NaCl$$

Both these molecules are common in the human body.

Although over 100 different elements are known, most are rather rare. Over 95% of the earth and its atmosphere consists of only a dozen elements. Similarly, oxygen, hydrogen, carbon, and nitrogen compose over 95% of the human body. Water molecules make up about 70% of the mass of the human body.

A measurable quantity of one type of molecule is called a **chemical compound.** The contents of a vial of sodium chloride constitute a chemical compound. Sodium, hydrogen, carbon, and oxygen atoms can combine to form a molecule of sodium bicarbonate ($NaHCO_3$). A measurable quantity of sodium bicarbonate constitutes a chemical compound commonly called baking soda.

The interrelations between atoms, elements, molecules, and compounds should now be clear. The smallest portion of an element is an atom; the smallest portion of a compound is a molecule. This organizational scheme is what the ancient Greeks were trying to describe by their substances and essences. The chart in Fig. 3-4 is a diagram of this orderly modern scheme of matter.

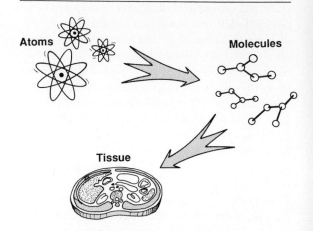

Fig. 3-4. Matter has many levels of organization. Atoms combine to make molecules, and molecules combine to make structures. Atoms are the smallest particle of an element; molecules are the smallest particle of a chemical compound.

MAGNITUDE OF MATTER

From inner space, the atom, to outer space, the universe, an enormous range of size is encompassed. Over forty orders of magnitude, or powers of ten, are needed to measure objects as small as an electron and as large as the universe. Fig. 3-5 depicts some objects and their relative sizes and shows why power-of-ten notation is necessary.

One meter (10^0 m) is about 3 feet. One hundred meters (10^2 m) is about the length of a football field. One centimeter (10^{-2} m) is this long _____. Other prefixes for large and small powers of ten are shown in Table 1-3. The following example should emphasize the value of power-of-ten notation.

EXAMPLE: Measured in English units, the wavelength of a 50 keV x ray is about 0.00000000117 inches. In metric units this is approximately

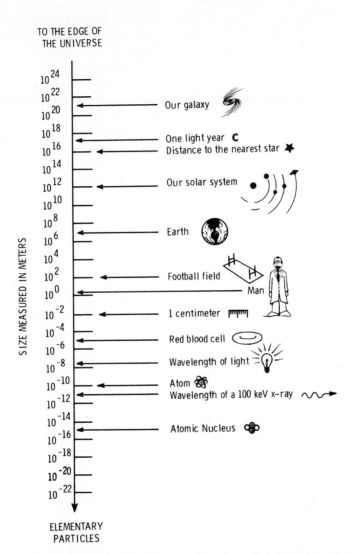

TO THE EDGE OF
THE UNIVERSE

ELEMENTARY
PARTICLES

Fig. 3-5. Matter in our surroundings is composed of objects whose size varies enormously. So wide is the size range that it could hardly be represented with arithmetic nomenclature. Power-of-ten notation is used because over forty orders of magnitude are necessary to encompass the range of matter as we know it.

0.00000000003 m, or 3×10^{-11} m, or 30 pm. A useful calculation in x-ray physics involves dividing the speed of light ($c = 3 \times 10^8$ m/s) by the x-ray wavelength. This results in the x-ray frequency. What is the result of this calculation?

ANSWER:

$$\frac{3 \times 10^8}{0.00000000003} = \frac{300000000}{0.00000000003}$$

$$= 10000000000000000000$$

Using power-of-ten notation:

$$\frac{3 \times 10^8}{30 \times 10^{-12}} = \frac{3}{30} \times 10^{20}$$

$$= \frac{1}{10} \times 10^{20}$$

$$= 10^{-1} \times 10^{20}$$

$$= 10^{19}$$

EXAMPLE: Referring to Fig. 3-5 if necessary, what is the approximate size of
a. An atom?
b. A pencil (length)?
c. The distance from New York to Los Angeles?

ANSWER:
a. Diameter of an atom $\cong 10^{-10}$ m $= 10^{-1}$ nm $= 0.1$ nm
b. Length of a pencil $\cong 6$ in $\cong 15$ cm $= 0.15$ m
c. Distance from New York to Los Angeles $\cong 3000$ miles
   One mile $\cong 1500$ m $= 1.5 \times 10^3$ m
   Thus distance $\cong (1.5 \times 10^3$ m/mile) $\times (3 \times 10^3$ miles) $= 4.5 \times 10^6$ m or 4500 km

FUNDAMENTAL PARTICLES

Our understanding of the atom today is essentially that which Bohr theorized over a half century ago. With the development of high-energy **particle accelerators,** or "atom smashers" as some call them, the structure of the nucleus of an atom is slowly being mapped and identified. Over thirty subatomic particles have been detected and described by physicists working with these machines. However, these particles are of little consequence to radiology. Only the three primary constituents of an atom, the **electron,** the **proton,** and the **neutron,** will be considered here. They are the **fundamental particles.**

The atom can be viewed as a miniature solar system whose sun is the nucleus and whose planets are the electrons. The arrangement of the electrons around the nucleus determines the manner in which atoms interact. Electrons are very small particles carrying one unit of negative electric charge. Their mass is only 9.1×10^{-31} kg. They revolve about the nucleus at nearly the speed of light in precisely fixed orbits, like the planets in our solar system revolve around the sun. Because atomic particles are extremely small, their masses are sometimes expressed in **atomic mass units (amu)** for convenience. One amu is equal to one twelfth the mass of a carbon-12 atom. The electron mass is 0.000549 amu. When preciseness is not necessary, a system of whole numbers called **atomic mass numbers** is employed. The atomic mass number of an electron is 0.

The nucleus contains particles called **nucleons,** of which there are two types: protons and neutrons. Both have nearly 2000 times the

Table 3-1. Important characteristics of the fundamental particles

Particle	Location	Mass Relative	Mass Kilograms	Mass amu	Number	Charge	Symbol
Electron	Shells	1	9.109×10^{-31}	0.000549	0	−1	⊖
Proton	Nucleus	1836	1.673×10^{-27}	1.00728	1	+1	⊕
Neutron	Nucleus	1838	1.675×10^{-27}	1.00867	1	0	◯

mass of an electron. The mass of a proton is 1.673×10^{-27} kg, and the neutron is just slightly heavier at 1.675×10^{-27} kg. The atomic mass number of each is 1. The primary difference between a proton and a neutron is electric charge. The proton carries one unit of positive electric charge. The neutron carries no charge; it is electrically neutral.

Table 3-1 summarizes the more important characteristics of these fundamental particles and includes the symbols employed throughout this text.

ATOMIC STRUCTURE

One might be tempted to visualize the atom as a beehive of subatomic activity, since classical representations of it generally appear like that shown in Fig. 3-2, *D*. Because of the space limitations of the printed page, Fig. 3-2, *D*, is greatly oversimplified. In fact, the atom is mostly empty space, like our solar system. The nucleus of an atom is very small but contains nearly all the mass of the atom.

If a basketball whose diameter is 9.6 in (0.23 m) represented the size of the uranium nucleus, the largest naturally occurring atom, the path of the orbital electrons would take them over 8 miles (12.8 km) away. The size of an electron is approximately equal to the size of the nucleus, and therefore less than 0.001% of the volume of an atom is occupied by matter. The atom is indeed empty space. Since it contains all the neutrons and protons, the nucleus of the atom contains most of its mass. For example, the nucleus of a uranium atom contains 99.998% of the entire mass of the atom.

Atoms of the same element have identical structures and are called **isotopes.** Atoms of different elements differ in the number of nucleons and electrons they contain and in the arrangement of the electrons in shells about the nucleus.

The periodic table of the elements (Fig. 3-3) lists all the elements in order of increasing complexity, beginning with hydrogen (H). An atom of hydrogen contains one proton in its nucleus and one electron outside the nucleus. Helium (He), the second atom in the table, contains two protons, two neutrons, and two electrons. The third atom, lithium (Li), contains three protons, four neutrons, and three electrons. Two of these electrons are in the same orbital shell, the *K* shell, as are the electrons of hydrogen and helium. The third electron is in the next farther shell from the nucleus, the *L* shell. Electrons can exist only in certain **shells,** which represent different **electron binding energies,** or **energy levels.** For identification purposes the electron shells are given the code *K, L, M, N,* . . . to represent the relative binding energies of electrons from closest to the nucleus to farthest from the nucleus, respectively. The closer an electron is to the nucleus, the higher its binding energy.

The next atom on the periodic table, beryllium (Be), has four protons and five neutrons in the nucleus. Two electrons are in the *K* shell, and two are in the *L* shell. The complexity of the electron configuration of atoms increases as one progresses through the periodic table to the most complex naturally occurring element, uranium (U). Uranium has 92 protons and 146 neutrons. The electron distribution is as follows: two in the *K* shell, eight in the *L* shell, eighteen in the *M* shell, thirty-two in the *N* shell, twenty-one in the *O* shell, nine in the *P* shell, and two in the *Q* shell. Fig. 3-6 is a schematic representation of four of these atoms. Although these atoms are mostly empty space, they have been diagramed on one page. If the actual size of the helium nucleus were that in Fig. 3-6, the *K*-shell electrons would be several city blocks away!

Some additional general observations about the structure of the atom are in order. In their normal state, atoms are electrically neutral; that is, the electric charge on the atom is 0, since the total number of electrons in the orbital shells is exactly equal to the number of protons in the nucleus. If an atom has an extra electron or has had an electron removed, it is said to be **ionized.** An ionized atom is not electrically neutral but

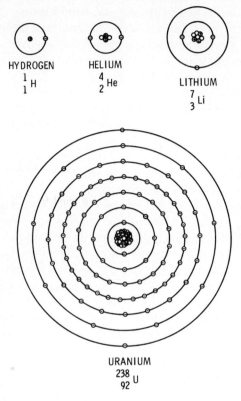

HYDROGEN
$^1_1$H

HELIUM
$^4_2$He

LITHIUM
$^7_3$Li

URANIUM
$^{238}_{92}$U

Fig. 3-6. Atoms are composed of neutrons and protons in the nucleus and electrons in specified orbits surrounding the nucleus. In the normal state of the atom, the number of protons equals the number of electrons. Shown here are the three smallest atoms and the largest naturally occurring atom, uranium.

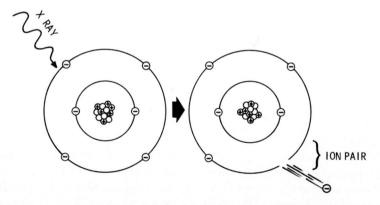

X RAY

ION PAIR

Fig. 3-7. Ionization of a carbon atom by an x ray leaves the atom with a net electric charge of +1. The ionized atom and the released electron are called an ion pair.

carries a charge equal in magnitude to the difference between the number of electrons and protons. One might theorize that atoms could be ionized by changing the number of positive charges as well as the number of negative charges, but atoms are not ionized by the addition or subtraction of a proton, since that type of atomic manipulation changes the atom from one elemental type to another. Similarly, an alteration in the number of neutrons does not ionize an atom, since the neutron is electrically neutral.

Fig. 3-7 represents the interaction between an x ray and a carbon atom, a primary constituent of the human body. The x ray transfers its energy to an orbital electron and ejects that electron from the atom. The x ray may cease to exist, and an ion pair is formed. The remaining atom is a positive ion, since it contains one more positive charge than negative charge.

In all except for the lightest atoms, the number of neutrons is always greater than the number of protons. The larger the atom, the greater the abundance of neutrons over protons. Mendeleev's original periodic table was based on atomic mass. The deviation from sequential mass in this early table was presumed to be caused by inaccurate measurements. The varying neutron/proton ratio of the nucleus accounts for this deviation from sequential mass numbers.

Table 3-2. Maximum number of electrons that can occupy each electron shell

Shell number	Shell symbol	Number of electrons
1	K	2
2	L	8
3	M	18
4	N	32
5	O	50
6	P	72
7	Q	98

Electron arrangement

The maximum number of electrons that can exist in each shell, shown in Table 3-2, increases with distance of the shell from the nucleus. These numbers need not be memorized, since the electron limit per shell can be calculated from the expression

$$(3\text{-}1)$$

$$2n^2$$

where n is the shell number.

EXAMPLE: What is the maximum number of electrons that can exist in the O shell?

ANSWER: The O shell is the fifth shell from the nucleus; therefore

$$n = 5$$
$$2n^2 = 2(5)^2$$
$$= 2(25)$$
$$= 50$$

Physicists call the shell number n the **principal quantum number.** Every electron in every atom can be precisely identified by a set of four quantum numbers, the most important of which is the principal quantum number. The other three quantum numbers represent the existence of subshells, which are unimportant to radiology and need not be considered further.

The observant reader may have noticed a relationship between the number of shells in an atom and its position on the periodic table of the elements. Oxygen has eight electrons; two occupy the K shell, and six occupy the L shell. Oxygen is in the second period and the sixth group of the periodic table (Fig. 3-3). Aluminum has the following electron configuration: K shell, two electrons; L shell, eight electrons; M shell, three electrons. Therefore aluminum is in the third period (M shell) and third group (three electrons) of the periodic table. The general relationship is that the number of the outermost occupied electron shell of an atom is equal to its period in the periodic table, and the number of electrons in the outermost shell is equal to its group.

EXAMPLE: Referring to Fig. 3-3, what are the period and group for barium?

ANSWER: Period 6 and group II.

Why does the periodic table show elements repeating similar chemical properties in groups of eight? In addition to the limitation on the maximum number of electrons allowed in any shell, there is a maximum number of electrons allowed in the outermost shell. **No outer shell can contain more than eight electrons.** All atoms having one electron in the outer shell lie in group I of the periodic table; atoms with two electrons in the outer shell fall in group II; and so on. When eight electrons are in the outer shell, the shell is filled. Atoms with filled outer shells lie in group VIII, the noble gases, and are very stable chemically.

The orderly scheme of atomic progression from smallest to largest atom is interrupted in the fourth period. Instead of a sequential ordering of electrons into the next shell there is some skipping around in filling the two outermost shells. The atoms associated with this phenomenon are called the **transitional elements.** Even in the transitional elements, however, no outer shell ever contains more than eight electrons. The chemical properties of the transitional elements are dependent on the number of electrons in the two outermost shells.

The shell notation of the electron arrangement of an atom not only identifies the relative distance of an electron from the nucleus, but also indicates the relative energy by which the electron is attached to the nucleus. One might expect that an electron would spontaneously fly off from the nucleus, just as a ball twirling on the end of a string does when the string is cut. This type of force is called **centripetal force,** or "center-seeking" force, and results from a basic law of electricity which states that opposite charges attract one another and like charges repel. One might therefore expect that the electrons would drop into the nucleus because of the strong electrostatic attraction. In the normal atom the centripetal force just balances the force created by the electron velocity so that they maintain their distance from the nucleus traveling in a circular or elliptical path. Fig. 3-8 is a representation of this state of affairs for a small atom. In more complex atoms the same balance of force exists, and each electron can be considered separately.

Electron binding energy

The strength of attachment of an electron to the nucleus is called the electron binding energy, usually designated E_b. The closer an electron is to the nucleus, the more tightly it is bound. K-shell electrons have higher binding energies than L-shell electrons, L-shell electrons are more tightly bound to the nucleus than

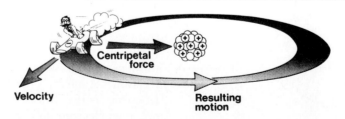

Fig. 3-8. Electrons revolve about the nucleus in fixed orbits, or shells. The electrostatic attraction produces a centripetal force that just matches the force of motion or velocity, resulting in a specific electron path about the nucleus. For a hydrogen atom the path is circular. For more complex atoms various elliptical orbits are possible.

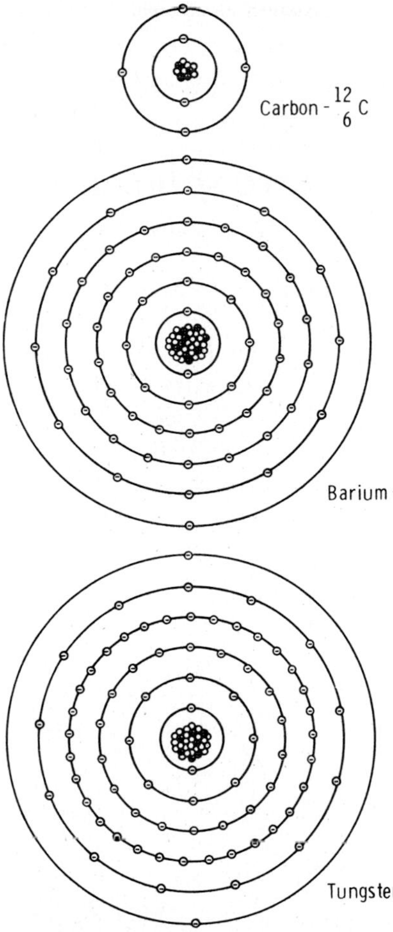

	Shell	Number of Electrons	Approximate Binding Energy (keV)
Carbon – $^{12}_{6}$C	K	2	0.28
	L	4	0.01
Barium – $^{137}_{56}$Ba	K	2	37.44
	L	8	5.99
	M	18	1.29
	N	18	0.25
	O	8	0.04
	P	2	
Tungsten – $^{184}_{74}$W	K	2	69.53
	L	8	12.10
	M	18	2.82
	N	32	0.60
	O	12	0.08
	P	2	

Fig. 3-9. Atomic configurations and approximate electron binding energies for three radiologically important atoms: carbon, barium, and tungsten. In all atoms, inner-shell electrons are more tightly bound than are outer-shell electrons. As atomic complexity increases, electrons in each shell are more tightly bound.

M-shell electrons, and so on. Not all *K*-shell electrons of all atoms are bound with the same binding energy. The greater the total number of electrons in an atom, the more tightly each is bound. To put it differently, the larger and more complex the atom, the higher the E_b for electrons in any given shell. Since electrons of large atoms are more tightly bound to the nucleus than those of small atoms, it takes more energy to ionize a large atom than a small atom.

Fig. 3-9 is a representation of the binding energies of electrons of several atoms of radiologic importance. The metal tungsten (W) is the primary constituent of the target of an x-ray tube. Barium (Ba) is employed extensively as the active ingredient in material used for radiographic and fluoroscopic contrast studies. Carbon (C) is a main and important component of the human body. The following examples refer to Fig. 3-9.

EXAMPLE: How much energy is required to ionize tungsten by removal of a *K*-shell electron?

ANSWER: The minimum energy must equal E_b, or 69.5 keV. A *K*-shell W electron will continue to be bound to the nucleus if energy less than 69.5 keV is transferred to it.

EXAMPLE: How much more energy is necessary to ionize barium than to ionize carbon by removal of *K*-shell electrons?

ANSWER:

$$E_b \text{ (Ba)} = 37,441 \text{ eV}$$
$$E_b \text{ (C)} = \underline{284 \text{ eV}}$$
$$\text{Difference} = 37,157 \text{ eV}$$
$$= 37.2 \text{ keV}$$

ATOMIC NOMENCLATURE

Often an element is indicated by an alphabetic abbreviation. Such abbreviations are called chemical symbols. Table 3-3 lists some of the radiologically more important elements and their chemical symbols. Other properties that will be considered later are also included in the table.

Table 3-3. Characteristics of some radiologically important atoms

Element	Chemical symbol	Atomic number (Z)	Atomic mass number (A)*	Number of naturally occurring isotopes	Elemental mass (amu)†	K-shell electron binding energy (keV)
Beryllium	Be	4	9	1	9.0122	0.111
Carbon	C	6	12	3	12.0111	0.284
Oxygen	O	8	16	3	15.9994	0.532
Aluminum	Al	13	27	1	26.9815	1.560
Calcium	Ca	20	40	6	40.080	4.038
Iron	Fe	26	56	4	55.847	7.112
Copper	Cu	29	63	2	63.546	8.979
Molybdenum	Mo	42	98	7	95.940	20.00
Ruthenium	Ru	44	102	7	101.07	22.12
Silver	Ag	47	107	2	107.868	25.68
Tin	Sn	50	120	10	118.69	29.20
Iodine	I	53	127	1	126.91	33.17
Barium	Ba	56	138	7	137.34	37.44
Tungsten	W	74	184	5	183.85	69.53
Gold	Au	79	197	1	196.97	80.73
Lead	Pb	82	208	4	207.19	88.00
Uranium	U	92	238	3	238.03	115.6

*Most abundant isotope.
†Average of naturally occurring isotopes.

The chemical properties of an element are determined by the number and arrangement of electrons around the nucleus. In the neutral atom the number of electrons equals the number of protons. The number of protons is called the **atomic number,** often represented by Z. Table 3-3 shows that the atomic number of barium is 56, thus indicating that fifty-six protons are in the barium nucleus.

The number of protons plus the number of neutrons in the nucleus of an atom is called the **atomic mass number,** often symbolized by A. As shown in Table 3-3, the atomic mass number is always a whole number. The use of atomic mass numbers is helpful in many areas of radiologic science. It must be understood that the atomic mass number and the precise mass of an atom are not equal. An atom's atomic mass number is a whole number equal to the number of nucleons in the atom. The actual **atomic mass** of an atom is determined by experimental measurements and rarely is a whole number. ^{135}Ba has $A = 135$, since its nucleus contains fifty-six protons and seventy-nine neutrons. The atomic mass of ^{135}Ba is 134.91 amu. Only one atom, ^{12}C, has an atomic mass equal to its atomic mass number. This occurs because the ^{12}C atom is the arbitrary standard for atomic measure.

Many elements in their natural state are composed of various proportions of atoms having different atomic mass numbers and different atomic masses, but identical atomic numbers. The characteristic mass of an element, the **elemental mass,** is determined by the relative abundance of the constituent atoms and their respective atomic masses. Barium, for example, has an atomic number of 56. The atomic mass number of its most abundant atom is 138. However, barium consists of seven different atoms with atomic mass numbers of 130, 132, 134, 135, 136, 137, and 138; the elemental mass is determined by the weighted average of all these atoms. The elemental mass of some of the radiologically important atoms is shown in Table 3-3.

A shorthand symbolic notation that incorporates the chemical symbol with subscripts and superscripts is employed to identify atoms. The chemical symbol (X) is positioned between two subscripts and two superscripts. The subscript and superscript to the left of the chemical symbol represent the atomic number and atomic mass number, respectively. The subscript and superscript to the right are values for the number of atoms per molecule and the valence state of the atom, respectively.

$$_{Z}^{A}X_{\text{Number of atoms}}^{\text{Valence}}$$

In this text we will be concerned only with the scripts to the left of X.

With this nomenclature the atoms identified in Fig. 3-6 would have the following symbolic representation:

$$_{1}^{1}\text{H}, \, _{2}^{4}\text{He}, \, _{3}^{7}\text{Li}, \, _{92}^{238}\text{U}$$

Since the chemical symbol also indicates the atomic number, the subscript is often omitted, as follows:

$$^{1}\text{H}, \, ^{4}\text{He}, \, ^{7}\text{Li}, \, ^{238}\text{U}$$

Atoms that have the same atomic number but different atomic mass numbers are called **isotopes.** Isotopes of a given atom contain a fixed number of protons but varying numbers of neutrons. As Table 3-3 shows, most elements have more than one stable isotope. The seven natural isotopes of barium are as follows:

$$_{56}^{130}\text{Ba}, \, _{56}^{132}\text{Ba}, \, _{56}^{134}\text{Ba}, \, _{56}^{135}\text{Ba}, \, _{56}^{136}\text{Ba}, \, _{56}^{137}\text{Ba}, \, _{56}^{138}\text{Ba}$$

EXAMPLE: How many protons and neutrons are in each of the seven naturally occurring isotopes of barium?

ANSWER: The number of protons in each isotope is 56. The number of neutrons is equal to $A - Z$. Therefore

^{130}Ba:	$130 - 56 =$	74 neutrons
^{132}Ba:	$132 - 56 =$	76 neutrons
^{134}Ba:	$134 - 56 =$	78 neutrons

and so on.

Table 3-4. Characteristics of various nuclear arrangements

Arrangement	Atomic number	Atomic mass number	Neutron number
Isotope	Same	Different	Different
Isobar	Different	Same	Different
Isotone	Different	Different	Same
Isomer	Same	Same	Same

Atomic nuclei that have the same atomic mass number but different atomic numbers are called **isobars.** Isobars are atoms that have different numbers of protons and different numbers of neutrons but the same total number of nucleons.

Atoms that have the same number of neutrons but different numbers of protons are called **isotones.** Isotones are atoms with different atomic numbers and different atomic mass numbers but a constant value for the quantity $A - Z$.

The final category of atomic configuration is the **isomer.** Isomers have the same atomic number and the same atomic mass number. In fact, isomers are identical atoms except that they exist at different energy states because of differences in nucleon arrangement.

Table 3-4 is a summary of the characteristics of these nuclear arrangements.

EXAMPLE: From the following list of atoms pick out those that are isotopes, isobars, and isotones.

$$^{131}_{54}\text{Xe}, \ ^{130}_{53}\text{I}, \ ^{132}_{55}\text{Cs}, \ ^{131}_{53}\text{I}$$

ANSWER: ^{130}I and ^{131}I are isotopes. ^{131}I and ^{131}Xe are isobars. ^{130}I, ^{131}Xe, and ^{132}Cs are isotones.

RADIOACTIVITY

Some atoms have nuclei that contain excess energy. Such an atom exists in an abnormally excited state, characterized by an unstable nucleus. To reach stability, the nucleus spontaneously emits particles and energy and trans-

forms itself into another atom. This process is called **radioactive disintegration** or **radioactive decay.** The atoms involved are **radionuclides.** Any nuclear arrangement is called a **nuclide;** only those nuclei that undergo radioactive decay are radionuclides.

Radioisotopes

Many factors affect nuclear stability. Perhaps the most important is the number of neutrons. When a nucleus contains either too few or too many neutrons, the atom undergoes radioactive decay, the end result being to bring the number of neutrons and protons into a stable and proper ratio. In addition to the stable isotopes that characterize all elements, radioactive isotopes, or **radioisotopes,** also occur. These are usually artificially produced in machines such as particle accelerators or nuclear reactors. Seven radioisotopes of barium have been discovered, all of which are artifically produced. In the following list of barium isotopes, the radioisotopes are in boldface:

$^{127}\textbf{Ba}, \ ^{128}\textbf{Ba}, \ ^{129}\textbf{Ba}, \ ^{130}\text{Ba}, \ ^{131}\textbf{Ba}, \ ^{132}\text{Ba}, \ ^{133}\textbf{Ba},$
$^{134}\text{Ba}, \ ^{135}\text{Ba}, \ ^{136}\text{Ba}, \ ^{137}\text{Ba}, \ ^{138}\text{Ba}, \ ^{139}\textbf{Ba}, \ ^{140}\textbf{Ba}$

Artificially produced radioisotopes have been identified for nearly all elements. A few elements have naturally occurring radioisotopes as well. There are two primary sources of these naturally occurring radioisotopes. Either they were formed at the time of the earth's formation and are decaying very slowly, or they are continuously being produced in the upper atmosphere by the action of cosmic radiation. Table 1-1 identifies the more prominent naturally occurring radioisotopes.

There are many ways by which radioisotopes can decay to stability, but only two, **beta emission** and **alpha emission,** are of particular importance here.

During beta emission, an electron-like particle is ejected from the nucleus with considerable kinetic energy and escapes from the atom. The

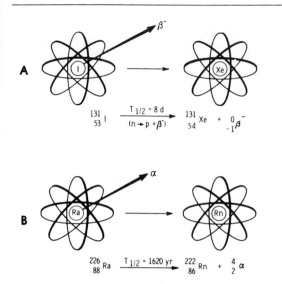

Fig. 3-10. A, ^{131}I decays to ^{131}Xe with the emission of a beta particle. **B,** The decay of ^{226}Ra to ^{222}Rn is accompanied by alpha emission.

chemically different, but is also lighter by 4 amu. An example of this type of radioactive decay is shown in Fig. 3-10, *B*.

Beta emission occurs much more frequently than alpha emission. Virtually all radioisotopes are capable of transformation by beta decay, but only heavy radioisotopes are capable of alpha emission. Some radioisotopes are pure beta emitters or pure alpha emitters, but most emit gamma rays simultaneously with the particle emission.

EXAMPLE: $^{139}_{56}$Ba is a radioisotope that decays via beta emission. What will be the value of *A* and *Z* for the atom that results from this emission?

ANSWER: In beta emission a neutron is converted to a proton and a beta particle: n → p + β; therefore $^{139}_{56}$Ba → $^{139}_{57}$?. Lanthanum is the element with Z = 57; thus, $^{139}_{57}$La is the result of the beta decay of $^{139}_{56}$Ba.

Radioactive half-life

Radioactive material is not here one day and gone the next. Rather, radioisotopes disintegrate into stable isotopes of different elements at an ever-decreasing rate, but the rate and consequently the quantity of radioactive material never quite reach zero. Remember from Chapter 1 that radioactive material is measured in curies (Ci) and that 1 Ci is equal to 3.7×10^{10} atoms disintegrating each second (3.7×10^{10} Bq). The rate of radioactive decay and the quantity of material present at any given time is described mathematically by a formula known as the **radioactive decay law.** From this formula we obtain a quantity known as **half-life** ($T_{1/2}$). **The half-life of a radioisotope is the period of time required for a quantity of radioactivity to be reduced to one half its original value.** Half-lives of radioisotopes are measured in periods of time ranging from less than a second to many years. Each radioisotope has a unique, characteristic half-life.

In Fig. 3-10 the half-life of ^{131}I is shown to be 8 days by $T_{1/2} = 8$ days. If 100 mCi (3.7×10^9

result is that a small quantity of mass and one unit of negative electric charge are removed from the nucleus of the atom. Simultaneously, a neutron undergoes conversion to a proton. The net result of beta emission is to increase the atomic number by one, while the atomic mass number remains the same. This nuclear transformation therefore results in an atom changing from one type of element to another. Fig. 3-10, *A*, shows an example of radioactive decay by beta emission.

Radioactive decay by alpha emission is a much more violent process. The alpha particle consists of two protons and two neutrons bound together; its atomic mass number is 4. A nucleus must be extremely unstable to emit an alpha particle, but when it does, it loses two units of positive charge and four units of mass. The transformation is significant because the resulting atom is not only

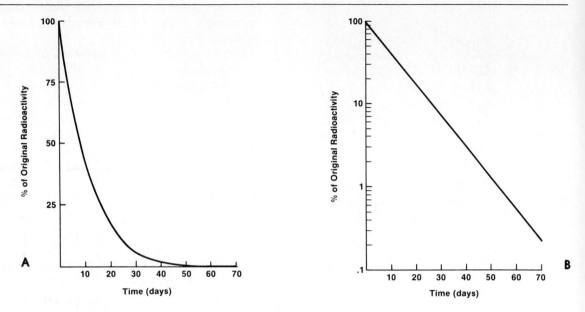

Fig. 3-11. ^{131}I decays with a half-life of 8 days. The linear graph, **A,** allows estimation of the activity remaining following a short decay time. The semilog graph, **B,** is useful for longer decay times.

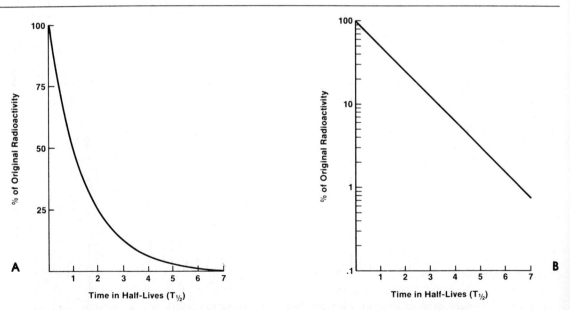

Fig. 3-12. Quantity of any radioactive material remaining after any period of time can be estimated from either the linear, **A,** or the semilog, **B,** graph. The original quantity is assigned a value of 100%, and the time of decay is expressed in units of half-life

Bq) of ^{131}I were present on January 1 at noon, then at noon on January 9 only 50 mCi $(1.85 \times 10^9$ Bq) would remain; on January 17, 25 mCi $(9.25 \times 10^8$ Bq) would remain, and on January 25, 12.5 mCi $(4.63 \times 10^8$ Bq) would be left. Fig. 3-11 is a plot of the radioactive decay of ^{131}I. This type of curve allows one to determine the amount of radioactivity remaining after any given time.

However, after about 25 days, approximately three half-lives, the linear-linear plot of the decay of ^{131}I becomes very difficult to read and interpret. Consequently, such graphs are usually presented in linear-logarithmic or semilogarithmic form, as in Fig. 3-11, *B*. With a presentation such as this, one can estimate remaining radioactivity after a very long time.

EXAMPLE: On Monday at 8 AM 100 µCi $(3.7 \times 10^6$ Bq) of ^{131}I is present. How much will remain on Friday at 5 PM?

ANSWER: The time period of decay is $4\frac{1}{3}$ days. According to Fig. 3-11, at $4\frac{1}{3}$ days approximately 63% of the original activity will remain. Therefore 63 µCi $(2.33 \times 10^6$ Bq) will be present on Friday at 5 PM.

Theoretically, all the radioactivity of a radioisotope never disappears. After each period of time equivalent to one half-life, one-half the activity present at the beginning of that time will remain. Therefore, although the quantity of radioisotope progressively decreases, it never quite reaches zero, regardless of how long a period is observed.

Fig. 3-12 shows graphs used to estimate the quantity of any radioisotope that remains after any period of time, given the half-life and initial radioactivity of the radioisotope. In these graphs the percent of radioactivity remaining is plotted against time, measured in units of half-life. To use these graphs, one must express the initial radioactivity as 100% and convert the time of interest into units of half-life. For decay times exceeding three half-lives, the logarithmic form is easier to use.

EXAMPLE: 65 mCi $(2.4 \times 10^9$ Bq) of ^{131}I are present at noon on Wednesday. How much will remain 1 week later?

ANSWER: 7 days $= \frac{7}{8}$ $T_{1/2} = 0.875$ $T_{1/2}$. Fig. 3-12 shows that at 0.875 $T_{1/2}$ approximately 55% of the initial radioactivity will remain; $55\% \times 65$ mCi $(2.4 \times 10^9$ Bq) $= 0.55 \times 65 = 35.8$ mCi $(1.32 \times 10^9$ Bq).

^{14}C is a naturally occurring radioisotope with $T_{1/2} = 5730$ years. The concentration of ^{14}C in the environment is constant, and ^{14}C is incorporated into living material at a constant rate. Trees of the petrified forest contain less ^{14}C than living trees because the ^{14}C of living trees is in equilibrium with the atmosphere; the carbon in a petrified tree was fixed many thousands of years ago, and the fixed ^{14}C is reduced with time by radioactive decay. Fig. 3-13 is a representation of this situation.

EXAMPLE: If a piece of petrified wood contains 25% of the ^{14}C that a tree living today contains, how old is the petrified wood?

ANSWER: The ^{14}C in living matter remains constant as long as the matter is alive because it is constantly exchanged with the environment. In this case the petrified wood has been dead long enough for the ^{14}C to decay to 25% of its original value. That time period represents two half-lives. Consequently, we can estimate that the petrified wood sample is approximately $2 \times 5730 = 11,460$ years old.

EXAMPLE: How many half-lives are required before a quantity of radioactive material has decayed to less than 1% of its original value?

ANSWER: The simplest approach to this type of problem is to count half-lives.

Half-life number	Radioactivity remaining
1	50%
2	25%
3	12.5%
4	6.25%
5	3.12%
6	1.56%
7	0.78%

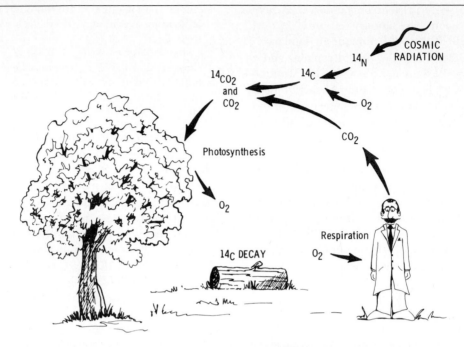

Fig. 3-13. Carbon is a biologically active element. A small fraction of all carbon is the radioisotope ^{14}C. As a tree grows, ^{14}C is incorporated into the wood in proportion to the amount of ^{14}C in the atmosphere. When the tree dies, further exchange of ^{14}C with the atmosphere does not take place. If the dead wood is preserved by petrification, the ^{14}C content diminishes as it radioactively decays. This phenomenon is the basis for radiocarbon dating.

The concept of half-life is essential to radiology. It is used daily in nuclear medicine and has an exact parallel in x-ray terminology, the **half-value layer.** The better half-life is understod now, the clearer the meaning of half-value layer will be later.

TYPES OF IONIZING RADIATION

Table 3-5 demonstrates that all ionizing radiation can be conveniently classified into the two categories **particulate radiation** and **electromagnetic radiation.** No other types of ionizing radiation are known. The types of radiation employed in diagnostic ultrasound and in magnetic resonance imaging are not ionizing.

Although all ionizing radiation acts on biologic tissue in the same manner, there are fundamental differences between various types of radiation. These differences can be analyzed according to five physical characteristics: mass, energy, velocity, charge, and origin.

Particulate radiation

Any subatomic particle in motion is capable of causing ionization. Consequently, electrons, protons, neutrons, and even rare nuclear fragments can all be classified as particulate ionizing radiation if they are in motion and possess sufficient kinetic energy. At rest, ionization cannot occur. There are two principal types of partic-

Table 3-5. General classification of ionizing radiation

Type of radiation	Symbol	Atomic mass number	Charge	Origin
Particulate				
Alpha radiation	α	4	+2	Nucleus
Beta radiation	β	0	−1	Nucleus
Other particles	*	*	*	Nucleus
Electromagnetic				
Gamma rays	γ	0	0	Nucleus
X rays	X	0	0	Electron cloud

*Variable.

ulate radiation—**alpha particles** and **beta particles**—both of which are associated with radioactive decay.

The alpha particle is equivalent to a helium nucleus. It contains two protons, two neutrons, and no associated orbital electrons. Its mass is approximately 4 amu, and it carries two units of positive electric charge. Compared with a target electron about to be stripped from its atom by ionization, the alpha particle is enormous and exerts a fantastically large electrostatic attraction. (Recall that opposite electrostatic charges attract and like charges repel.) Alpha particles are emitted only from the nuclei of heavy elements. Light elements are incapable of alpha particle emission, since they do not have enough excess mass (excess energy!).

Once emitted from a radioactive atom, the alpha particle travels with enormous velocity through matter. However, because of its great mass and charge, it easily transfers this kinetic energy to orbital electrons of target atoms. Ionization frequently accompanies alpha radiation. The average alpha particle possesses 4 to 7 MeV of kinetic energy and ionizes approximately 40,000 atoms for every centimeter of travel through air. This ionization rate is called **specific ionization.** Specific ionization is usually specified in ion pairs per centimeter of air or per micrometer of water.

Because of this rapid transfer of energy, the energy of an alpha particle is quickly dissipated and thus has a very short range through matter. In air alpha particles can travel about 5 cm, whereas in soft tissue the range may approach 100 μm. Consequently, alpha radiation from an external source is nearly harmless, since the radiation energy is deposited in the superficial layers of the skin. As an internal source of radiation, just the opposite is true. If an alpha-emitting radioisotope is deposited in the body, it can severely irradiate the local tissue. When an alpha particle finally loses all its kinetic energy, it comes to rest, attracts two free electrons, and becomes an atom of helium gas.

Beta particles differ from alpha particles in both mass and charge. They are light particles with an atomic mass number of 0, carry one unit of negative charge, and are emitted from the nucleus of radioactive atoms. The only difference between electrons and beta particles is that beta particles originate in the nuclei of radioactive atoms, and electrons exist in shells outside the nuclei of all atoms. Once emitted from a radioisotope, beta particles traverse air with a specific ionization of several hundred ion pairs per centimeter. Their range is longer than that of an alpha particle. Depending on its energy, a beta particle may traverse 10 to 100 cm of air and about 1 to 2 cm of soft tissue. Once a beta particle has transferred all its kinetic energy, it comes to rest and combines with an atom deficient in electrons.

Electromagnetic radiation

X rays and gamma rays are forms of electromagnetic ionizing radiation. Since this type of radiation will be covered more completely in the next chapter, the treatment here is necessarily brief. X rays and gamma rays are often called **photons.** They have no mass and no charge, trav-

el at the speed of light ($c = 3 \times 10^8$ m/s), and may be considered energy disturbances in space.

Just as the only difference between beta particles and electrons is their origin, so the only difference between x rays and gamma rays is their origin. Gamma rays are emitted from the nucleus of a radioisotope and are usually associated with alpha and beta emission. X rays are produced outside the nucleus in the electron cloud.

Table 3-6. Characteristics of several types of ionizing radiation

Type of radiation	Approximate energy	Specific Ionization (ip/cm of air)	Approximate range		Origin
			In air	In soft tissue	
Particulate					
Alpha particles	4-7 MeV	20,000-60,000	1-10 cm	Up to 0.1 mm	Heavy radioactive nuclei
Beta particles	0-7 MeV	100-400	0-10 m	0-2 cm	Radioactive nuclei
Electromagnetic					
X rays	0-10 MeV	Up to 500	0-100 m	0-30 cm	Electron cloud
Gamma rays	0-5 MeV	Up to 500	0-100 m	0-30 cm	Radioactive nuclei

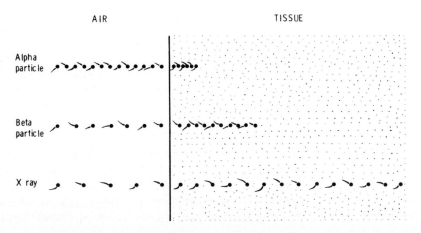

Fig. 3-14. Various types of radiation ionize matter with different efficiencies. Alpha particles are highly ionizing radiation with a very short range in matter. Beta particles do not ionize so readily and have a longer range. X rays have low specific ionization and a very long range.

X rays and gamma rays exist either at the speed of light or not at all. Once emitted, they traverse air with a specific ionization of approximately 100 ion pairs per micrometer, about equal to that for beta particles. Unlike beta particles, however, x rays and gamma rays have an unlimited range in matter. Photon radiation decreases in intensity as it traverses matter, but it never quite reaches zero as does particulate radiation.

Table 3-6 summarizes the more important characteristics of each of these types of ionization radiation. In nuclear medicine technology, beta and gamma radiation are most important. In x-ray technology, only x rays are of prime importance. The difference in the manner in which these types of ionizing radiation interact with matter is schematically diagramed in Fig. 3-14. The penetrability and low specific ionization of x rays make them particularly useful for medical imaging.

REVIEW QUESTIONS

1. Define or otherwise identify the following:
   a. The Thomson, Rutherford, and Bohr atoms
   b. Specific ionization
   c. Nucleons
   d. The arrangement of the periodic table of the elements
   e. Isobars
   f. Half-life
   g. W (chemical symbol for what element?)
   h. Centripetal force
   i. Chemical compound
   j. Alpha particle

2. Fig. 3-4 shows the following approximate sizes: an atom, 10^{-10} m; the earth, 10^7 m.
   a. By how many orders of magnitude do these objects differ?
   b. Write each size in decimal form.
3. How many protons, neutrons, electrons, and nucleons are in the following?

$$^{17}_{8}O, \ ^{27}_{13}Al, \ ^{60}_{27}Co, \ ^{226}_{88}Ra$$

4. Using the data in Table 3-1, determine the mass of $^{99}_{43}Tc$ in atomic mass units and in grams.
5. Diagram the expected electron configuration of $^{40}_{20}Ca$.
6. If atoms large enough to have electrons in the *T* shell existed, what would be the maximum number allowed in that shell?
7. How much more tightly bound are *K*-shell electrons than (a) *L*-shell electrons, (b) *M*-shell electrons, (c) free electrons? (Refer to Fig. 3-9 [Tungsten].)
8. From the following list of nuclides, identify sets of isotopes, isobars, and isotones.

		$^{60}_{28}Ni$	$^{61}_{28}Ni$	$^{62}_{28}Ni$
	$^{59}_{27}Co$	$^{60}_{27}Co$	$^{61}_{27}Co$	
$^{58}_{26}Fe$	$^{59}_{26}Fe$	$^{60}_{26}Fe$		

9. $^{90}_{38}Sr$ has a half-life of 29 years. If 10 Ci (3.7×10^{11} Bq) were present in 1950, approximately how much would remain in (a) 1979, (b) 1990, (c) 2100?
10. Complete the following table with relative values.

Type of radiation	Mass	Energy	Charge	Origin
α				
β				
γ				
X				

4

Electromagnetic radiation

PHOTONS EVERYWHERE

ELECTROMAGNETIC SPECTRUM

RADIOLOGICALLY IMPORTANT PHOTONS

ENERGY AND MATTER: A REVIEW

PHOTONS EVERYWHERE

Ever present all around us is a field, or state, of energy, called **electromagnetic energy,** which exists over a wide range of magnitudes, called an energy **continuum.** A continuum is an uninterrupted (continuous) ordered sequence. A free-flowing river or a sidewalk might represent a continuum. If the river is dammed or the sidewalk curbed, then the continuum is interrupted and is no longer a continuum. Only an extremely small segment of the electromagnetic energy continuum—the visible-light segment—is apparent to us.

The ancient Greeks recognized the unique nature of light. It was not one of their four basic essences but was given entirely separate status. They called an atom of light a **photon.** Today many types of electromagnetic radiation in addition to visible light are recognized, but the term "photon" is still used. A photon is the smallest quantity of any type of electromagnetic radiation, just as an atom is the smallest quantity of an element. A photon may be pictured as a small bundle of energy, sometimes called a

quantum, traveling through space at the speed of light. We speak of x-ray photons, light photons, and other types of electromagnetic radiation as photon radiation.

Velocity and amplitude

The physics of visible light has always been a subject of investigation quite apart from other areas of science. Nearly all the classical laws of optics were described hundreds of years ago. Late in the nineteenth century Maxwell showed that visible light has both electric and magnetic properties, hence the term **electromagnetic radiation.** By the beginning of the twentieth century, other types of electromagnetic radiation had been described and a uniform theory evolved. The theory of electromagnetic radiation is best explained by reference to a visible model, in much the same way that the atom is described by the Bohr model.

Photons are energy disturbances moving through space at the speed of light (c). Some sources give the speed of light as 186,000 miles per second, but in the SI system of units $c = 3 \times 10^8$ m/s.

EXAMPLE: What is the precise value of c in miles per second, given $c = 3 \times 10^8$ m/s?

ANSWER: $c = \dfrac{3 \times 10^8 \text{ m}}{\text{s}} \times \dfrac{\text{mile}}{5280 \text{ ft}} \times \dfrac{3.2808 \text{ ft}}{\text{m}}$

$\quad = \dfrac{3 \times 3.2808 \times 10^8 \text{ m-mile-ft}}{5.280 \times 10^3 \text{ s-ft-m}}$

$\quad = 1.864 \times 10^5$ mile/s

$\quad = 186,400$ mile/s

Although photons have no mass and therefore no easily identifiable form, they do have electric and magnetic fields that are continuously changing in a sinusoidal fashion. The term **field** is used by physicists to describe the interaction between different energies, forces, or masses that can otherwise be described only mathematically. For instance, we can understand the gravitational field; even though we cannot see it, we know the gravitational field exists because we are held to the earth by it. The gravitational field governs how different masses interact. Similarly, the electric field governs the interaction of electrostatic charges, and the magnetic field, the interaction of magnetic poles.

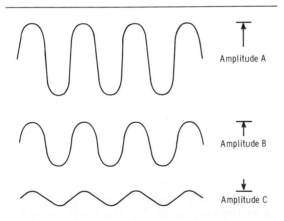

Fig. 4-1. These three sine waves are identical except for their amplitudes. Wave A has the highest amplitude; wave C, the lowest.

Fig. 4-1 shows three examples of a sinusoidal variation. This type of variation is usually called a **sine wave** or **sine curve.** Sine waves can be described by a mathematical formula and therefore find much application in physics. They also exist in nature associated with many familiar objects as shown in Fig. 4-2. Alternating electric current consists of electrons moving back and forth sinusoidally through a wire. A long rope fastened at one end vibrates in a sine wave if the free end is moved up and down in whiplike fashion. The arms of a tuning fork vibrate in sinusoidal fashion after being struck with a hard object. The weight on the end of a coil spring varies sinusoidally up and down after the spring has been stretched.

The sine waves in Fig. 4-1 are identical except for their amplitude, sine wave A having the largest amplitude, and sine wave C the smallest. **Amplitude** is the range from crest to valley over which the sine wave varies. Amplitude is an important property of some sine waves, such as those in Fig. 4-2, but it is relatively unimportant for electromagnetic radiation. Sine-wave amplitude will be discussed later in connection with high-voltage generation in an x-ray machine.

Frequency and wavelength

The sine-wave model of electromagnetic radiation describes the variations of the electric and magnetic fields as the photon travels with velocity c. The important properties of this model are **frequency,** represented by the Greek letter nu, ν, and **wavelength,** represented by the Greek letter lambda, λ. Fig. 4-3 is another interpretation of the vibrating rope in Fig. 4-2 and includes a technologist observing the motion of the rope from a point midway between the fastened end and the scientist. What does the technologist see? If she moves her field of view along the rope, she will observe the crest of the sine wave traveling along the rope to the end. If she fixes her attention on one segment of the rope, such as point A, she will see the rope rise and fall harmonically as the waves pass. The more

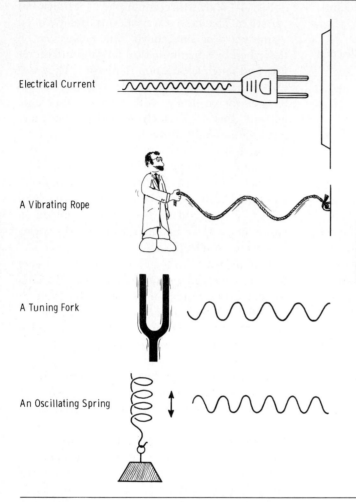

Electrical Current

A Vibrating Rope

A Tuning Fork

An Oscillating Spring

Fig. 4-2. Sine waves are associated with many naturally occurring phenomena in many systems in addition to electromagnetic radiation. A few examples of sine wave generation are shown here.

rapidly the scientist holding the loose end moves the rope up and down, the faster the sequence of rise and fall.

This rate of rise and fall is called frequency. It is usually identified as oscillations per second or cycles per second. the unit of measurement is the **hertz (Hz).** One Hz is equal to 1 cycle per second. The number of crests or the number of valleys that pass the point of an observer per unit time is the frequency. If the observer, using a stopwatch, counts twenty crests passing in 10 seconds, then the frequency would be 2 Hz. If the scientist doubles the rate at

which he moves the rope up and down, the observer would count forty crests passing in 10 seconds, and the frequency would be 4 Hz.

The distance from one crest to another, from one valley to another, or from any point on the sine wave to the next corresponding point, is called the wavelength. Fig. 4-4 shows sine waves of three different wavelengths. With a meter rule, one can verify that wave A repeats every 1 cm and therefore has a wavelength of 1 cm. Similarly, wave B has a wavelength of 0.5 cm, and wave C of 1.5 mm. As may be clear from

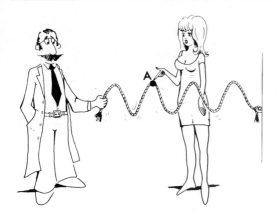

Fig. 4-3. Someone moving one end of a rope in a whiplike fashion will set into motion sine waves that travel down the rope to the fastened end. An observer, midway, can determine the frequency of oscillation by counting the crests (A) or valleys that pass a point per unit time. The wavelength is the distance measured from one crest to another.

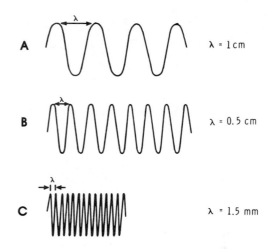

Fig. 4-4. Three sine waves shown have different wavelengths. The shorter the wavelength, the higher the frequency.

Figs. 4-3 and 4-4, as the frequency is changed, the wavelength is also changed. The wave amplitude is not related to these parameters of wavelength and frequency.

Three wave parameters—velocity, frequency, and wavelength—are nearly all that need be known to fully describe a photon of electromagnetic radiation. The interrelationship among these parameters is an important concept. A change in one affects the value of one or both of the others.

Suppose a radiologic technologist is positioned so that she can observe the flight of the sine-wave arrows to determine their frequency (Fig. 4-5). The first is measured and found to have a frequency of 60 Hz, that is, one full oscillation of the sine wave passes every $\frac{1}{60}$ second. The unknown archer now puts an identical sine-wave arrow into his bow and shoots it with less force so that this second arrow has only half the velocity of the first arrow. The observer correctly measures the frequency at 30 Hz, even though the wavelength of the second arrow was

the same as that of the first arrow. In other words, as the velocity changes, the frequency changes proportionately. Now the archer shoots a third sine-wave arrow with precisely the same velocity as the first had but with a wavelength twice as long as that of the first. What should be the observed frequency? Thirty hertz is correctly observed. Otherwise stated, the wavelength and frequency are inversely proportional if the velocity is constant.

This brief analogy demonstrates how the three parameters associated with a moving sine wave are interrelated. A simple mathematic formula, called **the wave equation,** expresses this relationship:

Velocity = Frequency × Wavelength

or

(4-1)

$$v = \nu\lambda$$

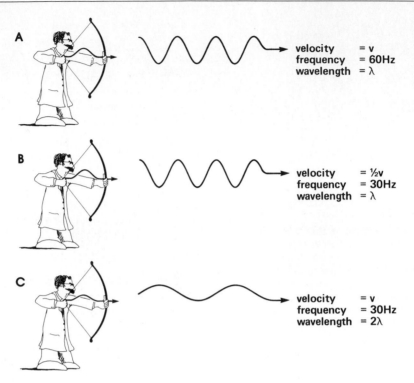

Fig. 4-5. Relationship between velocity *(v)*, frequency *(ν)*, and wavelength (λ). If sine-wave arrows have contstant λ (**A** and **B**), **an increase in *v* will cause a proportionate increase in *ν*.** If *v* is **constant (A** and **C)**, an increase in λ will cause a proportionate decrease in *ν*. If *ν* is constant (**B** and **C**), *v* will increase directly with λ.

EXAMPLE: The speed of sound in air is approximately 340 m/s. The highest treble tone that man can hear is about 20 kHz. What is the wavelength of this sound?

ANSWER: $v = \nu\lambda$

$$\lambda = \frac{v}{\nu}$$

$$= \frac{340 \text{ m/s}}{20 \text{ kHz}}$$

$$= \frac{3.40 \times 10^2 \text{ m}}{\text{s}} \times \frac{\text{s}}{2 \times 10^4 \text{ cycle}}$$

$$= 1.7 \times 10^{-2} \text{ m}$$

$$= 1.7 \text{ cm}$$

When dealing with electromagnetic radiation, we can simplify equation 4-1 because all such radiation travels with the same velocity, *c*:

(4-2)

$$c = \nu\lambda$$

The product of frequency and wavelength always equals the velocity of light for electromagnetic radiation. Stated differently, **for electromagnetic radiation, frequency and wavelength are inversely proportional.** The following are alternate forms of equation 4-2:

$$(4\text{-}2a)$$

$$\nu = \frac{c}{\lambda}$$

and

$$(4\text{-}2b)$$

$$\lambda = \frac{c}{\nu}$$

As the frequency of electromagnetic radiation increases, the wavelength decreases, and vice versa.

EXAMPLE: Yellow light has a wavelength of about 580 nm. What is the frequency of a photon of yellow light?

ANSWER: $\nu = \dfrac{c}{\lambda}$

$$= \frac{3 \times 10^8 \text{ m/s}}{580 \text{ nm}}$$

$$= \frac{3 \times 10^8 \text{ m}}{\text{s}} \times \frac{1}{580 \times 10^{-9} \text{ m}}$$

$$= \frac{3 \times 10^8 \text{ m}}{\text{s}} \times \frac{1}{5.8 \times 10^{-7} \text{ m}}$$

$$= 0.517 \times 10^{15} \text{ cycle/s}$$

$$= 5.17 \times 10^{14} \text{ Hz}$$

EXAMPLE: The shortest x-ray wavelength produced at 100 kVp has a frequency of 2.42×10^{19} Hz. What is its wavelength?

ANSWER: $\lambda = \dfrac{c}{\nu}$

$$= \frac{3 \times 10^8 \text{ m}}{\text{s}} \times \frac{\text{s}}{2.42 \times 10^{19} \text{ cycle}}$$

$$= 1.24 \times 10^{-11} \text{ m}$$

$$= 12.4 \text{ pm}$$

ELECTROMAGNETIC SPECTRUM

The frequencies of electromagnetic radiation as we know it extend from approximately 10 to 10^{24} Hz and perhaps higher. The photon wavelengths associated with these radiations are approximately 10^7 to 10^{-16} m, respectively. This wide range of values covers many types of electromagnetic radiation, most of which are familiar to us. Grouped together, these radiations make up the electromagnetic continuum, or the **electromagnetic spectrum.** Fig. 4-6 shows the known electromagnetic spectrum and emphasizes the three portions of the spectrum most important to radiologic technology: visible light, x-radiation, and high-frequency radio waves. Other portions of the spectrum include ultraviolet and infrared light, microwave radiation, and the radio-broadcast region. Photons of each of these various radiations are essentially the same in that each can be represented as a bundle of energy consisting of varying electric and magnetic fields traveling at the speed of light. The only difference among photons of these various portions of the electromagnetic spectrum is in frequency and wavelength.

Measurement of electromagnetic spectrum

The electromagnetic spectrum shown in Fig. 4-6 contains three different scales of values, one each for frequency, wavelength, and energy. Since the velocity of all electromagnetic radiation is constant, not only are wavelength and frequency inversely related, but the energy contained in each photon is directly proportional to the photon frequency as well. Although the segments of the electromagnetic spectrum are generally considered to have precise ranges, there is overlap because of the methods of production and techniques for detection of these various radiations. For example, by definition ultraviolet light has a shorter wavelength than violet light and cannot be sensed by the eye. However, what is visible violet light to one observer may be ultraviolet to another. Similarly, microwaves and infrared radiation are indistinguishable in their common region of the spectrum. The method of production is the identifying characteristic.

Radio emissions

Because the scientific investigation of the electromagnetic spectrum occurred over hundreds of years, three units of measure for photon

THE ELECTROMAGNETIC SPECTRUM

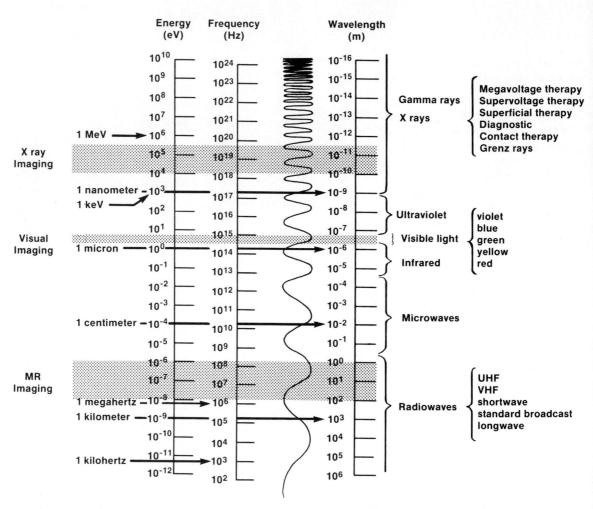

Fig. 4-6. Electromagnetic spectrum extends over more than twenty-five orders of magnitude. This chart shows the values of energy, frequency, and wavelength and identifies some common values and regions of the spectrum.

radiation have developed. Scientists working with radiation at one portion of the spectrum were often unaware of others investigating another portion. Consequently, there is no generally accepted, single dimension for measuring photon radiation. A radio or television engineer describes photon emissions in terms of their frequency. For example, radio station WIMP might broadcast at 960 kHz, and its associated television station WIMP-TV might broadcast at 63.7 MHz. Communications broadcasts are usually identified by their frequency of transmission and are called radiofrequency emissions or **RF.**

RF comprises a considerable portion of the electromagnetic spectrum. Photons of RF have very low energies and very long wavelengths. Only long electrical oscillations produce photon radiation of longer wavelength. Ham operators speak of broadcasting on the 10 m band or the 30 m band; these numbers refer to the approximate wavelength of emissions. Standard AM broadcast has a wavelength of about 100 m. Television and FM broadcasting occur at a much shorter wavelength. Because microwaves are also used for communication, there is considerable overlap between what are identified as RF and as microwaves.

Visible light

An optic physicist describes photons of visible light in terms of their wavelength. When sunlight passes through a prism (Fig. 4-7), it emerges not as white sunlight but as the colors of the rainbow. Although photons of visible light travel in straight lines, their course can be deviated when they pass from one transparent medium to another. This deviation in line of travel, called **refraction,** is the cause of many peculiar but familiar phenomena, such as a rainbow or the apparent bending of a straw in a glass of water. White light passing through a prism is refracted because it is composed of photons of a range of wavelengths, and the prism acts to separate and group the emerging light according to wavelength. The component colors of white light have wavelength values ranging from approximately 400 nm for violet to 700 nm for red.

Visible light occupies the smallest segment of the electromagnetic spectrum, and yet it is the only portion that we can sense directly. Sunlight refracted through a prism, as in Fig. 4-7, also contains two types of invisible light: infrared and ultraviolet. **Infrared light** consists of photons with wavelengths longer than those of visible light but shorter than those of microwaves. Infrared light heats any substance on which it shines. **Ultraviolet light** is located in the electromagnetic spectrum between visible light and ionizing radiation. It is responsible for molecular interactions that can result in sunburn.

Ionizing radiation

Unlike radio emissions or visible light, ionizing electromagnetic radiation is usually characterized by the energy contained in a photon. When an x-ray machine is operated at 80 kVp, the x rays it produces contain energies varying from 0 to 80 keV. An x-ray photon contains considerably more energy than a visible-light photon or a photon of a radio broadcast. The fre-

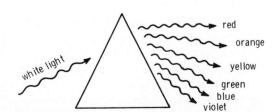

red
orange
yellow
green
blue
violet

Fig. 4-7. When it passes through a glass prism, white light is refracted into its component colors. These colors have wavelengths extending from approximately 400 to 700 nm.

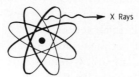 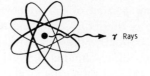

Fig. 4-8. X rays are produced outside the nucleus of artificially excited atoms; gamma rays are produced inside the nucleus of radioactive atoms.

quency and wavelength of x-radiation are much higher and shorter, respectively, than for other types of electromagnetic radiation.

The distinction is sometimes made between x-ray and gamma-ray photons that gamma-ray photons have higher energy. In the early days of radiology this was true because of the limited capacity of the available x-ray machines. Today, with large particle accelerators available, it is possible to produce x rays with energies considerably higher than those of gamma-ray emissions. Consequently, the distinction by energy is not appropriate. **The only difference between x rays and gamma rays is their origin.** As indicated in Fig. 4-8, x rays are emitted from the electron cloud of an atom that has been artificially stimulated; gamma rays, on the other hand, come from inside the nucleus of a radioactive atom. X rays are produced in electrical machines, whereas gamma rays are emitted spontaneously from radioactive material. Nevertheless, given an x ray and a gamma ray of equal energy, one could not tell them apart.

This situation is analogous to the difference between beta particles and electrons. These particles are the same, except that beta particles come from the nucleus and electrons come from outside the nucleus.

RADIOLOGICALLY IMPORTANT PHOTONS

Three regions of the electromagnetic spectrum are particularly important to radiologic technology. Naturally the x-ray region is fundamental to producing a high-quality radiograph. The visible-light region is also important

because the conditions under which a radiographic or fluoroscopic image is viewed are critical to the ultimate description of diagnostic information. More recently, with the introduction of magnetic resonance imaging (MRI), the radiofrequency region has taken on added importance to radiology.

A photon of x-radiation and a photon of visible light appear exactly the same, except that the former has a much higher frequency, hence a shorter wavelength, than the latter. These differences result in differences in the way in which these photons interact with matter. Visible-light photons tend to exhibit more wave nature than particle nature. The opposite is true of x-ray photons, which behave more like particles than waves. In fact, both types of photons exhibit both types of behavior, a phenomenon known as the **wave-particle duality** of radiation.

Another general way to consider the interaction of electromagnetic radiation with matter is as a function of wavelength. Photons most frequently interact with matter when the matter is approximately the same size as the photon wavelength. Consequently, photons of radio broadcast, which have wavelengths measured in meters, interact with metal rods or wires called antennae. Microwaves, with wavelengths measured in centimeters, interact most easily with objects of the same size, such as hot dogs, hamburgers, and rolled roasts. Visible light has wavelengths measured in micrometers and interacts with living cells, such as the rods and cones of the eye. Ultraviolet light interacts with molecules, and x rays interact with atoms and

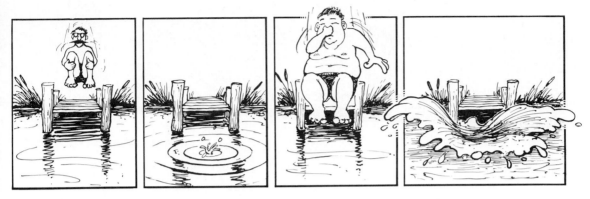

Fig. 4-9. A small object dropped into a smooth pond will create waves of short wavelength. A large object will create waves of much longer wavelength.

subatomic particles. All radiation with wavelength longer than that of x-radiation interacts primarily as a wave phenomenon. X rays behave as though they were particles.

Wave model: visible light

One of the unique features of animal life is the sense of vision. It is interesting that we have developed organs that sense only a very narrow portion of the enormous spread of the electromagnetic spectrum. This narrow portion is called **visible light.** The visible-light spectrum extends from short-wavelength violet radiation through green and yellow to long-wavelength red radiation. On both sides of the visible-light spectrum are similar radiations, ultraviolet and infrared, that cannot be detected by the human eye but can be detected by other means, such as a photographic emulsion.

Visible light interacts with matter very differently from x rays. When a photon of light strikes an object, it sets molecules of the object into vibration. The orbital electrons of some atoms of some molecules are excited to a higher energy level than normal. This energy is immediately reirradiated as another photon of light. The atomic and molecular structures of the object determine which wavelengths of light are reir-

radiated. A leaf in the sunlight appears green because all the visible-light photons are absorbed by the leaf, but only photons with wavelengths in the green region are re-emitted. Similarly, a balloon may appear red by absorbing all visible photons and reirradiating only the long-wavelength red ones.

Many familiar phenomena of light, such as reflection, absorption, and transmission, are most easily explained by using the wave model of electromagnetic radiation. When a pebble is dropped into a still pond, ripples radiate from the center of the disturbance like miniature waves. This situation is similar to the wave nature of visible light. Fig. 4-9 shows the difference in the water waves between an initial disturbance caused by a large object and one caused by a small object. The distance between the crests of the waves caused by the large object is much longer than that of those caused by the small object. The difference in wavelength of these water waves is proportional to the energy introduced into the system. With light, the opposite is true. **The shorter the photon wavelength, the greater is the photon energy.**

If the analogy of the pebble in the pond is extended to a continuous, harmonious succession of pebbles dropped into a smooth ocean,

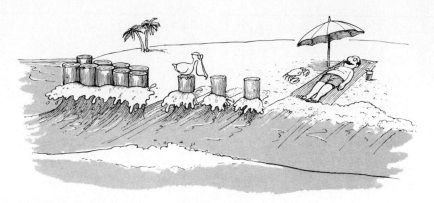

Fig. 4-10. Energy is reflected when waves crash into a bulkhead. It is absorbed by a beach. It is partially absorbed, or attenuated, by a line of pilings. Similarly, light is reflected, absorbed, or attenuated, depending on the composition of the surface on which it is incident.

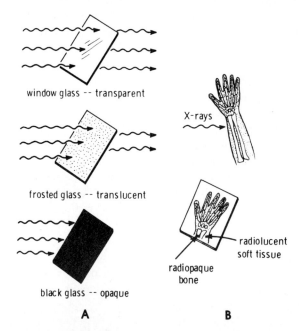

Fig. 4-11. Objects absorb light in three degrees: not at all (transmission), partially (attenuation), and completely (absorption). **A,** The objects associated with these degrees of absorption are called transparent, translucent, and opaque, respectively. **B,** Structures that absorb x rays are described as radiolucent or radiopaque, depending on the relative degree of x-ray transmission or absorption, respectively.

then at the edge of the ocean the waves will appear straight rather than circular. Light waves behave as though they were straight rather than circular because the relative distance from the source is great. The manner in which light is reflected from or transmitted through a surface is a consequence of this straight wavelike motion.

When the water waves of the ocean crash into a vertical bulkhead, as in Fig. 4-10, the reflected waves rebound from the bulkhead at the same angle that the incident waves struck it. When the bulkhead is removed and replaced with a beach, the water waves simply crash onto the beach, dissipate their energy, and are absorbed. When an intermediate condition exists in which the bulkhead has been replaced by a line of pilings, the energy of the waves is partially absorbed. Partial absorption of energy is called **attenuation.**

Visible light can similarly interact with matter. **Reflection** from the silvered surface of a mirror is common. Examples of **transmission, absorption,** and attenuation of light are equally easy to identify. When light waves are absorbed, the energy deposited in the absorber reappears as heat. A black asphalt road reflects very little visible light but absorbs a considerable amount. In so doing, the road surface can become quite hot.

Just a slight modification can change the manner in which or the extent to which some materials transmit or absorb light. Fig. 4-11, A, shows three degrees of interaction between light and an absorbing material: transparency, translucency, and opacity.

Window glass is **transparent;** it allows light to be transmitted almost unaltered. One can see through it because the surface of the glass is smooth and the molecular structure is tight and orderly. Incident light waves cause molecular and electronic vibrations within the glass. These vibrations are transmitted through the glass and reirradiated almost without change.

When the surface of the glass is roughened with sandpaper, light is still transmitted through the glass but is greatly altered and reduced in intensity. Instead of seeing clearly, one sees only shadows. Such glass is **translucent.**

When the glass is painted black, the characteristics of the pigment in the paint are such that no light can pass through. Any incident light is totally absorbed in the paint. Such glass is **opaque** to visible light.

The terms **radiolucent** and **radiopaque** are used routinely in x-ray diagnosis to describe the visual appearance of anatomic structures. Structures that absorb x rays are called **radiopaque.** Structures that attenuate x rays to a relatively small degree are called **radiolucent.** As Fig. 4-11, B, shows, bone is radiopaque; air and, to some extent, soft tissue are radiolucent.

Inverse square law

Another property of visible light is the manner in which its intensity decreases with distance from the source. When light is emitted from a point source such as the sun or a light bulb, the intensity decreases rapidly with the distance from the source. X rays exhibit precisely the same property. Fig. 4-12 shows that as a book is removed farther from a light source, the intensity of light is inversely proportional to the square of the distance of the object from the source. Mathematically this is called the **inverse square law** and is expressed as

(4-3)

$$\frac{I_1}{I_2} = \frac{d_2{}^2}{d_1{}^2}$$

or

(4-3a)

$$\frac{I_1}{I_2} = \left(\frac{d_2}{d_1}\right)^2$$

where I_1 is the intensity at distance d_1 from the source, and I_2 is the intensity at distance d_2 from the source.

The reason for the rapid decrease in intensity

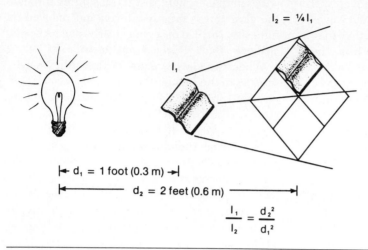

$I_2 = \frac{1}{4} I_1$

I_1

$d_1 = 1$ foot (0.3 m)

$d_2 = 2$ feet (0.6 m)

$$\frac{I_1}{I_2} = \frac{d_2{}^2}{d_1{}^2}$$

Fig. 4-12. Inverse square law describes the relationship between radiation intensity and distance from the radiation source.

is that the total light emitted is spread out over an increasingly large area as it moves farther from the source. The equivalent of this phenomenon in the water-wave analogy is that with increasing distance from the point of disturbance the waves lose their intensity while maintaining a fixed wavelength.

If the source of radiation is not a point but rather a line, such as a fluorescent light tube or a plane (for example, a flood-field radioisotope source), the inverse square law does not hold at distances close to the source. At great distances from the source, the inverse square law can be applied. As a rule, **the inverse square law can be applied to distances greater than seven times the longest dimension of the source.**

To apply the inverse square law, one must know three of the four parameters. The usual siltuation involves a known intensity at a fixed distance from the source and an unknown intensity at a greater distance.

EXAMPLE: The intensity of the headlamp of a diesel locomotive is 100 millilumens (mlm) at a distance of 20 ft (6.1 m). (The lumen is a unit of light intensity.) What is the intensity of light 40 ft (12.2 m) down the track?

ANSWER:
$$\frac{I_1}{I_2} = \frac{d_2{}^2}{d_1{}^2}$$

$$\frac{I_1}{100 \text{ mlm}} = \frac{20^2}{40^2}$$

$$I_1 = (100 \text{ mlm}) \left(\frac{20}{40}\right)^2$$

$$= (100 \text{ mlm})(0.25)$$
$$= 25 \text{ mlm}$$

This relationship between radiation intensity and distance from the source applies equally well to x-ray intensity.

EXAMPLE: The exposure from an x-ray tube operated at 70 kVp, 200 mAs is 400 mR (103 µC/kg) at 36 in (90 cm). What will the exposure be at 72 in (180 cm)?

ANSWER:
$$\frac{I_1}{I_2} = \left(\frac{d_2}{d_1}\right)^2$$

$$I_1 = I_2 \left(\frac{d_2}{d_1}\right)^2$$

$$= (400 \text{ mR}) \left(\frac{36 \text{ in}}{72 \text{ in}}\right)^2$$

$$= (400 \text{ mR})(\tfrac{1}{2})^2$$
$$= (400 \text{ mR})(\tfrac{1}{4})$$
$$= 100 \text{ mR}$$

This example illustrates a relationship that can be easily recalled by remembering that when the distance from the source is doubled, the intensity of radiation is reduced by one fourth,

Table 4-1. Some of the wide range of x rays produced by application in medicine, research, and industry

Type of x ray	Approximate energy	Application
Diffraction	Less than 10 kVp	Research: structural and molecular analysis
Grenz rays	10 to 20 kVp	Medicine: dermatology
Superficial	50 to 100 kVp	Medicine: therapy of superficial tissues
Diagnostic	30 to 150 kVp	Medicine: imaging anatomic structures and tissues
Orthovoltage*	200 to 300 kVp	Medicine: therapy of deep-lying tissues
Supervoltage*	300 to 1000 kVp	Medicine: therapy of deep-lying tissues
Megavoltage	Greater than 1 MV	Medicine: therapy of deep-lying tissues
		Industry: checking integrity of welded metals

*These radiation therapy modalities are slowly being phased out of use.

and, conversely, when the distance is halved, the intensity is increased by a factor of four.

EXAMPLE: For a given technique, the x-ray intensity at 40 in (100 cm) from the tube is 450 mR (116 µC/kg). What is the intensity at the edge of the control booth, a distance of 10 ft (3.05 m), if the tube head is directed toward the booth? (This, of course, should never be done.)

ANSWER: $\dfrac{I_1}{I_2} = \left(\dfrac{d_2}{d_1}\right)^2$

$I_1 = I_2 \left(\dfrac{d_2}{d_1}\right)^2$

$\quad = (450 \text{ mR})\left(\dfrac{40 \text{ in}}{10 \text{ ft}}\right)^2$

$\quad = (450 \text{ mR})\left(\dfrac{40 \text{ in}}{120 \text{ in}}\right)^2$

$\quad = (450 \text{ mR})(\tfrac{1}{3})^2$

$\quad = (450 \text{ mR})(\tfrac{1}{9})$

$\quad = 50 \text{ mR}$

Often it is necessary to determine the distance from the source at which the radiation has a given intensity. This type of problem is common in designing radiographic facilities.

EXAMPLE: A temporary chest unit is to be set up in an outdoor area. The technique used results in an exposure intensity of 25 mR (6.5 µC/kg) at 72 in (180 cm). The area behind the chest stand in which the exposure intensity exceeds 1 mR (0.3 µC/kg) is to be cordoned off. How far from the x-ray tube will this area extend?

ANSWER: $\dfrac{I_1}{I_2} = \dfrac{d_2^2}{d_1^2}$

$d_2^2 = d_1^2 \left(\dfrac{I_1}{I_2}\right)$

$d_2 = \left[d_1^2\left(\dfrac{I_1}{I_2}\right)\right]^{1/2}$

$\quad = \left[(72^2)\left(\dfrac{25}{1}\right)\right]^{1/2}$

$\quad = (72^2)^{1/2}(25)^{1/2}$

$\quad = (72)(5)$

$\quad = 360 \text{ in}$

$\quad = 30 \text{ ft}$

Quantum theory: x-ray photons

Unlike other portions of the electromagnetic spectrum, x rays are usually identified by their energy, measured in electron volts. The energies of x-ray photons range from approximately 1 keV to 50 MeV and higher. The associated wavelength for this range of x-radiation is approximately 10^{-9} to 10^{-12} m. The frequency of these photons varies from approximately 10^{18} to 10^{21} Hz. Table 4-1 describes the various types of x-ray photons produced and the general use made of each. We are primarily interested in the diagnostic range of x-radiation, though what is

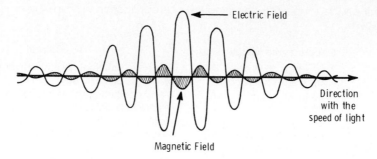

Fig. 4-13. An x-ray photon can be visualized best as two sine waves positioned at 90 degrees to each other and traveling in a straight line at the speed of light. One of the sine waves represents an electric field and the other a magnetic field.

said for that range holds equally well for other types of x-radiation. The maximum x-ray energy possible is limited only by how large an x-ray machine is available. Grenz-ray machines are quite small, whereas some megavoltage units require space equivalent to several rooms.

An x-ray photon can be thought of as containing an electric field and a magnetic field that vary sinusoidally at right angles to each other. The x-ray photon is a discrete bundle of energy, and therefore its beginning and end are sometimes described as diminished amplitude variations, as diagramed in Fig. 4-13. The wavelength of an x-ray photon is measured like that of any electromagnetic radiation; it is the distance from any position on either sine wave to the next corresponding position. The frequency of an x-ray photon is calculated like the frequency of any electromagnetic photon, by use of equation 4-1.

That x-ray photons are created at the speed of light and either exist with velocity c or do not exist at all is one of the substantive statements of **Planck's quantum theory.*** Another more im-

portant consequence of this theory is the relationship between energy and frequency: the photon energy is directly proportional to the photon frequency. The constant of proportionality, known as **Planck's constant** and symbolized by h, has a numeric value of 4.15×10^{-15} eV-s. Mathematically, the relationship between energy and frequency is expressed as

(4-4)

$$E = h\nu$$

where E is the photon energy in eV, h is Planck's constant in eV-s, and ν is the photon frequency in hertz.

EXAMPLE: What is the frequency of a 70 keV x-ray photon?

ANSWER: $E = h\nu$

$$\nu = \frac{E}{h}$$

$$= \frac{7 \times 10^4 \text{ eV}}{4.15 \times 10^{-15} \text{ eV-s}}$$

$$= 1.69 \times 10^{19}/\text{s}$$

$$= 1.69 \times 10^{19} \text{ Hz}$$

EXAMPLE: What is the energy contained in one photon of radiation from radio station WIMP, which has a broadcast frequency of 960 kHz?

ANSWER: $E = h\nu$

$$= (4.15 \times 10^{-15} \text{ eV-s})(9.6 \times 10^5/\text{s})$$

$$= 3.98 \times 10^{-9} \text{ eV}$$

---

*Max Planck was a German physicist whose mathematical and physical theories synthesized our understanding of electromagnetic radiation into a uniform model; for this work he received the Nobel Prize in 1918.

An extension of Planck's equation is the relationship between photon energy and photon wavelength; this relationship is useful in computing equivalent wavelengths of x rays and other types of radiation. By equations 4-4 and 4-2a, $E = h\nu$ and $\nu = c/\lambda$; thus, $E = h(c/\lambda)$, or

(4-5)

$$E = \frac{hc}{\lambda}$$

In other words, photon energy is inversely proportional to photon wavelength. In this relationship the constant of proportionality is a combination of two constants, Planck's and the speed of light. It should be clear that the longer the wavelength of radiation, the lower the energy of each photon.

EXAMPLE: What is the energy in one photon of green light whose wavelength is 550 nm?

ANSWER: $E = \dfrac{hc}{\lambda}$

$= \dfrac{(4.15 \times 10^{-15} \text{ eV-s})(3 \times 10^8 \text{ m/s})}{550 \times 10^{-9} \text{ m}}$

$= \dfrac{12.45 \times 10^{-7} \text{ eV-m}}{5.5 \times 10^{-7} \text{ m}}$

$= 2.26 \text{ eV}$

ENERGY AND MATTER: A REVIEW

This book began with the statement that everything in existence can be classified as matter or energy. It was further stated that matter and energy are really manifestations of each other. According to classical physics, matter can be neither created nor destroyed, a law known as the **law of conservation of matter.** A similar law, the **law of conservation of energy,** states that energy can be neither created nor destroyed. Planck and Albert Einstein greatly extended these theories. According to quantum physics and the physics of relativity, matter can be transmuted into energy, and vice versa. Nuclear fission, the basis for nuclear generation of electricity, is an increasingly familiar example of converting mass into energy. In radiology, a process known as pair production (Chapter 9) is an example of the conversion of energy into mass.

A simple equation introduced in Chapter 1 (equation 1-1) allows the calculation of the energy equivalence of mass and the mass equivalence of energy. This equation is a consequence of Einstein's theory of relativity and is familiar to all:

$$E = mc^2$$

E in the equation is the energy measured in joules, m is the mass measured in kilograms, and c is the velocity of light measured in meters per second.

Like the electron volt, the joule (J) is a unit of energy. One joule is equal to 6.24×10^{18} eV.

EXAMPLE: What is the energy equivalent of an electron (mass = 9.109×10^{-31} kg), measured in joules and in electron volts?

ANSWER: $E = mc^2$

$= (9.109 \times 10^{-31} \text{ kg})(3 \times 10^8 \text{ m/s})^2$

$= 81.972 \times 10^{-15}$ J

$= (8.1972 \times 10^{-14} \text{ J})\left(\dfrac{6.24 \times 10^{18} \text{ eV}}{\text{J}}\right)$

$= 51.15 \times 10^4$ eV

$= 511.5$ keV

The problem might be stated in the opposite direction.

EXAMPLE: What is the mass equivalent of a 70 keV x ray?

ANSWER: $E = mc^2$

$m = \dfrac{E}{c^2}$

$= \dfrac{(70 \times 10^3 \text{ eV})\left(\dfrac{\text{J}}{6.24 \times 10^{18} \text{ eV}}\right)}{(3 \times 10^8 \text{ m/s})^2}$

$= \dfrac{11.2 \times 10^{-15} \text{ J}}{9 \times 10^{16} \text{ m}^2/\text{s}^2}$

$= 1.25 \times 10^{-31}$ kg

By using equation 1-1 in conjunction with the two equations that relate to electromagnetic radiation, equations 4-2 and 4-4, one can calculate the mass equivalence of a photon when only the photon wavelength or photon frequency is known.

THE ELECTROMAGNETIC SPECTRUM

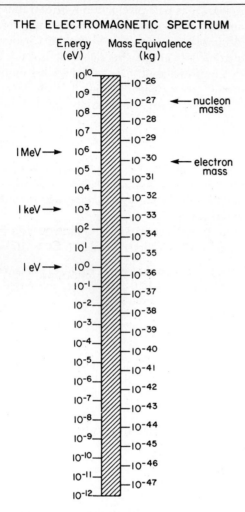

EXAMPLE: What is the mass equivalence of one photon of 1000 MHz microwave radiation?

ANSWER: $E = h\nu = mc^2$

$$m = \frac{h\nu}{c^2}$$

$$= \frac{(6.626 \times 10^{-34}\text{J-s})(1000 \times 10^6 \text{ Hz})}{(3 \times 10^8 \text{ m/s})^2}$$

$$= 0.736 \times 10^{-41} \text{ kg}$$

$$= 7.36 \times 10^{-42} \text{ kg}$$

EXAMPLE: What is the mass equivalence of a 330 nm photon of ultraviolet light?

ANSWER: $E = \frac{hc}{\lambda} = mc^2$

$$m = \left(\frac{hc}{\lambda}\right)\left(\frac{1}{c^2}\right) = \frac{h}{\lambda c}$$

$$= \frac{6.626 \times 10^{-34} \text{ J-s}}{(330 \times 10^{-9} \text{ m})(3 \times 10^8 \text{ m/s})}$$

$$= 0.00669 \times 10^{-33} \text{ kg}$$

$$= 6.69 \times 10^{-36} \text{ kg}$$

Calculations of this type can be employed to set up a scale of mass equivalence for the electromagnetic spectrum (Fig. 4-14). This scale can be used to check the answers to the above examples and to some of the problems at the end of this chapter.

Fig. 4-14. Mass and energy are actually two forms of the same medium. The equivalence of one to the other is described by Einstein's theory of relativity. This scale shows the equivalence of mass measured in kilograms to energy measured in electron volts.

REVIEW QUESTIONS

1. Define or otherwise identify the following:
   a. Photon
   b. Radiolucency
   c. The inverse square law
   d. Frequency
   e. The law of conservation of energy
   f. Gamma rays
   g. Electromagnetic spectrum
   h. Sinusoidal (sine)
   i. Quantum
   j. Visible light
2. Accurately diagram one photon of orange light (λ = 620 nm) and identify its velocity, electric field, magnetic field, and wavelength.
3. A thunder clap associated with lightning has a frequency of 800 Hz. If its wavelength is 50 cm, what is its velocity? How far away is the thunder if the time interval between seeing the lightning and hearing the thunder is 6 seconds?
4. What is the frequency associated with a photon of microwave radiation with a wavelength of 10^{-4} m?
5. Radio station WIMP-FM broadcasts at 104 MHz. What is the wavelength of this radiation?
6. In mammography 40 keV x rays are used. What is the frequency of this radiation?
7. Xeroradiography of bony structures calls for high-kVp technique. Many of these photons have energies of 110 keV. What is the frequency and wavelength of this radiation?
8. What is the energy of the 110 keV x ray of question 7 when expressed in joules? What is its mass equivalence?
9. The output intensity of a normal radiographic unit is 3 mR/mAs at 40 inches. What is the output intensity of such a unit at 80 inches? at 72 inches?
10. A portable x-ray machine has an output intensity of 4 mR/mAs at 40 inches. Conditions require that a particular examination be conducted at 30 in TFD (75 cm SID). What will be the output intensity at this distance?

WE PLAN TO PRODUCE GASTROINTESTINAL LAVAGE SOLUTIONS, POSITRON EMITTING RADIONUCLIDES, AND NONIONIC CONTRAST MEDIA, BUT JUST TO BE SURE, WE'RE STARTING WITH MOUTHWASH.

5

Electricity and magnetism

ELECTRIC TO ELECTROMAGNETIC
ENERGY

ELECTROSTATICS

ELECTRODYNAMICS

MAGNETISM

ELECTRIC TO ELECTROMAGNETIC ENERGY

In Chapter 1 various types of energy known today were briefly discussed. Two of these energies are particularly important in radiologic technology: electric and electromagnetic.

The primary function of an x-ray machine (Fig. 5-1, *A*) is to convert electric energy into electromagnetic energy. Electric energy is supplied to the x-ray machine in the form of a well-controlled electric current. A conversion takes place in the x-ray tube, where some of this electric energy is transformed into x rays. Before discussing the operation of an x-ray tube, or even the nature of the x-ray beam, we must consider some basic information regarding electricity and magnetism.

Fig. 5-1 shows other, more familiar, examples of electric energy conversion. When an automobile battery runs down, an electric charge restores the chemical energy of the battery.

Electric energy is converted into mechanical energy with a device known as an electric motor, which can be used to drive a table saw. A kitchen toaster or electric range converts electrical energy into thermal energy. There are, of course, many other examples of the conversion of electrical energy.

ELECTROSTATICS

Matter has been described as having mass, form, and an energy equivalence. Another fundamental property of matter is electric charge.

Electric charge comes in discrete units and is either positive or negative. The smallest unit of electric charge is associated with the electron and the proton. The electron has one unit of negative charge; the proton has one unit of positive charge. **Thus the electric charges associated with an electron and a proton have the same magnitude but opposite signs.**

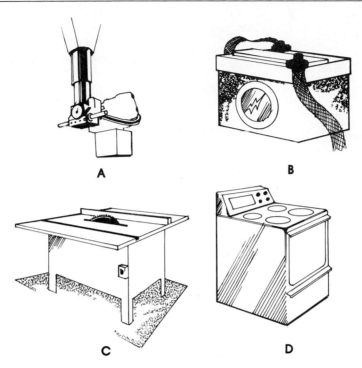

Fig. 5-1. Electric energy can be converted into other forms by various devices such as the following. **A,** X-ray machine for conversion to electromagnetic energy. **B,** A battery for chemical energy. **C,** A motor for mechanical energy. **D,** A kitchen range for thermal energy.

Because of the way atoms are constructed, electrons are free to travel from the outermost shell of one atom to the next. Protons, on the other hand, are fixed inside the nucleus of an atom and are not free to move. Consequently nearly all discussions of electric charge deal with negative electric charges, those associated with the electron. **Electrostatics** is the study of fixed, or stationary, electric charges. The most familiar example of a fixed electric charge is **static electricity.**

On touching a metal doorknob after having walked across a deep-pile carpet in winter, one gets a shock. Such a shock occurs because electrons are rubbed off the carpet onto one's shoes, causing one to become electrified. An object is said to be **electrified** if it has an insufficiency or an excess of electrons. Electrification can be cre-ated by contact, friction, or induction. It is an abnormal state relieved by providing some other object—the doorknob, for example—to or from which excess electrons can be transferred. Similarly, when one runs a comb through one's hair, electrons are removed from the hair and deposited on the comb; the comb becomes electrified with an excess of negative charges. In Fig. 5-2 such an electrified comb is shown picking up tiny pieces of paper as though it were a magnet. Because the comb is negatively electrified (excess electrons), it repels some electrons in the paper, causing that end of the paper to become slightly positively charged. This results in a small electrostatic attractive force. Similarly, one's hair is electrified because it has an abnormally low number of electrons and may stand on end because of mutual repulsion.

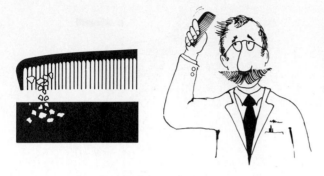

Fig. 5-2. Running a comb briskly through one's hair may cause both hair and comb to become electrified through the transfer of electrons from hair to comb. This electrified condition may make it possible to pick up small pieces of paper with the comb and may cause one's hair to stand on end.

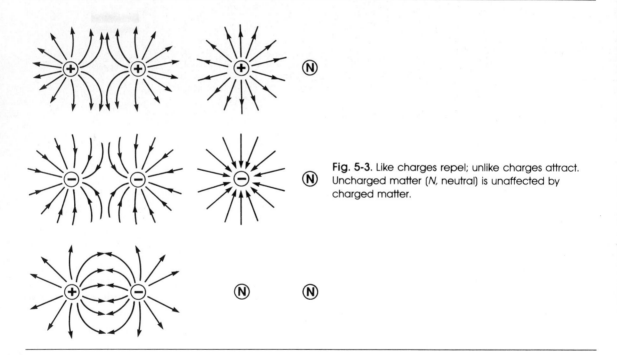

Fig. 5-3. Like charges repel; unlike charges attract. Uncharged matter (*N*, neutral) is unaffected by charged matter.

These phenomena demonstrate a principal law of electrostatics: **like charges repel; unlike charges attract.** Uncharged particles or objects exert no electrostatic force and are not acted on by charged particles (Fig. 5-3).

Viewed collectively, matter is electrically neutral because in all the universe the total number of negative charges equals the total number of positive charges. The outer-shell electrons of some types of atoms, however, are loosely bound to the nucleus and can easily be removed. In some molecules, electrons usually tightly bound become loosely bound. Removal of these electrons electrifies the substances from which they were removed and results in the phenomena associated with static electricity.

Another law of electrostatics states that **electrification occurs because of the movement**

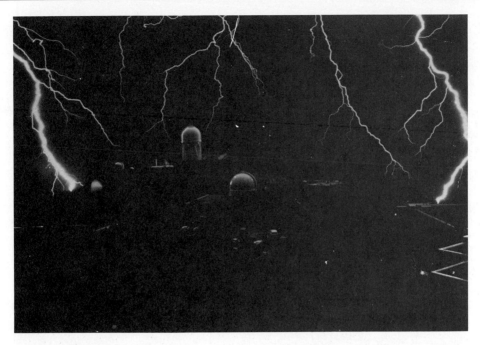

Fig. 5-4. Electrified clouds are the source of lightning in a storm. Lightning is the streaming of electrons, usually from a cloud to the ground, but sometimes from cloud to cloud. Shown here is a summer storm over Kitt Peak National Observatory. (Courtesy Gary Ladd.)

of negative electric charges. Positive electric charges do not move. The transfer of electrons from one object to another causes the first to be positively electrified and the second to be negatively electrified.

When a negatively electrified object is brought into contact with an electrically neutral object, the electric charges of the electrified object may be transferred to the neutral object. If the transfer is sufficiently violent, there will be a spark. One neutral object always available to accept electric charges from an electrified object is the earth. The earth behaves as a huge reservoir for deposit of stray electric charges. In this capacity it is called an **electric ground.** During a thunderstorm, wind and cloud movement can remove electrons from one cloud and deposit them on another. Both such clouds become

electrified, one negatively and one positively. If the electrification becomes great enough, if enough electronic charges are transferred, then a breakdown between the clouds can occur so that electrons are rapidly transported back to the cloud that is deficient in electrons. This phenomenon is called lightning. Although lightning can occur between clouds, it most frequently occurs between an electrified cloud and the earth. Fig. 5-4 illustrates this.

Another familiar example of electrification is that seen in every Frankenstein movie. Usually Dr. Frankenstein's laboratory is filled with electric gadgets, wire, and large steel balls with sparks flying in every diretion. An example of such a scene is shown in Fig. 5-5. The sparks are created because the various objects—wires, steel balls, and so on—are electrified by large

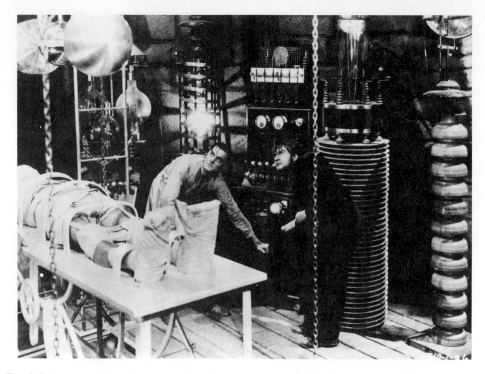

Fig. 5-5. This scene from the original *Frankenstein* movie in 1931 shows examples of static electricity. Dr. Frankenstein, on the left, was played by Colin Clive, and Dwight Frye played the role of Fritz, his assistant. (Courtesy The Bettmann Archive, Inc.)

numbers of electrons. Eventually the number of electric charges becomes so great that the electrification of the object is too great to be sustained. A breakdown occurs by the rapid movement of electrons through the air to an unelectrfied object, resulting in the spark, which is in effect a miniature lightning bolt.

Electrostatic laws

Four general laws of electrostatics describe the way in which electric charges interact with each other and with unelectrified objects. The first of these has already been introduced.

Unlike charges attract; like charges repel. Associated with each electric charge is an elec-

tric field. For a negative electric charge this electric field can be considered to exert a force radiating inward toward the electic charge. Positive electric charges can be considered similarly with the lines of electric field radiating outward from the charge. When two similar electric charges, negative and negative or positive and positive, are brought close together, their electric fields are in opposite direction and cause the electric charges to be repelled from each other. When unlike charges, one negative and one positive, are close to each other, the electric fields radiate in the same direction and cause the two charges to be attracted to each other. The force of attraction between unlike charges or repulsion between like charges is called an **electrostatic force.**

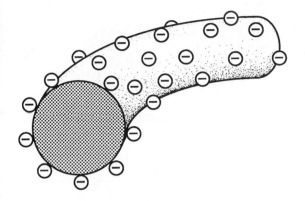

Fig. 5-6. Cross section of an electrified copper wire, showing that the electrostatic charges reside on the surface of the wire.

Coulomb's law. The magnitude of the electrostatic force is given by Coulomb's law, represented mathematically as

(5-1)

$$F = k\frac{Q_A Q_B}{d^2}$$

where F is the electrostatic force, Q_A and Q_B are quantities of electrostatic charge, d is the distance between the charges, and k is a constant of proportionality that depends on the units employed. According to Coulomb's law, the electrostatic force is directly proportional to the product of the electrostatic charges and inversely proportional to the square of the distance between them. The greater the electrostatic charge on either object, the greater the electrostatic force. As electrified objects are brought closer together, the electrostatic force increases not simply with the distance between the charges but much more rapidly. The electrostatic force is very strong when objects are close but decreases rapidly as objects are removed one from the other. This inverse square relationship for electrostatic force is the same as that for x-ray intensity (Chapter 4). The equation for electrostatic force has the same form as that for gravitational force, but electrostatic forces act only over short distances, whereas gravitational forces act over very long distances. The electrostatic force between two charges is unaffected by the presence of a third charge; similarly, the gravitational force between two masses is unaffected by the presence of a third mass.

Electric-charge distribution. When a diffuse nonconductor object becomes electrified, the electric charges are distributed throughout the object, such as the thunder cloud in Fig. 5-4. An electrified copper wire or other conductor has its excess electrons spread over the outer surface (Fig. 5-6).

Electric-charge concentration. In addition to being distributed along the outside surfaces of conductors, electric charges are concentrated along the sharpest curvature of the surface. An electrified cattle prod (Fig. 5-7) has electric charges equally distributed on the surface of the two electrodes except at each tip where electric charge is concentrated. "Our business is shocking" is the motto of the manufacturer of this cattle prod.

Electrostatic charge

The smallest unit of electric charge is that associated with an electron. This charge is much too small to be useful; consequently, the fundamental unit of electric charge is the coulomb, equivalent to 6.3×10^{18} electron charges.

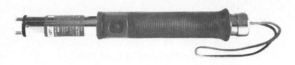

Fig. 5-7. Electrostatic charges are concentrated on surfaces of sharpest curvature. The cattle prod is a device that takes advantage of the electrostatic law. (Courtesy Hotshot Products Company, Inc.)

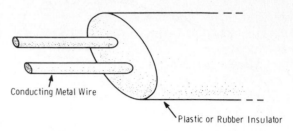

Conducting Metal Wire

Plastic or Rubber Insulator

Fig. 5-8. Conventional electrical wire usually consists of two parts, the metal conductor and the insulator.

EXAMPLE: What is the electrostatic charge on one electron?

ANSWER: One coulomb (C) is equivalent to 6.3×10^{18} electron charges; therefore

$$\frac{1\ C}{6.3 \times 10^{18}\ \text{electron charges}} =$$

$$1.6 \times 10^{-19}\ \text{C/electron charge}$$

EXAMPLE: The electrostatic charge transferred between two people after one has scuffed his feet across a nylon rug is about a microcoulomb. How many electrons are transferred?

ANSWER: $1\ C = 6.3 \times 10^{18}$ electrons
$1\ \mu C = 6.3 \times 10^{12}$ electrons

Electric potential

An earlier discussion of potential energy (Chapter 1) emphasized its relationship to work. A system possessing potential energy (stored energy) has the ability to do work when this energy is released. Electric potential is similarly defined. When positioned close to each other, like electric charges possess electric potential because they have the ability to do work when the electric potential is released and they fly apart. Electrons bunched up at one end of a wire possess electric potential because the electrostatic repulsive force will cause some electrons to move along the wire, and work can then be extracted.

The unit of electric potential is the **volt (V).** Electric potential is sometimes termed **electro-** motive force **(EMF).** The higher the voltage, the higher the potential to do work. The electric potential in homes and offices is 110 V. X-ray machines usually require 220 V or higher.

ELECTRODYNAMICS

The study of electrostatic charges in motion is called **electrodynamics;** we recognize electrodynamic phenomena as electricity. If an electric potential is applied to an electrified object, such as a copper wire, then the resting electric charges will move along the wire. This is called an **electric current** or **electricity.** An electric current is the flow of electrons. Electric currents occur in many types of objects and range from the very small currents of the human body measured by electrocardiograms to the very large currents of cross-country transmission lines.

Conductors and insulators

Basically, two types of material are involved in electricity. Any substance through which electrons easily flow is called an electric **conductor.** Substances that inhibit the flow of electrons are called electric **insulators.** A section of conventional household electric wire consists of a metal conducting wire coated with a rubber or plastic insulating material (Fig. 5-8). The insulator confines the electron flow to the conductor. Touching the insulator does not result in a shock; touching the conductor does. A rule of thumb:

good heat conductors are usually good electric conductors. Most metals are good electric conductors, copper being the best, although aluminum is also used. Water is also a good electric conductor because of the salts and other impurities it contains, which is why one should avoid water when operating power tools. Glass, clay, and other earthlike materials are usually good electric insulators.

In recent years materials have been discovered that exhibit two entirely different electric characteristics. In 1946 William Shockley demonstrated semiconduction. **A semiconductor** is a material that under some conditions behaves as an insulator, whereas under other conditions it acts as a conductor. The principal semiconductor materials are silicon (Si) and germanium (Ge). This development led first to the transistor, then to integrated circuits, and finally to the present very-large-scale integrated (VLSI) circuits that are the basis for the explosion in computer technology.

In the early 1960s the property of **superconductivity** was discovered. Superconducting materials such as niobium and titanium allow the flow of electrons without any resistance. Ohm's law, described in the next section, does not hold for superconductors. One might view a superconducting circuit as a perpetual motion machine since current flows without an electric potential or voltage. In order for material to behave as a superconductor, however, it must be made very cold, which requires energy. Table 5-1 summarizes the four electric states of matter.

Electric circuits

When electrons flow along a wire, they flow along its outer surface. Modifying the wire in some ways can cause it to resist the flow of electrons in certain regions. When this resistance is controlled and the conductor is made into a closed path, the result is an **electric circuit.**

In some respects an electric circuit is similar to a public water system. In such a system (Fig. 5-9) the first step is supplying the water with potential energy by pumping it into a water tow-

Table 5-1. Four electric states of matter

State	Material	Characteristics
Superconductive	Niobium Titanium	No resistance to electron flow No electric potential required Must by **very** cold
Conductive	Copper Aluminum	Variable resistance Obeys Ohm's law Requires a voltage
Semiconductive	Silicon Germanium	Can be conductive Can be resistive Basis for computer technology
Insulator	Rubber Glass	Does not permit electron flow Extremely high resistance Necessary with high voltage

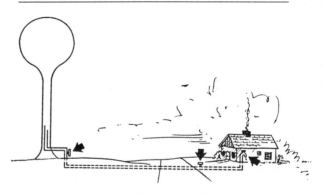

Fig. 5-9. In some respects a municipal water system is like an electric circuit. Water represents electric current; the water tank represents electric potential; and the valves represent electric resistors.

er. As the water flows through pipe with successively smaller diameters, resistance to its flow increases. Similarly, small-diameter wires resist the flow of electric current more than large-diameter wires do. A defect somewhere along the water line, such as a faulty valve, creates a large resistance to flow. This is similar to resistive elements built into electric circuits. When the valve is operating properly in the water line, the resistance to the flow of water can be controlled. Similarly, variable resistors in an electric circuit allow control of the flow of electrons. Increasing the resistance decreases the electric current. After the water has been distributed to homes and used, it is conveyed along waste water pipes back to the ground. Similarly, electric currents, after use, can be conducted back to ground, the earth.

Electric currents are measured in **amperes (A).** The ampere measures the number of electrons flowing in the electric circuit. One ampere is equal to an electric charge of one coulomb flowing through a conductor each second. Electric potential is measured in **volts (V),** and electric resistance is measured in **ohms (Ω).** Electrons powered by high voltage have high potential energy and high capacity to do work. If electrons are inhibited in their flow, the circuit resistance is said to be high.

The manner in which electric currents behave in an electric circuit is described by a relationship known as **Ohm's law.** Ohm's law states that **the voltage across the total circuit or any portion of the circuit is equal to the current times the resistance,** or mathematically,

(5-2)

$$V = IR$$

where V is the electric potential in volts, I is the electric current in amperes, and R is the electric resistance in ohms. Variations of this relationship are

(5-2a)

$$R = \frac{V}{I}$$

and

(5-2b)

$$I = \frac{V}{R}$$

EXAMPLE: If a current of 0.5 A flows through a conductor that has a resistance of 6 Ω, what is the voltage between the ends of the conductor?

ANSWER: $V = IR$
$= (0.5 \text{ A})(6 \text{ Ω})$
$= 3V$

EXAMPLE: A kitchen toaster draws a current of approximately 2.5 A. If the household voltage is 110 V, what is the electric resistance of the toaster?

ANSWER: $V = \frac{V}{I}$

$= \frac{110 \text{ V}}{2.5 \text{ A}}$

$= 44 \text{ Ω}$

Most electric circuits, such as those representing radio, television, or other electronic devices, are very complicated. X-ray circuits are complicated and contain a number of different types of circuit elements. Table 5-2 identifies some of the more important types of circuit elements, the functions of each, and their symbols. Usually electric circuits can be reduced to one of two basic kinds: a series circuit or a parallel circuit.

In a **series circuit** all circuit elements are connected in a line along the same conductor (Fig. 5-10). Rules for series circuits are summarized on p. 80.

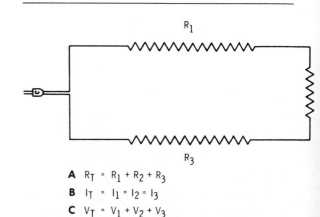

A $R_T = R_1 + R_2 + R_3$
B $I_T = I_1 = I_2 = I_3$
C $V_T = V_1 + V_2 + V_3$

Fig. 5-10. Series circuit and its basic rules.

Table 5-2. Electric circuit elements: their symbol and function

Circuit element	Symbol	Function
Resistor		Inhibits flow of electrons
Battery		Provides electric potential
Capacitor (condenser)		Momentarily stores electric charge
Ammeter	A	Measures electric current
Voltmeter	V	Measures electric potential
Switch		Turns circuit off by providing infinite resistance
Transformer		Increases or decreases voltage by fixed amount
Rheostat		Variable resistor
Diode		Allows electrons to flow in only one direction

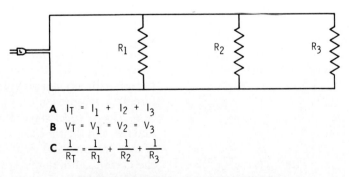

A $I_T = I_1 + I_2 + I_3$

B $V_T = V_1 = V_2 = V_3$

C $\dfrac{1}{R_T} = \dfrac{1}{R_1} + \dfrac{1}{R_2} + \dfrac{1}{R_3}$

Fig. 5-11. Parallel circuit and its basic rules.

1. The total resistance is equal to the sum of the individual resistances (Fig. 5-10, *A*).
2. The current through each circuit element is the same and is equal to the total circuit current (Fig. 5-10, *B*).
3. The sum of the voltages across each circuit element is equal to the total curcuit voltage (Fig. 5-10, *C*).

A **parallel circuit** contains elements that bridge the circuit rather than lie in a line along the conductor (Fig. 5-11). The basic rules for a parallel circuit are summarized as follows:

1. The sum of the currents through each circuit element is equal to the total circuit current (Fig. 5-11, *A*).
2. The voltage across each circuit element is the same and is equal to the total circuit voltage (Fig. 5-11, *B*).
3. The total resistance is inversely proportional to the sum of the reciprocals of each individual resistance (Fig. 5-11, *C*).

EXAMPLE: A series circuit contains three resistive elements having values of 8, 12, and 15 Ω. If the circuit potential is 110 V, what is the total circuit resistance and current, the current through each resistor, and the voltage across each resistor?

ANSWER: Refer to Fig. 5-10; let $R_1 = 8\ \Omega$, $R_2 = 12\ \Omega$, $R_3 = 15\ \Omega$.

$R_T = 8\ \Omega + 12\ \Omega + 15\ \Omega = 35\ \Omega$
$I_T = I_1 = I_2 = I_3 = V/R = 110/35 = 3.14\ A$
$V_1 = (3.14\ A)(8\ \Omega) = 25.12\ V$
$V_2 = (3.14\ A)(12\ \Omega) = 37.68\ V$
$V_3 = (3.14\ A)(15\ \Omega) = 47.10\ V$

EXAMPLE: Suppose the previous example were a parallel circuit rather than a series circuit. What would be the correct values for total circuit resistance and current, the current through each resistor, and the voltage across each resistor?

ANSWER: Refer to Fig. 5-11.

$$\frac{1}{R_T} = \frac{1}{8\ \Omega} + \frac{1}{12\ \Omega} + \frac{1}{15\ \Omega} =$$

$$\frac{15}{120} + \frac{10}{120} + \frac{8}{120} = \frac{33}{120}$$

$$R_T = \frac{120}{33} = 3.6\ \Omega$$

$I_T = 110\ V/3.6\ \Omega = 30.2\ A$
$I_1 = 110\ V/8\ \Omega = 13.6\ A$
$I_2 = 110\ V/12\ \Omega = 9.2\ A$
$I_3 = 110\ V/15\ \Omega = 7.3\ A$
$V_1 = V_2 = V_3 = V_T = 110\ V$

Christmas lights are a good example of the difference between series and parallel circuits. Christmas lights wired in series have only one wire connecting each lamp; when one lamp burns out, the entire string of lights goes off. Christmas lights wired in parallel, on the other hand, have two wires connecting each lamp; when one lamp burns out, the rest remain lit.

Most electric circuits are much more complicated than this. A television receiver has more than a thousand elements wired into a giant circuit consisting of many subcircuits, each of which is series or parallel or an combination of both.

Alternating current and direct current

Electric current, or electricity, is the flow of electrons through a conductor. These electrons can be made to flow in one direction along the electric conductor, in which case the electric current is called **direct current,** or **DC.** Most applications of electricity require that the electrons be controlled so that they flow first in one direction and then in the other. Current in which electrons oscillate back and forth is called **alternating current,** or **AC.**

Figs. 5-12 and 5-13 diagram the phenomena of DC and AC, respectively, and show how these phenomena are described by graphs called **waveforms.** The horizontal, or *x*, axis of the electric waveform represents time; the vertical, or *y*, axis represents the amplitude of the electric current. For DC, the electrons always flow in the same direction with the same velocity; therefore DC is represented by a second horizontal line. The vertical separation between this second line and the time axis represents the velocity of the electrons and therefore the magnitude of the current. If the line representing the current is above the time axis, it represents the flow of electrons in the positive direction. Electron flow

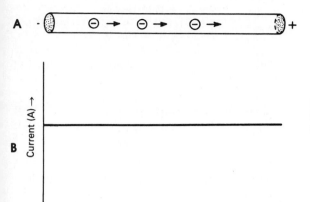

Fig. 5-12. Representation of direct current. **A,** Electrons flow in one direction only. **B,** The graph of the associated electric waveform is a straight line.

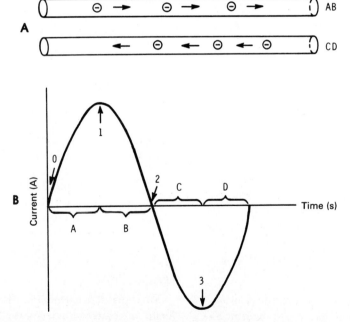

Fig. 5-13. Representation of alternating current. **A,** Electrons flow alternately in one direction and then the other. **B,** Alternating current is represented graphically by a sinusoidal electric waveform.

in the opposite direction is shown by a current line below the time axis. When the current line coincides with the time axis, the magnitude of the current is zero, indicating that no electrons flow.

The representation for AC, as shown in Fig. 5-13, should be familiar. It is a sine curve, representing electron flow first in a positive direction and then in a negative direction. At one instant in time (point *0* in Fig. 5-13) in an AC circuit, all electrons will be at rest. They then commence to move, first in the positive direction with increasing velocity (segment *A*). Once they reach maximum velocity, represented by the vertical distance from the time axis (point *1*), the electrons begin to slow down (segment *B*). They come to rest again momentarily (point *2*) and then reverse motion and flow in the negative direction (segment *C*), increasing in velocity until the magnitude of their velocity in the negative direction equals the magnitude of their maximum velocity in the positive direction (point *3*). There follows a reduction in velocity to zero (segment *D*). This oscillation in electron direction occurs in a sinusoidal fashion with each oscillation, or cycle, requiring $\frac{1}{60}$ second. Consequently, AC is identified as 60 Hz current (50 Hz in Europe and much of the rest of the world).

Electric power

Electric power is measured in **watts (W)**. One watt is equal to 1 A of current flowing through an electric potential of 1 V. Common household electric appliances such as toasters, blenders, mixers, and radios generally require from 500 to 1500 W of electric power. Light bulbs require from 30 to 150 W of electric power. An x-ray machine may require from 20 to 100 kW of electric power.

EXAMPLE: If the cost of electric power is 10 cents per kilowatt hour, how much does it cost to operate a 100 W light bulb an average of 5 hours per day for 1 month?

ANSWER:

$$\text{Total on time} = (30 \text{ days/mo})(5 \text{ hr/day})$$
$$= 150 \text{ hr/mo}$$

$$\text{Total power consumed} = (150 \text{ hr/mo})(100 \text{ W})$$
$$= 15,000 \text{ W-hr/mo}$$
$$= 15 \text{ kW-hr/mo}$$
$$\text{Total cost} = (15 \text{ kW-hr/mo})(10 \text{ cents/kW-hr})$$
$$= \$1.50/\text{mo}$$

The basic equation for the computation of electric power is

(5-3)

$$P = IV$$

where P is the power in watts, I is the current in amperes, and V is the electric potential in volts. However, since $V = IR$, then

(5-4)

$$P = I^2R$$

Either equation, 5-3 or 5-4, can be used to compute power.

EXAMPLE: An x-ray machine that draws 80 A of current, is supplied with 220 V. What is the power of consumption?
ANSWER: $P = IV$
$$= (80 \text{ A})(220 \text{ V})$$
$$= 17,600 \text{ W}$$
$$= 17.6 \text{ kW}$$

EXAMPLE: The overall resistance of a portable x-ray machine is 10 Ω. When plugged in to a 110 V receptacle, how much current does it draw and how much power is consumed?
ANSWER: $I = \dfrac{V}{R} = \dfrac{110}{10} = 11 \text{ A}$
$$P = IV$$
$$= (11 \text{ A})(110 \text{ V})$$
$$= 1210 \text{ W}$$

MAGNETISM

Magnetism is a fundamental property of some forms of matter. Such matter has the ability to attract iron and is said to be **magnetic.** This property is perhaps more difficult to understand than other characteristic properties of matter, such as mass, energy, and electric charge, because magnetism is difficult to detect and measure. We

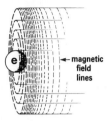

Fig. 5-14. A moving charged particle will induce a magnetic field in a plane perpendicular to its motion.

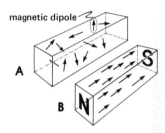

Fig. 5-15. A, In ferromagnetic material, the magnetic dipoles are randomly oriented. **B,** This changes when they are brought under the influence of an external magnetic field.

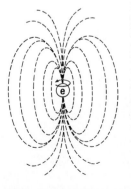

Fig. 5-16. An electric charge spinning on its own axis will create a magnetic field.

can feel mass, visualize energy, and be shocked by electricity, but we cannot sense magnetism.

The nature of magnetism

Any charged particle in motion will create a magnetic field, as shown in Fig. 5-14. The magnetic field is perpendicular to the motion of the charged particle, and its intensity is represented by imaginary lines. If the motion is a closed loop, as with an electron circling a nucleus, the magnetic field will be induced perpendicular to the plane of motion. Atoms having an odd number of electrons in their outer shell or shells therefore will exhibit a net magnetic field. Such a condition creates a magnetic domain that at the atomic level is called a **magnetic dipole.** In a hydrogen atom there is a strong magnetic dipole because of the unpaired electron, but in a hydrogen molecule the magnetic domains of the two electrons cancel one another so that there is no magnetic dipole. Under normal circumstances, magnetic dipoles are randomly distributed, as shown in Fig. 5-15, *A*. However, when acted on by an external magnetic field, such as the earth in the case of naturally occurring ores or an electromagnet in the case of artificially induced magnetism, the randomly oriented dipoles will line up along the magnetic field, as seen in Fig. 5-15, *B*. This is what happens when ferromagnetic material is made into a permanent magnet.

Spinning electric charges also induce a magnetic field, as shown in Fig. 5-16. The proton in a hydrogen nucleus spins on its axis and creates a nuclear magnetic dipole called a **magnetic moment.** This is the basis for magnetic resonance imaging (MRI), which will be discussed in Chapters 23 and 24.

The magnetic dipoles in a bar magnet generate imaginary lines of magnetic field, as illustrated in Fig. 5-17. If a nonmagnetic material is brought near such a magnet, there will be no disturbance in these field lines. However, if ferromagnetic material such as soft iron is brought near the bar magnet, the magnetic field lines will be deviated and concentrated into the fer-

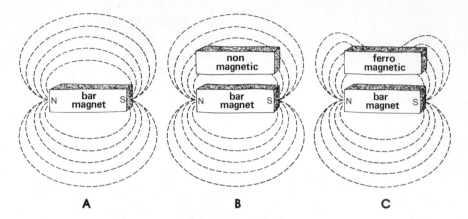

Fig. 5-17. A, Imaginary lines of force. **B,** These lines of force are undisturbed by nonmagnetic material. **C,** They are deviated by ferromagnetic material.

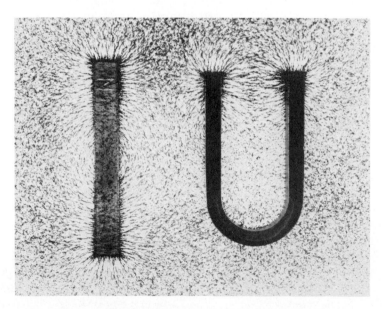

Fig. 5-18. Demonstration of magnetic lines of force with iron filings.

romagnetic material. Fig. 5-18 is a photograph of the magnetic fields of a bar magnet and a horseshoe magnet as demonstrated with iron filings.

Classification of magnets

Magnets are classified according to the origin of the magnetic property. Alternatively, all material can be classified according to the manner in which it interacts with an external magnetic field. There are three principal types of magnets: naturally occurring magnets, artifically induced permanent magnets, and electromagnets. The best example of a natural magnet is the earth itself. Some ores in the earth called **lodestones** consist of an iron oxide and exhibit strong magnetism, presumably because they have remained undisturbed for a long time in the earth's magnetic field. Artificially produced permanent magnets are available in many sizes and shapes but principally as bar or horseshoe-shaped magnets. A compass is a prime example of an artifical permanent magnet. Such permanent magnets don't necessarily stay permanent. One can destroy the magnetic property of a magnet by heating it or even by hitting it with a hammer. Either act causes the individual dipoles to be jarred from their alignment. They thus again become randomly aligned, and magnetism is lost.

Most materials are unaffected when brought into a magnetic field. Such materials are said to be **nonmagnetic.** They cannot be artifically magnetized, and they are not attracted to a magnet. Examples of nonmagnetic materials are wood, glass, and plastic. **Ferromagnetic** materials are iron, cobalt, and nickel. These are strongly attracted by a magnet and can usually be permanently magnetized by exposure to a magnetic field. An alloy of aluminum, nickel, and cobalt called **alnico** is one of the more powerful artificially induced magnets produced from ferromagnetic material. **Paramagnetic** materials lie somewhere between ferromagnetic and nonmagnetic. They are very slightly attracted to a magnet and loosely influenced by an external magnetic field.

Magnetic laws

The physical laws of magnetism are similar to those of electrostatics and gravity. If a magnet is placed on a surface with small iron filings as in Fig. 5-18, the filings will attach most strongly and with greater concentration to the ends of the magnet. These ends are called poles, and every magnet has two poles. Magnetic poles exist in two forms: a **north pole** and a **south pole,** analogous to positive and negative electrostatic charges. A basic law of magnetism states that **like magnetic poles repel and unlike magnetic poles attract.**

The second principal law of magnetism relates to the magnetic force of attraction or repulsion. **This force is proportional to the product of the magnetic pole strengths divided by the square of the distance between them.** This is similar to electrostatic and gravitational forces that also are inversely proportional to the square of the distance between the objects under consideration. If the distance between two bar magnets is halved, the magnetic force will be increased by four times. The SI unit of magnetic force is the tesla. Another common unit is the gauss. One tesla (T) = 10,000 gauss (G).

Some characteristics of the three fundamental forces in nature are shown in Table 5-3. Note the similarities in the formulation of the forces and the fields through which they act. There is considerable activity among theoretic physicists attempting to combine these fundamental forces with two others, the strong nuclear force and the weak interaction, to formulate a grand **unified field theory.**

A curious property of magnets is that they cannot exist without both a north and a south pole. Fig. 5-19 shows that when a magnet is broken into smaller and smaller pieces, one creates smaller and smaller magnets.

The earth behaves as though it has a large bar magnet embedded in it. At the equator, the north pole of a compass will point to the earth's North Pole (which is actually the earth's south magnetic pole!). As one travels toward the North Pole as in Fig. 5-20, the attraction of the compass

Table 5-3. Three fundamental forces in nature

	Gravitational	Electric	Magnetic
The force:	Attracts only	Attracts and repels	Attracts and repels
It acts in:	A mass, m	A charge, q	A pole, p
Through an associated field:	A gravitational field, g	An electric field, E	A magnetic field, B
With intensity:	$F = mg$	$F = qE$	$F = pB$
The source of the field is:	A mass, M	A charge, Q	A pole, P
The intensity of the field at a distance from the source is:	$g = \dfrac{GM}{d^2}$	$E = \dfrac{kQ}{d^2}$	$B = \dfrac{kP}{d^2}$
The force between fields is given by:	Newton's law	Coulomb's law	Gauss' law
	$F = -G\dfrac{Mm}{d^2}$	$F = k\dfrac{Qq}{d^2}$	$F = k\dfrac{Pp}{d^2}$
where:	$G = 6.678 \times 10^{-11}\dfrac{Nm^2}{kg^2}$	$k = 9.0 \times 10^9\dfrac{Nm^2}{C^2}$	$k = 10^{-7}\dfrac{W}{A^2}$

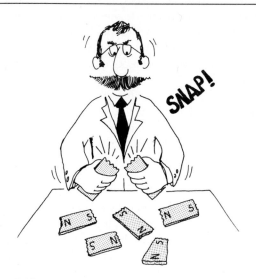

Fig. 5-19. If one breaks a single magnet into smaller and smaller pieces, one produces baby magnets.

will become more intense until the compass needle points directly into the earth not at the geographic North Pole but at a region in northern Canada—the magnetic pole. The magnetic pole in the southern hemisphere is in Australia.

There the direction of the compass is into space.

The use of a compass might suggest that the earth has a strong magnetic field, but it does not. The earth's magnetic field is about 100 μT (1 G), far less than the magnet on a door latch, which is about 0.1 T (1000 G).

REVIEW QUESTIONS

1. Define or otherwise identify the following:
   a. Electric charge and its smallest unit
   b. Electrodynamics
   c. Ohm's law
   d. Magnetism
   e. AC
   f. Electric circuit
   g. Insulator
   h. Electrostatics
2. If the distance between two charged bodies is doubled, what will be the change in electrostatic force?
3. If the distance between two magnetic poles is doubled, what will be the change in magnetic force?
4. A lightning bolt carries about 25 C of charge. How many electrons is this? Calculate the total mass of electrons involved.
5. What is the total circuit resistance when resistive elements of 5, 10, 15, and 20 Ω are connected in (a) series and (b) parallel?

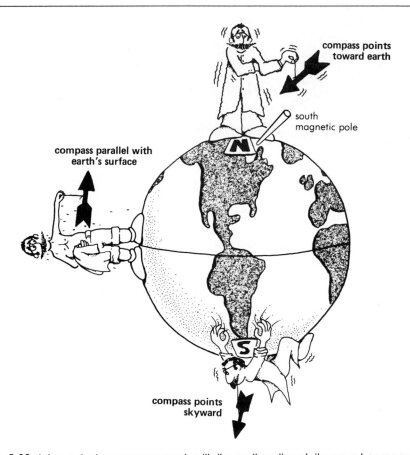

compass points
toward earth

south
magnetic pole

compass parallel with
earth's surface

compass points
skyward

Fig. 5-20. A free-swinging compass reacts with the earth as though it were a bar magnet.

6. If the resistive circuits in question 5 are connected to a 110 V source, what will be the total circuit current for (a) series and (b) parallel operations?
7. If the resistive circuits in question 5 each draw 7 A, what will be the voltage across the 10 Ω resistor for (a) series and (b) parallel operation?
8. How much electric power is consumed by the circuit in question 6?

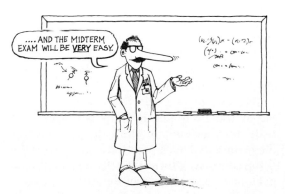

.... AND THE MIDTERM
EXAM WILL BE **VERY** EASY.

6

Electromagnetism

ELECTROMAGNETIC EFFECT

ELECTROMAGNETIC INDUCTION

ELECTRIC GENERATORS AND
MOTORS

THE TRANSFORMER

RECTIFICATION

ELECTROMAGNETIC EFFECT

We now know that electricity and magnetism are intimately connected. They are both different aspects of the same basic force—the electromagnetic force, one of the four fundamental forces of nature (gravity, the electromagnetic force, the strong nuclear force, and the weak interaction). Up until the nineteenth century, however, electricity and magnetism were viewed as separate effects. Although many scientists suspected an interconnection between the two, their research was hampered by the lack of any convenient way of producing and controlling electricity.

Magnetic fields could be generated and detected using various naturally occurring magnetic minerals such as the lodestone. Perhaps the earliest and most practical application of this is the compass, which is simply a piece of magnetic metal used to detect the earth's magnetic field. The north pole of the magnetic needle always points to the North Pole of the earth. European seafarers began using a compass as a navigational aid in the century before Columbus discovered America, but the compass was apparently known to Chinese navigators even earlier.

The study of electricity at this time was basically limited to the investigation of static charges, those which could be produced by friction (for example, those produced by rubbing fur on a rubber rod). Charges could be induced to move but only in a sudden discharge, as with a spark jumping a gap. It was the development of methods for producing a steady flow of charges (that is, an electric current) during the last century that stimulated investigations of both electricity and magnetism, which led to an increased understanding of electromagnetic phenomena. This, of course, ultimately precipitated the electronic revolution that is so much the basis of today's technology.

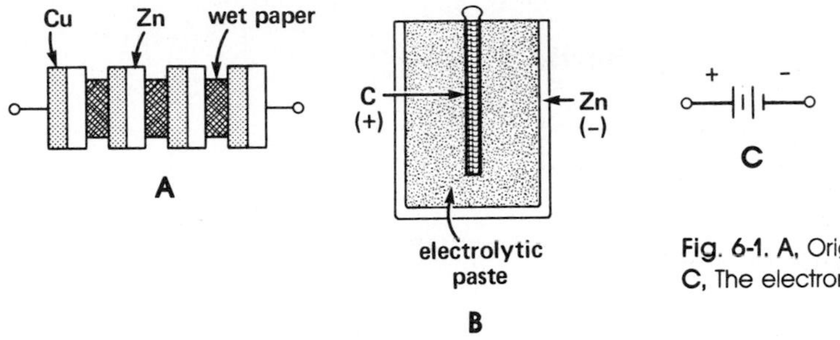

Fig. 6-1. A, Original Voltaic pile. **B,** A modern dry cell. **C,** The electronic symbol for a battery.

The battery and electromotive force

In the late 1700s an Italian anatomist made a discovery quite by accident. He discovered that a dissected frog leg could be made to twitch when touched by two dissimilar metals, just as if it had been touched by an electrostatic charge. This stimulated another Italian, a physicist by the name of Alessandro Volta, to question if an electric current might be produced when two dissimilar metals are brought into contact. Using zinc and copper plates, he succeeded in producing an electric current, although it was feeble. To increase the current, he stacked the copper-zinc plates like a Dagwood sandwich to form what was called the **Voltaic pile,** a precursor of the modern battery. Each zinc-copper sandwich is called a **cell of the battery.**

Modern dry cells use a carbon rod as the positive electrode surrounded by an electrolytic paste housed in a negative zinc cylindrical can. The Voltaic pile, modern battery, and the electronic symbol for the battery are shown in Fig. 6-1.

Both of these devices are examples of sources of electromotive force (EMF). Any device that converts some form of energy directly into electric energy is said to be a source of EMF. Although still commonly used, this somewhat archaic term is a little misleading. Electromotive force is not really a force, such as gravity, but rather it refers to stored **electric energy. EMF has units of joules per coulomb, or volts.**

Oersted's experiment

When scientists had a source of constant electric current to experiment with, there began extensive investigations into the possibility of a link between electric and magnetic forces. The first such link was discovered in 1820 by Hans Oersted, a Danish physicist. His experiment is illustrated in Fig. 6-2. A long straight wire was supported near a free-rotating magnetic compass. With no current flowing through the wire, the magnetic compass aligned itself with the earth's magnetic field as one would expect. However, when a current was passed through the wire, the compass needle swung to point straight at the wire. Here we have evidence of a direct link between electric and magnetic phenomena. The electric current evidently produced a magnetic field strong enough to overpower the earth's magnetic field and cause the magnetic compass to point toward the wire.

Further investigation showed that any charge in motion generates a magnetic field. A charge at rest produces no magnetic field. Thus electrons flowing through wires that make up an electric circuit generate a magnetic field about each wire. The magnetic field is represented by imaginary lines that form concentric circles centered on the wire, as shown in Fig. 6-3. The direction of the magnetic field lines can be determined by using what is called the **right-hand rule.** Imagine gripping the wire with the right hand. If the thumb is pointed in the direction

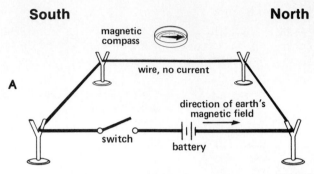

South   **North**

magnetic
compass

A

wire, no current

direction of earth's
magnetic field

switch   battery

Fig. 6-2. Oersted's experiment. **A,** With no current in the
wire the compass points north. **B,** With current flowing
the compass points toward the wire.

S   **N**

B

wire, current flow

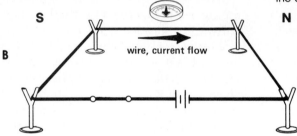

wire

magnetic
field lines

current

Fig. 6-3. Magnetic field lines form concentric circles
around the current-carrying wire.

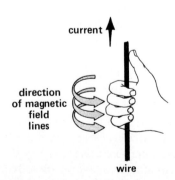

current

direction
of magnetic
field
lines

wire

Fig. 6-4. Determining the direction of the magnetic
field around the wire using the right-hand rule.

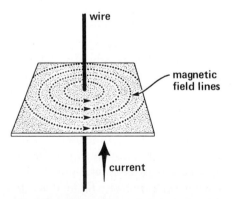

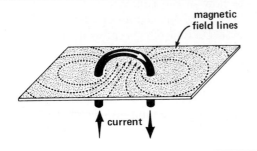

Fig. 6-5. Magnetic field lines are concentrated on the inside of the loop.

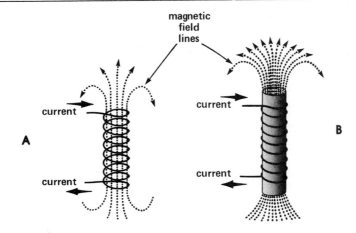

Fig. 6-6. A, Magnetic field lines around a solenoid. B, Magnetic field lines around an electromagnet.

of the current flow, the fingers of your hand will then curl in the direction of the magnetic field lines, as shown in Fig. 6-4.

The solenoid

These same rules apply if the current is flowing in a circular loop. Magnetic field lines form concentric circles around each tiny section of the wire. However, because the wire is curved, these field lines overlap inside the loop. In particular, at the very center of the loop, all the field lines add together, making the magnetic field strong (Fig. 6-5). Stacking more loops on top of each other increases the intensity of the

magnetic field running through the center, or axis, of the stack of loops. Thus, for a coil of wire called a **solenoid,** the magnetic field tends to be concentrated through the center of the coil (Fig. 6-6, A).

The magnetic field can further be intensified by wrapping the coil of wire around a ferromagnetic material such as iron. The iron core concentrates the magnetic field. In this case, almost all of the magnetic field lines are concentrated inside of the core, escaping only near the ends of the coil. This type of device, shown in Fig. 6-6, B, is called an **electromagnet.**

The magnetic field produced by an electromagnet is the same as that produced by a bar magnet. That is, if both were hidden from view behind a piece of paper, the pattern of magnetic field lines revealed by iron filings sprinkled on the paper surface would be the same. Of course, the advantage of the electromagnet is that its magnetic field can be adjusted or turned on and off simply by varying the current flow through its coil of wire.

ELECTROMAGNETIC INDUCTION

Oersted's experiment demonstrated that electricity can be used to generate magnetic fields. It is obvious, then, to wonder whether the reverse is true: can magnetic fields somehow be used to generate a current flow? It took Michael Faraday, a self-educated British experimenter, 6 years to find the answer to that question.

Induced currents

From a series of experiments, Faraday surmised that an electric current cannot be induced in a circuit merely by the presence of a magnetic field. For example, consider the situation illustrated in Fig. 6-7. A coil of wire is connected to a current-measuring device called an **ammeter.** If a bar magnet were set next to the coil, the meter would indicate that no current is flowing through the coil. However, Faraday discovered that, if the magnet is moved, a current will begin

to flow in the coiled wire, indicated by a deflection of the ammeter needle. Therefore to induce a flow of current using a magnetic field, the magnetic field cannot be constant but must be changing.

This observation is summarized in what is called Faraday's law, or the first law of electromagnetic induction: **an electric current will be induced to flow in a circuit if some part of that circuit is in a changing magnetic field.** The magnitude of the induced current depends on four factors:

1. The strength of the magnetic field
2. The velocity of the conductor as it moves through the magnetic field
3. The angle of the conductor to the magnetic field
4. The number of turns in the conductor

The changing magnetic field can be produced in many ways. For example, a bar magnet or an electromagnet can be moved near a coil of wire. Or, conversely, the magnet can be held stationary and the coil of wire moved near it. Alternatively, there need not be any relative motion. An electromagnet can be fixed near a coil of wire. If the current in the electromagnet is then either increased or decreased, its magnetic field will likewise change and induce a flow of current in the coil. A prime example of electromagnetic induction is radio reception. As emitted, RF sig-

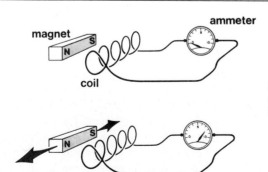

Fig. 6-7. Schematic description of Faraday's experiment shows how a moving magnetic field induces an electric current.

nal has an alternating magnetic component which induces a signal in an antenna.

The essential point in all these examples is that the intensity of the magnetic field at the coil must be changing to induce a current flow. If the magnetic field intensity is constant, there will be no induced current.

Lenz's law

In 1834 a Russian scientist, Heinrich Lenz, expanded on Faraday's work. He established the principle for determining the direction that the induced current would flow. This principle, the second law of electromagnetics, or Lenz's law, follows: **the induced current will flow in a direction such that it opposes the action that induces it.**

This principle may seem a little confusing at first and can perhaps be best illustrated by an example. Consider the situation diagramed in Fig. 6-8. The north pole of a magnet is being pushed into a coil of wire. Which direction will the current flow around the coil of wire? Because the magnet is being moved near the coil of wire, we know from the first law of electromagnetics that an induced current will flow through the coil of wire. We further know that a coil of wire with a current flowing in it acts like a tiny magnet. One end of the coil will be like a north pole of a magnet, and the other end will be like a

south pole, but which end will be which? Lenz's law answers this question. The action that induces the current in the coil is the motion of the north pole of the magnet toward the coil. According to Lenz's law, to oppose this action, the coil of wire will induce a north magnetic field at its left end (since the coil's north pole will repel, that is, "oppose," the inward motion of the magnet's north pole). To induce a north magnetic pole at the left end of the coil or wire, the induced current must flow as shown in Fig. 6-8.

These electromagnetic laws govern the induction of electric currents by magnetic fields of changing intensity. There are two basic types of induction—**self-induction** and **mutual induction**—and these form the bases for transformers, electric motors, and generators.

Self-induction

Consider the situation illustrated by Fig. 6-9. If a constant source of EMF is connected to a coil, a steady current of electricity will flow through the coil relatively unimpeded, and a constant magnetic field will be produced by the coil.

What will happen, however, if a varying source of EMF such as alternating current is connected to the coil? The current flow through and the magnetic field produced by the coil will

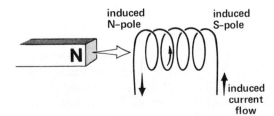

Fig. 6-8. Demonstration of Lenz's law shows that the current induced in a coil by a moving magnet produces a magnetic field opposing the motion of the magnet.

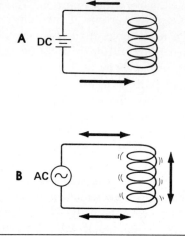

Fig. 6-9. Demonstration of self-induction. **A,** A coil passes constant current unimpeded. **B,** It will resist the passage of a changing current because of self-induction.

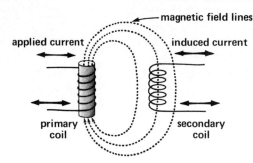

Fig. 6-10. Inducing a current in the secondary coil by mutual induction.

no longer be constant. By Lenz's law an opposing action in the coil will be induced by this changing magnetic field. In this case an induced EMF will be set up opposing the source EMF. If the source EMF increases, the induced-coil EMF opposes it by trying to reduce it. If, on the other hand, the source EMF is falling, then the induced-coil EMF will increase to oppose it. This induction of an opposing EMF in a single coil by its own changing magnetic field is called self-induction. The opposing EMF is sometimes called a **back EMF.** The self-induction of AC circuit components such as **choke coils** and **transformers** is an important consideration for design of equipment.

In summary, a coil will pass a steady direct current relatively unimpeded but will impede the passage of an alternating current flow because of self-induction in the coil.

Mutual induction

Faraday showed that it was not necessary to physically move a magnet near a coil to induce a current flow. All that is necessary is that the intensity of the magnetic field change. This can be accomplished by fixing an electromagnet near the coil and varying the current flow through the electromagnet, as shown in Fig. 6-10. The varying current flow in the electromagnet cre-

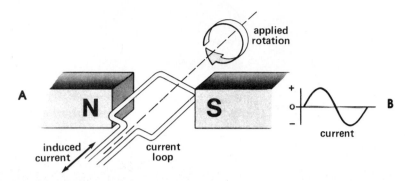

Fig. 6-11. A, Simple electric generator. **B,** Its output waveform.

ates a varying magnetic field, which, when it passes through the coil, induces a current flow in that coil. The first coil through which the varying current is passed is called the **primary.** The coil in which the induced current flows is called the **secondary.** This process of inducing a current flow through a secondary coil by passing a varying current through the primary coil is called mutual induction. Mutual induction will be considered in more detail under discussion of the transformer.

ELECTRIC GENERATORS AND MOTORS

Electric motors and generators are actually expanded practical applications of Oersted's and Faraday's experiments. In one case an electric current produced a mechanical motion (the motion of the compass needle). This is the basis of the electric motor. In the other experiment mechanical motion (the motion of a coil of wire near a magnet) induced a current flow in a coil of wire. This is the principle on which the electric generator operates. Let us now examine these two important **electromechanical devices** in more detail.

The electric generator

A simple electric generator is diagramed in Fig. 6-11, *A*. A coil of wire is placed in a strong magnetic field between two poles of a magnet. The coil is rotated by mechanical energy (for example, by hand, by water flowing past a water wheel, or by steam flowing over the vanes of a turbine blade in an atomic power plant). Because the coil of wire is moving in the magnetic field, a current is induced in the coil of wire. The induced current, however, is not constant. It varies according to the orientation of the coil's wire in the magnetic field. The induced current flows first in one direction and then the other, following a sinusoidal pattern, as shown in Fig. 6-11, *B*. Thus this type of simple electric generator produces an **alternating current (AC).**

A **direct current (DC)** generator can be constructed by adding a simple device called a **commutator ring,** as shown in Fig. 6-12. The commutator ring acts like a switch changing the polarity of the contact on the loop of wire at precisely those points when the current flow through the loop would reverse. The resulting reversed current, flowing out of the commutator

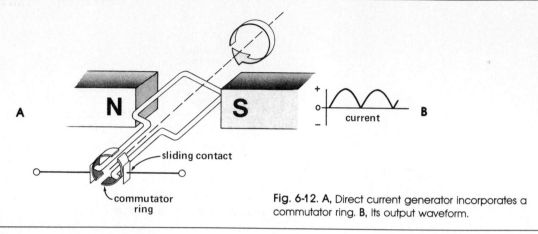

Fig. 6-12. A, Direct current generator incorporates a commutator ring. **B,** Its output waveform.

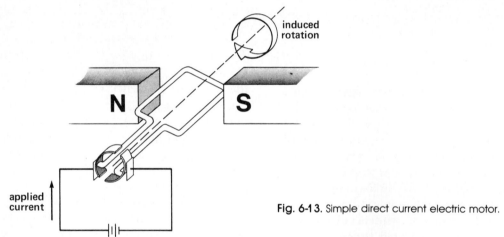

Fig. 6-13. Simple direct current electric motor.

ring assembly, is humped out always in one direction. Although in one direction (DC), it still does not produce a constant current.

The net effect of an electric generator is to convert mechanical energy into electric energy. The conversion process is, of course, not 100% efficient because of frictional losses in the mechanical moving parts and heat losses caused by resistances in the electric components.

The electric motor

A simple electric motor, as shown in Fig. 6-13, has basically the same components as an electric generator. In this case, however, electric energy is supplied to the current loop to produce a mechanical motion, that is, a rotation of the loop in the magnetic field.

When a current is passed through the wire loop, a magnetic field is produced, making it

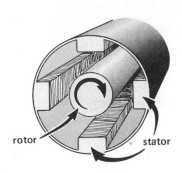

Fig. 6-14. Principal parts of an induction motor.

like a tiny electromagnet. Being free to turn, the electromagnet-current loop rotates as it attempts to align itself with the stronger magnetic field produced by the exterior bar magnet. Just as the current loop becomes aligned with the exterior magnetic field, the commutator ring switches the direction of current flow through the loop and therefore reverses the coil's required alignment. Because of the switch in current flow, the electromagnet is now no longer aligned with the exterior magnetic field of the bar magnet. It is now opposed to it. The electromagnet-current loop rotates 180 degrees in an attempt to realign itself once again with the bar magnet field. As the electromagnet again nears alignment, the commutator switches the direction of current flow and forces the loop to rotate again. This procedure repeats itself over and over, the electromagnet-current loop never quite being able to align itself with the magnetic field of the bar magnets. The net result is that the current loop continuously rotates.

In a practical electric motor many turns of wire are used for the current loop, and more than one pair of bar magnets are used to create the external magnetic field. However, the prin-

ciple of operation is basically the same. This type of electric motor is called a **direct current motor.**

The type of motor used in some x-ray tubes is called an **induction motor** (Fig. 6-14). In this type of motor the rotating rotor is still a series of wire loops; however, the exterior magnetic field is supplied by several electromagnets. No current is passed to the rotor. Instead, current flow is produced in the rotor windings by induction. The electromagnets surrounding the rotor are energized in sequence, producing a changing magnetic field. The induced current flow produced in the rotor windings generates a magnetic field. Just as in a conventional electric motor, this magnetic field attempts to align itself with the magnetic field of the exterior electromagnets. Because these electromagnets are being energized in sequence, the rotor begins to rotate, trying to bring its magnetic field in alignment. The net result is the same as in a conventional electric motor, that is, the rotor rotates continuously. The difference, however, is that the electric energy is supplied to the exterior magnets rather than the interior rotor windings.

THE TRANSFORMER

Both electric motors and generators make use of interacting electromagnetic fields produced by electric currents. They convert mechanical to electric energy (the generator) or electric to mechanical energy (the motor). Another device that makes use of the interacting magnetic fields produced by changing electric currents is the **transformer.** It, however, does not convert one form of energy to another but rather transforms the electric potential and current into higher or lower values.

Recall from the discussion of mutual induction that if two coils are placed near each other and a changing current is applied to one of them (the primary), then a current will be induced to flow in the other coil (the secondary). Recall also that placing a core of magnetic material in the center

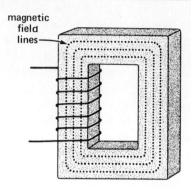

Fig. 6-15. Electromagnet that incorporates a closed iron core produces a closed magnetic field primarily confined to the core.

of the coil will greatly increase the strength of the magnetic field passing through its center. The magnetic field lines tend to be concentrated in the magnetic material of the core, escaping mainly at the ends. Imagine, however, that this magnetic core is bent around so that it forms a continuous loop (Fig. 6-15). There are no end surfaces from which the magnetic field lines can escape. Therefore the magnetic field tends to be confined to the loop of magnetic core material. If the secondary coil is then wound around the other side of this loop of core material, almost all the magnetic field produced by the primary windings will also pass through the center of the secondary winding. Thus there is a good **coupling** between the magnetic field produced by the primary winding and the secondary coil. A changing current passed through the primary will therefore induce a strong current flow in the secondary winding. This type of device is called a transformer.

It is essential to remember that because a transformer operates on the principle of mutual induction, **it will only operate with a changing electric current (AC).** A direct current applied

to the primary windings will induce no current flow in the secondary winding.

The transformer law

The transformer is used to change the magnitude of current and voltage in a circuit. This change is directly proportional to the ratio of the number of turns of the secondary winding (N_s) to the number of turns in the primary winding (N_p). If there are ten turns on the secondary winding for every turn on the primary winding, then the voltage generated in the secondary circuit (V_s) will be ten times the voltage supplied to the primary circuit (V_p). Mathematically, the transformer law is represented as follows:

(6-1)

$$\frac{V_s}{V_p} = \frac{N_s}{N_p}$$

The quantity N_s/N_p is known as the **turns ratio** of the transformer. The voltage change across the transformer is proportional to the turns ratio. A transformer with a turns ratio greater than 1 is said to be a **step-up transformer** because the voltage is increased, or stepped up, from the primary to the secondary side. When the turns ratio is less than 1, the transformer is called a **step-down transformer.**

Because the voltage changes across a transformer, the current (I) must necessarily change also; the transformer law may therefore be written

(6-2a)

$$\frac{I_s}{I_p} = \frac{N_p}{N_s}$$

or

(6-2b)

$$\frac{I_s}{I_p} = \frac{V_p}{V_s}$$

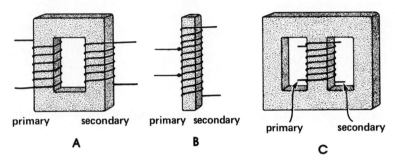

Fig. 6-16. Types of transformers. **A,** Closed-core transformer. **B,** Autotransformer. **C,** Shell-type transformer.

The magnitude of the current change across a transformer is in the opposite direction from the voltage change but in the same proportion. In a step-up transformer the current on the secondary side (I_s) is smaller than the current on the primary side (I_p); in a step-down transformer the secondary current is larger than the primary current.

The transformer is not 100% efficient. There are some losses in power from the primary to the secondary side, but for our purposes these losses can be considered negligible.

EXAMPLE: There are 125 turns on the primary side of a transformer and 90,000 turns on the secondary side. If 110 V AC is supplied to the primary winding, what will be the voltage induced in the secondary winding?

ANSWER: $\dfrac{V_s}{V_p} = \dfrac{N_s}{N_p}$

$$V_s = V_p\left(\frac{N_s}{N_p}\right)$$

$$= (110\ \text{V})\left(\frac{90,000}{125}\right)$$

$$= (110)(720)\ \text{V}$$
$$= 79,200\ \text{V}$$
$$= 79.2\ \text{kV}$$

EXAMPLE: The turns ratio of a filament transformer is 0.125. What will be the filament current if the current flowing through the primary winding is 0.8 A?

ANSWER: $\dfrac{I_s}{I_p} = \dfrac{N_p}{N_s}$

$$I_s = I_p\left(\frac{N_p}{N_s}\right)$$

$$= (0.8\ \text{A})\left(\frac{1}{0.125}\right)$$

$$= 6.4\ \text{A}$$

Types of transformers

There are many ways to construct a transformer. Several types are illustrated in Fig. 6-16.

The type of transformer discussed thus far, built about a square donut of magnetic material, is called a **closed-core transformer.** The core is not a single piece but rather is built up of laminated layers of iron. This is done to help reduce energy losses caused by heating in the core produced by the transformer's changing magnetic field.

Another type of transformer shown in Fig. 6-16 is called an **autotransformer.** It consists of an iron core with only one winding of wire about

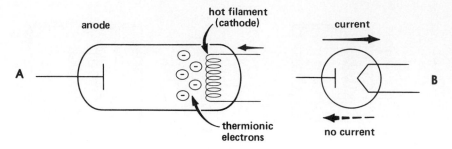

Fig. 6-17. **A,** Basic vacuum tube. **B,** Its electronic symbol.

it. This single winding acts as both the primary and the secondary windings. Connections are made at different points on the coil for both the primary and secondary sides. An autotransformer is generally smaller, and because both the primary and the secondary sides are connected to the same wire, its use is generally restricted to those cases where only a small step up or step down in voltage is required. Thus it would not be suitable for use as the high-voltage transformer in an x-ray machine.

The third type of transformer shown in Fig. 6-16 is called a **shell-type transformer.** Because this type of transformer traps even more of the magnetic field lines of the primary winding, it is more efficient than the closed-core transformer. Most transformers in modern use have this type of construction.

RECTIFICATION

The electrical devices we have discussed thus far are important components of modern x-ray systems. Induction motors are used to spin the anodes in most x-ray tubes, and step-up transformers provide the high voltage necessary for the production of x rays. The specific roles these components play in the x-ray system are discussed in more detail in later chapters. There is, however, one further important concept that will also be related to x-ray production in later

chapters. This is the concept of **rectification.**

The current from a common wall plug is AC. The current switches direction back and forth sixty times per second. However, as will be seen later, an x-ray tube requires a DC current, that is, electron flow in only one direction. Therefore some means must be provided for converting AC to DC. This process of converting AC to DC is called rectification.

An electronic device that allows current in only one direction is called a **rectifier.** There are two principal types of rectifiers: valve tube rectifiers and solid-state rectifiers.

Tube rectifiers

Consider an evacuated glass tube with a small coil of wire, **the filament,** at one end (Fig. 6-17). If a large current is passed through this filament, it will heat up and "boil" electrons off its surface. This process is called **thermionic emission.** (*Therm* refers to heat, *ion* refers to a charged particle, and *emission,* of course, means to give off; thus thermionic emission refers to the giving off of electrons from the surface of a heated metal.) This emitter of electrons is called the **filament** and constitutes the **cathode,** or negative side of the tube. A cold metallic plate is placed at the other end of the glass envelope. This is called the **anode,** or positive side. This combination of hot electron-emitting cathode

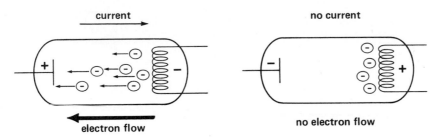

Fig. 6-18. Vacuum tube diode will conduct electrons in only one direction, from cathode to anode.

and cold anode enclosed in a vacuum-sealed glass tube is the basis for most electronic tubes, including the x-ray tube.

An electric current is made up of a flow of electrons. Therefore the electrons, thermionically boiling off the hot filament of a vacuum tube, offer the opportunity for a current. If a higher voltage is placed on the anode rather than the cathode, the electrons at the cathode will be attracted to the anode. They stream across the length of the tube, causing an electron flow through the tube (Fig. 6-18). Thus there can be electrons conducted through an electron tube from the cathode to the anode. If, however, a higher voltage is placed on the cathode than the anode, the electrons will remain attracted to the cathode. There are no free electrons at the anode end available to stream across the gap. Therefore no electrons will flow across the tube from the anode to the cathode.

In summary, then, a simple vacuum tube will conduct electrons in only one direction: from the cathode to the anode and not from the anode to the cathode. This type of vacuum tube is therefore a rectifier.

Unfortunately, there is that bothersome concept of the direction of electric current to keep in mind. Because Benjamin Franklin's early interpretations of electric currents assumed positive moving electric charges, by convention **the direction of electric current is always opposite that of electron flow.**

Solid-state rectifiers

Vacuum tube devices were first developed in the early part of this century. In the 1950s an entirely new class of electronic devices was developed—**solid state, or semiconductor, devices.** It has long been known that metals are good conductors of electricity and that some other materials such as glass or plastics are poor conductors of electricity. There is a third class of materials, called **semiconductors,** lying between the range of insulators and conductors in their ability to conduct electricity. Tiny crystals of these semiconductors were found to have some useful electrical properties, and they are the basis of transistors and the whole host of solid-state integrated marvels available today.

Semiconductors are classed into two types: **n type** and **p type.** N-type semiconductors have loosely bound electrons that are relatively free to move about inside the material. P-type semiconductors have electron traps, spaces for electrons to be bound into. These positive traps, called **holes,** can also be viewed as being free to migrate through the material.

Consider a tiny crystal of n-type material placed in contact with a p-type crystal to form what is called a **p-n junction** (Fig. 6-19). If a

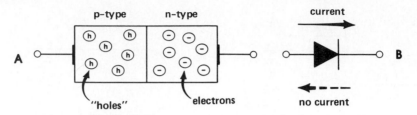

Fig. 6-19. A, P-n junction semiconductor shown as a solid-state diode. B, Its electronic symbol.

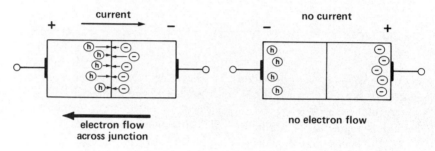

Fig. 6-20. Solid-state diode will conduct electrons in only one direction.

higher potential is placed on the p side of the junction (Fig. 6-20), then the electrons and holes will both migrate toward the junction and wander across it. This flow of electrons constitutes a current. Thus, in this case, there will be an electric current. If, however, a positive potential is placed on the n side of the junction, both the electrons and holes will be swept away from the junction, and there will be no electrons at the junction surface available to form a current. Thus, in this case, there will be very little current through the p-n junction.

In summary, a solid-state p-n junction will tend to conduct electricity in one direction while conducting very little current in the opposite direction. This type of p-n junction is called a **solid-state diode.** As can be seen, solid-state diodes, like tubes, are rectifiers because they pass currents easily in only one direction. The electronic symbol for a diode is shown in Fig.

6-19; the arrowhead in the symbol indicates the direction of the electirc current.

Half-wave rectification

Rectifying devices, either vacuum tube or solid-state, can be assembled into electronic circuits capable of converting alternating current into direct current electricity necessary for the operation of an x-ray tube. One such simple circuit is schematically diagramed in Fig. 6-21. The source of EMF is AC, varying from positive to negative. During the positive portion of the cycle, the vacuum tube conducts freely and allows current to pass through the load, which in this case is the x-ray tube, as shown in the upper portion of the diagram. During the negative cycle of the sources's oscillation, however, the tube will not conduct, and thus no current is allowed through the load. The resulting current is a series of positive humps separated by gaps where

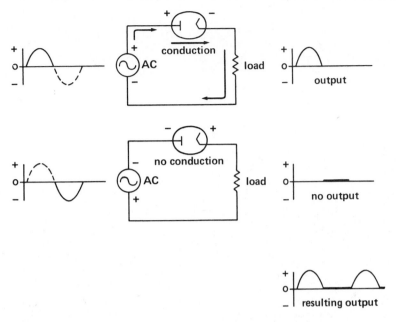

Fig. 6-21. Half-wave rectification and the resulting waveform.

the negative current has been cut off.

This output electric current is a rectified current, since electrons flow in only one direction. It is called half-wave rectification because the tube conducts during only half the cycle of the AC source. The negative portion of the cycle has been deleted.

A solid-state diode could have been substituted for the tube in this circuit with the same result.

Full-wave rectification

One shortcoming of half-wave rectification is that it wastes half the cycle of the source. It is possible, however, to devise a circuit that will rectify the entire AC source signal. Such a circuit is diagramed in Fig. 6-22 and is called a **full-wave rectifier.** The circuit is shown using solid-state diodes, but vacuum tube diodes could have also been used.

The current through the circuit is shown during both the positive and the negative phases of the input source signal. Note that in both cases the output signal across the load is positive. Also, there are no gaps in the output signal. All the input source signal is rectified into usable output. This is the preferred circuit for use in x-ray devices, since it does not waste any of the input source energy.

Three-phase power

All the voltage waveforms previously discussed are produced by single-phase electric power. Single-phase power results in a pulsating x-ray beam. This is caused by the alternate swing in voltage from zero to maximum potential 120 times each second under full rectification. The x rays produced when the single-phase voltage waveform has a value near zero are of little diagnostic value because of their low energy and

RADIOLOGIC SCIENCE FOR
TECHNOLOGISTS: PHYSICS, BIOLOGY,
AND PROTECTION

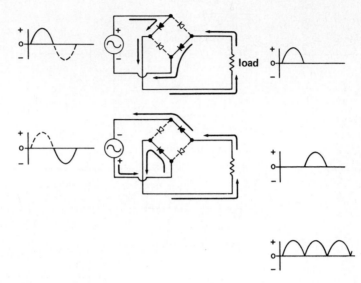

Fig. 6-22. Full-wave rectification circuit, employing four rectifiers, and the resulting waveform.

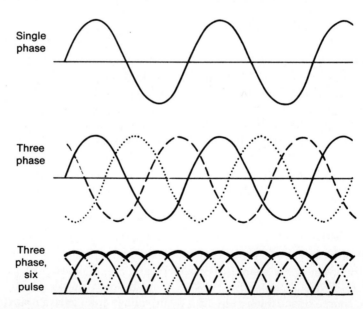

Fig. 6-23. Three-phase power is a more efficient way to produce x rays than is single phase. Shown here are the voltage waveforms for unrectified, single phase, three phase, and that for the associated rectified three phase.

therefore low penetrability. One method to overcome this deficiency is to employ some sophisticated electrical engineering principles to generate three simultaneous voltage waveforms out of step with one another. Such a manipulation results in **three-phase power.**

The engineering manipulations required to produce three-phase power involve the delivery of power from the utility and the manner in which the high-voltage step-up transformer is wired into the circuit. A discussion of these manipulations is unnecessary for our requirements. Fig. 6-23 shows the voltage waveform for single-phase power, for three-phase power, and for three-phase power when full-wave rectified. The latter voltage waveform shows that, with three-phase power, multiple voltage waveforms are superimposed on one another and result in an effective waveform that maintains a nearly constant high voltage showing six pulses per 1/60 second, compared to the two pulses characteristic of single-phase power (Fig. 6-22). With three-phase power, the voltage impressed across the x-ray tube is nearly constant, never dropping to zero during exposure.

Another way to characterize these voltage waveforms is by identification of the **ripple.** Single-phase power exhibits a **100% voltage ripple;** the voltage varies from zero to its maximum value. Three-phase, six-pulse power produces voltage with only approximately **13% ripple;** consequently, the voltage supplied to the x-ray tube never falls below approximately 87% of the maximum value. A further improvement on three-phase power results in twelve pulses per cycle rather than six. Twelve-pulse, three-phase power results in a voltage supply showing only **3.5% ripple,** and therefore the voltage supplied to the x-ray tube does not fall below 96.5%.

REVIEW QUESTIONS

1. Define or otherwise identify the following:
   a. Voltaic pile
   b. Electromotive force
   c. Solenoid
   d. Mutual induction
   e. Commutator ring
   f. Autotransformer
   g. Thermionic emission
   h. Rectification
   i. Shell-type transformer
   j. Lodestone
2. State the two principal laws of electromagnetics.
3. How does an electric motor work?
4. A transformer has 220,000 turns on the secondary winding and 200 turns on the primary winding. If 220 V are supplied to the primary side, what will be the voltage on the secondary side?
5. If 30 A are supplied to the primary side of the transformer in question 4, what will be the secondary current?
6. What is the electric power resulting from the 220 V and 30 A applied to the transformer in the previous question? From the information given, will the power be the same on the secondary side?
7. A portable x-ray machine is designed to operate on conventional 110 V AC power. Its maximum capacity is 110 kV and 100 mA. What is the high-voltage transformer turns ratio?
8. What should be the primary current in the previous question to produce a secondary current of 100 mA?
9. In a full-wave–rectified waveform, how many half-cycles occur in the following:
   a. 1 s
   b. 500 ms
   c. $1/120$ s
   d. 50 ms
   e. 8 ms
10. What voltage ripple is associated with the following waveforms:
   a. Half wave, single phase
   b. Full wave, single phase
   c. Full wave, three phase, six pulse
   d. Full wave, three phase, twelve pulse

7

The
x-ray
machine

SHAPES AND SIZES

When fast-moving electrons slam into a metal object, x rays are produced. The kinetic energy of the electron is transformed into electromagnetic energy. The function of the x-ray machine is to provide a sufficient intensity of electron flow in a controlled manner to produce an x-ray beam of desired quantity and quality.

The many different types of x-ray machines are usually identified according to either the energy of the x rays they produce or the purpose for which those x rays are intended. Diagnostic x-ray machines come in many different shapes and sizes, some of which are shown in Fig. 7-1. They are usually operated at maximum voltages ranging from 25 to 150 kVp and at tube currents from 25 to 1200 mA. Therapeutic x-ray machines, on the other hand, can be operated at higher or lower voltages but at tube currents not exceeding 20 mA.

The modern general purpose x-ray examination room usually contains a radiographic unit and a fluoroscopic unit with an electronic image intensifier. The fluoroscopic x-ray tube is usually located under the examining table. The head of the radiographic tube is attached to an overhead movable crane assembly that permits easy positioning of the tube and aiming of the x-ray beam. A room equipped in this fashion was described in Fig. 1-6. This type of equipment can be used for nearly all radiographic and fluoroscopic examinations. Rooms with a fluoroscopic examining table and two or more overhead radiographic tubes are generally employed for special vascular and neurologic examinations.

Every x-ray machine, regardless of its design, has three principal parts: the x-ray tube, the high-voltage section or generator, and the control console. In some types of x-ray apparatus, such as dental and portable machines, these

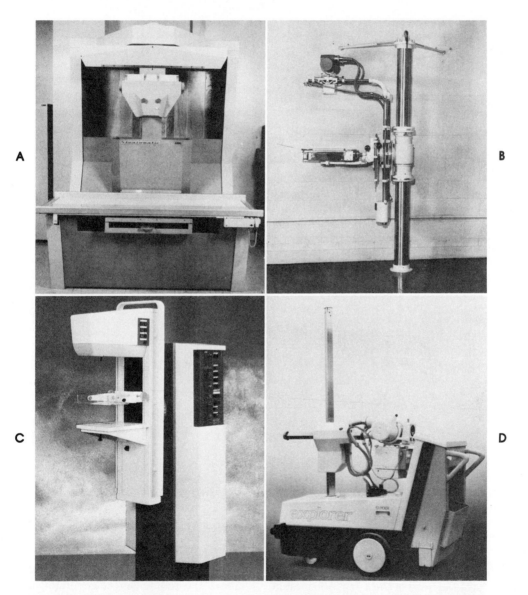

Fig. 7-1 Types of diagnostic x-ray machines. **A,** Tomographic. **B,** Head stand. **C,** Mammographic. **D,** Portable. (**A,** courtesy CGR Medical Corporation; **B,** courtesy Liebel-Flarsheim Co.; **C,** courtesy Lorad Medical Systems, Inc.; **D,** courtesy Picker International.)

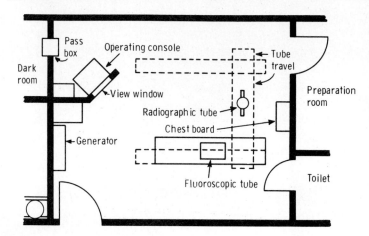

Fig. 7-2. Plan drawing of general purpose x-ray examining room showing location of the various x-ray apparatus. Chapter 25 considers the layout of such rooms in greater detail.

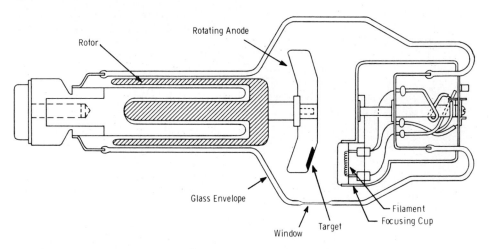

Fig. 7-3. Principal parts of a modern rotating-anode x-ray tube.

three components are housed compactly. Most, however, have the head of the x-ray tube located in one room, the control console in an adjoining room, and a protective barrier or wall, equipped with a viewing window, separating the two. The high-voltage generator is normally housed in a cubicle container, perhaps 1 m on a side, located in the corner of the examining room. Some newer installations take advantage of false ceil-ings and locate these generators out of sight above the room. Newer generator designs employing high-frequency circuits require even less room. Fig. 7-2 is a plan drawing of a conventional general purpose x-ray examining room.

X-RAY TUBE

The x-ray tube is a component of the x-ray machine rarely seen by the radiologic technol-

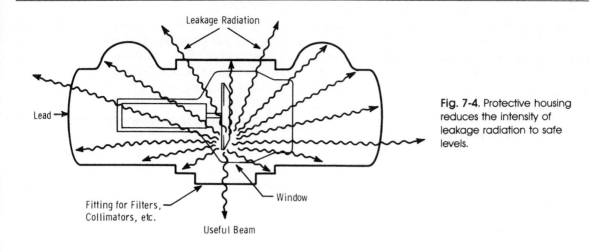

Leakage Radiation

Lead

Fitting for Filters,
Collimators, etc.

Window

Useful Beam

Fig. 7-4. Protective housing reduces the intensity of leakage radiation to safe levels.

ogist. It is contained in a protective housing and therefore is inaccessible. Fig. 7-3 is a schematic diagram of a modern rotating-anode diagnostic x-ray tube. Its components will be considered separately, but it should be clear that there are two primary parts: the **cathode** and the **anode.** Each of these is called an **electrode,** and any tube with two electrodes is called a **diode.** An x-ray tube is a special type of diode tube.

Protective housing

The x-ray tube is always mounted inside a lead-lined protective housing designed to control two serious hazards that plagued early radiology: **excessive radiation exposure** and **electric shock.**

When x rays are produced, they are emitted **isotropically,** that is, with equal intensity in all directions; we want to use only those emitted through the specially designed port, called the **window.** Fig. 7-4 diagrams this situation. Those x-rays emitted through the window are called the **useful beam.** Other x rays that penetrate through the protective housing are **leakage radiation;** they contribute nothing in the way of diagnostic information and result in unnecessary exposure of the patient and technologist. A prop-

erly designed protective housing reduces the level of leakage radiation to less than **100 mR/ hr at 1 m** (26 µC/kg-hr at 1 m) when operated at maximum conditions.

The protective housing incorporates specially designed high-voltage receptacles to protect against accidental **electric shock.** Death by electrocution was a very real hazard to early radiologic technologists. The protective housing also provides **mechanical support** for the x-ray tube and protects the tube from damage caused by rough handling. The protective housing around some x-ray tubes contains oil that serves as both an **electrical insulator** and a **thermal cushion.** Some protective housings have a cooling fan to air-cool the tube or the oil in which the tube is bathed.

In spite of its careful design, the protective housing should *never* be held during an x-ray examination. The high-voltage cables and terminals should *never* be used as handles for positioning the tube.

Glass envelope

An x-ray tube is an electronic vacuum tube like those contained in tube-type radios and televisions; the components of the tube are contained within a glass envelope. The x-ray tube, however, is a special kind of vacuum tube. It is considerably larger than most, perhaps 20 to 35 cm long and 15 cm in diameter. The glass envelope, usually made of Pyrex glass to enable it to withstand the tremendous heat generated, maintains a vacuum inside the tube. This vacuum allows for more efficient x-ray production and longer tube life. If the tube were filled with gas, the electron flow from cathode to anode would be hindered; fewer x rays would be produced, and more heat would be created.

Early x-ray tubes, modifications of the Crookes tube, were not vacuum tubes but rather contained controlled quantities of gas in their glass envelopes. The modern x-ray tube, the Coolidge tube, is a vacuum tube. If it becomes gassy, x-ray production will fall off and the tube will fail.

The tube window is a segment of the glass envelope, approximately 5 cm square, that contains a thin section of glass from which the useful beam of x rays is emitted. The thin window serves to allow maximum emission of x rays with minimum absorption in the glass envelope.

Cathode

The cathode is the negative side of the x-ray tube and has two primary parts: a filament and a focusing cup. Fig. 7-5 shows a photograph of a dual-filament cathode and a schematic drawing of its electrical supply.

Filament. The filament is a coil of wire similar to that in a kitchen toaster except much smaller. The coil is usually about 2 mm in diameter and 1 to 2 cm long. In the kitchen toaster an electric current is conducted through the coil, causing it to glow and emit a large quantity of heat. The filament emits electrons. When the current through the filament is sufficiently intense, approximately 4 A and above, the outer-shell electrons of the filament atoms are literally boiled off and ejected from the filament. This phenomenon is known as **thermionic emission.**

Filaments are usually made of **thoriated tungsten.** Tungsten provides for higher thermionic emission than other metals. Its melting point is 3410 °C, and therefore it is not likely to burn out like the filament of a light bulb. Also, tungsten does not vaporize easily. If it did, the tube

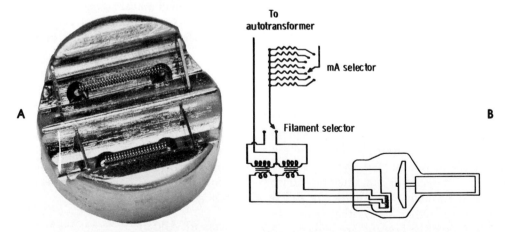

Fig. 7-5. A, Dual-filament cathode designed to provide focal spots of 0.5 mm and 1.5 mm. **B,** Electric schematic for dual-filament cathode. (**A** courtesy The Machlett Laboratories, Inc.)

would quickly become gassy and its internal parts coated with tungsten. Ultimately, however, tungsten metal does vaporize and plate out on internal components. This upsets some of the electrical characteristics of the tube and can lead to tube failure. Although not spectacular or sudden, **this is probably the most common cause of tube failure.** The addition of 1% to 2% thorium to the tungsten filament increases efficiency of thermionic emission and prolongs tube life.

Focusing cup. The filament is embedded in a metal shroud called the focusing cup. Since all the electrons accelerated from cathode to anode are electrically negative, the beam tends to spread out, and some electrons can even miss the anode altogether. The focusing cup is negatively charged so that it tends to condense the electron beam to a small area of the anode. Fig. 7-6 illustrates this property. The effectiveness of the focusing cup is determined by (1) its size and shape, (2) its charge, (3) the filament size and shape, and (4) the position of the filament within the focusing cup. In a **grid controlled x-ray tube** the focusing cup is the grid.

Filament current. When the x-ray machine is first turned on, a low current flows through the filament to warm it and prepare it for the thermal jolt necessary for x-ray production. At low filament current, no tube current flows because sufficient heating for thermionic emission has not been achieved. Once the filament current is high enough for thermionic emission, a small rise in filament current will result in a large rise in tube current. This relationship between filament current and tube current is dependent on the tube voltage, as shown in Fig. 7-7. **The x-ray tube current is adjusted by controlling the filament current.** Fixed stations of 100, 200, 300 mA, and so on usually correspond to discrete taps of the filament transformer.

When emitted from the filament, electrons remain in the vicinity of the filament momentarily before being accelerated to the anode. Since these electrons carry negative charges, they are mutually repulsive and tend to form a cloud about the filament. This cloud of electrons, called a **space charge,** makes it difficult for subsequent electrons to be emitted by the filament because of the electrostatic repulsion.

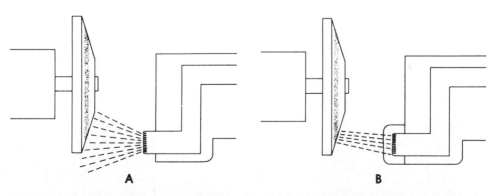

Fig. 7-6. A, Without a focusing cup, the electron beam would be spread beyond the anode because of mutual electrostatic repulsion among the electrons. **B,** With a focusing cup, which is negatively charged, the beam is condensed and directed to the desired area of the anode.

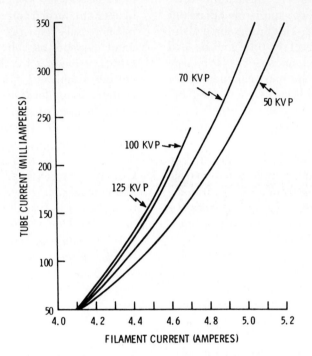

Fig. 7-7. X-ray tube current is actually controlled by changing the filament current. Because of thermionic emission, a small change in filament current results in a large change in tube current.

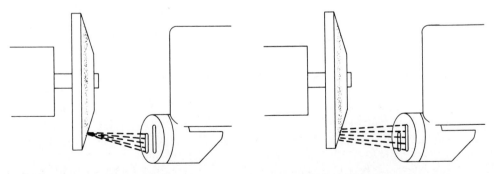

Fig. 7-8. In a dual-focus x-ray tube, focal spot size is controlled by heating one of the two filaments.

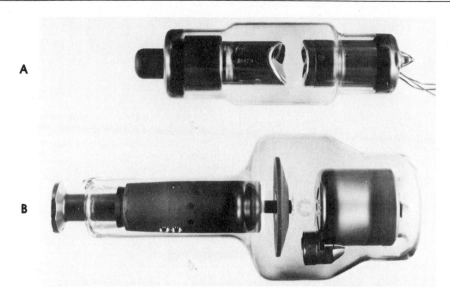

Fig. 7-9. All diagnostic x-ray tubes can be classified according to the type of anode they contain. **A,** Stationary anode. **B,** Rotating anode.

This phenomenon is called the **space-charge effect.** X-ray tubes under certain conditions of low kVp and high mA are said to be **space-charge limited.** A major obstacle in producing x-ray tubes with currents exceeding 1000 mA is the design of adequate space-charge–compensating devices.

Dual-focus tube. Most diagnostic x-ray tubes have two focal spots, one large and the other small. The small focal spot is used when high-resolution images are required. The large focal spot is used when techniques that produce high heat are required. The selection of one or the other is generally made with the mA-station selector on the control console. Small focal spots range from 0.3 to 1 mm; large focal spots usually range from 1 to 2.5 mm. Fig. 7-5, *A,* is a photograph of a modern dual-filament cathode assembly. Each filament is embedded in the focusing cup. The small focal spot size is associated

with the small filament, and the large focal spot size with the large filament. The electric current flows through the appropriate filament, as diagramed in Figs. 7-5, *B,* and 7-8.

Anode

The anode is the positive side of the x-ray tube. There are two types of anodes: **stationary** and **rotating** (Fig. 7-9). Stationary-anode x-ray tubes are used in dental x-ray machines, portable machines, and other special purpose units where high tube current and power are not required. Most general purpose x-ray tubes are the rotating-anode type because they must be capable of producing high-intensity x-ray beams in a short time.

The anode serves three functions in an x-ray tube. It receives electrons emitted by the cathode and conducts them through the tube to the connecting cables and back to the high-voltage section of the x-ray machine. The anode is an

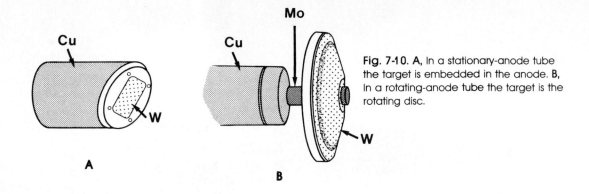

Fig. 7-10. A, In a stationary-anode tube the target is embedded in the anode. **B,** In a rotating-anode tube the target is the rotating disc.

electrical conductor. It provides **mechanical support** for the target. The anode must also be a good **thermal conductor.** When the electrons comprising the tube current slam into the anode, more than 99% of their kinetic energy is converted into heat. This heat must be conducted away quickly before it can melt the anode. Copper is the most common anode material. Adequate heat dissipation is the major engineering hurdle to higher-capacity x-ray tubes.

Target. The **target** is the area of the anode struck by the electrons from the cathode. In stationary-anode tubes the target consists of a tungsten-alloy metal embedded in the copper anode (Fig. 7-10, A). In rotating-anode tubes the entire rotating disc is the target (Fig. 7-10, B). Alloying the tungsten (usually with rhenium) gives it added mechanical strength to withstand the stresses of high rotation.

Tungsten is the material of choice for the target for three main reasons:

1. Atomic number—tungsten's high atomic number, 79, results in higher-efficiency x-ray production and in higher-energy x rays. The reason for this is discussed more fully in Chapter 8.

2. Thermal conductivity—tungsten has a thermal conductivity nearly equal to that of copper. It is therefore an efficient metal for dissipating the heat produced.

3. High melting point—any material, if heated sufficiently, will melt and assume a liquid state. Tungsten has a high melting point (3410° C compared with 1083° C for copper) and therefore can stand up under high tube current without pitting or bubbling.

Rotating anode. A major development in x-ray tube design that has resulted in higher tube currents is the **rotating anode.** The rotating-anode x-ray tube allows the electron beam to interact with a much larger target area, and therefore the heating of the anode is not confined to one small spot as in a stationary-anode tube. Fig. 7-11 compares the target areas of typical stationary-anode and rotating-anode x-ray tubes with 1 mm focal spots. The actual target area for the stationary tube is 1 mm × 4 mm = 4 mm². If the rotating-anode diameter is 7 cm, then the radius of the target area is approximately 3 cm (30 mm). The total target area of the rotating anode is $2\pi(30) \times 4$ mm = 754 mm². Thus the

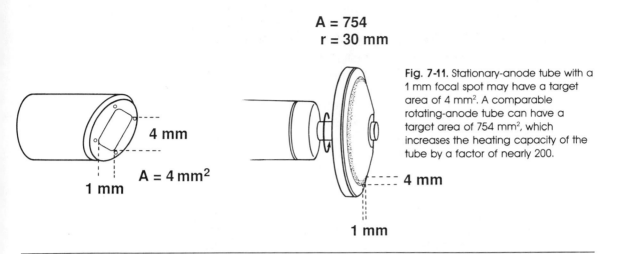

A = 754
r = 30 mm

A = 4 mm²

1 mm

4 mm

1 mm

4 mm

Fig. 7-11. Stationary-anode tube with a 1 mm focal spot may have a target area of 4 mm². A comparable rotating-anode tube can have a target area of 754 mm², which increases the heating capacity of the tube by a factor of nearly 200.

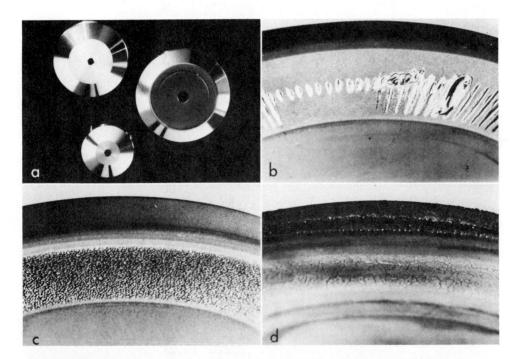

Fig. 7-12. Comparison of smooth, shiny appearance of rotating anodes when new, **a**, and their appearance after failure, **b** to **d**. Examples of anode separation and surface melting shown were caused by slow rotation caused by bearing damage (**b**), repeated overload (**c**), and exceeding of maximum heat storage capacity (**d**). (Courtesy The Machlett Laboratories, Inc.)

rotating-anode tube provides several hundred times more area for the electron beam to interact than a stationary-anode tube. Heating capacity can be further augmented by increasing the speed of rotation of the anode. Most rotating anodes revolve at 3400 rpm (revolutions per minute). The anodes of some high-capacity tubes rotate at 10,000 rpm. Occasionally the rotor mechanism of a rotating-anode tube fails. When this happens, the anode becomes overheated and pits or cracks, thereby causing tube failure. Fig. 7-12 shows some examples of rotating anodes that failed.

Induction motor. How does the anode rotate inside a glass envelope with no apparent driving mechanism? Most things that revolve are powered by chains or axles or gears of some sort.

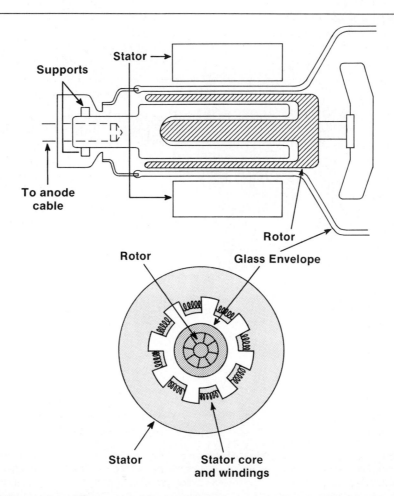

Fig. 7-13. Target of a rotating-anode tube is powered by an induction motor, the principal components of which are the startor and the rotor.

The rotating anode is driven by an electromagnetic **induction motor** (Fig. 7-13), which consists of two principal parts separated from each other by the glass envelope. The part outside the glass envelope, called the **stator,** consists of a series of electromagnets equally spaced around the neck of the tube. Inside the glass envelope is a shaft made of bars of copper and soft iron fabricated into one mass. This mechanism is called the **rotor.**

The induction motor works on a principle similar to that for a transformer. Current flowing in the stator develops a magnetic field that transverses the rotor. The stator windings are sequentially energized so that the induced magnetic field rotates on the axis of the stator. This magnetic field interacts with the rotor, causing it to rotate in synchrony with the activated stator windings.

After actuating the exposure switch of a radiographic unit, one must wait a short time, usually a second or two, before taking an exposure to allow the rotor to accelerate to its designed revolutions per minute. When the exposure is completed, one can hear the rotor slow down and stop within a minute or so. The rotor slows down this quickly because the induction motor is put into reverse. The rotor is a precisely balanced, low-friction device that if left alone might take 10 to 20 minutes to come to rest after use.

Line-focus principle. The **focal spot** is the area of the target from which x rays are emitted. It is the source of radiation. Radiology requires small focal spots because the smaller the focal spot, the sharper the radiographic image. Unfortunately, as the size of the focal spot decreases, the heating of the target is concentrated to smaller areas. This is the limiting factor to focal spot size.

Before the development of the rotating anode, another design was incorporated into x-ray tube targets to allow a large area for heating while maintaining a small focal spot. This design is known as the **line-focus principle.** By angling the target as shown in Fig. 7-14, one makes the effective area of the target much smaller than the actual area of electron interaction. The effective target area, or **effective focal spot size,** is the area projected onto the patient and the film. X-ray tubes have effective focal spots from 0.3 to 3 mm. The smaller the **target angle,** the

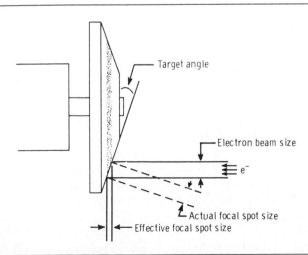

Fig. 7-14. The line-focus principle allows high anode heating with small effective focal spots. As the target angle decreases, so does the effective focal spot.

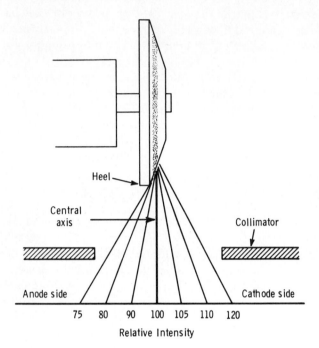

Fig. 7-15. Heel effect results in reduced x-ray intensity on the anode side of the useful beam because of absorption in the "heel" of the target.

smaller the effective focal spot size. Diagnostic x-ray tubes have target angles varying from about 7 to 18 degrees. The advantage of the line-focus principle is that it simultaneously provides the sharpness of image of a small focal spot and the heat accommodation of a large focal spot.

Heel effect. One unfortunate consequence of the line-focus principle is that **the radiation intensity on the cathode side of the x-ray field is higher than that on the anode side.** Electrons interact with target atoms at various depths into the target. The x rays produced are emitted isotropically, that is, with equal intensity in all directions. As shown in Fig. 7-15, the x rays that constitute the useful beam and are emitted from a depth in the target on the anode side must traverse a greater thickness of target material

than the x rays emitted in the cathode direction. Because of increased absorption, the intensity of the x rays that penetrate the "heel" of the target is lower than that of those that penetrate the "toe." This is the **heel effect.** Generally, the smaller the focal spot of an x-ray tube, the larger the heel effect.

The difference in radiation intensity across the useful beam of an x-ray field can vary as much as 45%. Fig. 7-15 graphically shows the typical variation in intensity across the x-ray field. If the radiation intensity along the **central axis** of the useful beam, the imaginary line generated by the centermost x ray in the beam, is designated as 100%, then the intensity on the cathode side may be as high as 120% and that on the anode side may be as low as 75%.

The heel effect should be considered when radiographing anatomic structures of greatly dif-

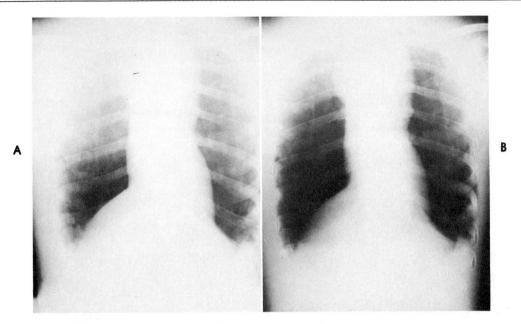

Fig. 7-16. PA chest radiographs demonstrating the heel effect. **A,** Radiograph taken with the cathode up (superior). **B,** Radiograph with cathode down (inferior). More uniform density is obtained with the cathode positioned to the thicker side of the anatomy, as in **B.**

ferent thicknesses or densities. In general, positioning the cathode side of the x-ray tube over the thicker part of the anatomy provides more uniform radiographic density on the film.* In chest radiography, for example, the cathode should be to the inferior side of the patient because the lower thorax, in the region of the diaphragm, is considerably thicker than the upper thorax and therefore requires higher radiation intensity if there is to be uniform exposure of the film. Abdominal films, on the other hand, should be taken so that the cathode is to the superior side of the patient. The upper abdomen is thicker than the lower abdomen and pelvis

and requires higher x-ray intensity for uniform film density. Fig. 7-16 shows two posterior-anterior (PA) chest radiographs, one taken with the cathode inferior, the other with the cathode superior. Can you tell the difference? Which do you think represents better radiographic quality? Resolve the difference before looking at the figure legend.

OPERATING CONSOLE

The operating console, the part of the x-ray machine most familiar to the radiologic technologist, is the apparatus that allows the technologist to control the x-ray tube current and voltage so that the useful x-ray beam is of proper intensity and penetrability for producing a good-quality radiograph. A typical x-ray operating console is shown in Fig. 7-17. The console usually provides for control of line compensation,

---

*The cathode and anode directions are usually indicated on the protective housing, sometimes near the cable connectors.

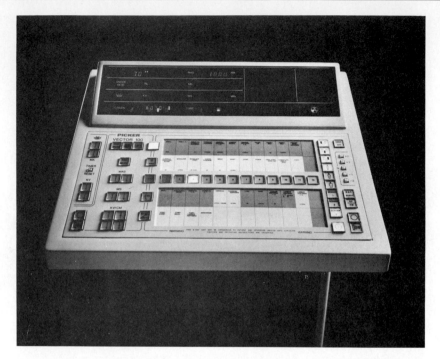

Fig. 7-17. Typical operating console. Number of meters and controls depends on the complexity of the console. (Courtesy Picker International.)

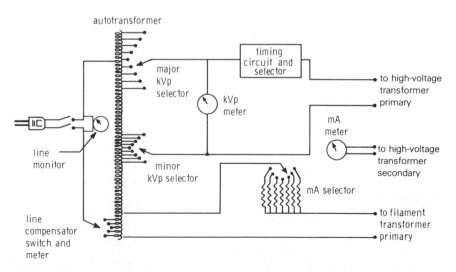

Fig. 7-18. Electric circuit diagram of the operating console identifies the controls and meters.

kVp, mA, and exposure time. Monitors in the form of meters are usually provided for kVp and mA. Sometimes a milliampere-second (mAs) meter is also provided. On newer equipment that incorporates phototiming, separate controls for mAs may be present.

All the electric circuits connecting the meters and controls located on the operating console are at a low voltage so that the possibility of hazardous shock is minimized. Fig. 7-18 is a simplified schematic diagram for a typical operating console. A look inside an operating console will indicate how simplified this schematic drawing is.

Line compensation

Most x-ray machines are designed to operate on a 220 V power source, although some can operate on 110 V or 440 V. Unfortunately, power companies are not capable of providing 220 V accurately and continuously. Because of variations in power distribution to the hospital and in power consumption by the various sections of the hospital, the voltage provided to an x-ray unit may easily vary by as much as 5%. Such variation in input voltage results in larger variation in x-ray output, which is unacceptable if high-quality radiographs are to be consistently produced. The line compensator incorporates a meter to measure the voltage provided to the unit and a switch to adjust that voltage to precisely 220 V. The switch is usually multistation and wired to the autotransformer, as shown in Fig. 7-18. On some machines the technologist must observe the meter and adjust the supply voltage with a control knob, but in most present day radiographic units line compensation is automatic, and a meter is not provided.

Autotransformer

The power supplied to the x-ray machine is first shunted to a special transformer called an **autotransformer.** The autotransformer is designed to supply voltage of varying magnitude to the several different circuits of the x-ray ma-

chine, most prominently the filament circuit and the high-voltage circuit. The voltage supplied to the high-voltage transformer is controlled and variable. It is much safer and easier in terms of engineering to vary a low voltage and then increase it than to increase a low voltage to the kilovolt level and then vary its magnitude.

The autotransformer works on the principle of electromagnetic induction but is very different from the conventional transformer. It has only one winding and one core. This single winding has a number of connections, or **electric taps,** located along its length, as shown in Fig. 7-19. Two of the taps, A and A′ as shown, conduct the input power to the autotransformer and are called primary taps. Some of the secondary taps, such as C, are located closer to one end of the winding than the primary taps. This allows the autotransformer to increase voltage as well as decrease it. The autotransformer can be designed to step up voltage to approximately twice the input voltage value.

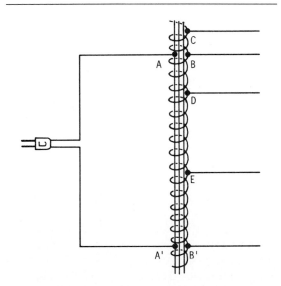

Fig. 7-19. Autotransformer in simplified form.

Because the autotransformer operates as an induction device, the voltage it receives (the primary voltage) and the voltage it provides (the secondary voltage) are in direct relation to the number of turns of the transformer enclosed by the respective taps. The **autotransformer law** is a modification of the transformer law and can be represented as

(7-1)

$$\frac{V_p}{V_s} = \frac{T_p}{T_s}$$

where V_p is the primary voltage; V_s, the secondary voltage; T_p, the number of windings enclosed by primary taps; and T_s, the number of windings enclosed by secondary taps.

EXAMPLE: If the autotransformer in Fig. 7-19 is supplied with 220 V to the primary taps AA', which enclose 500 windings, what will be the secondary voltage across BB' (500 windings), CB' (700 windings), and DE (200 windings)?

ANSWER:

BB': $\quad V_s = V_p\left(\dfrac{T_s}{T_p}\right) = (220\ V)\left(\dfrac{500}{500}\right) = 220\ V$

CB': $\quad V_s = (220\ V)\left(\dfrac{700}{500}\right) = (220\ V)(1.4) = 308\ V$

DE: $\quad V_s = (220\ V)\left(\dfrac{200}{500}\right) = (220\ V)(0.4) = 88\ V$

kVp adjustment

X-ray operating consoles usually have adjustments labeled **major kVp** and **minor kVp,** and by selecting a combination of these controls the technologist can provide precisely the required kVp. The major kVp adjustment and the minor kVp adjustment represent two separate series of taps of the autotransformer. Selection of the appropriate taps can be made by an adjustment knob or by a push button. If the primary voltage to the autotransformer is 220 V, the output of the autotransformer can be controlled from about 100 to 400 V depending on the design of the autotransformer. This low voltage becomes the input to the high-voltage step-up trans-

former and is subsequently increased in the high-voltage section to provide the kilovoltage required.

EXAMPLE: An autotransformer, connected to a 440 V supply, contains 4000 turns, all of which are enclosed by the primary taps. If 2300 turns are enclosed by secondary taps, what will be the voltage supplied to the high-voltage section?

ANSWER: $V_s = V_p\left(\dfrac{T_s}{T_p}\right)$

$\qquad = (440\ V)\left(\dfrac{2300}{4000}\right)$

$\qquad = (440\ V)(0.575)$
$\qquad = 253\ V$

The kVp meter is placed across the output terminals of the autotransformer and therefore reads voltage and not kilovoltage. There is a direct relationship between these two quantities, however, and the scale of the kVp meter reflects this proportionality factor so that the meter reading registers kilovolts.

On most operating consoles the kVp meter will register even though an exposure is not being made and no current is flowing in the circuit. This type of meter is known as a **pre-reading voltmeter.** It allows the voltage to be monitored before an exposure.

mA control

The x-ray tube current, the number of electrons crossing from cathode to anode, is measured in milliamperes (mA). The quantity of electrons emitted by the filament is determined by the temperature of the filament, and the temperature in turn is controlled by the filament current. As filament current increases, the filament becomes hotter, and more electrons are released by thermionic emission. Filaments normally operate at currents between 4 and 6 A.

X-ray tube current is controlled through a separate circuit called the filament circuit, shown in basic form in Fig. 7-20. Voltage for the filament circuit is provided from taps of the autotransformer. This voltage is dropped across pre-

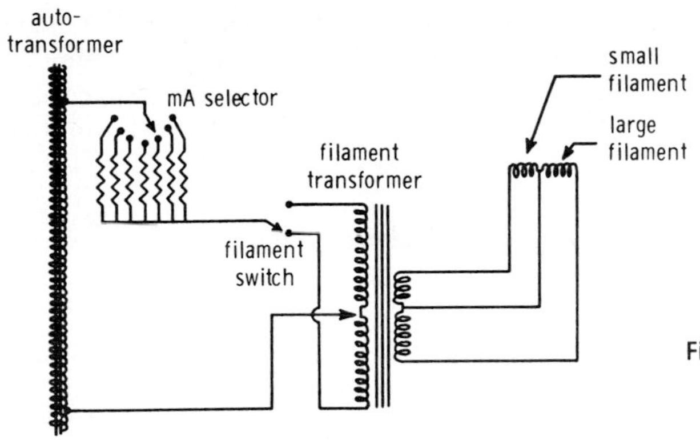

Fig. 7-20. Filament circuit for dual-filament x-ray tube.

cision resistors to a value corresponding to the mA station provided. X-ray tube current normally is not continuously variable; usually only currents of 50, 100, 200, 300 mA, and higher are provided. These fixed mA stations result from the precision resistors.

The voltage from the mA-selector switch is then delivered to the filament transformer. The filament transformer is a step-down transformer; therefore the voltage supplied to the filaments is lower, by a factor equal to the turns ratio, than the voltage supplied to the filament transformer. Similarly, the current is increased across the filament transformer in proportion to the turns ratio.

EXAMPLE: A filament transformer with a turns ratio of 1/10 provides 6.2 A to the filament. What is the current flowing through the primary coil of the filament transformer?

ANSWER: $\dfrac{I_p}{I_s} = \dfrac{N_s}{N_p}$

$$I_p = I_s \left(\frac{N_s}{N_p} \right)$$

$$= (6.2)\left(\frac{1}{10} \right)$$

$$= 0.62 \text{ A}$$

Tube current is monitored with an mA meter that must be placed in the tube circuit. The mA

meter usually is grounded from the center tap of the secondary winding of the high-voltage step-up transformer so that no part of the meter is in contact with the high-voltage section. Variations of this meter are sometimes provided so that mAs can be monitored in addition to mA.

Exposure timers

For any given radiographic examination the number of x rays reaching the film is directly related to the x-ray tube current and the time that the tube is energized. X-ray operating consoles provide a wide selection of beam-on times and, when used in conjunction with the appropriate mA station, an even wider selection of mAs values is possible.

EXAMPLE: A KUB examination (radiography of the *k*idneys, *u*reters, and *b*ladder) calls for 62 kVp, 80 mAs. If the technologist selects the 200 mA station, what exposure time should be used?

ANSWER: $\dfrac{80 \text{ mAs}}{200 \text{ mA}} = 0.4$ s, or ²⁄₅ s, or 400 ms

EXAMPLE: A lateral cerebral angiogram calls for 62 kVp, 90 mAs. If the generator has 1000 mA capacity, what is the shortest exposure time possible?

ANSWER: $\dfrac{90 \text{ mAs}}{1000 \text{ mA}} = 0.09$ s, or 90 ms

The timer circuit is separate from the other main circuits of the x-ray machine. Depending on the type of timer, it consists of mechanical or electronic devices whose action is to "make" and "break" the high voltage across the x-ray tube. This is nearly always done on the **primary side** of the high-voltage section. Devices called **relays** and **contactors** are the switch. There are five basic types of timing circuits. Four are technologist controlled, one is automatic. After studying this section, try to identify the types of timers on the equipment you use.

Mechanical timers. Mechanical timers are very simple devices now used only in some portable and dental units. The mechanical timer operates by clockwork. A preset exposure time is dialed by turning a knob that winds a spring. When the exposure button is depressed, the spring is released and unwinds. The time required to unwind corresponds to the exposure time. Mechanical timers are inexpensive but not very accurate. They can be used only for exposure times greater than about 250 millisecond.

Synchronous timers. In the United States electric current is supplied on a frequency of 60 Hz. (In Europe the frequency is 50 Hz.) A special type of electric motor, known as a synchronous motor, is a precision device designed to drive a shaft at precisely 60 rps or some whole subdivision thereof. In some x-ray machines synchronous motors are used as timing mechanisms. Machines with synchronous timers are easily recognizable because the minimum time possible is usually $\frac{1}{60}$ second (17 millisecond), and timing intervals increase by multiples thereof, for example $\frac{1}{30}$, $\frac{1}{20}$, and so on. Synchronous timers cannot be used for serial exposures because they must be reset after each exposure, which, even when done automatically, requires too much time.

Electronic timers. Electronic timers are the most sophisticated, most complicated, and most accurate of the x-ray timers. Electronic timers consist of rather complex circuitry based on the

time required to charge a capacitor through a variable resistance. They allow a wide range of time intervals to be selected and are accurate to intervals as small as 1 millisecond. Because they can be used for rapid serial exposures (up to 60 per second) they are particularly suitable for special procedures equipment. Most radiographic equipment produced today contains electronic timers.

mAs timers. Most x-ray apparatus is designed for accurate control of tube current and exposure time. However, the product of mA and time—mAs—determines the number of x rays emitted and therefore the density on the film. A special kind of electronic timer, called an mAs timer, monitors the product of mA and time and terminates the exposure when the desired mAs is attained. This mAs timer is usually designed to provide the highest safe tube current for the shortest time of exposure for any mAs selected. Since the mAs timer must monitor the actual tube current, it is located on the secondary side of the high-voltage section.

Phototimers. Unlike the four previous timing devices, the phototimer requires no operation by the technologist. A phototimer is a device that measures the quantity of radiation reaching the film and automatically terminates the exposure when sufficient radiation to provide the required film density has reached the film. Fig. 7-21 shows the operation of two types of phototimers.

The critical component of one type of phototimer is the photomultiplier sensing device. The photomultiplier views a fluorescent screen and converts the light therefrom into an electric charge. The intensity of fluorescence is directly proportional to the intensity of radiation incident on the film. The exposure is terminated when a preselected charge, corresponding to the desired film density, has been reached by the photomultiplier.

The type of phototimer employed by most

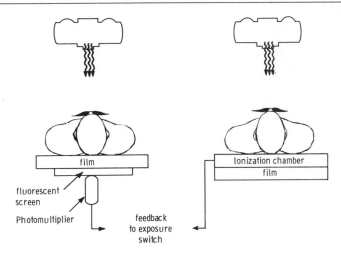

Fig. 7-21. Phototimer automatically terminates the x-ray exposure at the desired film density. This is done with either a photomultiplier or an ionization chamber sensing device.

manufacturers incorporates a flat, parallel plate ionization chamber between the patient and the film. The chamber is made radiolucent so that it will not interfere with the radiographic image. Ionization within the chamber creates a charge proportional to film density. When the appropriate charge has been reached, the exposure is terminated.

The operation of a phototimer is simple. When a phototimer unit is installed, it must be calibrated. This calls for making exposures of a phantom and adjusting the phototimer controls for the range of film densities required by the radiologist. Usually the service engineer takes care of this calibration. Once the photometer has been placed in clinical operation, the technologist simply selects the appropriate film density and places the timer in the phototime mode. When the electric signal from the phototimer sensing device reaches a preset level, a signal is returned to the operating console where the timer circuit is tripped to "off." Phototimers are now widely used and often are provided in addition to a manual timer. Care should be taken when using the phototime mode, especially at low KVp such as in mammography. Because of varying tissue thickness and composition the phototimer may not track well at low KVp, which can result in varying radiographic density. When radiographs are taken in the phototime mode, **the manual timer should be used as a backup timer** in case the phototimer fails to terminate. This precaution should be rigidly followed for the protection of patient and x-ray tube.

Checking a timer

It is absolutely essential that timers on x-ray machines function properly and accurately. Inaccurate or malfunctioning timers result in poor radiographs, unnecessary patient exposure, and retakes. As we shall see later in this chapter and in Chapter 8, x rays are emitted in pulses from all but three-phase equipment. Half-wave–rectified machines produce 60 pulses per second, and full-wave–rectified machines produce 120 pulses per second.

The **spinning top** is a simple device that can be used to check x-ray timers. Fig. 7-22 diagrams its use. It consists of a heavy metal disc, 5 to 25 cm in diameter. The disc rests on a low-

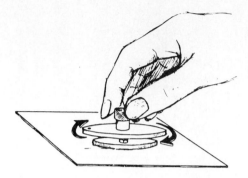

Fig. 7-22. Spinning top can be used to check x-ray exposure timers.

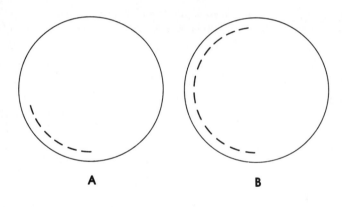

A   B

Fig. 7-23. A, A 0.1 s image of a spinning top should result in six dashes for half-wave—rectified operation. **B,** Image should result in twelve dashes for full-wave—rectified operation.

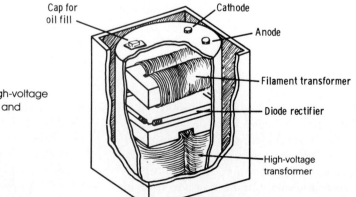

Cap for oil fill   Cathode

Anode

Filament transformer

Diode rectifier

High-voltage transformer

Fig. 7-24. Cutaway view of typical high-voltage section, showing oil-immersed diodes and transformers.

friction pedestal so that it can be rotated manually. Near the perimeter of the spinning top is a small hole. The spinning top is placed on an x-ray film and set spinning with a twist of thumb and forefinger. The x-ray timer is set for some short period (for example 100 ms), and an exposure of the spinning top is made. The resulting image consists of a series of dashes (Fig. 7-23). The number of dashes on the radiograph of the spinning top corresponds to the number of x-ray pulses emitted by the x-ray tube. A 100 ms exposure should produce six dashes on a half-wave–rectified machine and twelve dashes on a full-wave–rectified machine. If any other number of dashes appears, the timer is in error. Timer settings from about 50 to 500 ms are easily checked using the spinning top.

EXAMPLE: A spinning top is used to check the timer of a full-wave–rectified x-ray machine. The timer is set at 0.15 s, and a radiograph of the spinning top is made. How many dashes should appear on the image if the timer is set correctly?

ANSWER: 0.15 s × 120 pulses/s = 18 pulses

The spinning top cannot normally be used to check the timer of a three-phase or capacitor-discharge x-ray machine because these units do not produce pulsed radiation. The radiation output from such units is constant, and they are often capable of exposure times as short as 1 millisecond. Normally these exposure timers must be checked with an oscilloscope or with a solid-state radiation detector. The use of a **synchronous spinning top,** however, can be helpful in assessing timer accuracy for all but the shortest of exposure times with these units. A synchronous spinning top is powered by a synchronous motor turning at 1 rps. A half-second exposure would therefore produce an image of the hole in the top extending through half a circle, or 180 degrees. Similarly, a quarter-second exposure would result in a 90-degree image.

EXAMPLE: A synchronous spinning top, turning at 1 rps, is used to check the timer of a three-phase full-wave–rectified x-ray unit. Exposure time is set at 10 ms and the spinning top is imaged. Through what angle of a circle should the image appear?

ANSWER: 10 ms = 0.01 s. Since the synchronous spinning top revolves through 360 degrees/s, the resulting image should extend through

0.01 s × 360 degrees/s = 3.6 degrees

Solid-state radiation detectors are now used for most timer checks. These devices operate with a very accurate internal clock. They are capable of measuring exposure times as short as 1 ms. Such devices, however, are highly automated, so that the radiologic technologist only needs to know how to operate the instrument and record the data.

HIGH-VOLTAGE SECTION

The high-voltage section of an x-ray machine is responsible for converting the low-supply voltage into a kilovoltage of the proper waveform. The high-voltage section is usually enclosed in a large metal tank situated in the corner of the x-ray room. In some newer hospitals the high-voltage section, or **high-voltage generator,** is located in a false ceiling to conserve floor space. A cutaway view of a typical high-voltage generator is shown in Fig. 7-24. The high-voltage section contains three primary parts: the high-voltage step-up transformer, the filament transformer, and the **rectifiers,** all of which are immersed in oil. Although some heat is generated in the high-voltage section, the oil is used primarily for electrical insulation.

High-voltage transformer

The high-voltage transformer is a step-up transformer, that is, the secondary (induced) voltage is greater than the primary (supply) voltage because the number of secondary windings is greater than the number of primary windings. As detailed in Chapter 6, the ratio of the number of secondary windings to the number of primary windings is called the **turns ratio.** The voltage increase is proportional to the turns ratio, according to the transformer law (equation 6-1). Also, the current is reduced proportionately.

The turns ratio of a conventional high-voltage transformer is usually between 500 and 1000.

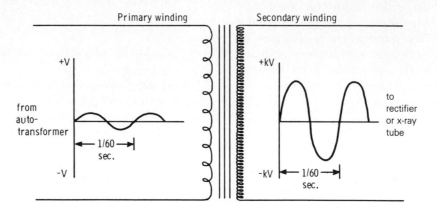

Fig. 7-25. Voltage induced in the secondary winding of a high-voltage step-up transformer is alternating like the primary voltage but has a higher value.

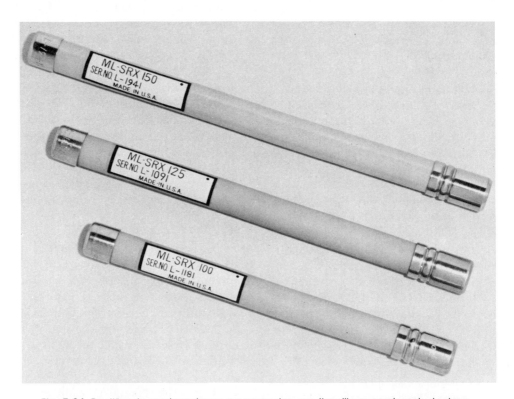

Fig. 7-26. Rectifiers in most modern x-ray generators are the silicon, semiconductor type. (Courtesy The Machlett Laboratories, Inc.)

Since transformers operate only on alternating current, the voltage waveform on both sides of a high-voltage transformer is sinusoidal. This is shown in Fig. 7-25, along with the transformer symbol. The only difference between the primary and secondary waveforms is their **amplitude.** The primary voltage is measured in volts, and the secondary voltage is measured in kilovolts.

EXAMPLE: The turns ratio of a high-voltage transformer is 700, and the supply voltage is peaked at 120 V. What is the secondary voltage supplied to the x-ray tube?

ANSWER: (120 Vp)(700) = 84,000 Vp
                              = 84 kVp

Voltage rectification

Although transformers operate on alternating current, x-ray tubes must be provided with direct current. X rays are produced by the acceleration of electrons from cathode to anode and cannot be produced by electrons flowing in the reverse direction, from anode to cathode. The construction of the cathode assembly is such that it could not withstand the tremendous heat generated by such operation even if the anode could emit electrons thermionically. It would be disastrous to the x-ray tube for electron flow to be reversed.

If the electron flow is to be only in the cathode-to-anode direction, the secondary voltage of the high-voltage transformer must be **rectified.** Rectification is the process of converting alternating voltage into direct voltage and therefore alternating current into direct current.

Diodes. Rectification is accomplished with devices called **diodes** (two electrodes). Until recently, all diode rectifiers were vacuum tubes, called **valve tubes,** and were very similar to x-ray tubes. Anodes and cathodes are constructed much differently, so that x rays are not emitted from valve tubes. The valve tube has been replaced in nearly all x-ray machines by solid-state rectifiers made of silicon. Fig. 7-26 shows examples of silicon rectifiers.

Unrectified voltage. Fig. 7-27, A, is a representation of unrectified voltage. This voltage waveform appears exactly as the voltage waveform supplied to the primary coil of the high-voltage transformer except for its amplitude.

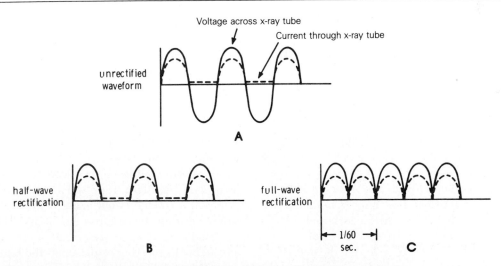

Fig. 7-27. Three degrees of rectification for typical x-ray circuit.

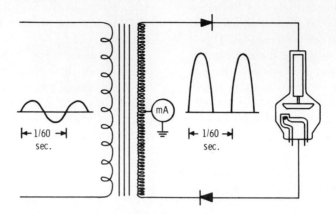

Fig. 7-28. A half-wave–rectified circuit usually contains two diodes, although some contain one or none.

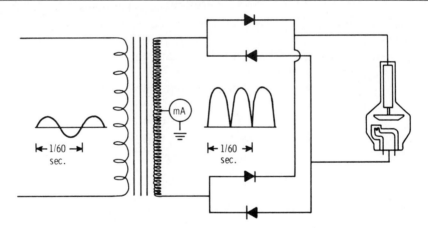

Fig. 7-29. A full-wave–rectified circuit contains at least four diodes. Current is passed through the tube at 120 pulses per second.

The current passing through the x-ray tube, however, exists only during the positive half of the cycle, when the anode is positive and the cathode negative. During the negative half of the cycle, current can flow only from anode to cathode, but this does not occur because the anode is not constructed to emit electrons. The voltage across the x-ray tube during the negative half-cycle is called **inverse voltage** and is harmful to the x-ray tube.

Half-wave rectification. The inverse voltage is removed from the supply to the x-ray tube by rectification. Half-wave rectification is shown in Fig. 7-27, *B*. This represents a condition in which the voltage is not allowed to swing negatively during the negative half of its cycle.

Usually half-wave rectification is accomplished with two diodes placed in the high-voltage section, as shown in Fig. 7-28. Sometimes only one diode is present. Some x-ray circuits

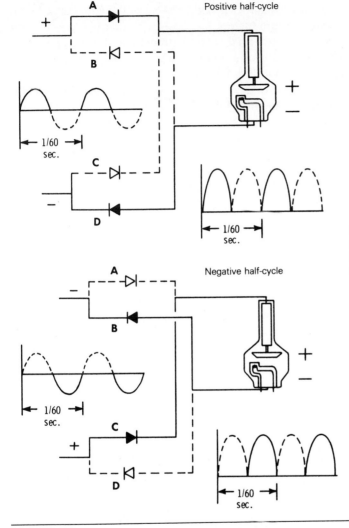

Positive half-cycle

Negative half-cycle

Fig. 7-30. In a full-wave–rectified circuit two diodes *(A* and *D)* conduct during the positive half-cycle and two *(B* and *C)* during the negative half-cycle.

are **self-rectifying;** that is, the x-ray tube itself serves as the rectifying diode, in which case no diodes are found in the high-voltage circuit. Many dental and low-power portable x-ray machines are self-rectified.

Half-wave–rectified circuits can always be recognized because they contain either zero, one, or two diodes. The x-ray output from a half-wave unit is pulsating, with sixty x-ray pulses produced each second.

Full-wave rectification. Full-wave-rectified x-ray machines contain at least four diodes in the high-voltage circuit, usually arranged as in Fig. 7-29. In a full-wave-rectified circuit the negative half-cycle corresponding to the inverse voltage is reversed so that a positive voltage is always impressed across the x-ray tube.

Fig. 7-30 helps explain how full-wave rectification works. During the positive half-cycle of the secondary voltage waveform, electrons flow from the negative side to diodes *C* and *D*. Diode *C* is unable to conduct electrons in that direction, but diode *D* can. The electrons flow through diode *D* and the x-ray tube. The electrons then butt into diodes *A* and *B*. Only diode *A* is positioned to conduct them, and they flow to the positive side of the transformer, thus completing the circuit. During the negative half-cycle, diodes *B* and *C* are pressed into service while diodes *A* and *D* block electron flow. Note that the **polarity** of the x-ray machine remains unchanged. The cathode is always negative, the anode always positive, even though the induced secondary voltage alternates between positive and negative.

Full-wave rectification is employed in nearly all stationary x-ray machines. Its main advantage is that the exposure time for any given technique is cut in half. As shown in Fig. 7-28, the half-wave–rectified x-ray tube emits x rays only half the time it is on. The pulsed x-ray output of a full-wave–rectified machine occurs 120 times each second instead of 60 times per second, as with half-wave rectification.

Three-phase power

There are many advantages to three-phase power. Table 7-1 lists some of these in comparison with single-phase power. The principal advantage is the higher radiation quantity and quality resulting from the nearly constant voltage supplied to the x-ray tube. The radiation quantity is higher because the efficiency of x-ray production increases with increasing x-ray tube potential. Stated differently, for any projectile electron emitted by the x-ray tube cathode, more x rays are produced when the electron energy is high than when it is low. The radiation quality is increased with three-phase power because there are no low-energy projectile electrons passing from cathode to anode to produce low-energy x rays. Consequently, the average x-ray energy is increased over that resulting from single-phase operation.

Because the x-ray output intensity and penetrability are greater for three-phase power than for single-phase power, technique charts developed for the latter cannot be used on the former. It is necessary to develop new technique charts when using three-phase equipment. With the same mAs employed as during single-phase operation, three-phase operation may require as much as a 10 kVp reduction to produce the same radiographic density. Contemporary three-phase radiographic equipment is manufactured with a capacity for tube currents as high as 1200 mA, and therefore exceedingly short, high-intensity exposures are possible. This capacity is particularly helpful in angiographic special procedures.

When three-phase power is provided for a radiographic/fluoroscopic room or for a special

Table 7-1. Comparison of single-phase and three-phase x-ray equipment

Characteristic	Single phase	Three phase
X-ray quantity	Variable	25% to 50% higher
X-ray quality	Variable	Slightly higher
Voltage ripple	100%	<15%
Heat capacity	Variable	Up to 35% higher
Supply power requirements	Moderate	High
Minimum exposure time	8 ms	1 ms
Usual anode speed	3400 rpm	3400-10,000 rpm
Minimum target angle	10½ degrees	6½ degrees
Capital cost	High	Higher
Operating cost	High	Lower

procedures room, all radiographic exposures are under three-phase control. The fluoroscopic mode, however, usually remains single phase. The exception is cineradiography, which is usually three phase.

The principal disadvantage of three-phase x-ray apparatus is its initial cost. The cost of installation and operation, however, can be lower than those associated with single-phase equipment. The overall capacity and flexibility provided by three-phase equipment are considerably greater than those for single-phase equipment. These advantages are responsible for the increasing specificiation of three-phase equipment for new radiologic facilities.

The newest development in high-voltage generator design uses a high-frequency electric circuit. Full-wave–rectified power at 60 Hz is converted to a higher frequency, usually 500 or 1000 Hz. Consequently, the voltage ripple is reduced to near zero. One advantage to the high-frequency generator is size; many such

generators can be placed within the x-ray tube housing. Portable x-ray machines especially benefit from this technology.

X-ray circuit

The three main sections of the x-ray machine—the x-ray tube, the operating console, and the high-voltage section—are represented in Fig. 7-31 by a simplified electric schematic. The locations of all meters, controls, and major components of importance are shown.

X-RAY TUBE RATING CHARTS

With careful use, x-ray tubes can provide long periods of service. With inconsiderate use, tube life may be shortened substantially, and they may even abruptly fail. The length of x-ray tube life is primarily under the control of the radiologic technologist. Basically, tube life is extended by employing the minimum radiographic factors of mA, kVp, and time that are appropriate for each examination. The use of faster image

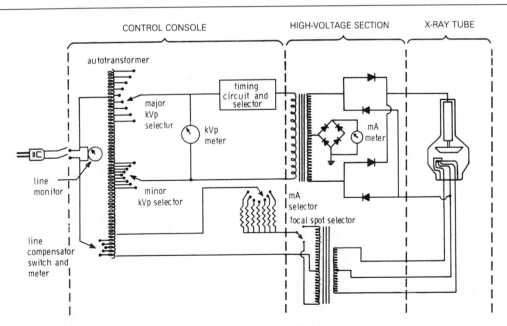

Fig. 7-31. Simplified electric circuit diagram for x-ray machine, showing three main sections: control console, high-voltage section, and x-ray tube.

receptors has resulted in much longer tube life.

Causes of tube failure

There are several causes of tube failure, all of which are related to the thermal characteristics of the x-ray tube. When the temperature of the anode is excessive during a single exposure, localized surface melting and pitting of the anode occurs. These surface irregularities result in variable and reduced radiation output. If the surface melting is sufficiently severe, the tungsten can be vaporized and can plate the inside of the glass envelope. This can cause filtering of the x-ray beam or interference with electron flow from cathode to anode. If the temperature of the anode increases too rapidly, the anode may crack, become unstable in rotation, and render the tube useless. This type of failure is particularly important with **three-phase operation. Maximum radiographic techniques should never be applied to a cold anode.** If maximum techniques are required for a particular examination, the anode should first be warmed with low-technique operation.

A second type of tube failure results from maintaining the anode at elevated temperatures for prolonged periods. During exposures lasting 1 to 3 seconds, the temperature of the anode may be sufficient to cause it to glow like an incandescent light bulb. Between exposures, this heat is dissipated, primarily through radiation, to the oil bath in which the tube is contained. Some heat is conducted through the narrow molybdenum neck to the rotor assembly, and this can cause subsequent heating of the rotor bearings. Excessive heating of the bearings results in increased rotational friction and in imbalance of the rotor-anode assembly. Bearing damage is another cause of tube failure.

If the thermal stress on the x-ray tube anode is maintained for prolonged periods, such as during fluoroscopy, the thermal capacity of the total anode system and of the x-ray tube housing is the limitation to operation. During fluoroscopy, the x-ray tube current is generally less than 5 mA rather than hundreds of mA, as in radiography. Under such conditions the rate of heat dissipation from the rotating target attains equilibrium with the rate of heat input, and this rate rarely is sufficient to cause surface defects in the target. The tube can fail, however, because of the continuous heat delivered to the rotor assembly, the oil bath, and the x-ray tube housing. Bearings can fail, the glass envelope can crack, and the tube housing can fail.

A final cause of tube failure involves the filament. Because of the high temperature of the filament, tungsten atoms are slowly vaporized and plate the inside of the glass envelope, even with normal use. This tungsten, along with that vaporized from the anode, disturbs the electrical balance of the x-ray tube, causing abrupt, intermittent changes in tube current, which often leads to arcing and tube failure. **This is perhaps the most frequent cause of tube failure.**

With excessive heating of the filament caused by high-mA operation for prolonged periods, more tungsten is vaporized. The filament wire becomes thinner and eventually severs, causing an **open filament.** This same type of failure occurs when an incandescent light bulb burns out.

The radiologic technologist is guided in the use of x-ray tubes by **x-ray tube rating charts.** It is absolutely essential that the technologist be able to read and understand these charts. There are several types of x-ray tube rating charts, but only three are particularly significant to the technologist: the radiographic rating chart, the anode cooling chart, and the housing cooling chart.

Radiographic rating chart

Of the three rating charts, the radiographic rating chart is perhaps the most important because it conveys which radiographic techniques are safe and which techniques are hazardous for tube operation. Fig. 7-32 shows four examples of radiographic rating charts. Each chart contains a family of curves representing the various tube currents in mA. The x axis and y axis show scales of the two other radiographic parameters,

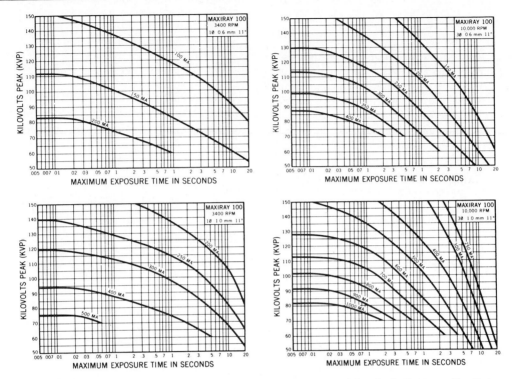

Fig. 7-32. Representative radiographic rating charts for given x-ray tube. Each chart specifies the conditions of operation to which it applies. (Courtesy General Electric Co.)

time and kVp. For a given mA, any combination of kVp and time that lies below the mA curve is safe. Any combination of kVp and time that lies above the curve representing the desired mA is unsafe; if an exposure were made, the tube might fail abruptly.

A series of radiographic rating charts accompanies every x-ray tube. These charts cover the various modes of operation possible with that tube. There are different charts for the filament in use (large or small focal spot), the speed of anode rotation (3400 rpm or 10,000 rpm), the target angle, and the voltage rectification (half wave, full wave, or three phase). **Be sure to employ the proper radiographic rating chart with each tube.** This is particularly important following the replacement of x-ray tubes. An appropriate radiographic rating chart is supplied

with each replacement x-ray tube and can be substantially different from that for the original tube.

The application of radiogrpahic rating charts is not difficult.

EXAMPLE: With reference to Fig. 7-32, which of the following conditions of exposure are safe, and which are unsafe?

a. 95 kVp, 150 mA, 1 s; 3400 rpm; 0.6 mm focal spot
b. 80 kVp, 400 mA, 0.5 s; 3400 rpm; 1 mm focal spot
c. 125 kVp, 500 mA, 0.1 s; 10,000 rpm; 1 mm focal spot
d. 75 kVp, 800 mA, 0.3 s; 10,000 rpm; 1 mm focal spot
e. 88 kVp, 400 mA, 0.1 s; 10,000 rpm; 0.6 mm focal spot

ANSWER:

   a. Unsafe   c. Safe   e. Unsafe
   b. Unsafe   d. Safe

EXAMPLE: Radiographic examination of the abdomen with a tube having a 0.6 mm focal spot and anode rotation of 10,000 rpm requires technique factors of 95 kVp, 150 mAs. What is the shortest possible exposure time for this examination?

ANSWER: Locate the proper radiographic rating chart (upper right in Fig. 7-32) and the 95 kVp line (horizontal line near middle of chart). Beginning from the left (shorter exposure times) determine the mAs for the intersection of each mA curve with the 95 kVp level.

   1. The first intersection is approximately 350 mA at 0.03 s = 10.5 mAs. Not enough.
   2. The next intersection is approximately 300 mA at 0.2 s = 60 mAs. Not enough.
   3. The next intersection is approximately 250 mA at 0.6 s = 150 mAs. This is sufficient.

Consequently, 0.6 s is the minimum possible exposure time.

Anode cooling chart

The anode assembly has a limited capacity for storing heat. Although heat is continuously dissipated to the oil bath and tube housing by conduction and radiation, it is possible through prolonged use or multiple exposures to exceed the heat storage capacity of the anode.

Thermal energy is conventionally measured in terms of calories, British thermal units (BTU), or joules. In x-ray applications thermal energy is measured in heat units (HU). The capacity of the anode and the housing to store heat is measured in heat units. One heat unit is equal to the product of 1 kVp, 1 mA, and 1 s.

(7-2)

$$HU = kVp \times mA \times s$$

EXAMPLE: Radiographic examination of the lateral lumbar spine requires 98 kVp, 120 mAs. How many heat units are generated by this exposure?

ANSWER: *Number of heat units* = 98 kVp × 120 mAs
                       = 11,760 HU

EXAMPLE: A fluoroscopic examination is performed at 76 kVp and 1.5 mA for 3½ minutes. How many heat units are generated?

ANSWER: *Number of heat units* = 76 kVp × 1.5 mA ×
                                    3½ min × 60 s/min
                              = 23,940 HU

More heat is generated for a given radiographic technique when three-phase equipment is used than when single-phase equipment is used. A modification factor is necessary for calculating heat units, so equation 7-2 becomes

(7-3)

$$HU = 1.35 \times kVp \times mA \times s$$

EXAMPLE: Six sequential skull films are exposed with a three-phase generator operated at 82 kVp, 120 mAs. What is the total heat generated?

ANSWER:

   Number of heat units/film = 1.35 × 82 × 120
                      13,284 HU
          Total HU = 6 × 13,284 HU
                 79,704 HU

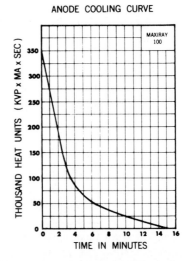

Fig. 7-33. Anode cooling chart showing time required for heated anode to cool. (Courtesy General Electric Co.)

The thermal capacity of an anode and its heat dissipation characteristics are contained in a tube rating chart called an anode cooling chart (Fig. 7-33). Unlike the radiographic rating chart, the anode cooling chart is not dependent on the filament size or the speed of rotation. The tube represented in Fig. 7-33 has a maximum anode heat capacity of 350,000 HU. The chart shows that if the maximum heat load were attained, it would take 15 minutes for the anode to completely cool. The rate of cooling is rapid at first and slows as the anode cools. In addition to determining the maximum heat capacity of the anode, the anode cooling chart is used to determine the length of time required for complete cooling following any level of heat input.

EXAMPLE: A particular examination results in 50,000 HU being delivered to the anode in a matter of seconds. How long will it take the anode to cool completely?

ANSWER: The 50,000 HU level intersects the anode cooling curve at approximately 6 minutes. From that point on the curve to complete cooling requires an additional 9 minutes (15 − 6 = 9). Therefore, 9 minutes are required for complete cooling.

Housing cooling chart

The cooling chart for the housing of the x-ray tube has a shape similar to that of the anode cooling chart and is used in precisely the same way. X-ray tube housings generally have maximum heat capacities in the range of 1 to 1.5 million HU. Complete cooling following maximum heat capacity requires from 1 to 2 hours. About twice that amount of time is required without auxiliary fan-powered air circulation.

REVIEW QUESTIONS

1. Define or otherwise identify the following:
   a. Leakage radiation
   b. Cathode
   c. Induction motor
   d. Spinning top
   e. Rectifier
   f. mA meter location
   g. Diode
   h. Thermionic emission
   i. Useful beam
   j. Autotransformer
2. Diagram a modern rotating-anode tube and identify the following: rotor, stator, target, window, focusing cup, filament, glass envelope, and protective housing.
3. Compare the actual target areas of a stationary-anode and a rotating-anode tube, both of which have effective focal spot sizes of 2 mm × 2 mm. The rotating target has a diameter of 6 cm.
4. Across 1200 windings of the primary coil of the autotransformer are supplied 220 V. If 1650 windings are tapped, what voltage will be supplied to the primary coil of the high-voltage transformer?
5. A kVp meter reads 86 kVp, and the turns ratio of the high-voltage step-up transformer is 1200. What is the true voltage across the meter?
6. The supply voltage from the autotransformer to the filament transformer is 60 V. If the turns ratio of the filament transformer is $1/12$, what is the filament voltage?
7. If the current in the primary of the filament transformer in question 6 were 0.5 A, what would be the filament current?
8. A spinning top is used to check a full-wave–rectified x-ray unit by exposing it for $5/20$ second. If all is working properly, what should the image look like?
9. The supply voltage to a high-voltage step-up transformer with a turns ratio of 550 is 190 V. What is the voltage across the x-ray tube?
10. Draw a complete x-ray circuit and locate the meters and controls found on the machine you operate.

8

X-ray production

ELECTRON-TARGET INTERACTION
X-RAY EMISSION SPECTRUM
FACTORS AFFECTING THE X-RAY EMISSION SPECTRUM

ELECTRON-TARGET INTERACTION

The x-ray machine was described in Chapter 7 with sufficient depth to emphasize that its primary function is to accelerate electrons from the cathode to the anode. The three principal segments of an x-ray machine—the control console, the high-voltage section, and the x-ray tube—are all designed to provide a large number of electrons focused to a small spot in such a manner that when the electrons arrive at the target, they have acquired high kinetic energy.

Kinetic energy is the energy of motion. Stationary objects have no kinetic energy; objects in motion have kinetic energy proportional to their mass and to the square of their velocity. For example, a 1000 kg automobile has four times the kinetic energy of a 250 kg motorcycle traveling at the same speed (Fig. 8-1). However, if the motorcycle were to double its velocity, it would have the same kinetic energy as the au-

tomobile. The equation used to calculate kinetic energy is

(8-1)

$$KE = \frac{1}{2}\,mv^2$$

where m is the mass in kilograms, v is the velocity in meters per second, and KE is the kinetic energy in joules. In determining the magnitude of the kinetic energy of a projectile, velocity is more important than mass. In an x-ray tube the projectile is the electron. As its kinetic energy is increased, both the intensity (the number of x rays) and the energy (their ability to pentrate) of the created x rays are increased.

The modern x-ray machine is a remarkable instrument. It conveys to the target an enormous number of electrons at a precisely controlled kinetic energy. At 100 mA, for example, 6×10^{17} electrons travel from the cathode to the anode of the x-ray tube every second. In an

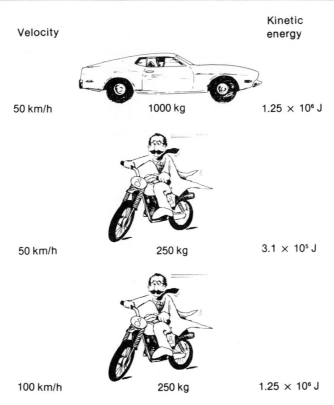

Velocity   Kinetic energy

50 km/h   1000 kg 1.25×10^6 J

50 km/h   250 kg 3.1×10^5 J

100 km/h   250 kg 1.25×10^6 J

Fig. 8-1. Kinetic energy is proportional to the product of mass and velocity squared. If the weight of a motorcycle is one fourth that of an automobile and the motorcycle is traveling twice as fast as the automobile, then the motorcycle and the automobile have equal kinetic energies.

x-ray machine operating at 70 kVp, each electron arrives at the target with a maximum kinetic energy of 70 keV. Since there are 1.6×10^{-16} J per keV, this energy is equivalent to

$$(70 \text{ keV})(1.6 \times 10^{-16} \text{ J/keV}) = 1.12 \times 10^{-14} \text{ J}$$

Inserting this energy into equation 8-1 and solving for the velocity of the electrons, we find

$$1.12 \times 10^{-14} \text{ J} = \tfrac{1}{2}(9.1 \times 10^{-31} \text{ kg})v^2$$

$$v^2 = \frac{(2)(1.12 \times 10^{-14} \text{ J})}{(9.1 \times 10^{-31} \text{ kg})}$$

$$= 0.25 \times 10^{17} \text{ m}^2/\text{s}^2$$
$$v = 1.6 \times 10^8 \text{ m/s}$$

EXAMPLE: At what fraction of the velocity of light do 70 keV electrons travel?

ANSWER: $\dfrac{v}{c} = \dfrac{1.6 \times 10^8 \text{ m/s}}{3.0 \times 10^8 \text{ m/s}}$

$$= 0.53$$

These calculations are not precisely correct; they do serve to illustrate the point and demonstrate the use of equation 8-1. Because of relativistic mass increase, the actual value of v/c is 0.47.

The distance between the filament and the target is only 1 to 3 cm. It is not difficult to imagine the intensity of the accelerating force required to raise the velocity of the electrons from zero to half the speed of light in so short a distance.

The electrons traveling from cathode to anode comprise the x-ray tube current and are sometimes called **projectile electrons.** When these projectile electrons impinge on the heavy metal atoms of the target, they interact with these atoms and transfer their kinetic energy to the target. These interactions occur within a very small depth of penetration into the target. As they occur, the projectile electrons slow down and finally come nearly to rest, at which time they can be conducted through the x-ray anode assembly and out into the associated electronic circuitry.

The projectile electron interacts with either the orbital electrons or the nuclei of target atoms. The interactions result in the conversion of kinetic energy into thermal energy and electromagnetic energy in the form of x rays.

Anode heat

By far, most of the kinetic energy of projectile electrons is converted into heat. Fig. 8-2 schematically illustrates how this occurs. The projectile electrons interact with the outer-shell electrons of the target atoms but do not transfer sufficient energy to these outer-shell electrons to ionize them. Rather, the outer-shell electrons are simply raised to an excited, or higher, energy level. The outer-shell electrons immediately drop back to their normal energy state with the emission of infrared radiation. The constant **excitation** and restabilization of outer-shell electrons are responsible for the heat generated in the anodes of x-ray tubes.

Generally, **more than 99% of the kinetic energy of projectile electrons is converted to thermal energy,** leaving less than 1% available for the production of x-radiation. One must conclude, therefore, that, sophisticated as it is, the x-ray machine is a very inefficient apparatus.

The production of heat in the anode increases

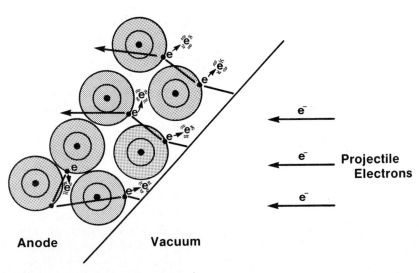

Fig. 8-2. Most of the kinetic energy of projectile electrons is transformed into heat energy by interactions with outer-shell electrons of target atoms. These interactions are primarily excitations rather than ionizations.

directly with increasing tube current. Doubling the tube current doubles the quantity of heat produced. Heat production also varies almost directly with varying kVp, at least in the diagnostic range. Although the relationship between varying kVp and varying heat production is approximate, it is sufficiently exact to allow the computation of heat units for use with anode cooling charts.

The efficiency of x-ray production is independent of the tube current. Consequently, regardless of what mA station is selected, the efficiency of x-ray production remains constant. The efficiency of x-ray production increases with increasing projectile-electron energy. At 60 keV, only 0.5% of the electron kinetic energy is converted to x rays; at 20 MeV, it is 70%.

Characteristic radiation

If the projectile electron interacts with an inner-shell electron of the target atom rather than an outer-shell electron, **characteristic x-radia-tion** can be produced. Characteristic x-radiation results when the interaction is sufficiently violent to ionize the target atom by total removal of the inner-shell electron. Excitation of an inner-shell electron does not produce characteristic x-radiation.

Fig. 8-3 illustrates how these characteristic x rays are produced. When the projectile electron ionizes a target atom by removal of a K-shell electron, a temporary electron hole is produced in the K shell. This is a highly unnatural state for the target atom and is corrected by an outer-shell electron falling into the hole in the K shell. Tungsten, for example, has electrons in shells out to the P shell (see Fig. 3-9), and when a K-shell electron is ionized, its position can be filled with electrons from any of the outer shells. The transition of an orbital electron from an outer shell to an inner shell is accompanied by the emission of an x-ray photon. The x ray has energy equal to the difference in the binding energies of the orbital electrons involved.

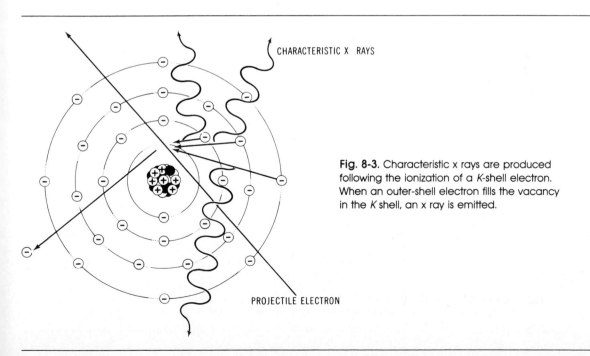

CHARACTERISTIC X RAYS

PROJECTILE ELECTRON

Fig. 8-3. Characteristic x rays are produced following the ionization of a K-shell electron. When an outer-shell electron fills the vacancy in the K shell, an x ray is emitted.

EXAMPLE: A *K*-shell electron is removed from a tungsten atom and is replaced by an *L*-shell electron. What is the energy of the characteristic x ray that is emitted?

ANSWER: Reference to Fig. 3-9 shows that for tungsten, *K* electrons have binding energies of 69.5 keV, and *L* electrons are bound by 12.1 keV. Therefore the characteristic x ray emitted has energy of

$$69.5 - 12.1 = 57.4 \text{ keV}$$

By the same procedure, the energy of x rays resulting from *M*-to-*K*, *N*-to-*K*, *O*-to-*K*, and *P*-to-*K* transitions can be calculated. All these x rays are called *K* x rays because they result from ionization of *K*-shell electrons.

Similar characteristic x rays are produced when the target atom is ionized by removal of electrons from shells other than the *K* shell. Fig. 8-3 does not show the production of x rays resulting from ionization of an *L*-shell electron; such a diagram would show the removal of an *L*-shell electron by the projectile electron. The vacancy in the *L* shell would be filled by an electron from any of the farther shells. X rays resulting from electron transitions to the *L* shell are called *L* x rays and are much less energetic than *K* x rays, since the binding energy of an *L*-shell electron is much lower than that of a *K*-shell electron.

Similarly, *M*-characteristic x rays, *N*-characteristic x rays, and even *O*-characteristic x rays can be produced in a tungsten target. Table 8-1 summarizes the production of characteristic x rays in tungsten. Although many characteristic x rays can be produced, it should be emphasized that they can be produced only at specific energies, equal to the difference in the electron binding energies for the various electron transitions. Except for *K* x rays, all the characteristic x rays have very low energy. The *L* x rays, with approximately 12 keV of energy, will penetrate only a few centimeters into soft tissue. Consequently, they are totally useless as diagnostic x rays, as are all the other low-energy–characteristic x rays. **Only the *K*-characteristic x rays, with an average energy of close to 70 keV,** are useful in this regard, and they contribute greatly to diagnostic radiographs. The last column in Table 8-1 shows the effective energy for each of the characteristic x rays of tungsten. These effective values will be referred to later.

In summary, characteristic x rays are produced by transitions of orbital electrons from outer to inner shells. Since the electron binding energy for every element is different, the characteristic x rays produced in the various elements are also different. This type of x-radiation is called characteristic radiation because it is **characteristic of the target element.** The effective energy of characteristic x rays increases with increasing atomic number of the target element.

Bremsstrahlung radiation

The production of heat and characteristic x rays involves interactions between the projectile

Table 8-1. Characteristic x rays of tungsten and their effective energies (keV)

| Characteristic x ray | Electron transition from | | | | | Effective energy |
	L shell	M shell	N shell	O shell	P shell	
K	57.4	66.7	68.9	69.4	69.5	69
L		9.3	11.5	12.0	12.1	12
M			2.2	2.7	2.8	2
N				0.52	0.6	0.6
O					0.08	0.08

electrons and the electrons of target atoms. A third type of interaction in which the projectile electron can lose its kinetic energy is an interaction with the nucleus of a target atom. In this type of interaction the kinetic energy of the projectile electron is converted into electromagnetic energy.

A projectile electron that completely avoids the orbital electrons on passing through an atom of the target may come sufficiently close to the nucleus of the atom to come under its influence, as shown in Fig. 8-4. Since the electron is negatively charged and the nucleus is positively charged, there is an electrostatic force of attraction between them. On approaching the nucleus closer, the projectile electron is influenced by a nuclear force much stronger than the electrostatic attraction. As it passes by the nucleus, it is slowed down and deviated in its course, leaving with reduced kinetic energy in a different

direction. This loss in kinetic energy reappears as an x-ray photon. This interaction is somewhat analogous to a comet in its course around the sun.

These types of x rays are called bremsstrahlung radiation, or **bremsstrahlung x rays.** Bremsstrahlung is a German word for slowing down or braking; bremsstrahlung radiation can be considered radiation resulting from the braking of projectile electrons by the nucleus.

A projectile electron can lose any amount of its kinetic energy in an interaction with the nucleus of a traget atom, and the bremsstrahlung radiation associated with the loss can take on a corresponding range of values. For example, an electron with kinetic energy of 70 keV can lose all, none, or any intermediate level of that kinetic energy in a bremsstrahlung interaction; the bremsstrahlung x ray produced can have an energy in the range of 0 to 70 keV. This is different

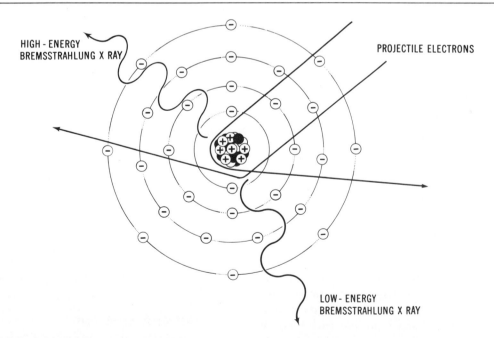

HIGH-ENERGY
BREMSSTRAHLUNG X RAY

PROJECTILE ELECTRONS

LOW-ENERGY
BREMSSTRAHLUNG X RAY

Fig. 8-4. Bremsstrahlung x rays result from an interaction between a projectile electron and a target nucleus. The electron is slowed down, and its course is shifted.

from the production of characteristic x rays, which have specified energies. Fig. 8-4 illustrates how one can consider the production of such a wide range of energies through the bremsstrahlung interaction. A low-energy bremsstrahlung x ray results when the projectile electron is barely influenced by the nucleus. A maximum-energy x ray occurs when the projectile electron loses all its kinetic energy and simply drifts away from the nucleus. Bremsstrahlung x rays with energies between these two extremes also occur.

Bremsstrahlung x rays can be produced at any projectile-electron energy; K-characteristic x rays require a tube potential of at least 70 kVp. In the diagnostic range most x rays are of bremsstrahlung origin. At 100 kVp, for example, only approximately 15% of the x-ray beam results from characteristic radiation.

X-RAY EMISSION SPECTRUM

Most of us have seen or heard of pitching machines, the devices used by baseball teams for batting practice so that the pitchers don't get worn out. There are similar machines for automatically ejecting bowling balls, tennis balls, and even Ping-Pong balls.

Suppose we had a device that could eject all these types of balls at random at a rate of one per second. The most straightforward way to determine how often each type of ball was ejected on the average would be to catch each ball as it was ejected, identify it, and drop it into a basket, so that at the end of the observation period the total number of each type of ball could be counted. Let us suppose that the results obtained for a 10-minute period are those in Fig. 8-5. A total of 600 balls were ejected. Perhaps the easiest way to graphically represent these results would be to plot the total number of each type of ball emitted during the 10-minute observation period and represent each total by a bar, as shown in Fig. 8-6.

The bar graph of Fig. 8-6 can be described as a discrete ball-ejection spectrum representative of the automatic pitching machine. It is a plot of the number of balls ejected per unit time as a function of the type of ball. It is called discrete because only five distinct types of balls are involved. Connecting the bars with a dashed curve as shown would indicate a large number of different types of balls. Such a curve is called a continuous ejection spectrum. The word **spectrum** refers to the range of types. The total number of balls ejected is represented by the sum of the areas under the bars, in the case of the discrete spectrum, and the area under the curve, in the case of the continuous spectrum.

Without regard to the absolute number of balls emitted, Fig. 8-6 could also be identified as a relative ball-ejection spectrum, since at a glance one can tell the relative frequency of ejection of each type of ball. Relatively speaking, baseballs are ejected most frequently, and basketballs least frequently. If the ball-ejection machine operated randomly, the results of this 10-minute observation would be characteristic of any time of observation.

This type of relationship is fundamental to describing the output of an x-ray machine. If one could stand in the middle of the useful x-ray beam, catch each individual x-ray photon, and measure its energy, one could describe what is known as the **x-ray emission spectrum,** the form of which is shown in Fig. 8-7. Here the relative number of x-ray photons emitted is plotted as a function of the energy of each individual photon. Although we cannot catch and identify each individual x-ray photon, there are instruments available that allow us to measure x-ray emission spectra. X-ray emission spectra have been described for all types of machines. Understanding x-ray emission spectra is a key to understanding how changes in kVp, mA, time, and filtration affect the density and contrast of a radiograph.

Discrete x-ray spectrum

We saw earlier that characteristic x rays have precisely fixed, or discrete, energies and that these energies are characteristic of the differences between electron binding energies of a

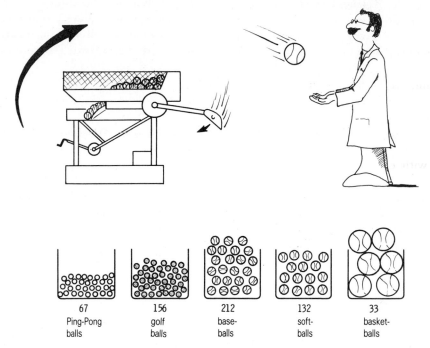

Fig. 8-5. In a 10-minute period an automatic ball-throwing machine might eject 600 balls, distributed as shown.

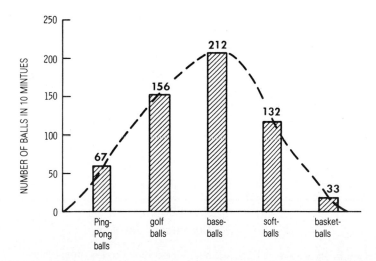

Fig. 8-6. Bar graph representing results of 10-minute observation of balls ejected by the automatic pitching machine in Fig. 8-5.

particular element. A characteristic x ray from tungsten, for example, can have one of fifteen energies (Table 8-1) and no others. A plot of the frequency with which characteristic x rays are emitted as a function of their energy would look like that shown for tungsten in Fig. 8-8. Such a plot is called the **discrete**, or **characteristic, x-ray emission spectrum**. There are five vertical

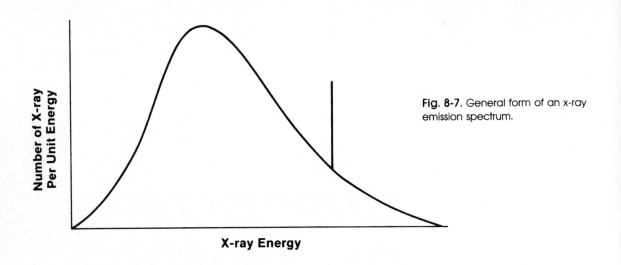

Fig. 8-7. General form of an x-ray emission spectrum.

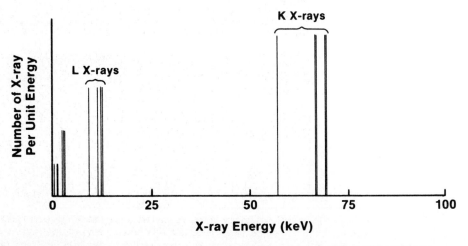

Fig. 8-8. Characteristic x-ray emission spectrum for tungsten contains fifteen different x-ray energies. The effective *K* x-ray energy of 69 keV is represented by the vertical bar.

lines representing *K* x rays and four vertical lines representing *L* x rays. The other, lower-energy lines represent characteristic emissions from the outer electron shells.

The relative intensity of the *K* x rays is greater than that of the lower-energy–characteristic x rays, as shown, because of the nature of the interaction process. *K* x rays are the only characteristic x rays of tungsten with sufficient energy to be of value in diagnostic radiology. Although there are five *K* x rays, it is customary to represent them as one, as has been done with a single vertical line at 69 keV. Only this line will be shown in later graphs.

Continuous x-ray spectrum

If it were possible to identify and quantitate the energy contained in each bremsstrahlung photon emitted from an x-ray tube, one would find that these energies extend from that associated with the peak electron energy all the way down to zero. In other words, when an x-ray tube is operated at 70 kVp, bremsstrahlung pho-

tons with energies ranging from 0 to 70 keV are emitted. A typical **continuous, or bremsstrahlung, x-ray emission spectrum** is shown in Fig. 8-9.

This emission spectrum is sometimes called the continous emission spectrum because, unlike in the discrete spectrum, the energies of the photons emitted may range anywhere from zero to some maximum value. The general shape of the continuous x-ray spectrum is the same for all x-ray machines. The maximum energy that an x ray can have is numerically equal to the kVp of operation. The greatest number of x-ray photons is emitted with energy approximately one third of the maximum photon energy. The number of x rays emitted decreases rapidly at very low photon energies and below 5 keV nearly reaches zero.

EXAMPLE: At what kVp was the x-ray machine represented in Fig. 8-9 operated?

ANSWER: Since the bremsstrahlung spectrum intersects the energy axis at about 90 keV, the machine must have been operated at 90 kVp.

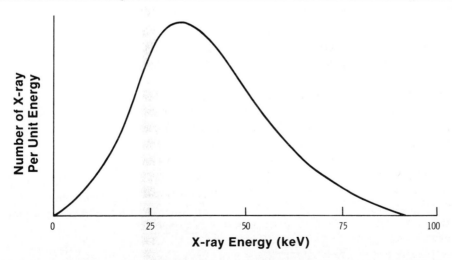

Fig. 8-9. Bremsstrahlung x-ray emission spectrum extends from zero to maximum projectile-electron energy, with the highest number of x rays having approximately one-third the maximum energy.

There are three primary reasons for the reduced intensity of x-ray emission at low energies:

1. The electrons accelerated from cathode to anode do not all have peak kinetic energy. Depending on the type of rectification and high-voltage circuitry, many of these electrons may have very low energies when they strike the target and hence can produce only low-energy x rays.
2. The conventional target of a modern diagnostic x-ray tube is relatively thick. Consequently, many of the bremsstrahlung x rays emitted result from multiple interactions of the projectile electrons, and for each successive interaction a projectile electron has less energy.
3. External filtration is nearly always added to the x-ray tube assembly. This added filtration serves to selectively remove low-energy photons from the beam.

EXAMPLE: Construct the expected emission spectrum for an x-ray machine with a pure molybdenum target (efective energy of K x ray equals 20 keV) operated at 94 kVp.

ANSWER: The spectrum should look something like the drawing below. THe curve intersects the energy axis at 0 and 95 keV and has the general shape shown in Fig. 8-7 except the bremsstrahlung spectrum is much lower. A line extends above the curve at 20 keV to represent the characteristic x rays.

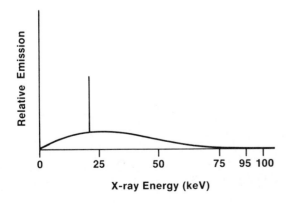

Minimum wavelength

As a result of early views of x-ray physics, x-ray emission spectra often are constructed as a function of x-ray photon wavelength rather than energy. This terminology, sometimes referred to as the Dwayne-Hunt law, has no application to radiology, but it does have relevance to x-ray diffraction and other analytical uses of x-radiation. It is reviewed here to provide some continuity with earlier textbooks and because questions of **minimum wavelength** (λ_{min}) sometimes appear on certification examinations.

The energy of an x-ray photon is directly proportional to the product of the photon frequency times Planck's constant. X-ray energy is also inversely proportional to the photon wavelength, as shown in equation 4-5: $E = hc/\lambda$. As photon wavelength increases, photon energy decreases and vice versa. Consequently, the minimum x-ray wavelength is associated with the maximum x-ray energy.

To calculate λ_{min}, one must solve equation 4-5 for λ:

(8-2)

$$\lambda = \frac{hc}{E}$$

Both h and c are constants ($h = 4.14 \times 10^{-15}$ eV-s, $c = 10^8$ m/s) and therefore

(8-3)

$$\lambda = \frac{12.4 \times 10^{-7} \; eV\text{-}m}{E}$$

Since the minimum wavelength of x-ray emission corresponds to the maximum photon energy, and the maximum photon energy is numerically equal to the kVp, equation 8-3 can be expressed as

$$\lambda_{min} = \frac{12.4 \times 10^{-10}}{kVp}$$

where λ_{min} is in meters.

To express λ_{min} in nanometers (nm) or Angstroms (Å), the following conversion factors are applied:

$$1 \text{ nm} = 10^{-9} \text{ m}$$
$$1 \text{ Å} = 10^{-10} \text{ m}$$

EXAMPLE: What is the minimum wavelength associated with the x rays emitted from a radiographic unit operated at 100 kVp?

ANSWER: At 100 kVp, the maximum photon energy will be 100 keV. Therefore

$$\lambda_{min} = \frac{12.4 \times 10^{-10}}{100 \text{ kVp}}$$
$$= 0.124 \times 10^{-10} \text{ m}$$
$$= 0.0124 \text{ nm}$$
$$= 0.124 \text{ Å}$$

FACTORS AFFECTING THE X-RAY EMISSION SPECTRUM

The total number of x-rays emitted from an x-ray tube could be determined by adding the number of x rays emitted at each energy over the entire spectrum, a process called **integration.** Graphically, the total number of x rays emitted is equivalent to the area under the curve. The general shape of an emission spectrum is always the same, but its relative position along the energy axis can change. The farther to the right a spectrum is, the higher the effective energy, or **quality,** of the x-ray beam. The greater the area under the curve, the higher the x-ray intensity, or **quantity.** A number of factors under the control of the radiologic technologist greatly influence the relative position and size of the x-ray emission spectrum. These factors are summarized in Table 8-2.

Influence of tube current

If one changes the mA station of an x-ray console from 200 to 400 mA while all other conditions remain constant, twice as many electrons will flow from cathode to anode. This operating change will produce twice as many x-ray photons at every photon energy. In other words, the photon emission spectrum will be changed in amplitude but not in shape, as shown in Fig. 8-10. Each point on the curve labeled 400 mA is precisely two times higher than the associated point on the 200 mA curve.

A change in x-ray tube current results in a proportionate change in the amplitude of the x-ray emission spectrum at all energies. This relationship also is true for changes in mAs. Thus the area under the x-ray emission curve varies proportionately with changes in mA or mAs, as does the output intensity of the x-ray machine.

EXAMPLE: Suppose the area under the 200 mA curve in Fig. 8-10 totals 4.2 cm², and that the output intensity of the associated machine is 325 mR/s (84 μC/kg-s). What would the area under the curve and the output intensity be if the tube current were increased to 400 mA while other operating factors remain constant?

ANSWER: In going from 200 to 400 mA, the tube current has been increased by a factor of two. The area under the curve and the output intensity are increased proportionately:

$$\text{Area} = 4.2 \text{ cm}^2 \times 2 = 8.4 \text{ cm}^2$$
$$\text{Intensity} = 325 \text{ mR/s} \times 2 = 650 \text{ mR/s}$$

Influence of tube potential

Unlike a change in tube current, a change in kVp affects both the amplitude and the position

Table 8-2. Factors affecting size and relative position of x-ray emission spectra

Factor	Effect
Tube current	Amplitude of spectrum
Tube voltage	Amplitude and position
Added filtration	Amplitude, most effective at low energy
Target material	Amplitude of spectrum and position of line spectrum
Voltage waveform	Amplitude, most effective at high energy

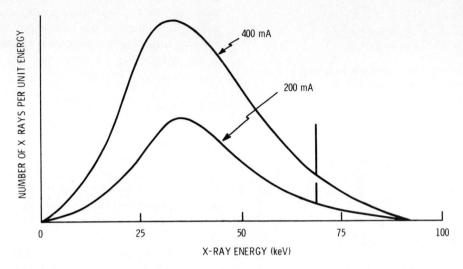

Fig. 8-10. Change in tube mA results in a proportionate change in the amplitude of the x-ray emission spectrum at all energies.

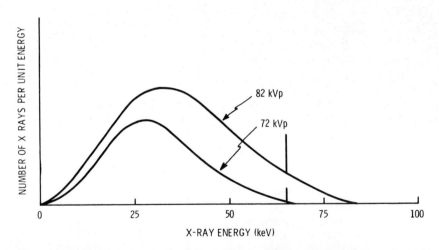

Fig. 8-11. Change in kVp results in an increase in the amplitude of the emission spectrum at all energies but a greater increase at high energies than at low energies. Therefore the spectrum is shifted to the right, or high-energy, side.

of an x-ray emission spectrum. As kVp is raised, the area under the curve approximately increases with the square of the factor by which kVp was increased. Accordingly, the output intensity increases with the square of this factor. When kVp is increased, the relative distribution of emitted x-ray photons shifts to the right, to higher x-ray energies. The maximum energy of emission is always numerically equal to the kVp.

Fig. 8-11 demonstrates the effect of increasing the kVp while other factors remain constant. The lower spectrum represents x-ray operation at 72 kVp, and the upper spectrum represents operation at 82 kVp, a 10 kVp increase. It can be seen that the area under the curve has approximately doubled while the relative position of the curve has been shifted to the high-energy side. More photons are emitted at all energies during operation at 82 kVp than during operation at 72 kVp. However, the increase is relatively greater for high-energy x-ray photons than for low-energy photons. Like a change in mA or mAs, a change in kVp does not shift the position of the discrete emission spectrum.

EXAMPLE: Suppose the curve labeled 72 kVp in Fig. 8-11 covers a total area of 3.6 cm and that this represents an output intensity of 125 mR/s (32 μC/kg-s). What area under the curve and output intensity would be expected for operation at 82 kVp?

ANSWER: The area under the curve and the output intensity are porportional to the **square** of the kVp. A ratio can be established.

$$\left(\frac{82}{72}\right)^2 (3.6 \text{ cm}) = (1.3)(3.6 \text{ cm})$$
$$= 4.7 \text{ cm}$$

and

$$(1.3)(125 \text{ mR/s}) = 163 \text{ mR/s}$$

This example helps explain the rule of thumb employed by radiologic technologists to relate the kVp and mA changes necessary to produce a constant film density. The rule states that **a 15% increase in kVp is equivalent to doubling the mAs.** At low kVp, for example, 50 to 60 kVp,

approximately a 7 kVp increase is equivalent to doubling the mAs. At tube potentials above about 100 kVp, a 15 kVp change may be necessary.

A 15% increase in voltage does not double the output intensity from an x-ray machine but is equivalent to doubling the mAs to obtain a given density on the film. To double the output intensity by increasing kVp, one would have to raise the kVp by as much as 40%. Radiographically, only a 15% increase in kVp is necessary because with increased kVp, the penetrability of the beam is increased and less radiation is absorbed by the patient, leaving proportionately more to blacken the film.

Influence of added filtration

Adding filtration to an x-ray machine has an effect on the relative position of the spectrum similar to that of increasing the kVp. This effect is shown in Fig. 8-12, where a tube is operated at 95 kVp with 2 mm aluminum (Al) added filtration, compared with the same operation with 4 mm Al added filtration. Added filtration more effectively absorbs low-energy x rays than high-energy x rays, and therefore the x-ray emission spectrum is reduced more on the left than on the right. **The overall result is an increase in the effective energy of the x-ray beam** (higher penetrability) with an accompanying reduction in beam intensity. The discrete spectrum is not affected nor is the maximum energy of x-ray emission. There is no simple method to calculate the changes in effective energy and intensity with change in added filtration.

Influence of target material

We have previously discussed how the atomic number of the target material affects both the number and the effective energy of x rays. Basically, as the atomic number of the target material increases, the efficiency of the production of bremsstrahlung radiation increases, and the high-energy photons increase in number more readily than the low-energy photons. The

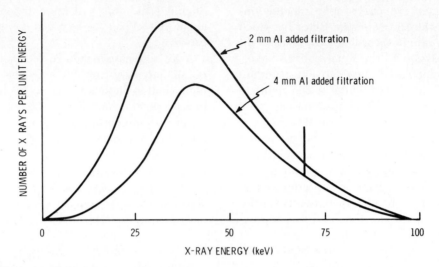

Fig. 8-12. Adding filtration to an x-ray tube results in reduced x-ray intensity but increased effective energy. The emission spectra represented here result from operation at the same mAs and kVp but with different filtrations.

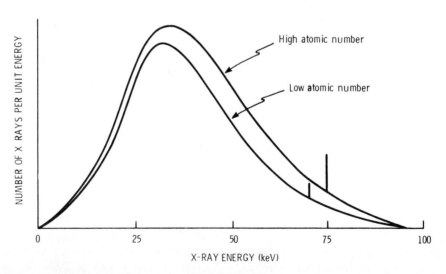

Fig. 8-13. Discrete emission spectrum shifts to the right with an increase in the atomic number of the target material. The continuous spectrum increases slightly in amplitude, particularly to the high-energy side, with an increase in target atomic number.

change in the continuous spectrum is not nearly so pronounced as the change in the discrete spectrum. Following an increase in the atomic number of the target material, **the discrete spectrum is shifted to the right,** representing the higher-energy–characteristic radiation. This phenomenon is a direct result of the higher electron binding energies associated with increasing atomic numbers.

These changes are shown schematically in Fig. 8-13. Tungsten is a primary component of most modern x-ray targets, but some specialty tubes employ gold as target material. The atomic numbers for tungsten and gold are 74 and 79, respectively.

Influence of voltage waveform

In Chapter 6 the various types of voltage waveforms produced by modern x-ray genera-

tors were discussed. There are principally four: half-wave rectification; full-wave rectification; three-phase, six-pulse power; and three-phase, twelve-pulse power. Half-wave– and full-wave– rectified voltage waveforms are the same except for the frequency of repetition. The difference between three-phase, six-pulse and three-phase, twelve-pulse power is simply the reduced ripple obtained with twelve-pulse generation compared wth six-pulse generation.

Fig. 8-14 shows an exploded view of a full-wave–rectified voltage waveform for an x-ray machine operated at 100 kVp. Recall that the amplitude of the waveform corresponds to the applied voltage and that the horizontal axis represents time. At $t = 0$, the voltage across the x-ray tube equals 0 V, indicating that at this instant no electrons are flowing and no x rays are being produced. At $t = 1$ ms, the voltage across

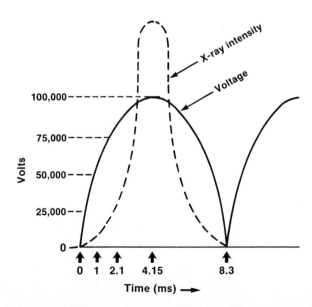

Fig. 8-14. As the voltage across the x-ray tube increases from zero to its peak value, the x-ray intensity increases, slowly at first and then rapidly as peak voltage is obtained.

the x-ray tube has increased from 0 to approximately 10,000 V; the x rays produced at this instant are of relatively low energy and intensity. At t = 2.1 ms, the tube voltage has increased to approximately 25,000 V and is rapidly approaching its peak value. At t = 4.2 ms, the maximum tube voltage is obtained, and the maximum energy and intensity of x-ray emission are produced. For the following one-quarter cycle between 4.2 ms and 8.3 ms, the x-ray intensity and effective x-ray energy decrease again at 0.

The number of x rays emitted at each instant through a cycle is not proportional to the voltage but rather inreases slowly and at low voltages and more rapidly at higher voltages. The resulting x-ray intensity will be similar to that diagramed in Fig. 8-14. The intensity of x-radiation is much higher at peak voltages than at lower voltages. Consequently, voltage waveforms of three-phase operation result in considerably more intense x-ray emission than those of full-wave–rectified operation.

This relationship between x-ray output and type of generator is the basis for another rule of thumb employed by radiologic technologists: **operation on three-phase equipment is equivalent to a 12% increase over single-phase equipment.** For example, if a lateral skull technique calls for 72 kVp on single-phase equipment, on three-phase equipment approximately 64 kVp will produce similar results.

This discussion is summarized in Fig. 8-15, where an emission spectrum from a full-wave–rectified unit is compared with that from a twelve-pulse, three-phase generator, both operated at 92 kVp and the same mAs. The x-ray emission spectrum resulting from three-phase operation is obviously much more efficient. The area under the curve is considerably greater, and the spectrum is shifted to the high-energy side. Note that the discrete emission spectrum representing characteristic x-ray production remains fixed in its position along the energy axis but increases slightly in magnitude because of

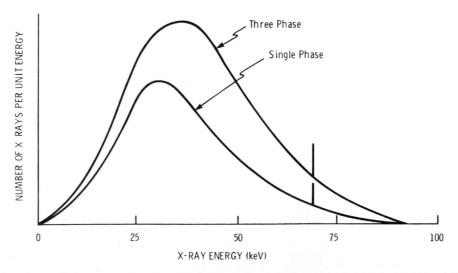

Fig. 8-15. Three-phase operation is considerably more efficient than single-phase operation. Both the x-ray intensity (area under the curve) and the effective energy (relative shift of amplitude) are increased. Here are shown representative spectra for 92 kVp operation.

the increased number of projectile electrons available for *K*-shell electron interaction. There is no simple way to calculate the differences in x-ray output between single-phase and three-phase operation.

EXAMPLE: What would be the difference in the x-ray emission spectra between a full-wave–rectified operation compared with a half-wave–rectified operation if the kVp and mA are held constant?

ANSWER: Under constant conditions of operation there should be no difference in the x-ray emission spectra. The x-ray intensity and effective energy should remain constant.

REVIEW QUESTIONS

1. Define or otherwise identify the following:
   a. Projectile electron
   b. Binding energy
   c. Characteristic x rays
   d. Bremsstrahlung x rays
   e. X-ray quantity
   f. X-ray quality
   g. Effective energy
   h. Rectification

2. Calculate the energy and wavelength of the characteristic x rays produced by the following electron transitions in a tungsten target (refer to Fig. 3-9):
   a. *K*-shell electron replaced by *M*-shell electron
   b. *L*-shell electron replaced by *O*-shell electron

3. What would be the fate of the photons in question 2 if the machine contained 2.5 mm Al filtration?

4. At what fraction of the velocity of light do 90 keV electrons travel?

5. Discuss what the discrete and continuous x-ray spectra represent.

6. Draw the x-ray emission spectrum for an x-ray machine with a tungsten target operated at 90 kVp.

7. What is the minimum wavelength, expressed in nanometers, for the machine in question 6?

8. When an x-ray machine is operated at 80 kVp, its emission spectrum covers a total area of 4.8 cm², and its output intensity is 350 mR/s. What will be the area under the curve and the output intensity be if the kVp is increased to 90 and the mA is doubled?

9. Discuss the effect the addition of three-phase power would have on the x-ray emission spectrum if the kVp and mA are held constant.

10. Explain the effect the addition of filtration to an x-ray machine would have on the discrete and continuous x-ray emission spectra.

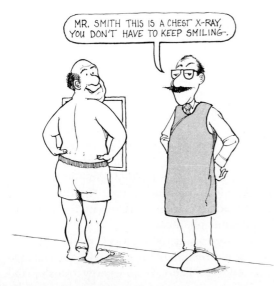
MR. SMITH THIS IS A CHEST X-RAY, YOU DON'T HAVE TO KEEP SMILING.

9

X-ray interaction with matter

FIVE BASIC INTERACTIONS
DIFFERENTIAL ABSORPTION
CONTRAST EXAMINATIONS
EXPONENTIAL ATTENUATION

FIVE BASIC INTERACTIONS

In Chapter 4 the interaction of electromagnetic radiation with matter was briefly described. The interaction was said to have wavelike and particle-like properties. A fundamental relationship was that electromagnetic radiation interacts with structures similar in size to the wavelength of the radiation.

X rays have very small wavelengths, no larger than approximately 10^{-8} to 10^{-9} m. The higher the energy of an x ray, the shorter is its wavelength. Consequently, low-energy x rays tend to interact with whole atoms, which have diameters of approximately 10^{-9} to 10^{-10} m; moderate-energy x rays generally interact with electron clouds; and high-energy x rays generally interact with nuclei. There are five basic mechanisms by which x rays interact at these various structural levels: classical scattering, Compton effect, photoelectric effect, pair production, and photodisintegration. The two of these of particular im-

portance to diagnostic radiology, the Compton effect and the photoelectric effect, will be dealt with in some detail.

Classical scattering

Low-energy x rays, those with energies below 10 keV, can interact with matter by **classical scattering,** sometimes called **coherent** or **Thompson scattering** (Fig. 9-1). In classical scattering the incident photon interacts with a target atom, causing it to become excited. The target atom immediately releases this excess energy as a secondary, or scattered, photon with wavelength equal to that of the incident photon ($\lambda = \lambda'$) and therefore of equal energy. The direction of the secondary photon is different from that of the incident photon.

The net result of classical scattering is a change in direction of the x ray without a change in its energy. There is no energy transfer and therefore no ionization. Most classically scattered x rays are scattered in the forward direction.

Classical scattering is of little importance to diagnostic radiology because it primarily involves low-energy x rays, which contribute little to the radiograph anyway. However, some classical scattering occurs throughout the diagnostic range. At 70 kVp perhaps a few percent of the x rays undergo classical scattering, which contributes slightly to **film fog,** the general graying of a radiograph by non-information-carrying photons.

Compton effect

Moderate-energy x rays, x rays throughout the diagnostic range, can undergo an interaction with outer-shell electrons that not only scatters the photon but reduces its energy and ionizes the atom as well. This interaction is called the **Compton effect,** or **Compton scattering,** and is shown schematically in Fig. 9-2. In this process

the incident x ray interacts with an outer-shell electron and ejects it from the atom, thereby ionizing the atom. The x ray continues in an altered direction with decreased energy. The energy of the Compton-scattered x ray is equal to the difference between the energy of the incident x ray and the energy imparted to the electron. The energy imparted to the electron is equal to its binding energy plus the kinetic energy with which it leaves the atom. Mathematically, this energy transfer is represented as

$$(9\text{-}1)$$

$$E_i = E_s + (E_b + E_{KE})$$

where E_i is the energy of the incident x ray; E_s, the energy of the scattered x ray; E_b, the electron binding energy; and E_{KE}, the kinetic energy of the electron.

EXAMPLE: A 30 keV x ray ionizes an atom of barium by ejecting an O-shell electron with 12 keV of kinetic energy. What is the energy of the scattered photon?

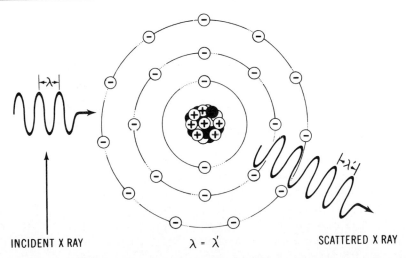

Fig. 9-1. Classical scattering is an interaction between low-energy x rays and atoms. The x ray loses no energy but changes direction slightly. The wavelength of the incident x ray is equal to the wavelength of the scattered x ray.

INCIDENT X RAY $\lambda = \lambda'$ SCATTERED X RAY

ANSWER: Fig. 3-9 shows that the binding energy of an O-shell electron of barium is 0.04 keV; therefore

$$E_s = 30 - (0.04 + 12)$$
$$= 30 - (12.04)$$
$$= 17.96 \text{ keV}$$

During a Compton interaction, most of the energy is divided between the scattered photon and the **secondary electron,** also called the Compton electron. Usually the scattered photon retains most of the energy. Both the scattered photon and the secondary electron may have sufficient energy to undergo many more ionizing interactions before losing all their energy. Ultimately, the scattered photon will be absorbed photoelectrically, and the secondary electron will drop into an atomic-shell hole previously created by some other ionizing event.

Compton-scattered photons can be deflected in any direction, including 180 degrees from the incident photon. The formulas relating to deflection angle are beyond the scope of this text. At a deflection of 0 degrees no energy is transferred. As the angle of deflection increases to 180 degrees, more energy is transferred to the secondary electron, but even at 180 degrees deflection the scattered x ray retains at least about two thirds of its original energy.

Photons scattered back in the direction of the incident x-ray beam, approximately 180 degrees, are called **backscatter radiation.** This type of radiation is of considerable importance to radiotherapy. In diagnostic radiology, backscatter is responsible for the cassette-hinge image sometimes seen on a radiograph even though the hinge was on the back side of the cassette.

The probability that a given x ray will undergo a Compton interaction is a complex function of the energy of the incident photon, but generally

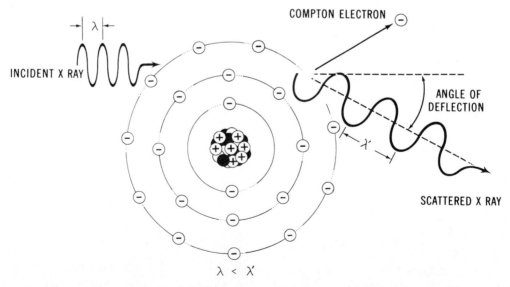

Fig. 9-2. Compton effect occurs between moderate-energy x rays and outer-shell electrons. It results in ionization of the target atom, change in photon direction, and reduction of photon energy. The wavelength of the scattered x ray is greater than that of the incident x ray.

the probability decreases as x-ray energy increases. The probability of Compton interaction is nearly independent of the atomic number of the target atom. Any given x ray is just as likely to undergo Compton interaction with an atom of soft tissue as with an atom of bone. Fig. 9-3 diagrams these relationships.

Compton scattering can occur with all diagnostic x rays and is therefore of considerable importance in radiology. Its importance is in a negative sense, however. Scattered x rays provide no useful information on the film. Rather, they contribute to film fog, which results in an inferior radiograph. There are ways of reducing scattered radiation, which will be discussed later, but none is totally effective, and therefore radiographs are not as clear as they might otherwise be.

The scattered x rays from Compton interactions can create a serious radiation exposure hazard in radiography and particularly in fluoroscopy. A large amount of radiation can be scattered from the patient during fluoroscopy. Such radiation is the source of most of the occupational radiation exposure that radiologic technologists receive. During radiography, the hazard is less severe because persons other than the patient are not normally in the examining room;

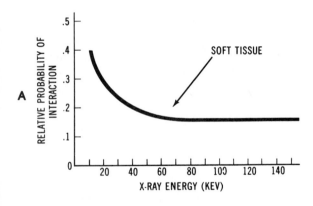

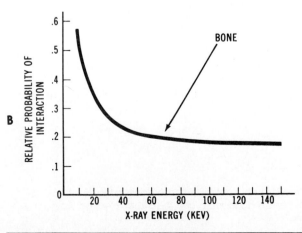

Fig. 9-3. The probability that an x ray will interact by Compton effect is about the same for target atoms of soft tissue and bone. This probability decreases with increasing photon energy. **A,** Probability for soft tissue. **B,** Probability for bone.

nevertheless, scattered radiation levels are sufficient to require protective shielding of the room.

Photoelectric effect

X rays in the diagnostic range can also undergo ionizing interactions with inner-shell electrons of target atoms, so that the x ray is not scattered but totally absorbed. This process, diagramed in Fig. 9-4, is called the photoelectric effect. **The photoelectric effect is a photon absorption interaction.** The electron removed from the atom, called a **photoelectron,** escapes with kinetic energy equal to the difference between the energy of the incident x ray and the binding energy of the electron. Mathematically, this is shown as

(9-2)

$$E_i = E_b + E_{KE}$$

where symbols are the same as in equation 9-1.

For low atomic number target atoms, such as in soft tissue, the binding energy of even K-shell electrons is low (0.284 keV for carbon, for instance), and therefore the photoelectron is released with kinetic energy nearly equal to the energy of the incident x ray. For higher atomic number target atoms, the electron binding energies are higher (37.4 keV for barium K-shell electrons), and therefore the kinetic energy of the photoelectron is proportionately lower.

Characteristic x rays are produced following a photoelectric interaction in a manner similar to that described in Chapter 8. The ejection of a K-shell photoelectron by the incident x ray results in a vacancy in the K shell, an unnatural state immediately corrected by an outer-shell electron, usually from the L shell, dropping into the vacancy. This electron transition is accompanied by the emission of an x ray whose energy is equal to the difference in the binding energies of the shells involved. These characteristic x rays are also **secondary radiation** and behave in the same manner as scattered radiation. They contribute nothing of diagnostic value and occur with insignificant intensity.

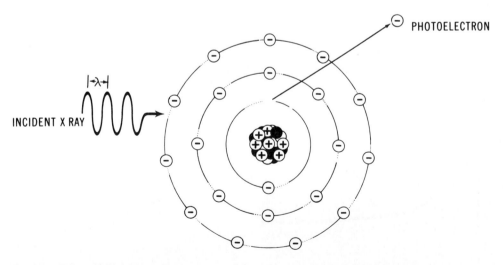

Fig. 9-4. Photoelectric effect occurs when an incident x ray is totally absorbed during the ionization of an inner-shell electron. The incident photon disappears, and the K-shell electron, now called a photoelectron, is ejected from the atom.

EXAMPLE: A 50 keV x ray interacts photoelectrically with (a) a carbon atom and (b) a barium atom. What is the kinetic energy of each photoelectron and each characteristic x ray if an L-to-K transition occurs? (See Fig. 3-9.)

ANSWER:

a. $E_{KE} = E_i - E_b$
$= 50 - 0.284$
$= 49.72$ keV
$E_X = 0.284 - 0.006$
$= 0.278$ keV

b. $E_{KE} = E_i - E_b$
$= 50 - 37.4$
$= 12.6$ keV
$E_X = 37.441 - 5.989$
$= 31.452$ keV

The probability that a given x ray will undergo a photoelectric interaction is a function of both the photon energy and the atomic number of the target atom.

A photoelectric interaction cannot occur unless the incident x ray has energy equal to or greater than the electron binding energy. A barium K-shell electron bound to the nucleus by 37.441 keV cannot be removed by a 25 keV photon. If the incident photon has sufficient energy, the probability that it will undergo a photoelectric interaction decreases with the cube of the photon energy: **the probability of photoelectric interaction is inversely proportional to the third power of the photon energy.** This relationship

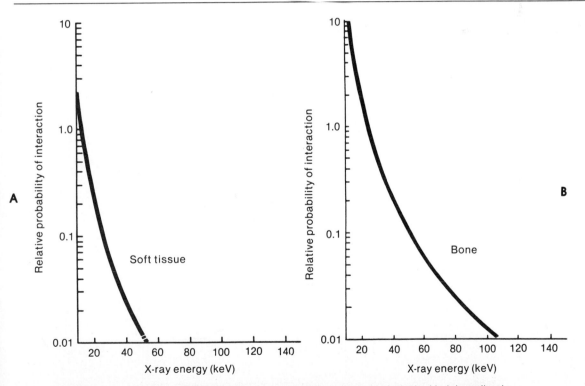

Fig. 9-5. The relative probability that a given x ray will undergo a photoelectric interaction is inversely proportional to the third power of the photon energy and directly proportional to the third power of the atomic number of the absorber. **A,** Relationship for soft tissue. **B,** Relationship for bone.

Table 9-1. Effective atomic numbers of various materials important to diagnostic radiology

Type of substance	Effective atomic number
Human tissue	
Muscle	7.4
Fat	6.3
Bone	13.8
Lung	7.4
Contrast material	
Barium	56
Iodine	53
Air	7.6
Other	
Concrete	17
Tungsten	74
Lead	82

is shown graphically in Fig. 9-5 for soft tissue and bone.

As the relative vertical displacement between the graphs of soft tissue and bone in Fig. 9-5 demonstrates, a photoelectric interaction is much more likely to occur with high-Z atoms than with low-Z atoms. In fact, **the probability of photoelectric interaction is directly proportional to the third power of the atomic number** of the absorbing material. Table 9-1 presents the effective atomic numbers of target materials of radiologic importance.

EXAMPLE: If an 80 keV x ray has a relative chance of one of interacting photoelectrically within the first centimeter of soft tissue, what is its relative probability of interacting with

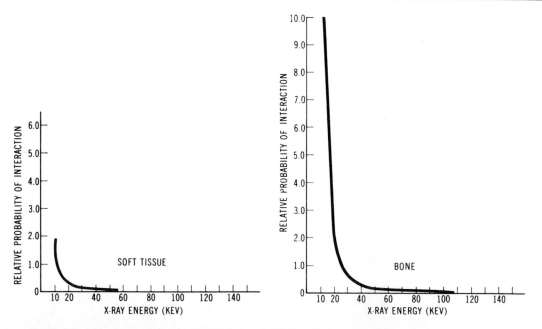

Fig. 9-6. Relative probability for photoelectric interaction ranges over several orders of magnitude. If it is plotted in the conventional arithmetic fashion, as here, one cannot estimate its value above an energy of about 20 keV.

a. Fat?
b. Barium?

ANSWER:

a. $\left(\dfrac{6.3}{7.4}\right)^3 = 0.62$

b. $\left(\dfrac{56}{7.4}\right)^3 = 4.33$

Semilog graphs. Fig. 9-5 is an example of a graph having a logarithmic (log, for short) scale. A review of Table 2-1 will show that whole log values represent orders of magnitude in power-

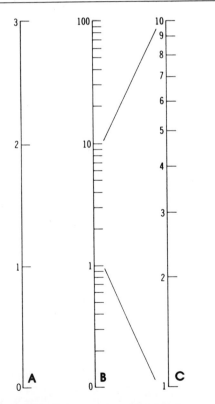

Fig. 9-7. Graphic scales can be arithmetic or logarithmic. **A,** Arithmetic scale. **B** and **C,** Log scales. The log scale is used to plot wide ranges of values.

of-ten notation. Therefore the difference between log 4 and log 2 is two orders of magnitude, or $10^4 - 10^2$.

A log scale is a power-of-ten scale used to plot data that cover several orders of magnitude. In Fig. 9-5, for example, the relative probability for photoelectric interaction with soft tissue varies from about 2 to less than 0.01 over the energy range from 10 to 60 keV. A plot of these data in conventional arithmetic form appears in Fig. 9-6. Clearly this type of graph is unacceptable because all probability values above 40 keV are so close to zero.

On an arithmetic scale equal intervals have equal numerical value, but on a log scale they do not. This difference in scales is shown in Fig. 9-7. All major intervals on the arithmetic scale have a value of 1, and the subintervals a value of 0.1. On the other hand, the log scale contains major intervals that each equal one order of magnitude and subintervals that are not equal in length. Fig. 9-7 also shows an exploded view of one major log interval.

Cubic relationships. A probability of interaction proportional to the third power changes rapidly. For the photoelectric effect this means that a small variation in atomic number or x-ray energy results in a large change in the chance that a given x ray will undergo such an interaction. This is unlike the situation that exists for the Compton interaction.

EXAMPLE: If the relative probability of photoelectric interaction with soft tissue for a 20 keV x ray is 1, how much less likely will an interaction be for a 50 keV x ray? How much more likely is interaction with iodine than with soft tissue for a 70 keV x ray?

ANSWER: $\left(\dfrac{20 \text{ keV}}{50 \text{ keV}}\right)^3 = \left(\dfrac{2}{5}\right)^3$

$= 0.064$

Atomic number of iodine = 53
Atomic number of soft tissue = 7.4

$\left(\dfrac{53}{7.4}\right)^3 = 368$

Pair production

If an incident x ray has sufficient energy, it may escape interaction with the electron cloud and come close enough to the nucleus of the target atom to come under the influence of the nuclear force field. The interaction between the photon and the nuclear force causes the photon to disappear, and in its place appear two electrons, one positively charged and called a **positron,** and one negatively charged. This process, called **pair production,** is diagrammed in Fig. 9-8.

In Chapter 4 we calculated that the energy equivalence of the mass of an electron was 0.51 MeV. Since two electrons are formed in a pair-production interaction, the incident photon must have at least 1.02 MeV of energy. An x ray with less than 1.02 MeV cannot undergo a pair-production event. Any energy in excess of 1.02 MeV is distributed equally between the two electrons as kinetic energy. Because pair pro-

duction involves only x rays with energies greater than 1.02 MeV, it is unimportant in diagnostic radiology.

Photodisintegration

High-energy x-ray photons, those with energies above 10 MeV, can escape interaction with the electron cloud and the nuclear force field and be absorbed directly by the nucleus, in which case the nucleus is raised to an excited state and instantaneously emits a nucleon or other nuclear fragment. This process is called **photodisintegration** and is shown schematically in Fig. 9-9. Because it involves only x rays with energies greater than approximately 10 MeV, photodisintegration, like pair production, is unimportant to diagnostic radiology.

DIFFERENTIAL ABSORPTION

Of the five ways an x ray can interact with matter, only two are particularly important to

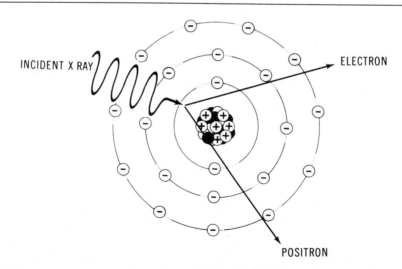

Fig. 9-8. Pair production occurs with x rays that have energies greater than 1.02 MeV. The photon interacts with the nuclear force field, and two electrons that have opposite electrostatic charge are created.

radiology: the Compton effect and the photo-electric effect. More important than the x rays resulting from these two effects, however, is a third type of x ray, the x ray transmitted through the body without interacting. Fig. 9-10 shows schematically how each of these three types of x rays contributes to a radiograph.

It should be clear that **the Compton-scattered x ray contributes no useful information** but in fact results in negative information that tends to fog the radiograph. When a Compton-scattered x ray interacts with the film, the film assumes that the x ray came straight from the x-ray tube target, as indicated by the wavy lines in Fig. 9-10. The film does not recognize the scattered x ray as representing an interaction off the straight line from the target. These scattered x rays result in **film fog,** a generalized dulling of the image on the radiograph by film densities not representing diagnostic information. To reduce this type of fog, we use techniques and apparatus to reduce the number of scattered x rays that reach the film.

X rays that undergo photoelectric interaction provide diagnostic information in a negative sense. Since they do not reach the film, these x rays are representative of anatomic structures with high x-ray absorption characteristics—such structures are **radiopaque.** The photoelectric absorption of x rays results in the bright areas of a radiograph, such as those corresponding to bone.

Other x rays penetrate the body and are transmitted with no interaction whatever. They result in the dark (high-density) areas of a radiograph. The anatomic structures through which these x rays pass are **radiolucent.**

Dependence on atomic number

Basically then, an x-ray image results from the difference between those x rays absorbed photoelectrically and those not absorbed at all. This

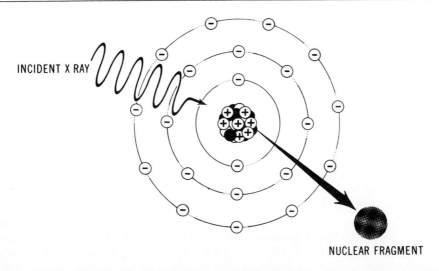

INCIDENT X RAY

NUCLEAR FRAGMENT

Fig. 9-9. Photodisintegration is an interaction between high-energy photons and the nucleus. The photon is absorbed by the nucleus, and a nuclear fragment is emitted.

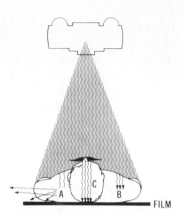

Fig. 9-10. Three types of x rays are important to the making of a radiograph: those scattered by Compton interaction *(A)*, those absorbed photoelectrically *(B)*, and those transmitted through the patient without interaction *(C)*.

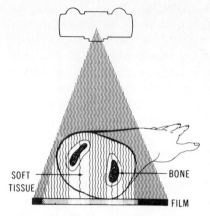

Fig. 9-11. Radiograph of bony structures results from the differential absorption between bone and soft tissue.

characteristic of the making of a radiograph is called **differential absorption.** Except at very low kVp, most x rays that interact do so by the Compton effect; this is one reason that radiographs are not as sharp and clear as photographs. A general rule of thumb is that for most radiographic examinations less than 5% of the x rays incident on a patient reach the film, and less than half these interact with the film to form the image. The radiographic image, then, results from approximately 1% of the x rays emitted by the machine. Consequently, careful control and selection of the x-ray beam is necessary to produce high-quality radiographs.

Producing a high-quality radiograph primarily requires the proper selection of kVp so that the effective x-ray energy will result in maximum differential absorption. **Differential absorption increases as the kVp is lowered,** but lowered kVp unfortunately results in increased patient dose. A compromise is necessary for each examination.

Consider a radiograph of the long bone shown in cross section in Fig. 9-11. An image of the bone is produced because many more x rays are absorbed photoelectrically in bone than in soft tissue. Recall that the probability of an x ray undergoing photoelectric absorption is proportional to the third power of the atomic number of the absorbing material. According to Table 9-1, bone has an atomic number of 13.8, whereas soft tissue has an atomic number of 7.4. Consequently, the probability that an x ray will undergo a photoelectric interaction is approximately seven times greater in bone than in soft tissue ($[13.8/7.4]^3 = 6.49$), as shown in the two graphs in Fig. 9-5. These graphs are combined in Fig. 9-12 so that the relative values of interaction are more apparent. Notice that the relative probability of interaction between bone and soft tissue (differential absorption) remains constant, while the absolute probability of each decreases with increasing energy. With higher x-ray energy fewer interactions occur, so more x rays are transmitted without interaction.

Compton scattering of x rays is independent

of the atomic number of the absorbing material, as shown in the two graphs in Fig. 9-3. These two graphs are combined in Fig. 9-13. The probabilities of Compton scattering for bone atoms and for soft tissue atoms are about equal and decrease with increasing x-ray energy. This decrease in scattering, however, is not so rapid as that occurring with photoelectric absorption. The probability of Compton scattering is approximately inversely proportional to the first power of the x-ray energy.

At low energies the majority of x-ray interactions are photoelectric, whereas at high energies Compton scattering predominates. Of course, as x-ray energy is increased, the chance of any interaction at all decreases. Consequently, as kVp is increased, more x rays get to the film, and therefore a lower x-ray output (lower mAs) is required. Fig. 9-14 combines all these factors into one graph. At 20 keV the probability of photoelectric effect equals the probability of Compton scattering in soft tissue. Below this energy most of the x rays that interact with soft tissue interact photoelectrically. Above this energy the predominate interaction with soft tissue is Compton scattering. **To image small differences in soft tissue, one must use low-kVp technique to get maximum differential absorption.** This is the basis for mammography.

The relative frequency of Compton interaction compared with photoelectric interaction increases with increasing energy. The crossover point between photoelectric effect and Compton scattering for bone is about 40 keV. Therefore high-kVp technique can be employed for examination of bony structures, resulting in much lower patient exposures. When high-kVp technique is used in this manner, the amount of scattered radiation from surrounding soft tissue is less than the differential absorption in bone. When the amount of scattered radiation becomes too high, grids are employed. Grids do not affect the magnitude of the differential absorption.

Differential absorption in bone and soft tissue,

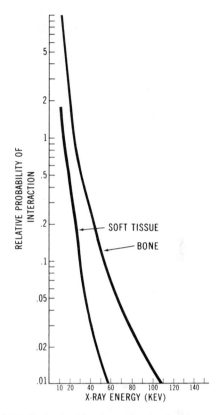

Fig. 9-12. Photoelectric absorption is about seven times greater in bone than in soft tissue regardless of energy. This is differential absorption.

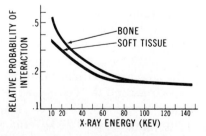

Fig. 9-13. Compton interaction occurs as readily with atoms of bone as with atoms of soft tissue.

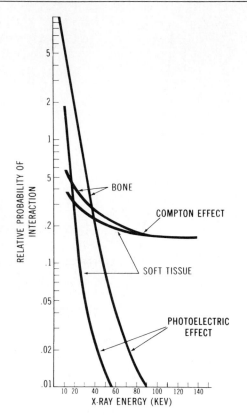

Fig. 9-14. Graph showing probabilities of photoelectric and Compton interaction with soft tissue and bone. The intersections of these curves indicate those x-ray energies at which the chance of photoelectric absorption equals the chance for Compton scattering.

Table 9-2. Densities (kg/m³ × 10³) of various materials important to diagnostic radiology

Type of substance	Density
Human tissue	
Muscle	1.00
Fat	0.91
Bone	1.85
Lung	0.32
Contrast material	
Barium	3.5
Iodine	4.93
Air	0.001293
Other	
Concrete	2.35
Tungsten	19.3
Lead	11.35

which results from the Z-related photoelectric interaction and the blurring and loss of contrast caused by Compton scattering, is the fundamental mechanism for making a radiograph; but two other factors are also important: the x-ray emission spectrum and the density of the target material.

The crossover energies of 20 keV and 40 keV assume a **monoenergetic** x-ray beam, that is, a single-energy beam. In fact, as we saw in Chapter 8, clinical x rays are **polyenergetic;** they are emitted over an entire spectrum of energies.

Therefore the correct selection of kVp for optimum differential absorption depends on the other factors discussed in Chapter 8 that affect the x-ray emission spectrum. For instance, in AP radiography of the lumbar spine, at 110 kVp, more x rays may be emitted above the 40 keV crossover for bone than below it. Less filtration or a grid may then be necessary.

Dependence on density

Intuitively, we know that we could image bone even if differential absorption were not Z related because bone has higher density than soft tissue. **Density** is the quantity of matter per unit volume, usually specified in units of kilograms per cubic meter. Table 9-2 gives the densities of several radiologically important materials. Density basically tells how tightly the atoms of a substance are packed. Water and ice are composed of precisely the same atoms, but ice occupies more volume. The density of ice is 917 kg/m³ compared with 1000 kg/m³ for water. Ice floats in water because of this difference in density.

The interaction between x rays and tissue is

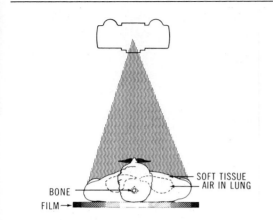

Fig. 9-15. Even if x-ray interaction were not related to atomic number (Z), differential absorption would occur because of differences in density.

proportional to the density of the tissue. When the density is doubled, the chance for x-ray interaction is doubled because there are twice as many electrons available for interaction. Therefore, even without the Z-related photoelectric effect, nearly twice as many x rays would be absorbed and scattered in bone as in soft tissue. The bone would be imaged.

Lungs are imaged on a chest radiograph primarily because of differences in density. According to Table 9-2, the density of soft tissue is 773 times that of air; for similar thicknesses, we can expect 773 times as many x rays to interact with the soft tissue as with air. The Z values of air and soft tissue are about the same—7.4 for soft tissue and 7.6 for air; thus differential absorption in air-filled soft tissue cavities is due primarily to density differences. Fig. 9-15 demonstrates differential absorption in air, soft tissue, and bone caused by density differences.

CONTRAST EXAMINATIONS

Because of their high atomic numbers and high densities compared with soft tissue, barium and iodinated compounds are used as an aid for imaging internal organs. The atomic number of barium is 56; that of iodine is 53. The probability that an x ray will undergo a photoelectric interaction in these contrast media is approximately 400 times greater than the probability of interaction in soft tissue ($[57/7.4]^3 = 367$). Consequently, when an iodinated compound fills the internal carotid artery or when barium fills the colon, these internal organs are readily visualized on the radiograph. Low-kVp technique (for example, below 80 kVp) will produce excellent, high-contrast radiographs of the organs of the gastrointestinal (GI) tract. Higher kVp operation (for example, above 90 kVp) can often be used in these examinations not only to outline the organ under investigation but also to penetrate the contrast media to more clearly visualize the lumen of the organ.

Air was previously used as a contrast medium in procedures such as pneumoencephalography and ventriculography. In these procedures the normal body fluids filling these internal cavities were replaced by air. Such procedures have become rare, however, since the introduction of computed tomography and magnetic resonance imaging.

EXPONENTIAL ATTENUATION

When a beam of x rays is incident on any type of absorbing material, the x rays can interact with the atoms of that material by any of the five mechanisms previously discussed. The relative frequency of interaction by each mechanism is dependent primarily on the atomic number of the target atom and the x-ray energy.

An interaction such as the photoelectric effect is called an absorption process because the x ray disappears. **Absorption** is an all-or-none condition for x-ray interaction. An interaction in which the x-ray photon is only partially absorbed, such as the Compton effect, is called a **scattering** process. Classical scattering, pair production, and photodisintegration also represent scattering events because the photons emerging from the interaction travel in a direction differ-

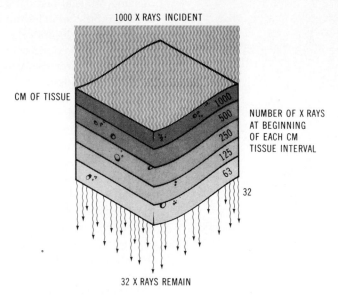

1000 X RAYS INCIDENT

CM OF TISSUE

1000
500
250
125
63
32

NUMBER OF X RAYS
AT BEGINNING
OF EACH CM
TISSUE INTERVAL

32 X RAYS REMAIN

Fig. 9-16. Interaction of x rays by absorption and scatter is called attenuation. In this example the x-ray beam has been attenuated 97%; 3% has been transmitted.

ent from that of the primary incident photon.

The total reduction in the number of x rays remaining in an x-ray beam following penetration through a given thickness of matter is called **attenuation.** When a broad beam of x rays is incident on any absorber, some of the x rays are absorbed and some are scattered. The result is a reduction in the number of x rays, a condition usually referred to as x-ray attenuation.

X rays are attenuated exponentially, which means that they do not have a fixed range of, for example, 1 cm or 1000 m, but rather are reduced in number by a given percentage for each incremental thickness of absorber they traverse.

For example, in the situation diagramed in Fig. 9-16, 1000 x rays are incident on tissue 5 cm thick. The x-ray energy and the atomic number of the tissue are such that 50% of the x rays are removed by attenuation for each centimeter traversed. Therefore in the first centimeter 500 x rays are removed, leaving 500 available to enter the second centimeter. By the end of the second centimeter 50% of the 500, or 250, additional x rays have been removed, leaving 250 x rays to enter the third centimeter of thickness. Similarly, entering the fourth centimeter of thickness will be 125 x rays, and entering the fifth centimeter will be 63. Half the sixty-three x rays will be attenuated in the last centimeter of tissue, and therefore only thirty-two will emerge. The total effect of these interactions is 3% transmission and 97% attenuation of the x-ray beam.

A plot of this hypothetical beam attenuation, which closely resembles the actual situation, appears in Fig. 9-17. It should be clear that, theoretically at least, the number of x rays emerging from any thickness of absorber will never reach zero. Each succeeding thickness can attenuate

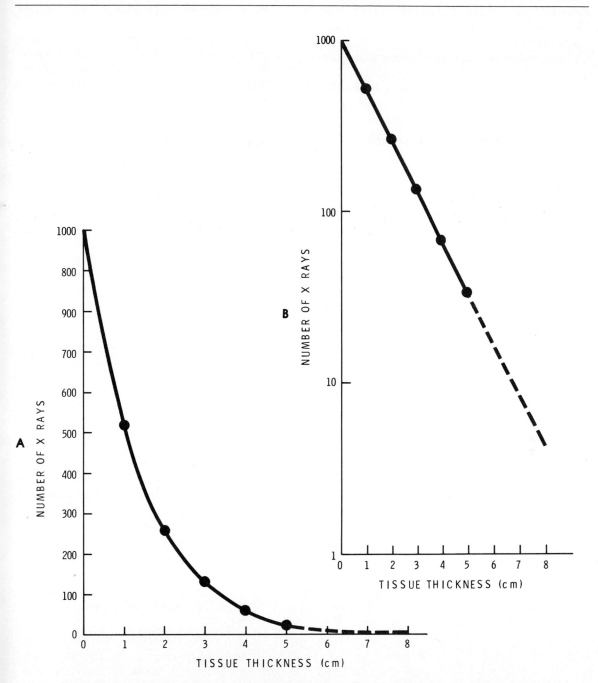

Fig. 9-17. A, Linear plot of exponential x-ray attenuation data in Fig. 9-16. **B,** Semilog plot of same data.

the x-ray beam only by a fractional amount, and a fraction of any positive number is always greater than zero.

This is unlike the manner in which alpha particles and beta particles interact with matter. Regardless of the energy of the particle and the type of absorbing material, these particulate radiations can penetrate only so far before they are all absorbed. For example, beta particles with 2 MeV of energy have a range of about 1 cm in soft tissue. Substantially, no beta particles of that energy can penetrate beyond that thickness. The exponential attenuation of photon radiation is due primarily to the fact that photons have no mass and no charge and travel with a constant velocity of c.

REVIEW QUESTIONS

1. Define or otherwise identify the following:
   a. Differential absorption
   b. Classical scattering
   c. Density
   d. 1.02 MeV
   e. Semilogarithmic graph
   f. Compton effect
   g. Z^3/E^3
   h. Monoenergetic
   i. Secondary electron
   j. Photoelectric effect
2. What are the three primary factors important to differential absorption? Discuss each.
3. A 28 keV x ray interacts photoelectrically with a K-shell electron of a calcium atom. What is the kinetic energy of the secondary electron? (See Table 3-3.)
4. Incident on bone and soft tissue of equal thickness are x rays with energy of 140 keV. If eighty-seven are scattered in soft tissue, approximately how many are scattered in bone?
5. Iodinated compounds are excellent agents for vascular contrast examinations because of which of the following qualities?
   a. Low vaporization
   b. Density
   c. Energy
   d. Atomic number
6. Diagram the Compton interaction and identify the incident photon, positive ion, negative ion, secondary radiation, and scattered photon.
7. Describe backscatter radiation. Can you think of examples in diagnostic radiology?
8. Tungsten is sometimes alloyed into the beam-defining collimators of an x-ray machine. If a 63 keV x ray undergoes a Compton interaction with an L-shell electron and ejects that electron with 12 keV of energy, what is the energy of the scattered x ray? What will be the possible energies of the subsequent L x rays? (See Fig. 3-9.)
9. Of the five basic mechanisms of x-ray interaction with matter, three are not important to diagnostic radiology. Which are they and why are they not important?
10. On average, 33.7 eV are required for each ionization in air. How many ion pairs would a 22 keV x ray probably produce in air, and about how many of these would be produced photoelectrically?

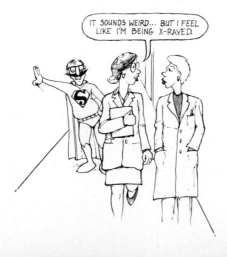

IT SOUNDS WEIRD... BUT I FEEL LIKE I'M BEING X-RAYED.

10

X-ray emission

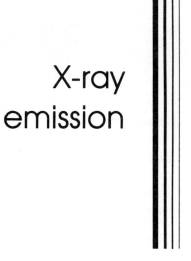

X-RAY QUANTITY
X-RAY QUALITY

X-RAY QUANTITY

The **output intensity** of an x-ray machine is measured in roentgens (R) or milliroentgens (mR) and is termed the **x-ray quantity.** Another term, **radiation exposure,** is often used instead of x-ray intensity or x-ray quantity. All have the same meaning, and all are measured in roentgens.

There is a subtle difference among the units roentgen, rad, and rem (Chapter 1). The rad (Gy) is the unit of energy absorbed and describes the radiation dose to the patient. The rem (Sv) is applicable only for occupational exposure. In diagnostic radiology these units have equal value, which sometimes leads to incorrect usage.

The roentgen (C/kg) is a measure of the number of ion pairs produced in air by a quantity of x-radiation. Ionization of air increases as the number of x rays in the beam increases. The relationship between the x-ray quantity as mea-

sured in roentgens and the number of x rays in the beam is not always one to one. There are some small variations related to the effective x-ray energy. These variations are unimportant over the x-ray energy range employed in radiology, and we can therefore assume that **the number of x rays in the useful beam is the radiation quantity.** Most general purpose radiographic tubes, when operated at approximately 70 kVp, produce x-ray intensities of from 3 to 6 mR/mAs (75 to 150 μC/kg-mAs) at 100 cm source–to–image receptor distance (SID). Fig. 10-1 is a nomogram for estimating x-ray intensity for a wide range of techniques. These curves apply only for single-phase, full-wave–rectified apparatus.

Factors affecting x-ray quantity

A number of factors affect x-ray quantity. Most were discussed in Chapter 8; consequently, this

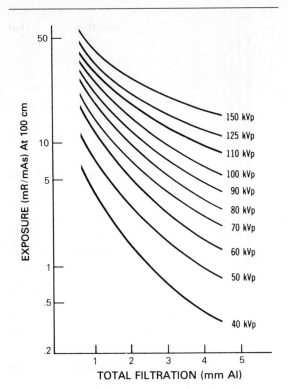

Fig. 10-1. Nomogram for estimating intensity of x-ray beams. From the position on the χ axis corresponding to the filtration of the machine draw a vertical line until it intersects with the appropriate kVp. A horizontal line from that point will intersect the γ axis at the approximate x-ray quantity for the machine. (Modified from McCullough, E., and Cameron, J., University of Wisconsin.)

section may serve primarily as a review. In Chapter 16 it will be shown that the factors affecting x-ray quantity are nearly the same as those controlling radiographic film density.

Milliampere-seconds. X-ray quantity is directly proportional to the mAs. When the mAs is doubled, the number of electrons striking the tube target is doubled, and therefore the number of x rays emitted is doubled.

(10-1)

$$\frac{I_1}{I_2} = \frac{mAs_1}{mAs_2}$$

EXAMPLE: A lateral chest technique calls for 100 kVp, 20 mAs, which results in an x-ray intensity of 32 mR (8.3 μC/kg) at the position of the patient. If the mAs is reduced to 15, what will the x-ray intensity be?

ANSWER: $\dfrac{x}{32 \text{ mR}} = \dfrac{15 \text{ mAs}}{20 \text{ mAs}}$

$$x = \frac{(15 \text{ mAs})(32 \text{ mR})}{20 \text{ mAs}}$$

$$= 24 \text{ mR}$$

Kilovoltage. X-ray quantity varies rapidly with changes in kVp. A rigorous mathematical exercise shows that the change in x-ray quantity is approximately proportional to the square of the ratio of the change in kVp; in other words, if kVp were doubled, the x-ray intensity would increase by a factor of four. Mathematically, this is expressed as

(10-2)

$$\frac{I_1}{I_2} = \left(\frac{kVp_1}{kVp_2}\right)^2$$

where I_1 and I_2 are the x-ray intensities at kVp_1 and kVp_2, respectively.

EXAMPLE: A lateral chest technique calls for 110 kVp, 20 mAs and results in an x-ray intensity of 32 mR (8.3 μC/kg). What will the intensity be if the kVp is increased to 125 and the mAs remains fixed?

ANSWER: $\dfrac{I}{32 \text{ mR}} = \left(\dfrac{125 \text{ kVp}}{110 \text{ kVp}}\right)^2$

$$I = \left(\frac{125 \text{ kVp}}{110 \text{ kVp}}\right)^2 (32 \text{ mR})$$

$$= (1.14)^2 (32 \text{ mR})$$
$$= (1.29)(32 \text{ mR})$$
$$= 41.3 \text{ mR}$$

In the clinic a slightly different situation prevails. X-ray technique must be selected from a relatively narrow range of values, from about 40 to 150 kVp. Theoretically, to double the x-ray intensity by kVp manipulation alone, one would have to increase the kVp by 41%. This relationship cannot be adopted clinically because as kVp is increased the penetrability of the x rays is increased and relatively fewer x rays are absorbed in the patient, that is, more traverse the patient and interact with the film. Consequently, to maintain a fixed exposure of the film and therefore constant film density, **an increase of 15% in kVp should be accompanied by a reduction of one half in mAs.**

Distance. Radiation exposure from an x-ray tube varies inversely with the square of the distance from the target. This relationship is known as the inverse square law (Chapter 4). If careful measurements are taken and the results plotted, this relationship can be verified, except at large distances where air attenuation can occur.

(10-3)

$$\frac{I_1}{I_2} = \frac{d_2^2}{d_1^2}$$

EXAMPLE: An examination with a portable x-ray machine is normally conducted at 100 cm SID and results in an exposure of 12.5 mR (3.2 μC/kg) at the film plane. If 91 cm is the maximum SID that can be obtained for a particular situation, what will the exposure be at the film plane? The technique factors remain constant.

ANSWER: $\dfrac{I}{12.5 \text{ mR}} = \left(\dfrac{100 \text{ cm}}{91 \text{ cm}}\right)^2$

$$I = (12.5 \text{ mR})\left(\frac{100 \text{ cm}}{91 \text{ cm}}\right)^2$$

$$= (12.5 \text{ mR})(1.1)^2$$
$$= (12.5 \text{ mR})(1.21)$$
$$= 15.1 \text{ mR}$$

Filtration. X-ray machines have metal filters, usually 1 to 3 mm aluminum (Al), positioned in the useful beam. The primary purpose of these filters is to reduce the number of low-energy x rays that reach the patient. Low-energy x rays contribute nothing to diagnostic quality and serve only to increase patient dose unnecessarily because they are absorbed in superficial tissues and do not penetrate to reach the film. When filtration is inserted in the x-ray beam, the patient dose is reduced because there are fewer low-energy x rays in the useful beam. Calculation of the amount of reduction in exposure requires a knowledge of half-value layer (HVL), discussed in the following section. An estimate

of exposure reduction can be made from the nomogram in Fig. 10-1, where it is shown that the reduction is not proportional to the thickness of added filter but is complexly related.

X-RAY QUALITY

As the effective energy of an x-ray beam is increased, the penetrability is also increased. **Penetrability** refers to the range of x-ray beams in matter; higher-energy x-ray beams are able to penetrate matter farther than low-energy beams. The penetrability, or penetrating power, of an x-ray beam is called the **x-ray quality.** X-ray beams with high penetrability are termed high-quality, or **hard,** beams; those with low penetrability are of low quality and are called **soft** beams.

X-ray quality is identified numerically by HVL. The HVL is affected by the kVp of operation and the amount of filtration in the useful beam. X-ray quality is thus influenced by kVp and filtration. As we shall see in Chapter 16, these factors that affect beam quality also influence radiographic film contrast. Distance and mAs do not affect radiation quality as they do radiation quantity.

Half-value layer

Although x-rays are attenuated exponentially, high-energy x rays are considerably more penetrating than low-energy x rays. Whereas a 100 keV x ray is attenuated approximately 3% per centimeter of soft tissue, a 10 keV x-ray beam is reduced approximately 15% per centimeter of soft tissue. X rays of any given energy are more penetrating in low atomic number material than in high atomic number material.

In radiology the quality of x rays is characterized by **half-value layer (HVL). The HVL of an x-ray beam is the thickness of absorbing material necessary to reduce the x-ray intensity to half its original value.** HVL therefore is a characteristic of the x-ray beam. A diagnostic x-ray beam usually has an HVL in the range of 3 to 5 mm Al, or 4 to 8 cm of soft tissue.

Half-value layers are determined experimen-

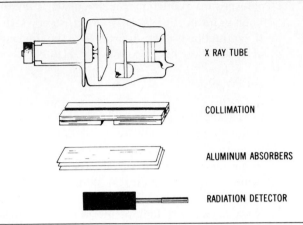

X RAY TUBE

COLLIMATION

ALUMINUM ABSORBERS

RADIATION DETECTOR

Fig. 10-2. Typical experimental arrangement for determination of half-value layer.

tally, using a setup similar to that shown in Fig. 10-2. There are three principal parts to this setup: the x-ray tube, a radiation detector, and graded thicknesses of filter, usually aluminum. First a radiation measurement is made with no filter between the x-ray machine and the detector. Then measurements of radiation intensity are made for successively thicker sections of filter. The thickness of filtration that reduces the x-ray beam intensity to half its original value is the HVL.

EXAMPLE: The following data are obtained with a radiographic tube operated at 70 kVp while the detector is positioned 100 cm from the target with 0.5 mm Al filters inserted halfway between the target and the detector. Estimate the HVL from a simple observation of these data; then plot the data to see how close you were.

Added mm Al	mR
None	94
0.5	79
1.0	67
1.5	57
2.0	49
2.5	42
3.0	38
3.5	33

ANSWER: One half of 94 is 47, and therefore the HVL must be between 2 and 2.5 mm Al. A plot of the data shows the HVL to be 2.12 mm Al.

HVL is the best method for specifying x-ray quality, mainly because variations in penetrability with changes in kVp and filtration are not simple relationships. Different combinations of added filtration and kVp can result in the same x-ray beam HVL. For example, measurements may show that a single machine has the same HVL when operated at 90 kVp with 2 mm Al total filtration as when operated at 70 kVp with 5 mm Al total filtration. In this case the beam penetrability remains constant, as does the HVL. It would be erroneous to specify beam quality by either kVp or filtration.

A number of methods can be employed to determine the HVL of an x-ray beam. Perhaps the most straightforward is to graph the results of x-ray intensity measurements made with an experimental setup like that in Fig. 10-2. The graph in Fig. 10-3 shows how this can be done when the following steps are completed. Sample numeric values are shown in the table accompanying Fig. 10-3.

1. Determine the x-ray intensity with no absorbing material.
2. Determine the x-ray intensity equal to half the original intensity and locate this value on the y, or vertical, axis of the graph (A).
3. Draw a horizontal line parallel with the x

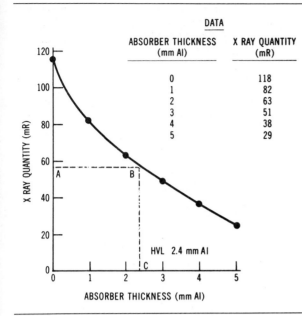

DATA

ABSORBER THICKNESS (mm Al)	X RAY QUANTITY (mR)
0	118
1	82
2	63
3	51
4	38
5	29

Fig. 10-3. Data in the table are typical for a half-value layer determination. The plot of these data shows a half-value layer of 2.4 mm Al. See text for the steps involved.

axis from the point identified in step 2 until it intersects the curve *(B)*.

4. From this point of intersection drop a vertical line to the x axis.
5. On the x axis read the thickness of absorber required to reduce the x-ray intensity to half its original value *(C)*. This is the half-value layer.

Factors affecting x-ray quality

Kilovoltage. As kVp is increased, so is beam quality and therefore HVL. An increase in kVp results in a shift of the x-ray emission spectrum toward the high-energy side, causing an increase in the effective energy of the beam, thus making it more penetrable. Table 10-1 shows the measured change in HVL as kVp is increased from 50 to 150 kVp for a representative x-ray machine. The total filtration of the beam is 2.5 mm Al.

Filtration. The primary purpose of adding filtration to an x-ray beam is to selectively remove low-energy x rays that have no chance of getting to the film. Fig. 10-4 shows emission spectra

Table 10-1. Relationship between kVp and HVL for fixed radiographic unit having 2.5 mm Al total filtration

kVp	HVL (mm Al)
50	1.90
75	2.80
100	3.7
125	4.55
150	5.45

representing unfiltered, normally filtered, and ideally filtered beams. The ideally filtered beam shows that it is desirable to totally remove all photons with energies below a level determined by the type of x-ray examination. Unfortunately, total removal is not possible. **As filtration is increased, so is beam quality.**

Almost any material could serve as an x-ray filter. Aluminum is chosen because it is efficient in removing low-energy x rays through photoelectric effect and because it is available, inexpensive, and easily shaped into filters.

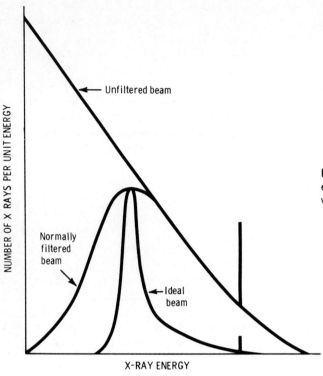

Fig. 10-4. Filtration is used to selectively remove low-energy x rays from the useful beam. Ideal filtration would remove all low-energy x rays.

Types of filtration

Filtration of diagnostic x-ray beams has two components: inherent filtration and added filtration.

Inherent filtration. The x-ray beam filtration we normally think of is that produced by thin sheets of aluminum attached between the protective tube housing and the collimator; this type of filtration is **added filtration.** The glass envelope of an x-ray tube also filters the emerging x-ray beam; this type of filtration is called **inherent filtration.** Inspection of an x-ray tube will reveal that the part of the glass envelope through which x rays are emitted—the window—is thin. This is to provide for low inherent filtration.

The inherent filtration of a general purpose x-ray tube is usually about 0.5 mm Al equivalent.

With age, inherent filtration tends to increase as some of the tungsten metal of both target and filament is vaporized and deposited on the inside of the glass envelope. Special purpose tubes, such as those employed in mammography, have very thin tube windows, sometimes made of beryllium rather than glass, and have inherent filtrations of approximately 0.1 mm Al.

Added filtration. The addition of a filter to an x-ray beam, called **added filtration,** attenuates x rays of all energies emitted by the tube, but it attenuates a higher percentage of low-energy x rays than high-energy x rays. This shifts the x-ray emission spectrum to the high-energy side, as was shown in Fig. 8-12. This shift in the emission spectrum results in a beam with higher effective energy and therefore greater penetrability and higher quality. **The addition of filtration results in an increased half-value layer.** The extent of increase in the half-value layer cannot be predicted even when the thickness of added filtration is known.

Because added filtration attenuates the x-ray beam, it affects x-ray quantity. This value can be predicted if one knows the half-value layer of the beam. The addition of filtration equal to the beam half-value layer reduces the beam quantity to half its prefiltered value and results in a harder x-ray beam.

EXAMPLE: A general purpose x-ray tube has a half-value layer of 2.2 mm Al. The exposure from this machine is 2 mR/mAs (0.5 µC/kg-mAs) at 100 cm SID. If 2.2 mm Al is added to the beam, what will be the approximate beam intensity?

ANSWER: This is an addition of one HVL; therefore the beam intensity will be 1 mR/mAs (0.25 µC/kg-mAs).

Added filtration usually has two sources and totals 2 to 3 mm of aluminum equivalent. First, 1 or 2 mm sheets of aluminum will be permanently installed in the port of the x-ray tube housing, between the housing and the collimator. If the collimator is a conventional light-localizing variable-aperture collimator, the collimator will contribute an additional 1 mm aluminum equivalent added filtration. This filtration results from the silver surface of the mirror in the collimator.

Compensating filters. One of the most difficult tasks facing the radiologic technologist is producing an image with a uniform average density when examining a body part that varies greatly in thickness or tissue composition. During PA chest radiography, for instance, if the left chest is relatively radiopaque because of fluid, consolidation, or mass, the image would appear with very low optical density on the left side of the chest and very high optical density on the right side of the chest. One could compensate for this density variation by inserting a wedge filter so that the thin part of the wedge is positioned over the left side of the chest. When a filter is employed in this fashion, it is called a **compensating filter** because it compensates for differences in subject radiopacity. Compensating filters can be fabricated for many procedures and therefore come in various sizes and shapes. They are nearly always constructed of aluminum, but plastic materials can also be employed. Fig. 10-5 contains some commonly employed compensating filters.

The wedge filter is principally used when radiographing a body part, such as the foot, that varies considerably in thickness. During an AP projection of the foot, the wedge would be positioned with its thick portion shadowing the toes and the thin portion toward the heel.

A bilateral wedge filter, or a **trough filter,** is sometimes employed in chest radiography. The thin central region of the wedge is positioned over the mediastinum, while the lateral thick portions shadow the lung fields. The result is a radiograph with more uniform optical density. Specialty compensating wedges of this type are generally employed with dedicated apparatus such as an x-ray machine employed exclusively for chest radiography.

Special "bow tie"–shaped filters are used with some CT scanners to compensate for the shape of the head or body. Conic filters, either concave or convex, find application in digital fluoroscopy where the image receptor, the image-intensifier tube, is round.

A step-wedge filter, diagrammed in Fig. 10-6, is an adaptation of the wedge filter. It is employed in some special procedures, usually where long sections of the anatomy are radiographed and imaged with two or three separate films. A common application of this technique employs a three-step aluminum wedge and three 14 × 17 in (30 × 36 cm) films in a rapid changer for translumbar and femoral arteriography and venography. These procedures call for careful selection of screens, grids, and radiographic technique.

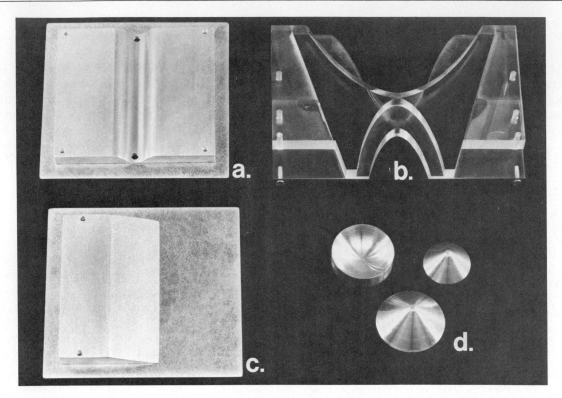

Fig. 10-5. Compensating filters. **a,** Trough filter. **b,** "Bow tie" filter for use in CT. **c,** Wedge filter. **d,** Conic filters for use in digital fluoroscopy.

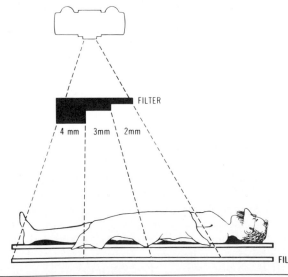

FILTER

4 mm   3 mm   2 mm

FILM

Fig. 10-6. Arrangement of apparatus employing an aluminum step wedge for serial radiography of the abdomen and lower extremities.

REVIEW QUESTIONS

1. Define or otherwise identify the following:
   a. Inherent filtration
   b. The unit of x-ray quantity
   c. A filtered x-ray spectrum
   d. A kVp change equal to twice mAs
   e. The choice of aluminum as a filter
   f. Half-value layer
   g. Wedge filter
   h. The unit of x-ray quality
   i. The approximate HVL of your machine
   j. X-ray intensity

2. Make a rough plot of the change in HVL with changing kVp (from 50 to 120 kVp) for an x-ray machine that has total filtration of 2.5 mm Al. Check your answer by plotting the data in Table 10-1.

3. Direct-exposure mammography requires 40 kVp, 1200 mAs and results in an exposure of 8 R (2.06×10^{-3} C/kg) at the entrance surface. Xeromammography technique calls for 40 kVp, 100 mAs. What is the skin exposure during xeromammography?

4. An abdominal film taken at 84 kVp, 150 mAs results in an exposure of 650 mR (1.68×10^{-4} C/kg). The film is too light and is remade at 84 kVp, 250 mAs. What is the exposure?

5. According to the rule of thumb, a 15% increase in kVp doubles the number of x rays reaching the film. In fact, the increase in x rays will not be twice but will be _____.

6. A film of the lateral skull taken at 68 kVp, 200 mAs has sufficient density but too much contrast. If the kVp is increased to 78, what should the new mAs be?

7. A chest film taken at 180 cm SID results in an exposure of 12 mR (3.1 μC/kg). What would the exposure be if the same radiographic factors were employed at (a) 90 cm SID? (b) 100 cm SID?

8. The following data were obtained with a fluoroscopic tube operated at 80 kVp. The exposure levels were measured 20 inches (50 cm) above the tabletop with aluminum absorbers positioned on the surface. Estimate the HVL by visual inspection of the data; then plot the data and determine the precise value of the HVL. What is the thickness of the second HVL?

Added mm Al	mR
none	65
1	48
2	37
3	30
4	25
5	21
6	18.5
7	16
8	14.5
9	13.0

9. When operated at 74 kVp, 100 mAs with 2.2 mm Al added filtration and 0.6 mm Al inherent filtration, the HVL of an x-ray machine is 3.2 mm Al and its output intensity at 100 cm SID is 350 mR (90 μC/kg). How much additional filtration is necessary to reduce the x-ray intensity to 175 mR?

10. The following technique factors have been shown to produce good-quality radiographs of the lateral skull with an x-ray machine having 3 mm Al total filtration. Refer to Fig. 10-1 and estimate the x-ray intensity at 100 cm SID for each.
   a. 62 kVp, 70 mAs
   b. 70 kVp, 40 mAs
   c. 78 kVp, 27 mAs

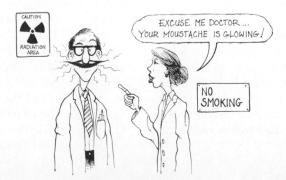

11

Beam-restricting devices

PRODUCTION OF SCATTER RADIATION

Two kinds of x-ray photons are responsible for the density, contrast, and image on a radiograph: those that pass through the patient without interacting and those that are scattered in the patient through a Compton interaction. Together these x rays that exit from the patient and intersect the film are called **remnant x rays.** This situation is diagramed in Fig. 11-1.

Proper collimation of the x-ray beam has the primary effect of reducing patient dose by restricting the volume of tissue irradiated. The corresponding reduction in scatter radiation, and the fogging it produces, is a secondary benefit. Ideally, only those photons that did not interact with the patient would reach the film.

As the number of scattered x rays increases, image clarity decreases. The radiograph loses contrast and looks dull and foggy, and the imaged structures appear blurred. There are three primary factors that influence the relative intensity of scatter radiation reaching the film, and two of these can be controlled by the radiologic technologist.

Factors affecting scatter radiation

Kilovoltage. As x-ray energy is increased, the relative number of x rays that undergo Compton interaction increases also. The absolute number of Compton interactions decreases with increasing x-ray energy, but the number of photoelectric interactions decreases much more rapidly. (These features of x-ray interaction were discussed in Chapter 9; a review of that material might be in order.)

Table 11-1 shows the percentage of x-ray photons incident on a 10 cm thickness of soft tissue that will undergo photoelectric interaction and Compton interaction at selected kVp's from 50 to 120. Kilovoltage is one of the factors that affects the level of scatter radiation and can be controlled by the radiologic technologist.

It would be easy enough to say that all radiographs should be taken at the lowest reasonable kVp, since this technique would result in minimum scatter and thus high image quality. Unfortunately, the situation is not that simple. Table 11-1 shows that the percentage of x rays that interact photoelectrically increases greatly as

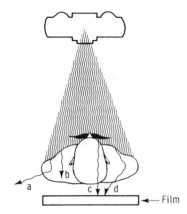

Fig. 11-1. Some x rays interact with the patient and are scattered away from the film, *a;* others interact with the patient and are absorbed, *b.* X rays that arrive at the film and produce a radiographic density are those transmitted through the patient without interacting, *c,* and those scattered in the patient, *d.* X rays of types *c* and *d* are called remnant radiation.

Table 11-1. Approximate percentages of x rays that interact by photoelectric and Compton processes and that are transmitted without interaction through a soft tissue body part 10 cm thick

	Percent interaction			
kVp	Photoelectric	Compton	Total	Percent transmission
50	78.9	21	99.998	0.002
60	69.9	30	99.9	0.1
70	59.8	39.8	99.6	0.4
80	46	52	98	2
90	38	59	97	3
100	31	63	94	6
110	23	70	93	7
120	18	83	91	9

kVp is lowered. This increase results in a considerable increase in patient dose. Also, fewer x rays reach the film at low kVp; this is usually compensated for by increasing the mAs. The result is still higher patient dose.

Some patients are so big that high kVp must be used to ensure adequate penetration of the portion of their body being radiographed. If, for example, the normal technique factors for an AP film of the abdomen are not sufficient to image the abdomen adequately, the technologist has a choice of increasing mAs or kVp. Increasing the mAs usually generates enough x rays to provide a satisfactory image on the film but may result in an unacceptably high patient dose. On the other hand, a much smaller increase in kVp is usually sufficient to provide an adequate number of incident x-ray photons on the film, and this can be done at a much lower patient dose. Unfortunately, when kVp is increased, the level of scatter radiation also increases, and therefore the radiographic contrast decreases.

Collimators and grids are employed to reduce the level of scatter radiation. Fig. 11-2 shows a series of radiographs of a skull phantom taken at 70, 80, and 90 kVp using appropriate colli-

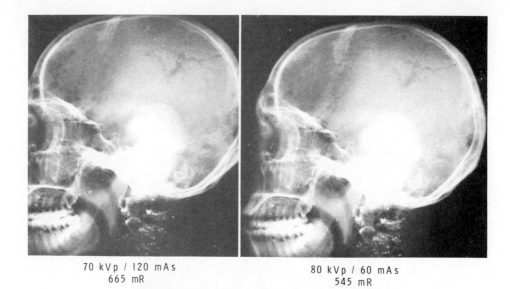

70 kVp / 120 mAs
665 mR

80 kVp / 60 mAs
545 mR

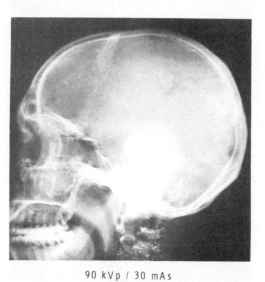

90 kVp / 30 mAs
230 mR

Fig. 11-2. All these skull radiographs are of acceptable quality. The technique factors for each are shown, along with the resulting patient exposure.

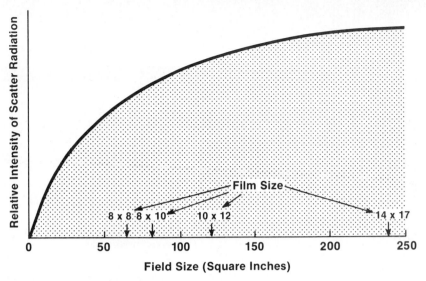

Fig. 11-3. This graph is representative of operation at 70 kVp with a patient 20 cm thick. The relative intensity of scatter radiation increases with increasing field size.

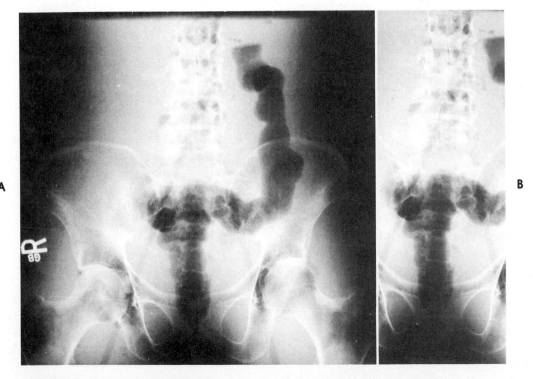

Fig. 11-4. Recommended technique for lumbar spine calls for collimation of the beam to the vertebral column. Unfortunately, the full-field technique is too often used and results in reduced image clarity. **A,** Full-field technique. **B,** Preferred technique with collimation of beam to vertebral column.

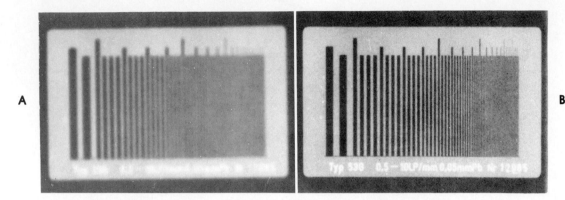

Fig. 11-5. Small field sizes are particularly important in fluoroscopy. These spot films of a test pattern embedded in the middle of 20 cm of tissue equivalent material were taken with full-field exposure and with the x-ray beam restricted to the area of the pattern. **A,** Full-field exposure. **B,** Beam restricted to area of pattern. The radiograph in **B** is clearer because the smaller field size resulted in less scatter radiation.

mators and grids with the mAs adjusted so as to produce radiographs of nearly equal density. Most radiologists would accept any of these radiographs. Notice that the patient dose at 90 kVp is approximately one third that at 70 kVp. In general, because of this reduction in patient dose, **high-kVp radiographic exposure is preferred to low-kVp technique.**

Field size. Another factor affecting the level of scatter radiation and under the control of the technologist is field size. In general, as the field size for a given radiograph is increased, the level of scatter radiation increases also. Changes in size are more important when the x-ray field is small than when the field is large. This relationship is shown graphically in Fig. 11-3. Fig. 11-4 shows two AP films of the lumbar spine. One was taken on a full-frame, 14 × 17 in (35 × 43 cm) film, and the other has a field size restricted to just the spinal column. There is a noticeable loss of contrast in the full-frame radiograph because of the increased scatter radiation that accompanies larger field size.

Restriction of beam size to improve image quality is perhaps even more important during fluoroscopy. Fig. 11-5 shows two spot films taken of a bar phantom embedded in the middle of a masonite phantom 20 cm thick. The first image was taken with a full-field exposure, the second with the x-ray beam restricted to the area of the bar phantom. The difference in image clarity is obvious.

Patient thickness. More scatter radiation results from taking x rays of thick parts of the body than thin parts of the body. A comparison of the clarity of bony structures in a radiograph of an extremity with the clarity of bone structures in a pelvic or chest radiograph will demonstrate this. Even when the two are taken with the same screen-film combination, the extremity radiograph will be much sharper because of the reduced amount of scatter radiation. Fig. 11-6 shows the relative intensity of scattered x rays as a function of thickness of soft tissue for an 8 × 10 in (20 × 25 cm) field. Exposing a 3 cm thick extremity at 70 kVp results in about 45%

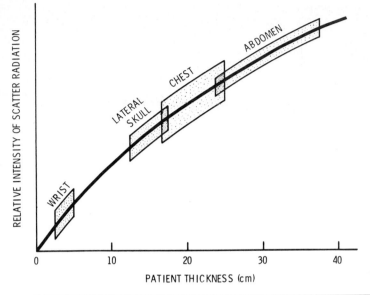

Fig. 11-6. Relative intensity of scatter radiation increases with increasing thickness of the irradiated part.

scatter radiation. Exposing a 30 cm thick abdomen results in nearly 100% of the x rays exiting the patient as scattered x rays. With increasing patient thickness, more x rays undergo multiple scattering, so that the average angle of scatter in the remnant beam is greater.

Unfortunately, patient thickness is not under the control of the technologist. However, if one recognizes that more x rays are scattered with increasing patient thickness, one can produce a high-quality radiograph by choosing the proper technique and using devices designed to reduce the amount of scatter radiation reaching the film. Compression devices, for example, improve image quality by reducing patient thickness and bringing the object closer to the image receptor.

CONTROL OF SCATTER RADIATION

The radiologic technologist has available two types of devices designed to reduce the amount of scatter radiation reaching the film. These are various types of **beam restrictors** and **grids**. Grids are discussed in Chapter 12. There are basically three types of beam-restricting devices: the aperture diaphragm, cones or cylinders, and the variable-aperture collimator.

Aperture diaphragm

An aperture diaphragm is the simplest of all beam-restricting devices. It is basically a lead or lead-lined metal diaphragm attached to the x-ray tube head. The opening in the diaphragm is usually designed to cover just less than the size of film employed in the particular examination. Fig. 11-7 shows schematically the relationship between the x-ray tube, an aperture diaphragm, and the x-ray film. A properly designed diaphragm projects onto the radiograph an image **1 cm smaller on all sides than the size of the radiograph.** Therefore, when a diaphragm is used, an unexposed border should be visible on each edge of the radiograph.

EXAMPLE: If a 20 cm square film is to be imaged at 100 cm SID and the diaphragm is placed 10 cm from the target, what should be the dimension of one side of the diaphragm opening? Note: To leave an unexposed border of

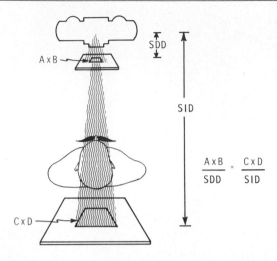

$$\frac{A \times B}{SDD} = \frac{C \times D}{SID}$$

Fig. 11-7. Aperture diaphragm is a fixed lead opening designed for a fixed film size and constant SID. SDD is the source-to-diaphragm distance.

1.0 cm on each side, we must reduce the beam size to 18 cm.

$$\text{ANSWER: } \frac{A}{10 \text{ cm}} = \frac{18 \text{ cm}}{100 \text{ cm}}$$

$$A = \frac{(18)(10) \text{ cm}}{100}$$

$$= 1.8 \text{ cm}$$

X-ray head stands present possibly the most familiar clinical example of the use of aperture diaphragms. The typical head stand has a fixed SID and is equipped with diaphragms to accommodate film sizes of 5 × 7 in (13 × 18 cm), 8 × 10 in (20 × 25 cm), and 10 × 12 in (25 × 30 cm). Fig. 11-8 is a photograph of a head stand and the diaphragms usually employed with it. When using a diaphragm, the technologist should take care that it is inserted into the tube head so that the long axis of the diaphragm is parallel to the long axis of the image receptor. If it is not, diaphragm cutoff can result, leaving large portions of the radiograph unexposed and causing unnecessary exposure to the patient because of possible repeat examinations.

Today many x-ray rooms being set up specifically for chest examinations are supplied with fixed-aperture diaphragms. Usually these dia-

phragms are securely fastened to the radiographic head and therefore are not easily removed. Diaphragms for chest rooms are designed for exposure of all but a 1 cm border of 14 × 17 in (35 × 43 cm) films.

Dental radiography is another area where aperture diaphragms are employed. Dental radiographs are customarily obtained at 20 or 40 cm SID. The diaphragm used in these techniques must provide a circular x-ray beam not exceeding 7 cm in diameter at the entrance surface of the patient. Typically, the diameter of an aperture diaphragm for 20 cm SID is 18 mm, and that for 40 cm SID is 9 mm. Some dental apparatus is supplied with rectangular collimation, which requires precise alignment and positioning of the x-ray tube head, the patient, and the film by the dental radiologic technologist.

Cones and cylinders

Radiographic cones and cylinders can be considered modifications of the aperture diaphragm. A typical cone and cylinder are diagramed in Fig. 11-9. In both, an extended metal structure restricts the useful beam to the required size. Unlike that produced by the aper-

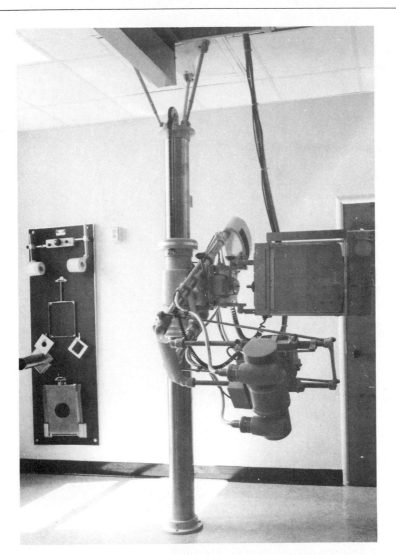

Fig. 11-8. Typical head stand used for imaging the skull and its internal organs. An array of the aperture diaphragms used with this unit can be seen on the wall.

ture diaphragm, the useful beam produced by a cylinder or cone is always circular. Both these beam restrictors are routinely called **cones,** even though the type used most widely is actually a cylinder. One difficulty of using cones is alignment. If the tube, cone, and film are not aligned on the same axis, one side of the radiograph may

not be exposed because the edge of the cone may interfere with the x-ray beam. Such interference is called **cone cutting.**

The same limitations that apply to aperture diaphragms apply to cones and cylinders. Their openings are fixed, and they are therefore appropriate for only specific types of examinations.

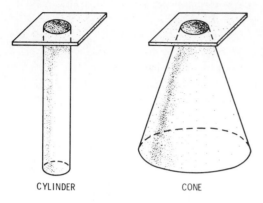

Fig. 11-9. Radiographic cones and cylinders produce restricted useful x-ray beams of circular shape.

CYLINDER   CONE

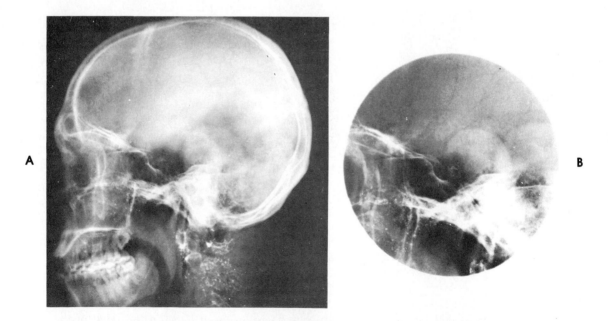

A   B

Fig. 11-10. A, View of the sella turcica made with open collimation. **B,** View made with cone collimation. Use of a cone reduces scatter radiation and improves image clarity.

At one time cones were used extensively in diagnostic radiology. Today they are reserved primarily for examinations of the head and spine. Fig. 11-10 shows the improvement in image clarity that results when a cone is used for examination of the sella turcica. In diagnostic radiology the light-localizing variable-aperture collimator has replaced the cone in many examinations.

Beam-defining cones are used extensively in dental radiology. Fig. 11-11 is a photograph of four typical dental cones. Dental cones are usually fabricated of plastic, and some are lead lined. The long lead-lined dental cones result in slightly less exposure to the patient than the other types. The 20 cm plastic pointer cones previously used on most dental x-ray machines have been shown to result in unnecessarily high patient exposure caused by scattering of the useful beam in the cone tip. Many dentists now use the long-cone technique. Proper alignment is a little more difficult, but the films produced have less distortion, and the patient dose is less. The dental cone and circular diaphragm are often fabricated as one accessory; together they provide rather good beam restriction.

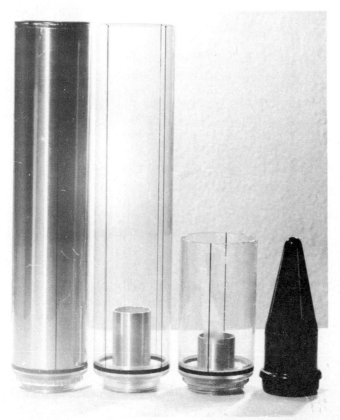

Fig. 11-11. Four typical dental cones. **A,** Long, lead-lined, plastic, open-end cone. **B,** Long, plastic, open-end cone. **C,** Short, plastic, open-end cone. **D,** Plastic pointer cone.

A   B   C   D

Variable-aperture collimator

The variable-aperture collimator is perhaps the most common beam-restricting device in diagnostic radiology. The photograph in Fig. 11-12, A, is an example of a modern automatic variable-aperture collimator. Fig. 11-12, B, identifies the principal parts of such a collimator.

Not all x rays are emitted precisely from the focal spot of an x-ray tube. Some x rays are produced when electrons stray and interact at positions on the anode other than the focal spot. Such radiation is called **off-focus radiation** and tends to diminish the sharpness of a radiograph. To control off-focus radiation, a first-stage entrance shuttering device consisting of multiple collimator blades protrudes from the top of the collimator into the x-ray tube housing.

The second-stage collimator shutter leaves are usually lead, at least 3 mm thick. They work in pairs and are independently controlled, thereby allowing for both rectangular and square fields. Early models of variable-aperture collimators employed several collimating leaves fabricated like the lens diaphragm of a photographic camera. This type of collimator, however, produced only circular fields, which resulted in more tissue being irradiated than was necessary.

Light localization in a typical variable-aperture collimator is accomplished with a small lamp and mirror. The mirror must be far enough on the tube side of the collimator leaves to project a sufficiently sharp light pattern through the collimator leaves when the lamp is on. The lamp, mirror, and collimator leaves must all be adjusted so that the projected light field coincides with the x-ray beam. If the light and x-ray beam do not coincide, adjustment of the mirror or lamp is usually necessary.

Today nearly all light-localizing collimators manufactured in the United States for fixed radiographic equipment are automatic. They are called **positive beam limiting** (**PBL**) devices. When a film-loaded cassette is inserted in the Bucky tray and clamped into place, sensing devices in the tray identify the size and alignment of the cassette. An electric signal is transmitted to the collimator housing and actuates synchronous motors that drive the collimator leaves to

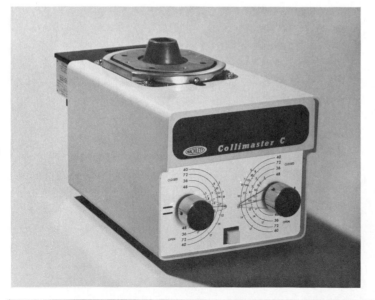

A

Fig. 11-12. **A,** Automatic collimator. The extensive mechanical and electrical components required for operation are not shown. An override switch for manual operation is provided. **B,** Simplified schematic drawing of automatic, light-localizing collimation. (**A** and **B** courtesy The Machlett Laboratories, Inc.)

SHUTTER OPERATION

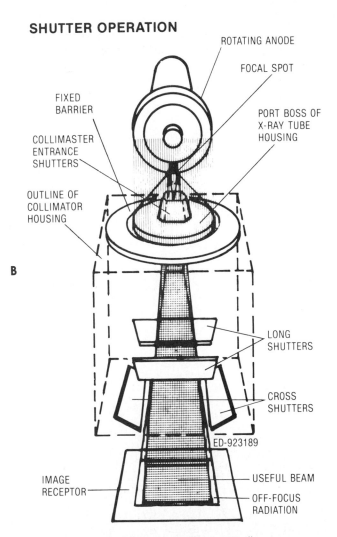

ROTATING ANODE

FOCAL SPOT

FIXED
BARRIER

PORT BOSS OF
X-RAY TUBE
HOUSING

COLLIMASTER
ENTRANCE
SHUTTERS

OUTLINE OF
COLLIMATOR
HOUSING

B

LONG
SHUTTERS

CROSS
SHUTTERS

ED-923189

IMAGE
RECEPTOR

USEFUL BEAM

OFF-FOCUS
RADIATION

Fig. 11-12, cont'd. For legend see opposite page.

a precalibrated position, so that the x-ray beam is restricted to the film size in use. When properly adjusted, the automatic collimator provides an unexposed border on all sides of the finished radiograph.

Collimator filtration

Because prescribed thicknesses of filtration, which vary with the tube potential, are needed to produce high-quality radiographs with minimum patient exposure, some collimator housings are designed to allow easy changing of the added filtration. Most commonly, filtration stations of 0, 1, 2, and 3 mm Al are provided. Even in the zero position, however, the added filtration to the x-ray tube is not zero because collimator structures intercept the beam. The exit portal, usually plastic, and the reflecting mirror provide filtration in addition to the inherent filtration of the tube. The added filtration of the collimator assembly is usually equivalent to approximately 1 mm Al.

This added filtration is one reason why high-quality screen-film mammograms cannot be produced through a collimator. The total filtration with the collimator may be too high. For screen-film mammography, therefore, the collimator and other added filtration should be removed and replaced with a cone or cylinder.

REVIEW QUESTIONS

1. Define or otherwise identify the following:
   a. Three factors affecting scatter radiation
   b. Approximate equivalent collimator filtration
   c. Aperture diaphragm
   d. Cone cutting
   e. Automatic collimation
2. Why should a radiograph of the lumbar vertebrae be well collimated?
3. A chest room is designed for only 14 × 17 in (35 × 43 cm) radiographs. If the SID is 180 cm and the SDD is 10 cm, what should the diaphragm opening be to allow an unexposed border of 1 cm around the film?
4. An acceptable intravenous pyelography (IVP) can be obtained with technique factors of 74 kVp, 120 mAs or 82 kVp, 80 mAs. Discuss possible reasons for selecting one technique over the other.
5. When radiographed, will a long bone in a wet cast result in more or less scatter than a long bone in a dry cast? Why?

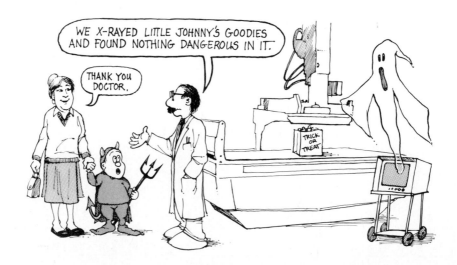

12

The grid

CONTROL OF SCATTER RADIATION

Scattered x rays are produced in the patient by the Compton effect and serve no useful purpose in diagnostic radiology. The relative intensity of scatter radiation was previously shown to be a complex function of many factors, primarily kVp, beam size, and patient thickness.

The amount of scatter radiation is reduced as kVp is lowered because reduction of kVp enhances differential absorption. However, there are a number of factors opposing the use of low kVp for making radiographs. The beam-restricting devices discussed in the previous chapter are very efficient in reducing the quantity of scattered x rays, but their effect is not enough, since even in the most favorable conditions more than half the **remnant x rays** (all x rays exiting the film side of the patient) will be scattered. Fig. 12-1 illustrates that scattered x rays are emitted in all directions from the patient. The

direction of the scatter radiation becomes slightly more forward as the kVp of the primary beam is increased.

Effect of scatter radiation on contrast

In a later chapter many characteristics that affect the quality of a radiograph will be discussed in detail. One of the most important characteristics of film quality is **contrast,** the degree of difference between the light and dark areas of a radiograph.

If one could radiograph a long bone in cross section using only primary-beam x rays, the image would be very sharp, as shown in Fig. 12-2, A. The change in density from dark to light corresponding to the bone–soft tissue interface would be very great, and therefore the radiographic contrast would be high. On the other hand, if the radiograph were taken with only scatter radiation and no primary-beam x rays

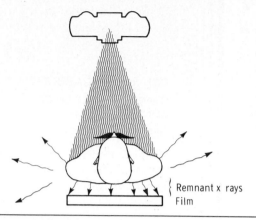

Fig. 12-1. When primary x rays interact with a patient, secondary, scattered x rays are emitted from the patient in all directions.

Fig. 12-2. Radiographs of a cross section of long bone. **A,** High contrast would result from using only primary photons. **B,** No contrast would result from using only scattered photons. **C,** Moderate contrast would result from using both primary and scattered photons.

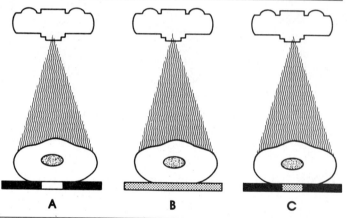

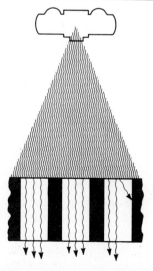

Fig. 12-3. The only x rays transmitted through a grid are those traveling in the direction of the interspace. X rays scattered obliquely through the interspace are absorbed.

reached the film, the image would be dull gray, as in Fig. 12-2, *B*. The radiographic contrast would be very low or perhaps even nonexistent. In the normal situation, however, the x rays arriving at the film consist of both primary and scattered x rays. If the radiograph were properly exposed, the image in cross-sectional view would appear as in Fig. 12-2, *C*. The image would be neither as sharp as that in Fig. 12-2, *A*, nor as dull as that in Fig. 12-2, *B*; it would have moderate contrast. The loss of contrast results from the presence of scattered x rays; **the more scattered x rays, the lower the contrast.**

How a grid works

Two general approaches to reducing the amount of scattered x rays in the remnant beam are possible.

The film could be treated so that the scattered x rays could not interact. Scattered x rays have lower energy than primary-beam x rays, but unfortunately radiographic film is nearly equally sensitive to x rays throughout the diagnostic range. To date no additive to the film emulsion has been effective in increasing film sensitivity to primary-beam x rays at the expense of scattered x rays. **The use of screens in conjunction with x-ray film increases the contrast of the image** but not because primary-beam x rays are preferentially absorbed over scattered x rays.

The second approach would be to reduce the number of scattered x rays arriving at the film plane. Since scattered x rays have lower energies than primary-beam x rays, a properly designed filter should be an effective device for reducing the amount of scattered x rays. **Selective filtration** has been investigated but unfortunately has been shown to be largely ineffective.

An extremely effective device for reducing the level of scatter radiation is the **grid,** a carefully fabricated series of sections of radiopaque material (**grid material**) alternating with sections of radiolucent material (**interspace material**). The grid is designed to transmit only those x rays whose direction is on a line from the source to the image receptor. X rays that travel obliquely (at an angle) are absorbed in the grid material. Fig. 12-3 is a schematic of how a grid **cleans up** scatter radiation. This technique for reducing the amount of scatter radiation reaching the film was first demonstrated in 1913 by Dr. Gustave Bucky. Over the years Dr. Bucky's grid has been improved by more precise manufacturing, but the basic principle is unchanged.

All x-ray photons exiting the patient that are incident on the radiopaque grid material are absorbed and do not reach the film. For instance, a typical grid may have grid strips approximately 50 μm thick separated by interspace material approximately 350 μm thick. Consequently, up to 12.5%* of all photons incident on the grid will interact with radiopaque grid material and be absorbed.

Primary-beam photons incident on the interspace material are transmitted through to the film. Scattered x-ray photons incident on interspace material may or may not be absorbed, depending on their angle of incidence and the physical characteristics of the grid. If the deviation of a scattered x ray is great enough to cause it to intersect the grid material, it will be absorbed. If the deviation is slight, the scattered x ray will be transmitted like a primary x ray. Laboratory measurements show that high-quality grids can be expected to attenuate 80% to 90% of the incident scatter radiation. Such a grid is said to exhibit good **cleanup.**

EXAMPLE: When viewed from the top, a particular grid shows a series of lead strips 40 μm wide separated by interspaces 300 μm wide. How much of the radiation incident on this grid should be absorbed?

ANSWER: If 300 + 40 represents the total surface area and 40 the surface area of absorbing material, then percent absorption is

$$\frac{40}{340} = 0.118$$

$$= 11.8\%$$

---

*(50/[350 + 50])(100) = 12.5%.

CHARACTERISTICS OF GRID CONSTRUCTION
Grid ratio

A number of characteristics of a grid are used to specify its radiographic properties; the grid ratio is perhaps the one most often employed. Grid ratio can best be understood by reference to Fig. 12-4. There are three important dimensions on a grid: (1) the thickness of the grid material (T); (2) the thickness of the interspace material (D); and (3) the height of the grid (h). The **grid ratio** is the height divided by the interspace thickness:

(12-1)

$$Grid\ ratio = \frac{h}{D}$$

Grids with high ratios are more effective in cleaning up scatter radiation than are grids with low ratios because the angle of deviation allowed by high-ratio grids is less than that permitted by low-ratio grids. Fig. 12-5 illustrates this property.

Unfortunately, grids with high ratios are more difficult to manufacture than are low-ratio grids. High-ratio grids are made by reducing the width of the interspace or increasing the height of the grid material or, as is usually the case, a combination of both. All these approaches require high exposure factors to get a sufficient number of x rays through the grid to the film; **the higher the grid ratio, the higher the patient exposure.** In general diagnosis, grid ratios range from 5:1 to 16:1, with the higher-ratio grids most often used in high-kVp radiography. An 8:1 or 10:1 grid is frequently used in general purpose examination rooms. A 5:1 grid will clean up approximately 85% of the scatter radiation, whereas a 16:1 grid may clean up as much as 97%.

EXAMPLE: A certain grid is made of lead 30 μm thick sandwiched between fiber interspace material 300 μm thick. The height of the grid is 2.4 mm. What is the grid ratio?

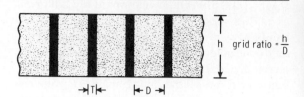

Fig. 12-4. Grid ratio is defined as the height of the grid strip divided by the thickness of the interspace material.

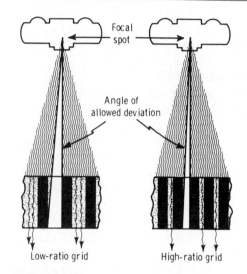

Fig. 12-5. High-ratio grids are more effective than low-ratio grids in cleaning up scatter radiation because the angle of deviation they allow is smaller.

ANSWER: $Grid\ ratio = \dfrac{h}{D}$

$$= \frac{2400}{300}$$

$$= 8:1$$

Grid frequency

The number of grid strips or grid lines per inch or per centimeter is called the grid frequency. Grids with high frequencies show less distinct grid lines on the x-ray film than grids with low frequencies. If the thickness of the grid strips is held constant, the higher the frequency of a grid, the thinner its strips of interspace material must be. In general, **the higher the grid frequency, the higher the radiographic technique required and the greater the dose to the patient,** because as grid frequency increases, there is relatively more grid material to absorb radiation. The disadvantage of the increased patient dose associated with high-frequency grids can be overcome by reducing the thickness of the grid strips, but this effectively reduces the grid ratio and therefore the cleanup.

Most grids have frequencies in the range of 60 to 110 lines per inch (25 to 45 lines per centimeter). It is easy to calculate grid frequencies if the thicknesses of the grid material and the interspace are known. Grid frequency is computed by dividing the thickness of one line pair $(T + D)$, expressed in μm, into 1 cm:

(12-2)

$$Grid\ frequency = \frac{10,000\ \mu m/cm}{(T + D)\ \mu m/line\ pair}$$

EXAMPLE: What is the grid frequency of the previously described grid that had a grid strip thickness of 30 μm and an interspace thickness of 300 μm?

ANSWER: If 1 line pair = 300 μm + 30 μm = 330 μm, how many line pairs are in 10,000 μm (10,000 μm = 1 cm)?

$$\frac{10,000\ \mu m/cm}{330\ \mu m/line\ pairs} = 30.3\ lines/cm$$

$$(30.3\ lines/cm)(2.54\ cm/in) = 77\ lines/in$$

Interspace material

The purpose of the interspace material is to maintain a precise separation between the delicate lead strips of the grid. The interspace material of most grids is either **aluminum** or **plastic fiber;** there are conflicting reports as to which is better. Aluminum has a higher atomic number than plastic and therefore may provide some selective filtration of scattered x rays not absorbed in the grid material. Aluminum also has the advantage of producing less visible grid lines on the radiograph. On the other hand, use of alu-

minum as interspace material increases the absorption of primary photons in the interspace, especially at low kVp, and results in higher patient dose. Above 100 kVp this property is unimportant, but at low kVp patient dose may be increased by 20% or more. For this reason fiber-interspace grids are usually preferred to aluminum-interspace grids. Still, aluminum has two additional advantages over fiber. It is non-hygroscopic; that is, it does not absorb moisture as plastic fiber will. Fiber-interspace grids can become warped because of their hygroscopicity. Also, aluminum-interspace grids are easier to manufacture with high quality because aluminum is easier to form and roll into sheets of precise thickness than fiber is.

Grid material

Theoretically, the grid strip should be infinitely thin and have high absorption properties. There are several possible materials out of which to form these strips. **Lead** may not be the best in terms of its interaction with x rays, but it is the most widely used because it is easy to shape and relatively inexpensive. The high atomic number and high density of lead also contribute to making it the material of choice in the manufacture of grids. Tungsten, platinum, gold, and uranium have all been tried, but none has the overall desirable characteristics of lead.

Regardless of its composition, the grid is encased completely by a thin cover of aluminum. The aluminum casing provides rigidity for the grid and helps to seal out moisture. Table 12-1 is a summary of the characteristics of the most popular commercially available grids.

MEASURING GRID PERFORMANCE

Perhaps the largest single factor responsible for poor diagnostic quality is scatter radiation. By removing scattered x rays from the remnant beam, the radiographic grid removes the source of dullness on the radiograph. This dullness has been previously described as loss of contrast,

Table 12-1. Construction characteristics of some of the more popular commercially available grids

Type	Interspace	Grid frequency (lines/in)	Grid ratio
Focused	Aluminum	103	12:1, 10:1, 8:1, 6:1
Parallel	Aluminum	103	6:1
Focused	Aluminum	85	12:1, 10:1, 8:1, 6:1, 5:1
Parallel	Aluminum	85	6:1, 5:1
Crossed-focused	Aluminum	85	6:1, 5:1
Crossed-parallel	Aluminum	85	6:1, 5:1
Focused	Fiber	80	12:1, 8:1, 5:1
Crossed-focused	Fiber	80	8:1, 5:1
Focused	Fiber	60	6:1
Parallel	Fiber	60	6:1

and thus **the principal function of a grid is to improve contrast.** The characteristics of grid construction previously described, especially the grid ratio, are usually specified when identifying a grid. However, grid ratio does not relate the ability of the grid to improve radiographic contrast. This property of the grid is specified by the **contrast improvement factor** *(k)*.

Contrast improvement factor

The contrast improvement factor is the ratio of the contrast of an x-ray film taken with the grid to the contrast of an x-ray film taken without a grid. A contrast improvement factor of 1 indicates no improvement whatsoever. Most grids have contrast improvement factors of between 1.5 and 2.5. In other words, the radiographic contrast is approximately doubled when grids are used. Mathematically, the contrast improvement factor *k* is expressed as follows:

(12-3)

$$k = \frac{Radiographic\ contrast\ with\ grid}{Radiographic\ contrast\ without\ grid}$$

EXAMPLE; An aluminum step wedge is placed between a plastic fiber phantom 20 cm thick and the film, and a radiograph is taken. Without a grid, analysis of the radiograph shows an average gradient (a measure of contrast) of 1.1. With a 12:1 grid, radio-

graphic contrast is 2.8. What is the contrast improvement factor of this grid?

$$\text{ANSWER: } K = \frac{2.8}{1.1}$$
$$= 2.55$$

The contrast improvement factor is usually measured at 100 kVp, but it should be realized that *k* is a complex function of the x-ray emission spectrum, the patient thickness and the area irradiated. Generally, **the contrast improvement factor is higher for high-ratio grids.** Other factors, such as lead content, also influence this measure of grid performance.

Bucky factor

Although the use of a grid improves contrast, thereby improving image quality, a penalty is paid in the form of patient dose. The amount of remnant radiation penetrating a grid is much less than the remnant radiation incident on the grid. Therefore, in order to produce the same radiographic density when using a grid, the technique must be increased. The amount of such increase is given by the **Bucky factor B:**

(12-4)

$$B = \frac{Incident\ remnant\ radiation}{Transmitted\ remnant\ radiation}$$

The Bucky factor is named for Gustave Bucky, the inventor of the grid. It is an attempt to measure the penetration of both primary and scatter radiation through the grid. Table 12-2 gives representative values of the Bucky factor for several popular grids.

Two generalizations can be made from the data presented in Table 12-2:

1. **The higher the grid ratio, the higher will be the Bucky factor.** The pentration of primary radiation through a grid is rather independent of grid ratio. Penetration of scatter radiation through a grid becomes less likely with increasing grid ratio, and therefore the Bucky factor increases.

2. **The Bucky factor increases with increasing kVp.** At high kVp more scatter radiation is produced. This scatter radiation has a more difficult time penetrating the grid, and thus the Bucky factor increases.

Whereas the contrast improvement factor measures an improvement in image quality when using grids, the Bucky factor measures how much of an increase in technique will be required compared with nongrid exposure. Bucky factor also indicates how much of an increase in patient dose accompanies the use of a particular grid. **With increasing Bucky factor, radiographic technique and patient dose increase proportionately.**

Selectivity (lead content)

The ideal grid would be constructed so that all primary x rays would be transmitted and all scattered x rays would be absorbed. The ratio of transmitted primary radiation to transmitted scatter radiation is called the **selectivity** of the grid and is usually identified by a Greek sigma (Σ):

(12-5)

$$\Sigma = \frac{\text{Primary radiation transmitted through grid}}{\text{Scatter radiation transmitted through grid}}$$

TABLE 12-2. Approximate Bucky factor values for popular grids

Grid ratio	Bucky factor at		
	70 kVp	90 kVp	120 kVp
No grid	1	1	1
5:1	2	2.5	3
8:1	3	3.5	4
12:1	3.5	4	5
16:1	4	5	6

Selectivity is primarily a function of the construction characteristics of the grid rather than the characteristics of the x-ray beam. This is not the case for the contrast improvement factor.

Selectivity is related to grid ratio, but the total mass of lead in the grid has a major influence on selectivity. Fig. 12-6 shows how two grids can have the same grid ratio yet greatly different masses of lead. This is usually accomplished with a small loss in grid frequency. The heavier a grid is, the more lead it contains, the higher its selectivity, and the more efficient it is in cleaning up scatter radiation. Of course, the lead must be properly arranged. A flat sheet of lead with high mass would make a very poor grid.

The radiologic technologist will normally select a grid based on its ratio. The radiologic engineer or radiologic physicist will take into account grid ratio, grid frequency, contrast improvement factor, and selectivity in setting up apparatus for a particular radiographic suite or procedure. The relationships among these grid characteristics are beyond the scope of this text; however, a few general rules regarding them follow:

1. **High-ratio grids have high contrast improvement factors.**
2. **High-frequency grids have low contrast improvement factors.**
3. **Heavy grids have high selectivity and high contrast improvement factors.**

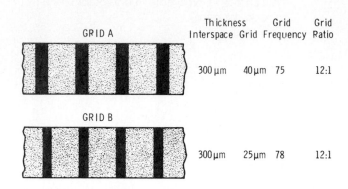

	Thickness Interspace	Grid	Grid Frequency	Grid Ratio
GRID A	300 μm	40 μm	75	12:1
GRID B	300 μm	25 μm	78	12:1

Fig. 12-6. Because grids *A* and *B* have the same height and interspace thickness, they have identical ratios. Grid *A* has 60% more lead but a slightly lower frequency. Grid *A* has higher selectivity.

TYPES OF GRIDS
Linear grid

The simplest type of grid, and perhaps that most often employed, is the linear grid, diagramed in cross section in Fig. 12-7. In the linear grid all lead grid strips are parallel. This type of grid is the easiest to manufacture, but it has some properties that are clinically undesirable.

Nearly all grids except those used with spot-filming devices are large enough to cover a 14 × 17 in (35 × 43 cm) film. As Fig. 12-7 illustrates, with these larger radiographs the attenuation of primary-beam x rays becomes greater as one approaches the edge of the film. The lead strips in 14 × 17 inch grids are 17 inches long. Across the 14-inch dimension a variation in density may be observed because of the primary-photon attenuation. The density reaches a maximum along the center line of the film and decreases toward the sides.

The undesirable absorption of primary-beam x rays in the grid is called **grid cutoff.** Grid cutoff may be partial or complete and result in reduced radiographic density or total absence of film exposure, respectively. The term is derived from the fact that the useful x rays are "cut off" from getting to the film. Grid cutoff can occur with any type of grid if the grid is improperly positioned, but it is most common with linear grids.

This characteristic of linear grids is most pro-

nounced when the grid is used at a short source-to–image receptor distance (SID). Fig. 12-8 demonstrataes the geometric relationship for attenuation of primary-beam x rays by a linear grid. The distance from the central axis at which complete cutoff will occur is given by the following equation:

(12-6)

$$Distance\ to\ cutoff = \frac{SID}{Grid\ ratio}$$

For instance, theoretically a 10:1 grid when used at 100 cm SID should completely absorb all primary x rays farther than 10 cm from the central axis. When this grid is used with a 14 × 17 inch film, film density should be apparent only over an 8 × 17 inch area of the film. The radiographs in Fig. 12-9 were taken with a 6:1 parallel grid at 76 and 61 cm SID (*A* and *B*, respectively). They demonstrate increasing degrees of grid cutoff with decreasing SID.

Crossed grid

Linear grids clean up scatter radiation in only one direction, along the axis of the grid. **Crosshatched grids** have been made to overcome this deficiency. These grids have lead grid strips running parallel to the long and short axes of the grid, as shown in Fig. 12-10. They are usually

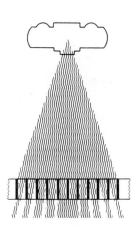

Fig. 12-7. Linear grid is constructed with parallel grid strips. At a short SID some grid cutoff may occur.

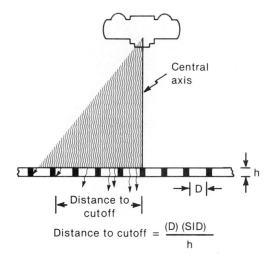

Distance to cutoff $= \dfrac{(D)\,(SID)}{h}$

Fig. 12-8. With a linear grid, film density decreases toward the edge of the film. Grid cutoff will occur according to equation 12-6.

made by sandwiching two linear grids together with their grid strips perpendicular to one another. They are not too difficult to manufacture and therefore are not excessively expensive. However, they have found restricted application in clinical radiology.

Crossed grids are much more efficient than linear grids in cleaning up scatter. In fact, a crossed grid has a higher contrast improvement factor than a linear grid of twice the grid ratio: a 6:1 crossed grid will clean up more scatter radiation than a 12:1 linear grid. This advantage of the crossed grid increases as the kVp of operation is lowered. A crossed grid identified as having a grid ratio of 6:1 is constructed with two 6:1 linear grids.

There are two serious disadvantages to using crossed grids. Positioning the grid is critical; the central axis of the x-ray beam must coincide with the center of the grid. Tilt-table techniques are possible only if the tube and table are properly aligned. If the table is horizontal and the tube angled, grid cutoff will occur.

Focused grid

The main disadvantage of linear and crossed grids is grid cutoff. The focused grid is designed to minimize this deficiency. The lead grid strips of a focused grid are angulated so that they lie on imaginary radius lines from the center of a circle. The x-ray tube target should be placed at the center of this imaginary circle when a focused grid is in use. Fig. 12-11 illustrates this property.

Focused grids are more difficult to manufacture than linear grids. They are characterized by all the properties of linear grids except they have less grid cutoff. The technologist must take care when positioning focused grids because of their geometric limitations. Every focused grid will be marked with its intended focal distance. If radiographs are made at distances other than those intended, grid cutoff will occur. A focused grid intended for use at 100 cm SID will usually have sufficient latitude to produce acceptable radiographs when used at an SID between 90 and 110 cm. **High-ratio grids have less posi-**

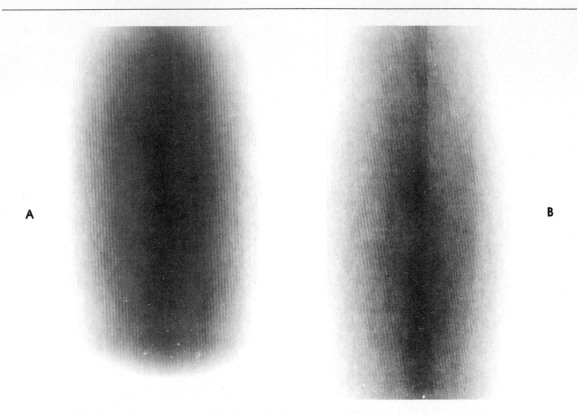

Fig. 12-9. A, Radiograph taken with a 6:1 parallel grid at an SID of 76 cm. **B,** Radiograph taken with 6:1 parallel grid at an SID of 61 cm. Radiographic density decreases from the center to the edge with complete cutoff occurring according to equation 12-6.

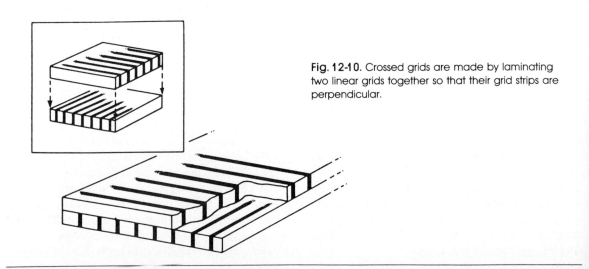

Fig. 12-10. Crossed grids are made by laminating two linear grids together so that their grid strips are perpendicular.

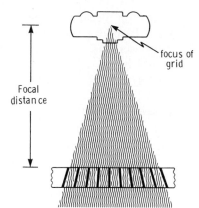

focus of
grid

Focal
distance

Fig. 12-11. Focused grid is made so that the grid strips are coincident with the primary x-ray path across the entire film.

tioning latitude than low-ratio grids. Use of a 100 cm SID 16:1 focused grid at 180 cm would produce severe grid cutoff.

Moving grids

An obvious and annoying shortcoming of the grids previously discussed is that they produce **grid lines** on the radiograph. Grid lines are the images made when primary-beam x rays are absorbed in the grid strips. Even though the grid strips are very small, their image is still observable. One can demonstrate the presence of grid lines simply by radiographing a grid. Generally, high-frequency grids present less obvious grid lines than low-frequency grids. This is not always the case, since the visibility of grid lines is directly related to the width of the grid strips.

A major improvement in grid development occurred in 1920. Dr. Hollis E. Potter hit on a very simple idea: move the grid while the x-ray exposure is being made. A device that does this is now called a **moving grid,** although the terms "Potter-Bucky diaphragm," "Bucky diaphragm," and "Bucky grid" are still widely used. Focused grids are usually employed as moving grids. They are placed in a holding mechanism that is moved at the time of x-ray exposure. There are three basic types of moving-grid mechanisms: single stroke, reciprocating, and oscillating.

Single-stroke grid. As its name implies, the single-stroke mechanism causes the grid to move continuously across the film while the x-ray exposure is being made. Usually it is spring loaded and requires a manual cocking of the mechanism before each exposure. Exposure times no shorter than perhaps 200 ms can be accommodated. The spring mechanism of the moving grid will be designed for the shortest posible exposure time. Longer exposure times are accommodated by damping the mechanism so that it moves more slowly.

Single-stroke moving grids are difficult to use because they require cocking before exposure. On some models the time of grid movement is not automatically adjusted by the exposure-time selector; these models require that the technologist select the appropriate grid-movement time also. Single-stroke moving grids are not employed in most modern radiographic equipment. The total grid movement is usually about 2 to 3 cm.

Reciprocating grid. A reciprocating grid is a moving grid that is motor driven back and forth several times during x-ray exposure. The total distance of drive is about that for the single-stroke grid: 2 to 3 cm. The main advantage this type of moving-grid mechanism has over the single-stroke grid is that it does not require resetting after each exposure.

Oscillating grid. An oscillating grid has some of the characteristics of both the single-stroke and the reciprocating grids. An oscillating grid is positioned in a frame with 2 to 3 cm tolerance on all sides between the frame and grid. Delicate springlike devices located in the four corners hold the grid centered in the frame. A powerful electromagnet pulls the grid to one side and releases it at the beginning of the exposure. Thereafter the grid oscillates in a circular fashion around the grid frame, coming to rest after 20 to 30 seconds.

The main difference between reciprocating and oscillating grids is their pattern of motion. The motion of a reciprocating grid is to and fro, whereas that of an oscillating grid is circular.

Disadvantages of moving grids. The grids available in the early days of radiology when the moving-grid mechanism was developed contained large, thick lead grid strips and therefore produced very objectionable grid lines. Because today's grids are of much higher quality, with thinner grid strips and grid frequencies of over 100 lines per inch (40 lines per centimeter), many radiologists find stationary grids perfectly acceptable.

Moving grids require a bulky mechanism that is subject to failure. The distance between the patient and the film is increased with moving grids because of this mechanism; that extra distance creates an unwanted increase in magnification and geometric unsharpness. Moving grids often introduce motion into the film-holding device, which can result in a blurred image. If not properly designed, moving grids can produce a stroboscopic effect when used with half- or full-wave–rectified x-ray generators because of synchronization between x-ray pulsation and grid movement. This effect results in the presence of pronounced grid lines. Also, the minimum exposure time is longer with moving grids than with stationary grids.

Fortunately, the advantages of moving grids far outweigh the disadvantages. The types of motion unsharpness discussed are for descriptive purposes only. The motion unsharpness generated by moving grids that are functioning properly is undetectable. Only malfunctioning moving-grid systems create problems, and those problems occur very infrequently. Moving grids are usually the technique of choice and therefore are rather universally employed.

USE OF GRIDS

The most frequent error in the use of stationary grids is improper positioning. For the grid to function correctly it must be precisely positioned relative to the x-ray tube target and to the central axis of the x-ray beam. There are basically four situations that must be prevented. All are characteristic of focused grids. Only one is a problem with linear and crossed grids.

Off-level grid

A properly functioning grid must lie in a plane perpendicular to the central-axis x-ray beam, as shown in Fig. 12-12. The central-axis x-ray beam is composed of the x rays traveling along the center of the useful x-ray beam. Despite its name, an **off-level grid** is in fact usually produced by having an improperly positioned radiographic tube head and not an improperly positioned grid. If the central-axis x ray is incident on the grid at an angle, then all incident x rays will be abnormally angulated and grid cutoff will occur across the entire radiograph, resulting in reduced density. The condition can be prevented by paying careful attention to the installation of grids and the positioning of the x-ray tube head. Grid cutoff caused by off-level grids can occur with all types of grids. It is the only positioning problem that occurs with linear and crossed grids.

Off-center grid

A grid can be perpendicular to the central x-ray beam and still produce grid cutoff if it is shifted laterally. This is a problem with focused

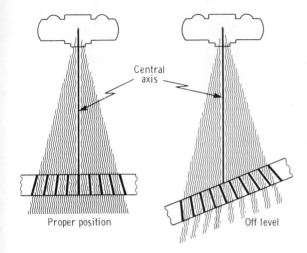

Fig. 12-12. If a grid is off level so that the central axis is not perpendicular to the grid, partial cutoff will occur over the entire film.

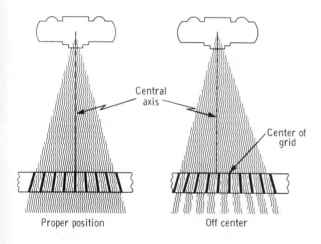

Fig. 12-13. When a focused grid is positioned off center, partial grid cutoff will occur over the entire film.

grids, as shown in Fig. 12-13, where an off-center grid is shown with a properly positioned grid. The center of a focused grid must be positioned directly under the x-ray tube target so that the central-axis x-ray beam passes through the centermost interspace of the grid. Any lateral shift will result in grid cutoff across the entire grid. This error in positioning is called **lateral decentering.** As with off-level grids, this condition is more a matter of positioning the tube head than the grid. In practice it means that the technologist must carefully line up the center of the

light-localized field with the center of the cassette holder. Marks on both, and sometimes on the table, are provided so that this can be done quickly and easily.

Off-focus grid

A major problem with using a focused grid arises when radiographs are taken at SIDs unspecified for that grid. Fig. 12-14 illustrates what happens when a focused grid is not used at the proper focal distance. The farther the grid is from the specified focal distance, the more se-

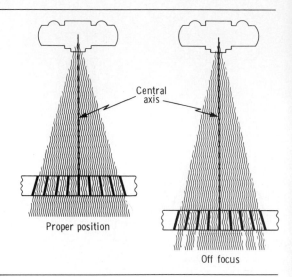

Fig. 12-14. If a focused grid is not positioned at the specified focal distance, grid cutoff will occur and the radiographic density will decrease with distance from the central axis.

vere will be the grid cutoff. In Fig. 12-14 the grid cutoff is not uniform across the film but rather is more severe to the periphery. This condition is not normally a problem if all chest radiographs are taken at 180 cm SID and all table radiographs at 100 cm SID. Occasionally, table radiographs are taken at an SID other than 100 cm, with a grid having a 100 cm focal distance. Positioning the grid at the proper focal distance is important with high-ratio grids. More positioning latitude is possible with low-ratio grids.

Upside-down grid

The explanation of an upside-down grid is obvious. It need occur only once and it will be noticed immediately. A radiographic image taken with an upside-down focused grid would show severe grid cutoff on either side of the central axis (Fig. 12-15). Every focused grid has a clear label on one side and sometimes on both. The label indicates the tube side or film side, or both, and the prescribed focal distance. With even moderate attention, upside-down grids will not occur.

GRID SELECTION

Modern grids are sufficiently well manufactured that many radiologists do not find the grid lines of stationary grids objectionable. However, moving-grid mechanisms rarely fail and image degradation rarely occurs. Therefore in most situations it is appropriate to design radiographic procedures around moving grids. When moving grids are employed, linear grids can be used, but focused grids are more common.

Focused grids are generally far superior to linear grids, but they require care and attention in use. When focused grids are used, the indicators on the x-ray apparatus must be in good adjustment and properly calibrated. The source–to–image receptor distance indicator, the source-to-tabletop distance indicator, and the light-localizing collimator must all be properly adjusted.

Selection of a grid with the proper ratio depends on an understanding of three interrelated factors: kVp, degree of cleanup, and patient dose. When using high kVp, one should employ high-ratio grids. Of course the choice of grid will also be influenced by the size and shape of the part of the anatomy being radiographed. As grid ratio increases, the amount of cleanup also increases. Fig. 12-16 shows as a function of grid ratio the approximate percentage of scatter radiation and primary radiation transmitted. Note that the difference between a grid ratio of 12:1

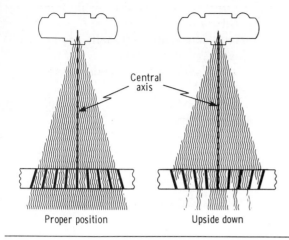

Fig. 12-15. Focused grid positioned upside down should be detected on the first radiograph. Complete grid cutoff will occur except in the region of the central axis.

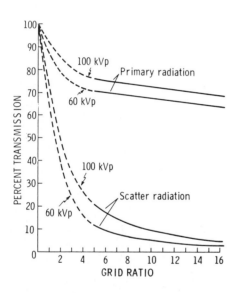

Fig. 12-16. As grid ratio increases, the transmission of scatter radiation and primary radiation decreases; therefore, as grid ratio increases, attenuation (cleanup) of scatter radiation also increases.

and a grid ratio of 16:1 is small. However, the difference in patient dose is large, and therefore 16:1 grids are not often used.

As a general rule of thumb, **grid ratios up to 8:1 are satisfactory at tube potentials below 90 kVp. Grid ratios above 8:1 find application when kVp exceeds 90.** Many general purpose x-ray examination facilities find an 8:1 grid a good compromise between the desired levels of scatter radiation cleanup and patient dose. The

use of one grid also reduces the likelihood of grid cutoff because improper grid positioning can easily accompany frequent changes of grids. In those facilities where high-kVp technique for chest radiography is employed, 16:1 grids can be used.

Patient dose with use of grids

One major disadvantage that accompanies the use of x-ray grids is the increased patient dose

Table 12-3. Approximate entrance doses (mrad) for examination of the adult pelvis with a 200-speed image receptor

	Entrance dose (mrad)		
Type of grid	70 kVp	90 kVp	110 kVp
No grid	85	70	50
5:1	270	215	145
8:1	325	285	205
12:1	425	395	290
16:1	520	475	365
5:1 crossed	535	405	295
8:1 crossed	585	530	405

required. For a given examination, using a grid may require several times more radiation to the patient than not using one. Use of a moving grid instead of a stationary grid with similar physical characteristics requires approximately 15% more radiation to the patient. Table 12-3 is a summary of approximate patient doses for various grid techniques with a 200-speed image receptor.

Low-ratio grids are increasingly used during screen-film mammography. All current dedicated mammographic equipment comes equipped with a 3:1 to a 6:1 ratio moving grid. Even at the low kVp employed for screen-film mammography, considerable scatter radiation occurs. Use of such grids greatly improves image contrast, with no loss of spatial resolution. **The only disadvantage is the increased patient dose,** which can be as much as twice that without a grid. With dedicated equipment and a grid, patient dose still is very low. Grids are not necessary and should not be used with xeromammography.

The concern about exposure to the patient is an important one. However, grid selection should not be compromised so far that the loss of contrast enhancement will interfere with diagnostic interpretation. The following three factors must be remembered when selecting a grid:

1. **Patient dose increases with increasing grid ratio.**
2. **High-ratio grids are usually employed for high-kVp examinations.**
3. **Patient dose at high kVp is less than that at low kVp.**

In general, compared with the use of low kVp and low-ratio grids, the use of high kVp and high-ratio grids will result in lower patient dose and radiographs of equal quality.

One additional disadvantage of using grids is the increased exposure time required. When a grid is used, the technique factors must be increased over what they were for nongrid examinations; either the time of exposure or the mA must be increased. Usually both are increased, and the increased time can result in image blurring caused by patient motion.

Air-gap technique

A clever technique that seems to be growing in application as an alternative to the use of radiographic grids is the **air-gap technique.** The use of the air-gap technique is another method of reducing scatter radiation, thereby enchaning radiographic contrast. In a typical air-gap technique, the film would be moved 10 to 15 cm from the patient, as illustrated in Fig. 12-17. A portion of the scattered x rays generated in the patient would be scattered away from the film and not be detected. Since fewer scattered x rays interact with the film, the contrast is enhanced. Generally, when employing an air-gap technique, the technique factors are about the same as those for a 7:1 grid. Therefore the patient dose is higher than nongrid technique and is approximately equivalent to that of an intermediate grid technique.

One disadvantage of the air-gap technique is image magnification with associated geometric unsharpness. The air-gap technique has found application particularly in areas of chest radiography and cerebral angiography. The magnification that accompanies these techniques is usually acceptable. However, in chest radiog-

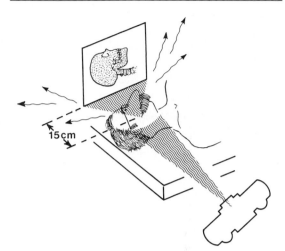

Fig. 12-17. To apply the air-gap technique, one positions the film 10 to 15 cm from the patient. A large fraction of the scattered x rays will not interact with the film, the exact amount depending on exposure factors.

raphy some technologists will increase the SID from 180 to 300 cm. This results in very little magnification and a sharper image. Of course, the technique factors must be increased, but the patient dose is not.

The air-gap technique is not normally as effective with high-kVp radiography, in which the direction of the scattered x rays is more forward. At tube potentials below approximately 90 kVp, the scattered x rays are directed more to the side and therefore have a higher probability of being scattered away from the film. Nevertheless, at some centers 120 to 150 kVp air-gap chest radiography is employed with good results.

The air-gap technique is sometimes called air filtration, but it should be obvious from Fig. 12-17 that air filtration is an improper name for this procedure. In the air-gap technique the **air does not act as a selective filter** of low-energy scattered x rays; rather, the distance between the patient and the film permits the scattered x rays to escape from the vicinity of the film without interaction.

REVIEW QUESTIONS

1. Define or otherwise identify the following:
   a. Contrast
   b. Remnant radiation
   c. Grid cutoff
   d. Lateral decentering
   e. Selectivity
   f. Air-gap technique
   g. Reciprocating grid
   h. Cleanup
   i. Grid focal distance
   j. Contrast improvement factor
2. With particular reference to materials employed and dimensions of various parts, discuss the construction of a grid.
3. Refer to Fig. 12-16 and approximate the (a) percent transmission and (b) percent attenuation of scatter radiation through 6:1, 10:1, and 14:1 grids at 80 kVp.
4. Referring to Table 12-3, determine the relative magnitude of patient dose from radiographs taken at (a) 70 kVp, no grid, (b) 90 kVp, 8:1 grid, and (c) 110 kVp, 12:1 grid, letting the dose at 70 kVp, 5:1 grid equal 1.
5. A focused grid has the following characteristics: 100 cm focal distance, 27.2 lines/cm, 2.8 mm height, 40 μm grid strips, and 350 μm interspace. What is the grid ratio?
6. A focused grid has the following characteristics: 180 cm focal distance, 12:1 grid ratio, 20 μm grid strips, and 280 μm interspace. What is the grid frequency?
7. A linear grid has the following characteristics: 100 cm focal distance, 14:1 grid ratio, 20 μm grid strips, and 250 μm interspace. What percentage of primary x rays will this grid absorb?
8. A focused grid has the following characteristics: 100 cm focal distance, 3.2 mm height, 22 μm grid strips, and 26 lines/cm grid frequency.
   a. What is the interspace thickness?
   b. What is the grid ratio?
   c. What percentage of primary x rays will the grid absorb?
9. A radiograph of a phantom skull overlying an aluminum step wedge shows an average gradient of 1.9. When a 10:1 grid is used, the average gradient is 3.4. What is the contrast improvement factor for the 10:1 grid?
10. A 16:1 linear grid is used with a 25 × 30 cm film at an SID of 100 cm. What area of the film will be exposed?

13

Radiographic film

FILM CONSTRUCTION
FORMATION OF LATENT IMAGE
TYPES OF FILM
HANDLING AND STORAGE OF FILMS

The primary purpose of diagnostic radiologic apparatus and techniques is to transfer information from an x-ray beam to the eye-brain complex of the radiologist. The useful beam emerging from the x-ray tube contains x rays rather uniformly distributed in space. After interaction with the patient, the beam of **remnant x rays** is not uniformly distributed in space but varies in number according to the characteristics of the anatomic structure through which it has passed. The information of diagnostic value in this remnant beam must be transferred to a form intelligible to the radiologist. X-ray film is one medium for this information transfer. Other media include the fluoroscopic screen, the image intensifier, the television monitor, and the multiformat camera, all of which are discussed later.

The construction and characteristics of x-ray film are similar to regular photographic film. X-ray film is manufactured with higher quality con-trol and has a spectral response different from that of photographic film, but its mechanism of operation is much the same. The discussion that follows concerns x-ray film, but with very few modifications it could be applied to photographic film.

FILM CONSTRUCTION

The manufacture of radiographic film is a precise, high-quality procedure. Manufacturing facilities are extremely clean, since the slightest bit of dirt or other contaminant in the film will limit the ability of the film to transfer the information of the x-ray beam. During the early 1960s, at the height of nuclear weapons testing, x-ray film manufacturers took extraordinary precautions to ensure that radioactive contamination from fallout did not invade their manufacturing environment. Such contamination could seriously **fog** the film.

Radiographic film basically has two parts, the

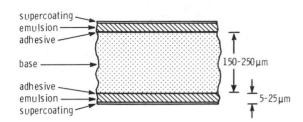

supercoating

emulsion

adhesive

base

150-250 μm

adhesive

emulsion

supercoating

5-25 μm

Fig. 13-1. Cross-sectional view of radiographic film. The bulk of the film is the base. The emulsion contains the diagnostic information.

base and the **emulsion** (Fig. 13-1). Most film has the emulsion coated on both sides and therefore is called **double-emulsion film.** Between the emulsion and the base is a thin coating of material, called the **adhesive layer,** to ensure uniform adhesion of the emulsion to the base. This adhesive layer allows the emulsion and base to maintain proper contact and integrity during use and processing. The emulsion is enclosed by a protective covering of gelatin, called the **supercoating.** This supercoating protects the emulsion from scratching, pressure, and contamination during use and processing and allows for relatively rough manipulation of x-ray film before exposure. Particularly careful handling of processed film is also unnecessary. The thickness of a sheet of radiographic film ranges from 200 to 300 μm (about 0.25 mm).

Base

The base is the foundation for radiographic film. Its primary purpose is to provide a rigid structure onto which the emulsion can be coated. The base is flexible and unbreakable to allow easy handling, but it is sufficiently rigid to be snapped into a view box. Conventional photographic film has a much thinner base than radiographic film and therefore is not as rigid. Can you imagine attempting to snap a 14 × 17 inch photographic negative into a view box?

The base of radiographic film maintains its size and shape during use and processing so that it does not contribute to image distortion. This property of the base is known as **dimensional stability.** The base is of uniform **lucency,** nearly transparent to light, so that there is no unwanted pattern or shading on the film caused by the base. During manufacture, dye is added to the base to slightly tint the film blue. Compared with untinted film, this coloring results in less eyestrain and fatigue for the radiologist and therefore is conducive to more efficient and accurate diagnoses.

The original radiographic film base was a glass plate. Some older radiologists still refer to radiographs as x-ray plates. During World War I, the availability of the high-quality glass used as the radiographic film base became severely limited, and at the same time the medical applications of x rays, particularly by the military, was greatly increasing. A substitute material, **cellulose nitrate,** soon became the standard base. Cellulose nitrate, however, has one serious deficiency: it is flammable. The improper storage and handling of some x-ray film files resulted in severe hospital fires during the 1920s and early 1930s. By the mid-1920s film employing a "safety base," **cellulose triacetate,** was introduced. Cellulose triacetate has properties similar to cellulose nitrate but is not as flammable. It has been the main radiographic film base since its introduction. In the early 1960s a **polyester** base was introduced. Polyester has taken the place of cellulose triacetate as the film base of choice and may be the only film base manufactured in the near future. Polyester is more resistant to warping with age and stronger than cellulose triacetate, permitting easier transport through automatic processors. Its dimensional stability is superior. Polyester bases are thinner than triacetate bases (approximately 175 μm compared with 200 μm, respectively) but are just as strong.

The polyester base is similar in composition to the polyester fibers in clothing. Principally two chemicals, ethylene glycol and dimethyl terephthalate, are formed into a molten polymer (a very large molecule made from two or more smaller ones) by mixing at high temperature and low pressure. For clothing the polyester is produced in thin strands like thread. For film it is formed into thin sheets of appropriate size. Cronar is the term used by E.I. du Pont de Nemours and Company, who invented this plastic, to identify their polyester-base film. Estar is used by Eastman Kodak Company.

Emulsion

The emulsion is the heart of the x-ray film. It is the material in which x rays or light photons from screens interact and transfer information. The emulsion consists of a homogeneous mixture of **gelatin** and **silver halide crystals.**

The gelatin is similar to that used in salads and desserts but is of much higher quality. It is clear, so that it transmits light, and is sufficiently porous for the processing chemicals to penetrate to the crystals of silver halide during processing. Its principal function is to provide mechanical support for the silver halide crystals by holding them uniformly dispersed in place.

The silver halide crystal is the active ingredient of the radiographic emulsion. In the typical emulsion 95% of the silver halide is **silver bromide;** the remainder is usually **silver iodide.** These atoms have relatively high atomic numbers ($Z_I = 53$, $Z_{Br} = 35$, $Z_{Ag} = 47$) compared with the gelatin and base (for both, $Z \approx 7$). The interaction of x-ray and light photons with these high-Z atoms ultimately results in the formation of an image on the radiograph.

The silver halide crystals are flat and triangular, approximately 1 μm on a side. The arrangement of atoms in the crystals is cubic, as shown in Fig. 13-2. The crystals are made by dissolving metallic silver (Ag) in nitric acid (HNO_3) to form silver nitrate ($AgNO_3$). The light-sensitive silver bromide (AgBr) crystals are

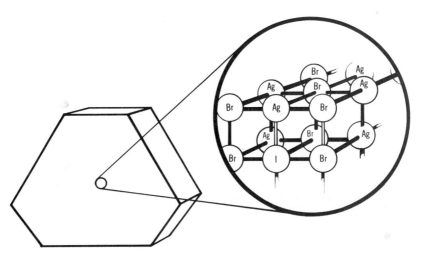

Fig. 13-2. Silver halide crystal is triangular. The arrangement of atoms in the crystal is cubic.

formed by mixing the silver nitrate with potassium bromide (KBr) in the following reaction:

$$AgNO_3 + KBr \longrightarrow AgBr \downarrow + KNO_3$$

The arrow $\downarrow$ indicates that the silver bromide is precipitated while the potassium nitrate, which is soluble, is washed away. The entire process takes place in the presence of gelatin, with the temperature, the pressure, and the rate at which ingredients are mixed being precisely controlled.

The shape and lattice structure of the silver halide crystals are not perfect, and some of the imperfections result in the imaging property of the crystals. The type of imperfection thought to be responsible is a chemical contaminant, usually silver sulfide (AgS), that either intrudes into the crystal lattice or, more frequently, resides on its surface. This contaminant has been given the name **sensitivity speck.** It has been shown that during the processing of the radiographic image the silver atoms are attracted to and concentrate at the location of the sensitivity speck.

The differences in speed, contrast, and resolution among various radiographic films are determined by the process by which the silver halide crystals are manufactured and by the mixture of these crystals into the gelatin. The number of sensitivity specks per crystal, the concentration of crystals in the emulsion, and the size and distribution of the crystals also affect the performance characteristics of radiographic film. Direct-exposure film, for example, contains a thicker emulsion layer with more silver halide crystals than screen film. **The concentration of silver halide crystals is the principle determinant of film speed.** The composition of the radiographic emulsion is a proprietary secret closely guarded by each manufacturer. The manufacture of radiographic film is conducted in total darkness. From the moment the emulsion ingredients are brought together until final packaging, no light is present. This presents special problems to the manufacturer.

FORMATION OF LATENT IMAGE

The remnant radiation exiting the patient and incident on the radiographic film deposits energy in the emulsion primarily by photoelectric interaction with the atoms of the silver halide crystal. This energy is deposited in a pattern representative of the object or part of the anatomy being radiographed. If one observed the film immediately after exposure, no image would be seen. There is, however, an image present, called a latent image. **The latent image is the undetectable change induced in the various silver halide crystals.** With proper chemical processing the latent image becomes a **manifest image.**

The interaction between photons and silver halide crystals is fairly well understood, as is the processing of the latent image into the manifest image. However, the formation of the latent image, sometimes called the **photographic effect,** is not well understood and continues to be the subject of considerable research. The following discussion is an extraction of the Gurney-Mott theory, the accepted, though incomplete, explanation of latent-image formation.

Silver halide crystal

The silver, bromine, and iodine atoms are fixed in the **crystal lattice** in ion form, as shown in Fig. 13-3. Silver is a positive ion, and bromine and iodine are negative ions. An ion is an atom that has either too many or too few electrons and therefore, as a whole, is not electrically neutral. When a silver halide crystal is formed, the silver atoms each release an outer-shell electron, which becomes attached to a halide atom (either bromine or iodine). Now the silver atom is missing an electron and therefore is a positively charged ion, identified as Ag^+. The bromine and iodine atoms each have one extra electron and therefore are negatively charged ions and identified as Br^- and I^-, respectively.

The silver halide crystal is not as rigid as some crystals (diamond crystals, for example, are very rigid), and under certain conditions both atoms

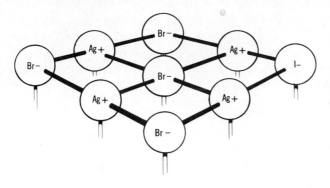

Fig. 13-3. Silver halide crystal lattice contains ions. Electrons from Ag atoms have been loaned to Br and I atoms.

Fig. 13-4. Model of silver halide crystal emphasizing sensitivity speck and concentration of negative ions on surface.

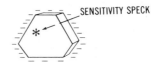

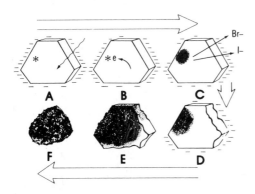

Fig. 13-5. Production of the latent image and the conversion of the latent image into a manifest image follow several simultaneous steps. **A,** Radiation interaction releases electrons. **B,** These electrons migrate to the sensitivity speck. **C,** At the sensitivity speck, atomic silver is formed. **D,** This process is repeated many times, resulting in the disappearance of the negative surface electrification and the buildup of silver atoms. **E,** The remaining silver halide is converted with processing. **F,** The resulting silver grain.

and electrons are free to migrate within the crystal. The halide ions, bromine and iodine, are generally in greatest concentration along the surface of the crystal. Therefore the crystal takes on a negative surface charge, which is matched by the positive charge of the **interstitial** silver ions, the silver ions inside the crystal. The sensitivity speck is believed to be located on or near the surface. A model of the silver halide crystal is shown in Fig. 13-4.

Photon interaction with silver halide crystal

When radiation interacts with film, it is the silver and halide atoms (Ag, Br, I) that respond to form the latent image even though most photon energy is transferred in nonphotographic interactions with the gelatin. If the x ray is totally absorbed (Fig. 13-5, A), its interaction is photoelectric. If it is partially absorbed, its interaction is Compton. In both cases a **secondary**

electron, either a photoelectron or Compton electron, is released with sufficient energy to travel a large distance in the crystal. While traversing the crystal, the secondary electron may have sufficient energy to dislodge additional electrons from the crystal lattice. Consequently, as a result of one x-ray interaction, a number of electrons are released and travel through the crystal lattice. The release of these secondary electrons is represented as follows:

$$Br^- + photon \longrightarrow Br + e^-$$

The result is the same if the interaction involves visible light from an intensifying screen, but because light photons have lower energy, many more are needed to produce an equal number of migrating secondary electrons.

Some of these migrating electrons pass near or through the sensitivity speck (Fig. 13-5, *B*). Here many of them are trapped by the positively charged silver ion. This reaction is represented as:

$$e^- + Ag^+ \longrightarrow Ag$$

Most of these electrons come from the bromine and iodine ions, since these negative ions have one extra electron. These negative ions therefore are converted to neutral atoms, and the loss of ionic charge results in a disruption of the crystal lattice. The bromine and iodine atoms are now free to migrate, since they are no longer bound by ionic forces. They migrate out of the crystal into the gelatin portion of the emulsion (Fig. 13-5, *C*). The deterioration of crystalline structure also makes it easier for remaining silver ions to migrate.

Latent image

The concentration of electrons at the sensitivity speck produces a region of negative electrification. As the halide atoms are removed from the crystal, the positive silver ions are electrostatically attracted to the sensitivity speck. After migrating to the sensitivity speck, the silver ions are neutralized by the electrons and converted to atomic silver (Fig. 13-5, *D*). In each crystal

less than 10 silver atoms are deposited at the sensitivity speck in this fashion. Consequently, this silver deposition is not observable, even microscopically. This group of silver atoms is called a **latent-image center.** It is here that visible quantities of silver will form during processing to create the radiographic image.

Crystals with silver deposited at the sensitivity speck will be developed into black grains. Crystals that have not been irradiated will remain crystalline and inactive. The unobservable information contained in radiation-activated and inactivated silver halide crystals constitutes the latent image. **Processing** is the term applied to the chemical reactions that transform the latent image into a manifest radiographic image. Because of its importance, this subject is dealt with separately in the following chapter.

TYPES OF FILM

Medical imaging, especially radiologic imaging, is becoming extremely technical and sophisticated, and this is reflected in the growth, number, and variety of the films employed. The major film manufacturers each produce over twenty-five different films for medical imaging. When considered in light of the various film formats offered, over 500 selections are possible. By far the most commonly employed film is that customarily referred to as **screen film.** However, even screen film comes in a variety of types.

In addition to screen film, there is **direct-exposure film,** sometimes called **nonscreen film,** and special application films such as those used in mammography, video recording, duplication, subtraction, cineradiography, and dental radiography. Each has particular characteristics that become more familiar to the technologist with use. The following is a brief summary of the characteristics of these various image receptors.

Screen film

Screen film is the most widely employed image receptor in radiology. In general, there are three characteristics to be considered when selecting a screen film: contrast, speed, and light absorption characteristics.

Most manufacturers provide screen films with two or more contrast levels. High-contrast film produces a very black-and-white image, while a low-contrast film image is more gray. Contrast is dealt with in more detail in Chapter 16. The contrast of an image receptor is inversely proportional to its exposure latitude, that is, the range of exposure techniques that will produce an acceptable image. Consequently, screen films are available in two or more latitudes. Usually the manufacturer will identify these as medium-, high-, or higher-contrast films. The difference is basically one of **silver halide crystal size and distribution.** A high-contrast emulsion will contain smaller silver halide grains with a relatively uniform grain size. Lower-contrast films, on the other hand, contain larger grains having a wider range of sizes.

Screen films are also available with different sensitivity, or speed, characteristics. Usually a manufacturer will offer two or three different films having different speeds because of different emulsions. In general, the thicker the emulsion, the more sensitive is the film and therefore the higher the speed. There is a limit, however, because the light from the intensifying screen will be absorbed very rapidly in the superficial layers of the emulsion. If the emulsion thickness is too great, that portion next to the base will remain unexposed. In general, large-grain emulsions are more sensitive than small-grain emulsions. However, this is less important because of newer silver technology developed by the manufacturers. Current emulsions contain less silver yet produce the same optical density per unit exposure. This more efficient use of silver is termed the **covering power** of the emulsion.

To optimize speed, screen films are almost always double emulsion, that is, an emulsion is layered on either side of the base. This provides for twice the speed that could be obtained with a single-emulsion film, even if the single emulsion were made twice as thick.

Perhaps the most important consideration in selecting a modern screen film is its spectral

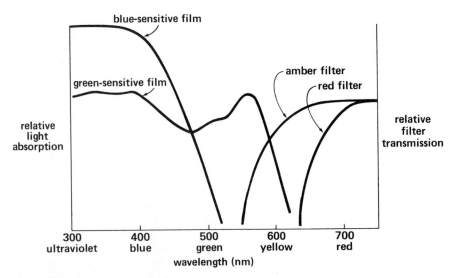

Fig. 13-6. Radiographic films are either blue sensitive or green sensitive, and they require amber and red filtered safelights, respectively.

absorption characteristics. Since the introduction of rare earth screens, one must be particularly cautious to use a film whose sensitivity to various colors of light, its **spectral reponse,** is properly matched to the spectrum of light emitted by the screen. Calcium tungstate screens emit blue and blue-violet light and therefore must be exposed only with standard silver halide film. These films respond to violet and blue light but not to green, yellow, or red. They are called **blue-sensitive** film. If rare earth screens are used, they should be matched with a film that is sensitive not only to blue light but also to green light. Such film is **orthochromatic,** or **ortho,** film and is called **green-sensitive film.** This is distinct from **panchromatic,** or **pan, film,** which is used in photography and is sensitive to the entire visible-light spectrum. Fig. 13-6 shows the spectral response of blue-sensitive and green-sensitive film. Blue-sensitive film should be used with calcium tungstate screens. Green-sensitive film is usually exposed with rare earth screens, although at least one phosphor, lanthanum oxybromide, emits in the blue-violet region of the spectrum. If there is an improper match of a screen with a film, the image-receptor speed will be greatly reduced, and patient dose will have to be increased.

The use of these films requires certain precautions in the darkroom. Safelights are incandescent lamps with a color filter to provide some minimum illumination in the darkroom. With blue-sensitive film, an amber filter is used. The amber filter only transmits light having wavelengths longer than about 550 mm, which is above the spectral response of blue-sensitive film. The use of an amber filter would fog green-sensitive film; therefore a red filter, which transmits only light above about 600 mm, must be used. A red filter suitable for use with green-sensitive film would also be suitable with blue-sensitive film. Fig. 13-6 shows the approximate transmission characteristics for an amber and a red safelight filter.

Direct-exposure film

When one uses radiographic intensifying screens with film, the radiographic technique is lower, the patient dose is less, but the image is less sharp than it would be following exposure without screens. In the past certain film was manufactured for use without screens, and it was employed for imaging thin body parts such as hands and feet that have high subject contrast. Today, however, it is rarely used for that purpose. This type of film is identified as **direct-exposure film.** The emulsion of a direct-exposure film is thicker than that of screen film and it contains a higher concentration of silver halide crystals to enhance direct x-ray interaction. Direct-exposure film is usually employed with a cardboard cassette, although some are available in individually packaged paper wrappings.

The extremity examinations that were earlier performed with direct-exposure film now employ fine-grain, high-detail screens and single-emulsion film as the image receptor. These films can be processed automatically.

Mammography film

Mammography was originally performed with an industrial-grade double-emulsion direct-exposure film. The radiation doses associated with such a technique are much too high and consequently specialty films have been developed—Lo Dose by E.I. duPont de Nemours and Company and Min-R by Eastman Kodak Company, for example.

These mammography films are fine-grain single-emulsion films designed to be exposed with a single intensifying screen. Lo Dose uses a calcium tungstate screen, and Min-R a rare earth screen. The spectral response of each emulsion is adjusted accordingly. These single-emulsion films are manufactured to be compatible with rapid processing techniques. Following processing, double-emulsion film is flat because the expansion and contraction characteristics of the two emulsion layers compensate for one another.

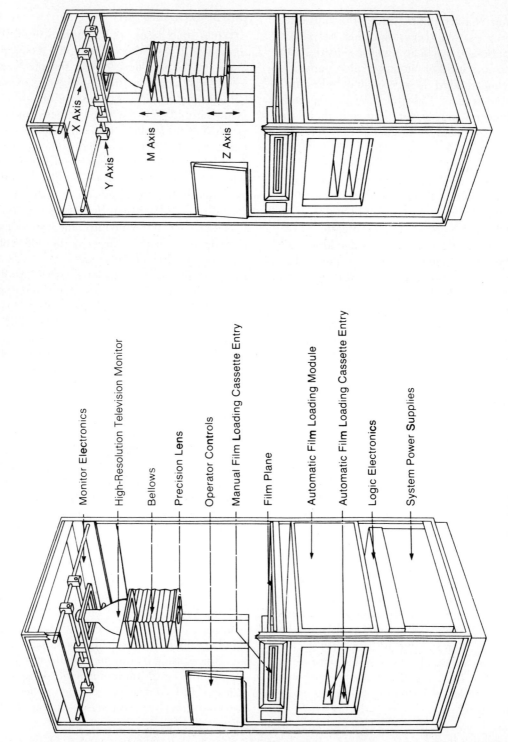

X Axis

Y Axis

M Axis

Z Axis

Monitor Electronics

High-Resolution Television Monitor

Bellows

Precision Lens

Operator Controls

Manual Film Loading Cassette Entry

Film Plane

Automatic Film Loading Module

Automatic Film Loading Cassette Entry

Logic Electronics

System Power Supplies

Fig. 13-7. A multiformat camera. (Courtesy of Matrix Instruments, Inc.)

With single-emulsion film, however, special attention must be paid to the swelling of the emulsion during processing and its shrinking during drying. The back side of the base is coated with clear gelatin, so that during processing the film will not curl and subsequently become distorted.

Video film

The use of video film is growing more rapidly than that of radiographic film because of the introduction and increasing use of computed tomogrpahy, digital radiography, ultrasound, and magnetic resonance imaging. In each of these types of imaging, the image receptor is not film but rather some type of radiation detector. The image is formed by electronic analysis, sometimes computer assisted, of detected radiation and is displayed on a video monitor for visualization. To provide the radiologist with a permanent image, a negative photograph of the television image is made. This is called video imaging or CRT imaging. The television picture tube is a **cathode-ray tube (CRT).** When used in office equipment, the CRT is the principal component of a video display terminal (VDT).

Patient dose is not a consideration in video imaging because it is totally independent of the manner in which the video image is obtained. What is important is that the video film be sufficiently sensitive, so that images can be obtained in a short time, and that it be properly matched to the spectral emission of the CRT. A conventional black-and-white television set uses a black-and-white CRT, and therefore panchromatic film should be used for image recording. Images are also obtained with what is known as a blue-dot or green-dot CRT phosphor. Such images must be recorded with blue-sensitive or green-sensitive film, respectively. Although some video-imaging films are spectrally matched for either blue or green CRT emission, most are orthochromatic films and therefore can be used with any type CRT. Panchromatic films are not used because they would become fogged with existing darkroom safelights.

Video-imaging films incorporate a single emulsion that is relatively thin. They are usually exposed in a device called a multiformat camera, such as that shown in Fig. 13-7, or a laser camera. These devices allow multiple images to be placed on a single sheet of film. The best cameras can accommodate many different film sizes and provide either a single image on the film or up to sixteen images per film. This multiimaging capacity is accomplished by a film mask and lens system on a multiformat camera and electronically on a laser camera.

Fig. 13-8 illustrates in cross section a representative sample of single-emulsion film such as that used for mammography and video imaging.

Specialty films

Occasionally a technologist will be requested to perform a different type of task that requires a different type of film. If one wants to duplicate an existing radiograph, **duplicating film** is used. Duplicating film is designed for same-size use; that is, the size of duplicating film is equal to the size of the film being duplicated. Duplicating film is a single-emulsion film that is exposed to ultraviolet light through the existing radiograph to produce a copy.

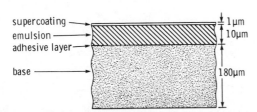

Fig. 13-8. Cross section of single-emulsion mammography film.

Subtraction film is sometimes employed in angiography, although with the increasing application of digital fluoroscopy, its use is declining. Subtraction film is single emulsion, and there are generally two types. One is designed to prepare the subtraction mask, and the other accommodates the superimposed image of the original radiograph and subtraction mask. Subtraction film has a high contrast to enhance the existing subject contrast.

Cinefluorography is a special examination reserved almost exclusively for the cardiac catheterization laboratory. The radiologic technologist who becomes involved in such procedures will use **cine films.** Cine film comes in two sizes, 16 mm and 35 mm, and is supplied in 100 to 500 foot rolls. Cine film is, in fact, movie-type film. Commercial movies are 35 mm and home movies 8 mm. Most cinefluorography employs 35 mm film, but some gastrointestinal studies can use 16 mm to good advantage. Although both have the same intrinsic resolution, when viewed with the proper projector, the perceived image obtained on 35 mm film will be better than that obtained on 16 mm film. Since the area of the 35 mm film is nearly four times that of a 16 mm film, the patient dose is increased proportionately.

Roll films from 70 to 105 mm in width are used in a number of different types of spot-film cameras. These films are similar in composition to cine film and are called **spot film.** Spot film is larger than cine film and therefore can be viewed directly on a conventional view box without resorting to a projector. Fig. 13-9 shows the format of the more popular sizes of cine and roll-type spot films.

Processing of cine film and spot film is critical to providing a quality image. Roll-type spot film can usually be adequately processed in the automatic processor used for conventional radiographs. Cine film, on the other hand, should be processed with specially designed movie film processing equipment, because when the image is magnified during projection, artifacts are likewise magnified.

Films for **dental radiography** are produced in two principal sizes—one for intraoral exposure and the other for panoramic exposure. The standard intraoral films are 1¼ × 1⅝ inches. They are double-emulsion films, but are exposed without screens. Each film is individually wrapped with a backing of lead foil to reduce

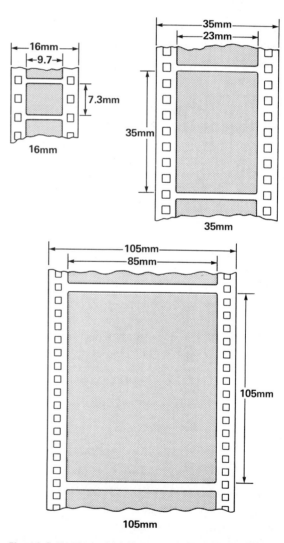

Fig. 13-9. The format of 16 mm and 35 mm cine film and 105 mm spot film.

patient dose. The panoramic films are single-emulsion screen films sized 5 × 12 inches. Although rapid processors are available, many dental films continue to be hand processed.

HANDLING AND STORAGE OF FILMS

Radiographic film is a sensitive radiation detector and must be handled accordingly. Improper handling and storage will result in poor radiographs with artifacts that interfere with diagnosis. For this reason it is essential that, when handling radiographic film, care is taken not to bend or crease it or otherwise subject it to rough handling, especially before processing. Clean hands are a must and hand lotions and creams should be avoided.

Improper handling or processing can cause **artifacts,** the marks or spurious images that sometimes appear on the processed radiograph. Artifacts can also be generated by the useful x-ray beam. Radiographic film is pressure sensitive, so rough handling or the imprint of any sharp object will be reproduced as an artifact in the processed radiograph. Creasing the film before processing will produce a linelike or fingernail-appearing artifact. Dirt on the hands or on intensifying screens will result in specular-type artifacts. In a dry environment, static electricity can cause characteristic artifacts. During automatic processing, wear or dirt on the transport system can cause artifacts that are usually identifiable by their repeating nature. Identifying artifacts and their cause is covered in Chapter 14.

Heat and humidity

Radiographic film is sensitive to the effects of elevated temperature and humidity, especially for long periods of time. Heat reduces contrast and increases the fog of a radiograph. Consequently, radiographic film should not be stored at temperatures in excess of about 20° C (68° F). If storage temperatures exceed this, the longer the time of storage, the more severe will be the loss of contrast and the increase in fog. Ideally, radiographic films should be stored under re-

frigeration. Storage for a year or longer is acceptable if the film is maintained at 10° C (50° F). Film should never be stored near steam pipes or other sources of heat. The basement is usually unsatisfactory as a storage area.

Storage under conditions of elevated humidity (for example, over 60%) will also reduce contrast and increase fog. Consequently, before use radiographic film should be stored in a cool dry place, ideally in a climate-controlled environment. Storage under too dry of conditions can be equally objectionable. If the relative humidity dips below about 40%, static artifacts are possible.

Light

Radiographic films must be stored and handled in the dark. No light can expose the emulsion before processing. If low-level, diffuse light exposes the film, fog will be increased. If bright light exposes or partially exposes the film, a gross, obvious artifact will be produced. The control of light is ensured by having a well-sealed darkroom and a lightproof storage bin for film that has been opened but not clinically exposed. The storage bin should have an electrical interlock that will prevent its being opened while the door to the darkroom is ajar or open.

Radiation

Ionizing radiation, other than the useful beam, will create an image artifact by reducing contrast and increasing fog. Darkrooms are usually located next to x-ray rooms and are lead lined. However, this is not always necessary. It is sometimes acceptable to lead-line only the storage shelf and film bin.

Radiographic film is far more sensitive to x-ray exposure than are people, and therefore more lead is required to protect film than people. The fog level for unprocessed film is approximately 0.2 mR (52 pC/kg), and therefore the thickness of lead will be designed to keep the total exposure of unprocessed film below this level. This, of course, requires some assumptions about the storage time of the film. If the turnover of film in an x-ray facility is monthly, then the required lead shielding would be four times more than if it were weekly.

Care should be taken to ensure that the receiving area for radiographic film is not the same as that for the radioactive material used in nuclear medicine. Even though the packaging of radioactive material ensures the safety of those who handle it, the low-level radiation emitted can fog film if the radioactive material and film are stored together for even a short period of time.

Shelf life

Most radiographic film is supplied in boxes of 100 sheets or more. Some film is packaged in an interleaved fashion with chemically treated protective paper between each sheet of film. Each box contains an expiration date indicating the maximum shelf life of the film. Under no circumstances should be film be stored for longer periods. It must be used before its expiration date, usually a year or so after purchase. The aging of film results in loss of speed and contrast and an increase in fog.

It is always wise to store boxes of film on edge rather than lying flat. When stored on edge, they are less apt to warp and, in the case of noninterleaved packaging, less apt to stick to one another.

The storage of film should be sequenced so that the oldest film is used first. A rotation of the film, much like the rotation of perishables in a supermarket, is appropriate. Most hospitals will receive film on a monthly basis and purchase enough film for 5 weeks of use. The extra few days above monthly use are necessary to cover civil emergencies when an unexpectedly large number of x-ray examinations would be necessary. Forty-five days should be the maximum storage time for radiographic film.

REVIEW QUESTIONS

1. Define or otherwise identify the following:
   a. Polyester
   b. Sensitivity speck
   c. Latent image
   d. Emulsion covering power
   e. Orthochromatic film
   f. Cathode-ray tube
   g. Spectral matching
   h. Artifact
   i. Radiation fog level
   j. Shelf life
2. Diagram the cross-sectional view of a radiographic film designed for use with a pair of intensifying screens, making sure to identify the base emulsion, adhesive layer, and supercoating and the composition and thickness of each.
3. What does the term dimensional stability mean when applied to radiographic film? Which part of the film is responsible for this characteristic?
4. List the principal ingredients in the radiographic emulsion and their individual atomic numbers.
5. Silver bromide crystals are made from silver nitrate and potassium bromide. Following exposure, some of the silver bromide is reduced to metallic silver. What are the chemical equations representing these interactions?
6. Describe the process whereby a latent image is created in one crystal of the emulsion.
7. What is the difference between panchromatic film and orthochromatic film, and what is the impact of their characteristics on diagnostic radiology?
8. The selection of a darkroom safelight is critical. What determines proper safelight selection?
9. What precautions are necessary when using films designed specifically for screen-film mammography?
10. What precautions are necessary when using and storing radiographic film?

14

Processing the latent image

PROCESSING CHEMISTRY
AUTOMATIC PROCESSING
QUALITY ASSURANCE
ARTIFACTS

The latent image is invisible because only a few silver ions have been changed to metallic silver and deposited at the sensitivity speck. Processing the film magnifies this action many millions of times until all the silver ions in an exposed crystal are converted to atomic silver (Fig. 13-5, *E* and *F*), thus converting the latent image into a manifest radiographic image. The exposed crystal then becomes a black grain that is visible microscopically. The silver contained in fine jewelry and tableware would also appear black except that it has been highly polished, which smooths out the surface and makes it more reflective.

Processing is as important as technique and positioning in making a quality radiograph. A change in processing conditions should never be a substitute for a poor radiographic exposure because that will always result in higher patient dose.

A number of steps are involved in the pro-cessing of radiographic film, and these are sum-marized in Table 14-1.

Nearly all radiographic processing is done au-tomatically today, and therefore the following discussion will not deal with manual processing except at those steps that are associated only with manual processing. The chemicals involved in both are basically the same. In automatic pro-cessing the times for each step are shorter, and the chemical concentrations and temperature are higher.

The first step in the processing sequence is to wet the film to loosen the emulsion so that subsequent chemical baths can reach all parts of the emulsion uniformly. This step is often omit-ted, and the wetting agent then is incorporated into the second step, development.

Development is the stage of processing in which the latent image is converted to a manifest image. After development, the film is rinsed in an acid solution designed to stop the develop-

Table 14-1. Sequence of events in processing a radiograph

Step	Purpose	Approximate time	
		Manual	Automatic
Wetting	Swelling of the emulsion to permit subsequent chemical penetration	15 s	—
Development	Production of a manifest image from the latent image	5 min	22 s
Stop bath	Termination of development and removal of excess chemicals from emulsion	30 s	—
Fixing	Removal of remaining silver halide from emulsion and hardening of gelatin	15 min	22 s
Washing	Removal of excess chemicals	20 min	20 s
Drying	Removal of water and preparation of radiograph for viewing	30 min	26 s
		>1 hr	90 s

ment process and remove excess developer chemicals from the emulsion. Photographers call this step **stop bath,** and in processing radiographs the stop bath is sometimes included in the next step, fixation. During **fixation,** the silver halide unexposed to radiation is dissolved and removed from the emulsion. The gelatin portion of the emulsion is **hardened** at the same time to make it structurally more sound. Fixation is followed by a vigorous **washing** of the film to remove any remaining chemicals from the previous processing steps. Finally, the film is **dried** to remove the water used to wash it and to make the film acceptable for handling and viewing.

The steps of development and fixation are the most important in the processing of radiographic film. The precise chemical reactions involved in these steps are not completely understood and are relatively unimportant for our purposes. However, a review of the general action is in order because of the importance processing plays in producing a high-quality radiograph.

PROCESSING CHEMISTRY
Wetting

The universal solvent is water, and water is the solvent for all the chemicals used in processing a radiograph. For these chemicals to penetrate through the emulsion, the radiograph must first be treated by a **wetting agent.** The wetting agent is water, and it penetrates through the gelatin of the emulsion, swelling it and causing it to expand. In automatic processing the wetting agent is in the developer.

Development

The principal action during development involves changing silver ions of the exposed crystals into metallic silver and concentrating this metallic silver in the region of the sensitivity speck. The developer is a chemical solution that performs this task. In addition to the solvent, it contains five basic ingredients: the developing agent, an activator, a restrainer, a preservative, and a hardener. The composition of the developer and the function of each component are outlined in Table 14-2.

For the ionic silver to be changed to metallic silver, an electron must be supplied to the silver ion. Chemically, the reaction is described as follows:

$$Ag^+ + e^- \rightarrow Ag$$

When an electron is given up by a chemical, the **developing agent** in this case, to neutralize a positive ion, the process is called **reduction.** The silver ion is said to be **reduced** to metallic silver,

Table 14-2. The components of the developer and their function

Component	Chemical	Function
Developing agent	Phenidone	Reducing agent; produces shades of gray rapidly
Developing agent	Hydroquinone	Reducing agent; produces black tones slowly
Activator	Sodium carbonate	Helps swell gelatin; produces alkalinity
Restrainer	Potassium bromide	Antifog agent; keeps unexposed crystals from being chemically attacked
Preservative	Sodium sulfite	Controls oxidation; maintains balance among developer components
Hardener	Glutaraldehyde	Controls emulsion swelling and aids archival quality
Solvent	Water	Dissolves chemicals for use

and the chemical responsible for this is called a **reducing agent.** The opposite of reduction is oxidation, a reaction that produces an electron. Oxidation and reduction occur simultaneously and are called **redox** reactions. To help recall the proper association, think of **EUR/OPE**—electrons are used in reduction/oxidation produces electrons.

The chemical composition of film developers are closely guarded proprietary secrets. The principal component is a compound called **hydroquinone.** Secondary constituents of the developing agent are **phenidone** and **metol.** Usually, hydroquinone and metol are combined for manual processing, and hydroquinone and phenidone are combined for rapid processing. As reducing agents, each of these molecules has an abundance of electrons that can be easily released to neutralize positive silver ions. These molecules are not ions but are constructed in such a way that many of their electrons are concentrated on their outside surface.

In Chapter 16 we will discuss certain aspects of film sensitometry. The density of a processed radiograph comes from the synergistic action of hydroquinone and phenidone, as shown in Fig. 14-1. **Synergism** means that the action of two agents working together is greater than the sum of the action of each agent working independently. The characteristic curve of a radiograph is shaped by the synergistic action of developing

agents. Hydroquinone is rather slow acting but is responsible for the very blackest shades. Phenidone acts rapidly and influences the lighter shades of gray. Phenidone controls the toe of the characteristic curve, and hydroquinone controls the shoulder, as shown in Fig. 14-2.

An unexposed silver halide crystal has a negative electrostatic charge distributed over its surface. An exposed silver halide crystal, on the other hand, has a negative electrostatic charge distributed over its surface except in the region of the sensitivity speck. The similar electrostatic charges on the developing agent and silver halide crystal makes it difficult for the developing agent to penetrate the crystal surface except in the region of the sensitivity speck in an **exposed crystal.** In such a crystal, the developing agent penetrates the crystal through the sensitivity speck and reduces the remaining silver ions to atomic silver. The difference between the development of unexposed and exposed crystals is illustrated in Fig. 14-3.

Development occurs over a period of time that depends on factors such as crystal size, developer concentration, and temperature. If one could observe the process in action, one would see a slow buildup of metallic silver at the site of the sensitivity speck. After complete development, exposed crystals have been destroyed, and a grain of black metallic silver is all that remains. Unexposed crystals remain unaffected.

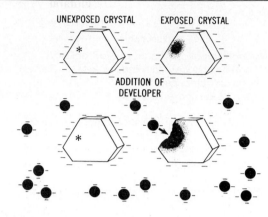

Fig. 14-1. Development is the chemical process that amplifies the latent image. Only crystals that contain a latent image are reduced to metallic silver by the addition of developer.

Fig. 14-2. The shape of the characteristic curve is controlled by the developing agents. Phenidone controls the toe and hydroquinone the shoulder.

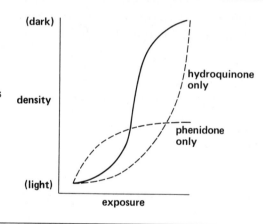

Fig. 14-3. Underdevelopment results in a dull radiograph because the crystals that contain a latent image have not been completely reduced. Overdevelopment produces a similar radiograph because of the partial reduction of unexposed crystals. Proper development results in maximum contrast.

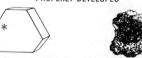

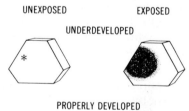

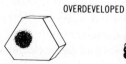

The reduction of a silver ion is accompanied by the liberation of a bromine ion. The bromine ion migrates through the remnant of the crystal into the gelatin portion of the emulsion. From there it is dissolved into the developer and removed from the film.

The developer contains alkali compounds, such as **sodium carbonate** and **sodium hydroxide,** to enhance the action of the developing agent by controlling the concentration of hydrogen ions, the pH. These compounds are called the **activator** in the developer. These alkali compounds are caustic; that is, they are very corrosive and can eat away at your skin. Sodium hydroxide is the strongest alkali and is commonly called **lye.** Be very cautious if you mix a developer solution containing sodium hydroxide. You should wear rubber gloves and, of course, never let it get near your mouth or eyes.

Potassium bromide and **potassium iodide** are added to the developer as **restrainers.** These compounds restrict the action of the developing agent only to those silver halide crystals that have been irradiated. Without the restrainer, even those crystals that had not been exposed would be reduced to metallic silver. This results in an increased fog that is termed **development fog.**

A **preservative** is also included in the developer to control the oxidation of the developing agent by air. Air is introduced into the chemistry when it is mixed, handled, and stored; when such oxidation occurs, it is called **aerial oxidation.** Mixed chemistry will last only a couple of weeks, and close-fitting floating lids on replenishment tanks therefore are essential for the control of aerial oxidation. Hydroquinone is particularly sensitive to aerial oxidation. Premixed chemistry, when stored at room temperature, will last a year. It is easy to tell when the developing agent has been oxidized because it will turn a brownish color. Addition of a preservative causes the developer to remain clear. **Sodium sulfite** is the usual preservative.

All developers used in automatic processors contain a **hardener,** usually glutaraldehyde. If the emulsion swells too much or becomes too soft, the film will not be transported properly through the system because of the very close tolerances of the transport system. The hardener controls the swelling and softening of the emulsion. Sometimes when films that drop from the processor are damp, the cause is depletion of the hardener. **Lack of sufficient glutaraldehyde may be the biggest cause of problems with automatic processing.**

Importance of proper development

Proper development implies that all exposed crystals containing a latent image are reduced to metallic silver, whereas those crystals unexposed are unaffected. However, the development process is not perfect; therefore some crystals containing a latent image remain undeveloped (unreduced), while other crystals that are unexposed may be developed. Both of these actions reduce the quality of the radiograph.

Film development is basically a chemical reaction. Like all chemical reactions, it is governed by three physical characteristics: time, temperature, and concentration (of the developer). Long development time leads to increased reduction of the silver in each grain and increased development of the total number of grains. High developer temperature has the same effect. Similarly, silver reduction is controlled by the concentration of the developing chemicals. With increased developer concentration, the reducing agent becomes more powerful and can more readily penetrate both exposed and unexposed silver halide crystals.

Manufacturers of x-ray film and developing chemicals have very carefully determined the optimum conditions of time, temperature, and concentration for proper development. Optimum conditions of contrast, speed, and fog (see Fig. 16-15) can be expected if the manufacturer's recommendations for development are followed. Deviation from the manufacturer's recommendations will result in loss of image quality and perhaps even a missed diagnosis. Fig. 14-3 illustrates three degrees of development for unexposed and exposed crystals. The importance of proper development is obvious.

The development of unexposed silver halide crystals is called **development fog.** The image of a fogged film is dull and washed-out and lacks proper contrast. The causes of fog are many, but perhaps the most important are those just enumerated: time, temperature, and developer concentration. An increase in any of these factors above manufacturer recommendations will result in increased development fog. Fog can also be produced by chemical contamination of the developer, **chemical fog,** by unintentional exposure to radiation, **radiation fog,** and by improper storage at elevated temperatures and humidity.

Fixing

Once development is complete, the film must be treated so that the image will not fade but will remain permanently. This stage of processing is termed **fixing.** The image is said to be fixed on the film, and this produces film of **archival quality.** Archival quality refers to the permanence of the radiograph. The image thus does not deteriorate with age but remains in its original state.

When the film is removed from the developer, some developer is trapped in the emulsion and continues its reducing action. If developing is not stopped, development fog will result. In manual processing the step following development is called **stop bath,** and its function is just

that: to neutralize the residual developer in the emulsion and stop its action. The chemical used in the stop bath is **acetic acid.**

In automatic processing a stop bath is not used because the rollers of the transport system squeeze the film clean. Furthermore, the fixer contains acetic acid that behaves as a stop bath. This acetic acid, however, is called an **activator.** It neutralizes the pH of the emulsion and stops developer action. Table 14-3 lists the additional chemical components of the fixer.

When referring to the fixer, one often hears the terms **clearing agent, hypo,** and **thiosulfate** used interchangeably. Ammonium thiosulfate is the clearing agent used in most fixer chemistries (sodium thiosulfate is seldom used anymore). Clearing agents remove unexposed and undeveloped silver halide crystals from the emulsion. They are said to clear the emulsion and are therefore called clearing agents. It is sodium thiosulfate that has been classically referred to as hypo. **Hypo retention** is a term used to describe the undesirable retention of the fixer in the emulsion. Excess hypo will slowly oxidize and cause the image to discolor to brown over a long period of time. Fixing agents retained in the emulsion will combine with silver to form silver sulfide, and **silver sulfide stain is the most common cause of poor archival quality.**

The fixer also contains chemical called **hardeners.** As the developed and unreduced silver bromide are removed from the emulsion during fixation, the emulsion shrinks. Hardeners accelerate this shrinking process and cause the emulsion to become more rigid, or hardened.

Table 14-3. The components of the fixer and their function

Component	Chemical	Function
Activator	Acetic acid	Neutralizes the developer and stops its action
Clearing agent	Ammonium thiosulfate	Removes undeveloped silver bromine from emulsion
Hardener	Potassium alum	Stiffens and shrinks emulsion
Preservative	Sodium sulfite	Maintains chemical balance
Solvent	Water	Dissolves other components

The purpose of hardeners is to ensure that the film is transported properly through the wash-and-dry section and also to ensure rapid and complete drying. The chemicals commonly employed as hardeners are **potassium alum, aluminum chloride,** and **chromium alum.** Normally, only one is used in a given formulation.

The fixer also contains a **preservative** that is of the same composition and that serves the same purpose as the preservative in the developer. The preservative is **sodium sulfite,** and it is necessary to maintain the chemical balance because of the carry-over of developer and fixer from one tank to another.

Finally, the fixer contains drinking-quality water as the solvent. Other chemicals might be applicable as a solvent, but they would be thicker and more apt to gum up the transport mechanism of the automatic processor.

Washing

The next stage in processing is to wash away any residual chemistry remaining in the emulsion, particularly hypo clinging to the surface of the film. Water is used as the wash agent. In automatic processing **the temperature of the wash water should be maintained at approxi-** **mately 5° F (2.8° C) below the developer temperature.** In this way the wash bath also serves to stabilize developer temperature. Inadequate washing will lead to excess hypo retention and the production of an image that will fade, turn brown with time, and be of generally poor archival quality.

Drying

The final step in processing is to dry the radiograph, and this is done by blowing warm dry air over both surfaces of the film as it is transported through the drying tank or chamber.

The total sequence of events involved in manual processing requires over 1 hour. Most modern automatic processors are identified as 90-second processors and require a total time from start to finish—dry-to-drop time—of just that, 90 s.

AUTOMATIC PROCESSING

With the introduction of automatic processors in the late 1950's, the efficiency of radiology services increased considerably. The time between exposure and the finished radiograph was shortened from an hour to a matter of minutes. The requirement for darkroom personnel dimin-

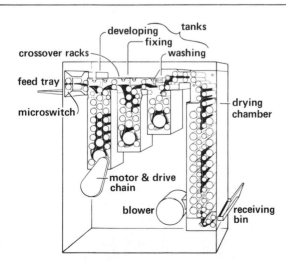

crossover racks

developing — tanks
fixing
washing

feed tray

microswitch

drying chamber

motor & drive chain

blower

receiving bin

Fig. 14-4. A cutaway view of an automatic processor with the major components identified.

ished proportionately. In addition to increased efficiency, automatic processing has resulted in better image quality because each radiograph is processed exactly the same way. The opportunity for human variation and error is nearly absent.

Fig. 14-4 is a cutaway view of an automatic processor. The principal component systems in an automatic processor are the transport system, the temperature-control system, the circulation system, the replenishment system, the dryer system, and the electrical system. The following is a brief description of each of these component systems of automatic processing.

Transport system

The transport system consists of three principal subsystems: **rollers, transport racks,** and **drive motor.** The transport system begins at the feed tray where the film to be processed enters the processor. Here, rollers grip the film to begin its trip through the processor. Here also is a **microswitch** that controls the replenishment rate of the processing chemicals. From the entrance rollers, the film is transported by rollers and racks through the wet chemistry tanks and drying chamber and finally is deposited in the receiving bin.

The transport system not only transports the film but also controls processing by controlling the time the film is immersed in each of the wet chemistries. The sequence of times for each step in processing is accomplished by moving the film through each stage at a carefully controlled rate.

Roller subassembly. There are basically two types of rollers employed in the transport system. **Transport rollers** are 1-inch diameter rollers that convey the film along its path. They either are positioned opposite one another in pairs or are offset from one another, as illustrated in Fig. 14-5. When the film makes a turn in the processor, and most of the turns are designed to reverse the direction of the film, a 3-inch diameter **master roller,** or solar roller, is used, as shown in Fig. 14-6. The master roller usually has positioned around it a number of **planetary rollers** and metal or plastic guide shoes.

Transport-rack subassembly. Except for the entering rollers at the feed tray, most of the rollers in the transport system are positioned on a rack assembly such as the one shown in Fig. 14-7. These racks are easily removable and provide for convenient maintenance and efficient cleaning of the processor. When the film is trans-

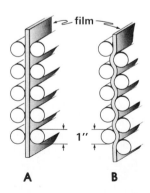

Fig. 14-5. A, Transport rollers positioned opposite each other. **B,** Transport rollers positioned offset from one another.

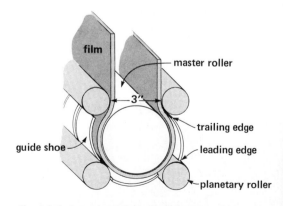

Fig. 14-6. A master roller with planetary rollers and guide shoes is used to reverse the direction of film in a processor.

ported in one direction along the rack assembly, only the 1-inch diameter rollers are required to guide and propel it. However, at each bend there is a curved metal lip with smooth grooves to guide the film around the bend. These are called **guide shoes.** For a 180-degree bend, the film would be positioned for the turn by the leading guide shoe, be propelled around the curve by the master roller and its planetary rollers, and leave the curve by entering the next straight run of rollers through the trailing guide shoe. Such as system of a master roller, planetary rollers, and guide shoes is called a **turnaround assembly.** The turnaround assembly is located at the bottom of the transport-rack assembly. Each wet-chemistry cycle has a transport-rack assembly positioned in the tank. When the film exits the top of the rack assembly, it is guided to the adjacent rack assembly through a **crossover rack.** The crossover rack is a smaller rack assembly composed of rollers and guide shoes.

Drive subsystem. Power for the transport system is provided by a fractional horsepower drive motor. The shaft of the drive motor is usually reduced to 10 to 20 rpm through a gear-reduction assembly. A chain, pulley, or gear assembly transfers power to the transport rack and drives the rollers. Fig. 14-8 illustrates the three principal mechanical devices—a belt and pulley, a chain and sprocket, and gears—used to connect the mechanical energy of the drive motor to the drive mechanism of the rack assembly.

The speed of the transport system is controlled by both the speed of the motor and the gear-reduction system employed. The tolerance on this mechanical assembly is quite rigid. **Film transport should not exceed ±2% of the time specified by the manufacturer.**

Temperature-control system

The three chemistries—developer, fixer, and wash—require precise temperature control. The developer temperature is most critical, and it is usually maintained at 95° F (35° C). Wash water temperature is maintained 5° F (2.8° C) lower. Temperature control in each tank is provided by a thermostatically controlled heating element.

Circulation system

Anyone who has manually processed a radiograph knows how important it is to agitate the film during processing. Agitation is necessary to continually mix the processing chemistry, to maintain a constant temperature throughout the

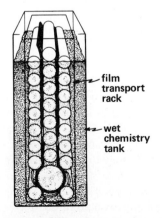

film
transport
rack

wet
chemistry
tank

Fig. 14-7. A transport-rack subassembly.

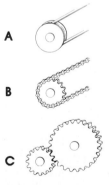

A

B

C

Fig. 14-8. A, Belt and pulley. **B,** Chain and sprocket. **C,** Gears. These are the three means by which transfer of power to the transport rack can be accomplished.

processing tank, and to aid in the exposure of the emulsion to the chemistry. Through proper replenishment and circulation of the chemistry, approximately 12 to 20 l/min (3 to 5 gal/min), the activity of the developer will be maintained. In automatic processing agitation is provided by a circulation system that continuously pumps the developer and the fixer, keeping each tank in constant agitation. A filter that will trap particles down to approximately 100 μm in size is required in the developer-circulation system to trap flecks of gelatin that are dislodged from the emulsion. The particles thus have less chance of becoming attached to the rollers, where they can produce artifacts. These filters are not 100% efficient, and therefore sludge can build up on the rollers. Consequently, cleaning of the tanks and the transport system should be a part of the routine maintenance of any processor.

Filtration in the fixer-circulation system is normally unnecessary, since the fixer hardens and shrinks the gelatin so that coating of the rollers does not occur. Furthermore, the fixer neutralizes the developer, and the products of this reaction will not affect the final radiograph.

Circulation of water through the wash tank is necessary to remove all of the processing chemicals from the surface of the film before drying to ensure archival quality. Rather than employ a closed-circulation system, this is usually done with an open system. Fresh tap water is piped into the tank at the bottom and overflows out the top, where it is collected and discharged directly to the sewer system. The minimum flow rate for the wash tank in most processors is 12 l/min (3 gal/min).

Replenishment system

Each time a film makes its way through the processor, it uses some of the processing chemistry. Some developer is absorbed into the emulsion, and then it is neutralized during fixing. The fixer, likewise, is absorbed during that stage of processing, and some is carried over into the wash tank. If neither the developer nor the fixer were replenished, they would quickly lose chemical balance, the level of solution in each tank would drop, and short contact times with the chemistry would result.

The replenishment system meters into each tank the proper amount of chemistry to maintain volume and chemical activity. Although the replenishment of the developer is more important, the fixer also has to be replenished. Wash water is not recirculated and therefore is continuously and completely replenished.

Replenishment rates are based on the amount of film processed. Usually the rate is established for every 14 inches of film travel. When a film is inserted into the feed tray with its widest dimension gripped by the leading rollers and its narrow side against the guide fence, a microswitch will be activated that will turn on the replenishment for as long as film travels through the microswitch. Replenishment rates are approximately 60 to 70 ml of developer and 100 to 110 ml of fixer for every 14 inches of film. **If the replenishment rate is increased, a slightly increased radiographic contrast will result. If the rate is too low, a significant decrease in contrast will occur.**

Dryer system

If a finished radiograph were at all wet or damp, then it would easily pick up dust particles in the air that could result in artifacts. Furthermore, a wet or damp film is difficult to handle in a view box. When stored, it can become sticky and be destroyed. The dryer system consists of a blower, ventilation ducts, drying tubes, and an exhaust system. It completely extracts all residual moisture from the processed radiograph so that it drops into the receiving bin dry.

The blower is usually a squirrel-cage type that sucks in room air and blows it across heating coils through ductwork to the drying tubes. The room air therefore should be at low humidity and dust free. Sometimes as many as three heating coils of approximately 2500 W capacity are used. The temperature of the air entering the drying chamber is thermostatically regulated.

The drying tubes are long hollow cylinders with a slitlike opening extending the length of the cylinder and facing the film. They are positioned on both sides of the film as it is transported through the drying chamber. The hot moist air is exhausted from the drying chamber and vented to the outside, much like the air in a clothes dryer. Some fraction of the exhaust air may be recirculated in the dryer system.

When damp films drop into the receiving bin, there is immediate suspicion that a malfunction of the dryer system has occurred. However, it seems that most processing faults leading to damp film occur because of a depletion of glutaraldehyde, the hardener in the developer.

Electrical system

Electrical power must be provided to the thermal and mechanical components of each of the previous systems. This is done, of course, through proper wiring of the automatic processor. Normally, each major electrical component will be fused, and the fuse box is the only part of the electrical system of importance to the technologist.

QUALITY ASSURANCE

Quality assurance in any activity refers to the routine and special procedures developed to ensure that the final product is of consistently high quality. Quality assurance in diagnostic radiology requires a planned, continuous program of evaluation and surveillance of radiologic equipment and procedures. When applied to automatic processing, such a program involves periodic cleaning, system maintenance, and daily monitoring.

Processor cleaning

The first automatic processor had a dry-to-drop time of 7 minutes. Soon this was shortened to 3 minutes by what is known as **double-capacity** (DC) processors. A further reduction in processing time was made with the **fast-access**

(FA) system, which is the current, popular 90-second processor.

Such a processor can handle up to 500 films per hour, but to do so it requires a high concentration of processing chemistry, a high development temperature (95° F [35° C]), and a developer immersion time of 22 s. The washwater temperature should be 87° F (30.5° C). Earlier automatic processors were supplied with hot and cold water, so the primary control of wash temperature was through a mixing valve. Nearly all new processors are supplied with only cold water. Temperature control is maintained with a thermostatically controlled heater.

This rapid activity carried on at high temperatures with concentrated chemistry tends to wear and corrode the mechanism of the transport system and contaminate the chemistry with processing soil. A deposit of sludge and debris on the rollers may result. This can severely affect film quality and cause artifacts if the processor is not properly cleaned at appropriate intervals.

In most facilities weekly cleaning is the appropriate frequency, and records of such cleaning should be maintained. The cleaning procedure is rather simple. One removes the transport and crossover racks and simply cleans them and the processing tanks. This takes no more than a few minutes and pays great dividends in reduced processor wear and the consistent production of high-quality radiographs that are artifact free.

Processor maintenance

As with any electromechanical device, maintenance is a must. If equipment is not properly maintained, then when least expected or when your workload is the highest, the processor will malfunction. There are three types of maintenance programs that should be a part of the quality-assurance program for an automatic processor.

Scheduled maintenance refers to those procedures that are applied on a routine basis, usually weekly or monthly. Such maintenance includes observation of all moving parts for wear; adjustment of all belts, pulleys, and gears; and application of proper lubrication to minimize wear. When lubricating a processor, it is especially important to keep the lubricant off of your hands, thereby keeping it away from film and rollers and, of course, out of processor chemistry.

Preventive maintenance is a planned program of parts replacement at regular intervals. Preventive maintenance requires that a part be replaced before its failure. With such a program, unexpected downtime should not occur.

Nonscheduled maintenance is, of course, the worst kind. When there is a failure in the system and the processor requires repair, that is a nonscheduled event. A proper program of scheduled maintenance and preventive maintenance will ensure that nonscheduled maintenance is kept to a minimum.

Processor monitoring

At least once per day, the operation of the processor should be observed and certain measurements recorded. The temperature of the developer and wash water should be noted. The developer and fixer replenishment rates should be observed and recorded.

The replenishment tanks should be checked to determine if the floating lids are properly positioned and if fresh chemistry is required. It is often appropriate to check the pH and specific gravity of the developer and fixer solutions. Residual hypo should be determined.

A sensitometric strip should be passed through the processor, and appropriate measures of fog, speed, and contrast should be determined and recorded. Most film suppliers will provide complete forms and assistance in establishing and conducting a program of processor monitoring. The written record of the results of such a program is important.

ARTIFACTS

An artifact is any irregular density on a radiograph that is not caused by the proper shadowing of the object by the primary x-ray beam. Artifacts therefore are undesirable densities or blemishes on the radiograph. They can interfere with the visualization of the radiographic image and lead to misdiagnoses. Artifacts can be controlled when their cause is identified. There are generally three areas in which artifacts can occur: exposure, processing, and handling. Fig. 14-9 provides a classification of artifacts one is likely to see.

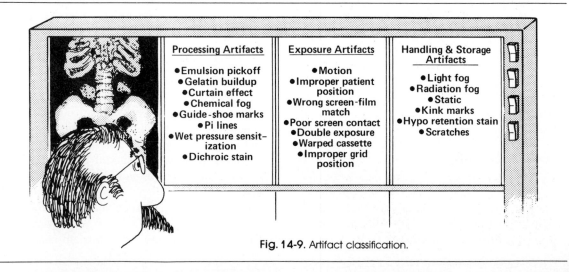

Processing Artifacts
- Emulsion pickoff
- Gelatin buildup
- Curtain effect
- Chemical fog
- Guide-shoe marks
- Pi lines
- Wet pressure sensitization
- Dichroic stain

Exposure Artifacts
- Motion
- Improper patient position
- Wrong screen-film match
- Poor screen contact
- Double exposure
- Warped cassette
- Improper grid position

Handling & Storage Artifacts
- Light fog
- Radiation fog
- Static
- Kink marks
- Hypo retention stain
- Scratches

Fig. 14-9. Artifact classification.

Exposure artifacts

Exposure artifacts are generally associated with the manner in which the technologist conducts the examination. Incorrect screen-film match, poor screen-film contact, warped cassettes, and improper positioning of the grid can all lead to gross artifacts. Improper patient position, patient motion, double exposure, and incorrect radiographic technique can result in very poor images that some would call artifacts. Such examples of poor technique have been shown to result in the largest number of repeat examinations. Exposure artifacts are usually easy to detect and correct.

Processing artifacts

During processing, any number of artifacts can be produced. Most are pressure-type artifacts caused by the transport system of the processor.

Guide-shoe marks occur when the guide shoes are sprung or improperly positioned. The ridges in the guide shoes press against the film, sensitize it, and leave a characteristic mark. Guide-shoe marks will occur before the fixing tank and can be found on the leading edge or the trailing edge of the film.

Pi lines occur at 3.1416-inch (π) intervals because of dirt or a chemical stain on a roller. Since the rollers are 1 inch in diameter, 3.1416 inches represent one revolution of a roller. Fig. 14-10 is an example of pi lines and guide-shoe marks appearing on the same film.

Dirty or warped rollers can cause **emulsion pickoff** and **gelatin buildup.** These artifacts usually appear as sharp areas of either increased or reduced density.

Improper or inadequate chemistry can result in chemical fog, dichroic stain, or a "curtain" effect. **Chemical fog** appears the same as light or radiation fog and is usually a uniform dull gray. **Dichroic stain** is a term generally applied

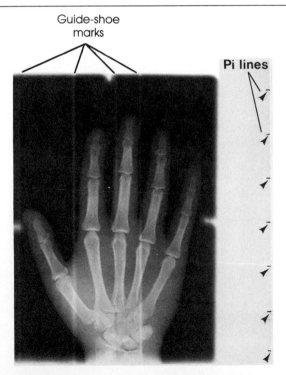

Fig. 14-10. Pi lines and guide-shoe marks on the same film. (Courtesy Charles Ahrens and William Hendee, University of Colorado Health Sciences Center, Denver, Colo.)

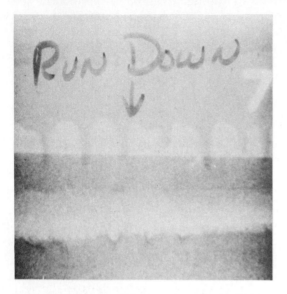

Fig. 14-11. Excess chemistry runs down the leading edge of the film creating a "curtain" effect. (Courtesy William McKinney, E.I. du Pont de Nemours & Co.)

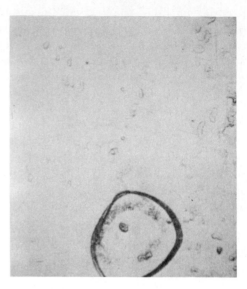

Fig. 14-12. Wet-pressure sensitization caused by a dirty processor. (Courtesy William McKinney, E.I. du Pont de Nemours & Co.)

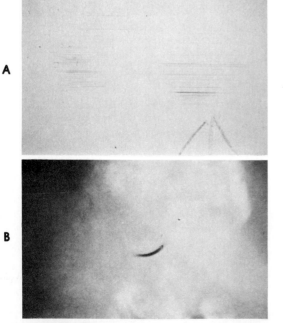

Fig. 14-13. Preprocessing pressure artifacts can appear as scratches caused by heavy finger pressure on the feed tray and as "fingernail" marks caused by kinking of the film. **A,** Scratches. **B,** "Fingernail" marks. (Courtesy William McKinney, E.I. du Pont de Nemours & Co.)

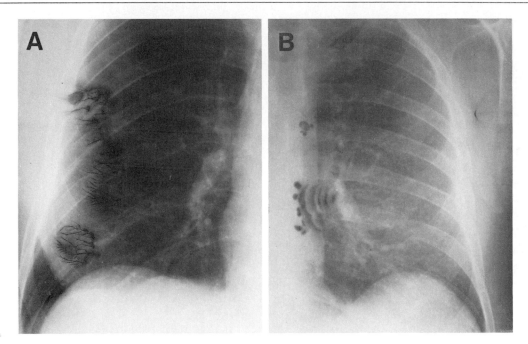

Fig. 14-14. A, Tree static. **B,** Smudge static. These are the two most common types of static artifacts. (Courtesy Joel Gray, Mayo Clinic, Rochester, Minn.)

to all chemical stains. Dichroic means two colors. The chemical stains seen on a radiograph can appear yellow, green, blue, or purple. In slow processors the chemistry may not be properly squeezed from the film, and it either "runs down" the leading edge of the film or "runs up" the trailing edge. Both are called a **curtain effect,** and such an artifact is shown in Fig. 14-11.

Wet-pressure sensitization, shown in Fig. 14-12, is a common artifact produced in the developer tank. Irregular or dirty rollers will cause pressure during development and produce small circular patterns of increased density.

Handling and storage artifacts

Characteristic artifacts can be caused by improper handling or storage either before or after processing. White-light leaks and improper safelight filters or intensities can cause fog. Rough handling before processing can cause scratches

and kink marks such as those shown in Fig. 14-13. Although the kink mark may appear as a fingernail mark, it is not. It is caused by the kinking or abrupt bending of film.

Static is probably the most obvious artifact. It is caused by the buildup of electrons in the emulsion and is most noticeable during the winter or during periods of extreme low humidity. There are three kinds of distinct patterns of static: crown static, tree static, and smudge static. The latter two are illustrated in Fig. 14-14.

Following processing, any debris in the viewbox can be mistaken for a film artifact. Mismatched bulbs in the viewbox can also simulate the appearance of fog.

If a yellowish stain slowly begins to appear on the radiograph with storage time, that indicates a problem with hypo retention. Not all of the residual thiosulfate was removed during washing, and silver sulfide slowly builds up.

REVIEW QUESTIONS

1. Define or otherwise identify the following:
   a. Solvent
   b. Glutaraldehyde
   c. Reducing agent
   d. Synergism
   e. Archival quality
   f. Planetary roller
   g. Guide shoe
   h. Preventive maintenance
   i. Pi line
   j. Wet-pressure sensitization
2. Identify the steps involved in the automatic processing of a radiograph and the time of each step for a 90-second processor.

3. Describe the action of phenidone and hydroquinone in producing optical density on a radiography.
4. By what other names is **fixer** known?
5. What is the difference between a fast-access and double-capacity processor?
6. Describe three types of artifacts and the necessary action to remove each.
7. What is the purpose of chemical filtration in an automatic processor, and at what stages is it necessary?
8. During the wash cycle, what restrictions are placed on temperature and flow rate?
9. What is a redox reaction?
10. Describe the organization of a quality-assurance program for an automatic processor.

DON'T YOU WORRY MR. WILSON, WE'VE PINPOINTED YOUR PROBLEM. ACCORDING TO THIS X-RAY YOU HAVE A TINY HAIRLINE FRACTURE RIGHT HERE.

15

Intensifying screens

SCREEN CONSTRUCTION
LUMINESCENCE
SCREEN CHARACTERISTICS
SCREEN-FILM COMBINATIONS
CARE OF SCREENS
FLUOROSCOPIC SCREENS

Using film to detect x rays and image anatomic structures is inefficient. In fact, less than 1% of the x rays incident on radiographic film interact with the film and contribute to the latent image. Most radiographs are taken with films in contact with intensifying screens because the use of film alone results in a high patient dose.

An intensifying screen is a device that converts the energy of the x-ray beam into visible light. This visible light then interacts with the radiographic film, forming the latent image. Approximately 30% of the x rays incident on an intensifying screen will interact with the screen. For each such interaction a large number of visible-light photons are emitted. Consequently, the intensifying screen acts as an amplifier of the remnant radiation reaching the screen-film cassette. Use of an intensifying screen results in considerably lower patient dose but has the disadvantage of causing a loss of image clarity. With modern intensifying screens, however, the loss of image clarity is not serious.

SCREEN CONSTRUCTION

X-ray intensifying screens resemble flexible sheets of plastic or cardboard. They come in sizes corresponding to film sizes. Usually the radiographic film is sandwiched between two screens; the film so used is double-emulsion film. In most screens there are four distinct layers, shown in cross section in Fig. 15-1.

Protective coating

The layer of the intensifying screen closest to the x-ray film is the **protective coating.** It is 15 to 25 μm thick and is applied to the face of the screen to make the screen resistant to abrasion and damage caused by handling. It also helps eliminate the buildup of static electricity and provides a surface for routine cleaning without

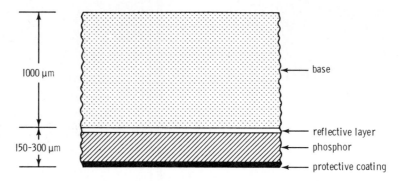

Fig. 15-1. Cross-sectional view of an intensifying screen, showing its four principal layers.

disturbing the active phosphor. Naturally, the protective layer must be transparent to light.

Phosphor

The active layer of the x-ray intensifying screen is the **phosphor.** The phosphor emits light during stimulation by x rays. Phosphor layers vary in thickness from perhaps 150 to 300 μm, depending on the type of screen. The active substance of most phosphors before about 1980 was crystalline calcium tungstate embedded in a polymer matrix. Rare earths are the phosphor material in newer, faster screens.

The phosphor has one purpose: **to convert the energy of the x-ray beam into visible light.** The action of the phosphor can be demonstrated by viewing an opened cassette in a darkened room through the protective barrier of the control booth. The screen will glow brightly when stimulated by x rays. There are many materials that react in this way, but to be satisfactory for use in radiography they must possess the following four characteristics:

1. The phosphor should have a **high atomic number** so that the probability of x-ray interaction is high. This is called **quantum detection efficiency** (QDE).
2. The phosphor should emit a large amount of light per x-ray interaction. This is called the x-ray **conversion efficiency.**

3. The light emitted must be of proper wavelength (color) to match the sensitivity of the x-ray film. This is called **spectral matching.**
4. Phosphor **afterglow,** the continuing emission of light after stimulation of the phosphor by x rays, should be minimum.

Through the years, four materials have been used as phosphors because they exhibit these characteristics. These materials are **calcium tungstate, zinc sulfide, barium lead sulfate,** and the **rare earths: gadolinium, lanthanum,** and **yttrium.**

Roentgen discovered x rays quite by accident. He observed the luminescence of **barium platinocyanide,** a phosphor that was never applied to diagnostic radiology with success.

Within a year of Roentgen's discovery of x rays, calcium tungstate was developed by the American inventor Thomas A. Edison. Although Edison demonstrated the use of screens before the beginning of the twentieth century, screen-film combinations did not come into general use until about the time of World War I. The phosphor employed at that time was calcium tungstate. For a time, barium lead sulfate screens were used, particularly with high-kVp techniques. Zinc sulfide was once used for low-kVp techniques but never gained wide acceptance. Calcium tungstate, because of improved man-

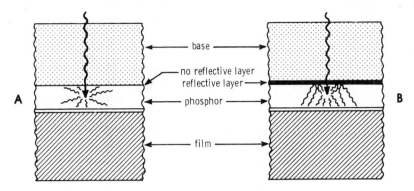

Fig. 15-2. A, Screen without reflective layer. **B,** Screen with reflective layer. Screens without reflective layers are not as efficient as those with reflective layers because fewer light photons reach the film when there is no reflective layer.

ufacturing techniques and quality-control procedures, proved superior for nearly all radiographic techniques and until recently was the phosphor used almost exclusively.

Some new rare earth screens have been introduced for use in diagnostic radiology. These screens are faster than those made of calcium tungstate, rendering them more useful for most types of radiographic imaging. Although they are more expensive, they have replaced calcium tungstate as the phosphor of choice.

Differences in screen imaging characteristics are basically caused by differences in the composition of the phosphor. The thickness of the phosphor layer and the concentration and size of the phosphor crystals influence the action of intensifying screens.

Reflective layer

Between the phosphor and the base is a reflective layer approximately 25 μm thick made of a shiny substance such as magnesium oxide or titanium dioxide. Its function is demonstrated in Fig. 15-2. When x rays interact with the active phosphor, light is emitted **isotropically,** that is, with equal intensity in all directions. Less than half the light is emitted in the direction of the film. The reflective layer intercepts light headed in other directions and redirects it to the film. The reflective layer increases the efficiency of

the x-ray intensifying screen, nearly doubling the number of light photons reaching the film.

Some screens incorporate special dyes in the phosphor layer to selectively absorb those light photons emitted at a large angle to the film. These light photons must travel a longer distance in the phosphor than those emitted perpendicular to the film, and therefore they are more easily absorbed by the dye. Unfortunately, this addition results in some reduction in screen speed.

Base

The layer farthest from the film is called the **base.** The base is perhaps 1 mm thick and serves principally as a mechanical support for the active phosphor layer. It is made of high-grade cardboard, polyester, or metal. Polyester is gaining popularity as a base material in screen construction just as it is as a base material for radiographic film. The requirements for a base material of high quality are as follows:

1. It must be **rugged** and moisture resistant.
2. It must not suffer radiation damage nor **discolor** with age.
3. It must be **chemically inert** and not interact with the phosphor layer.
4. It must be **flexible.**
5. It must not contain **impurities** that would be imaged by x rays.

LUMINESCENCE

Any material that emits light in response to some outside stimulation is called a **luminescent material,** or a **phosphor,** and the visible light so emitted is called **luminescence.** Materials can be caused to luminesce by a number of different stimuli, such as electric current (the fluorescent light), biochemical reactions (the lightning bug), visible light (a watch dial), and x rays (an intensifying screen).

Luminescence, shown schematically in Fig. 15-3, is a process somewhat analogous to characteristic x-ray formation. Luminescence involves **outer-shell electrons.** When a luminescent material is stimulated, the outer-shell electrons are raised to excited energy levels, somewhat more removed from the nucleus. This effectively creates a hole in the outer electron shell, which is an unstable condition for the atom. The hole is filled when the excited electron returns to its normal state, and this transition is accompanied by the emission of electromagnetic energy in the form of a visible-light photon. Energy is required to raise the outer-shell electron to an excited state, and this energy is released when the electron returns to its normal state. Only a narrow range of excited energy states for an outer-shell electron is possible, and these states depend on the structure of the luminescent material. The wavelength of the emitted light is determined by the level of excitation to which the electron was raised and is charac-

teristic of a given luminescent material. Consequently, luminescent materials emit light of characteristic color.

The physicist identifies two types of luminescence. If visible light is emitted only during the stimulation of the phosphor, the process is called **fluorescence.** If, on the other hand, the phosphor continues to emit light after stimulation, then the process is called **phosphorescence.** Some materials can phosphoresce for long periods following stimulation. For example, a light-stimulated watch dial will fade slowly in a dark closet. X-ray intensifying screens mainly fluoresce. Phosphorescence in an intensifying screen is called **screen lag,** or **afterglow,** and can be objectionable.

There is a precise distinction between fluorescence and phosphorescence related to the motion of the excited electron about its nucleus. If the electron returns to its normal state with the emission of light within one revolution following stimulation, then fluorescence has occurred. If more than one revolution is required, then the process is phosphorescence. The time required for an electron to make one revolution about the nucleus is 10 ns.

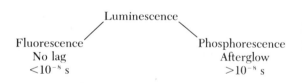

Fluorescence
No lag
$<10^{-8}$ s

Phosphorescence
Afterglow
$>10^{-8}$ s

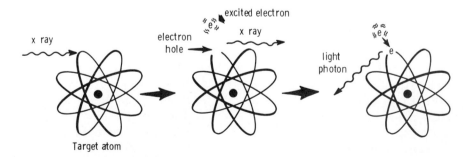

Fig. 15-3. Luminescence occurs when an outer-shell electron is raised to an excited state and returns to its ground state with the emission of a light photon.

SCREEN CHARACTERISTICS

Two primary characteristics of x-ray intensifying screens are important to the radiologic technologist. Since intensifying screens are used to reduce the patient dose, one characteristic is the magnitude of dose reduction obtained. This property is called the **intensification factor** and measures the speed of the screen. Unfortunately, when the remnant x-radiation is converted to visible light and the visible light in turn produces the latent image, some loss of image clarity occurs. The **resolution** of the screen is its ability to produce an accurate and clear image. Resolution is usually measured by the minimum line spacing that can be detected and imaged.

Screen speed

There are many types of x-ray intensifying screens, and each manufacturer uses different nomenclature to identify them. Collectively, however, x-ray intensifying screens usually can be identified according to three broad categories: par speed, high speed, and fine detail.

Screen speed is simply a relative number used to quantitate the efficiency of conversion of x-radiation into usable light. Par-speed screens are assigned a value of 100 and are the basis for comparison of all other screens. High-speed screens have speeds of 200 to 300, and fine-detail screens have speeds of approximately 50. Rare earth screens are manufactured in a variety of

speeds, ranging from 200 to 1200. These and other characteristics are summarized in Table 15-1.

The speed of a screen is relative to that of par-speed screens and thus conveys no information concerning dose reduction to the patient. This information is conveyed by the **intensification factor (IF)**. The intensification factor is defined as the ratio of the exposures required to produce the same film density with and without screens:

(15-1)

$$IF = \frac{Exposure\ required\ without\ screens}{Exposure\ required\ with\ screens}$$

The optical density chosen for comparing one screen with another is usually 1. The intensification factor value can be used to determine the dose reduction accompanying the use of an x-ray intensifying screen.

EXAMPLE: A pelvic examination using par-speed screens is taken at 75 kVp, 100 mAs and results in an exposure to the patient of 200 mR (52 μC/kg). A similar examination taken without screens would result in a patient exposure of 6400 mR (1.7 mC/kg). What is the approximate intensification factor of the screen-film combination?

ANSWER: $IF = \dfrac{6400}{200} = 32$

There are several factors influencing screen speed, some of which are under the control of the radiologic technologist. Ultimately, the

---

Table 15-1. Some characteristics of typical x-ray intensifying screens

Characteristic	Type of screen			
	Fine detail	Par speed	High speed	Rare earth
Type of phosphor	Calcium tungstate	Calcium tungstate	Calcium tungstate or barium lead sulfate	Oxysulfides and oxybromides of Y, La, Gd
Color of emission	Violet	Violet	Violet or ultraviolet	Green or blue
Approximate speed	50	100	200-300	200-1200
Intensification factor	20-35	30-60	80-100	80-400
Resolution (lp/mm)	15	10	7	7-15

screen speed is determined by the relative number of x rays interacting with the phosphor and the efficiency of conversion of x-ray energy into visible light that interacts with the film.

The following properties, listed in their relative order of importance, affect the intensification factor and cannot be controlled by the radiologic technologist:

1. **Phosphor composition.** Well-manufactured calcium tungstate efficiently converts x rays into usable light. Rare earth phosphors are even more efficient.
2. **Phosphor thickness.** The thicker the phosphor layer, the higher is the relative number of x rays converted into light. High-speed screens have thick phosphor layers; fine-detail screens have thin phosphor layers.
3. **Reflective layer.** The presence of a reflective layer increases screen speed but reduces resolution.
4. **Dye.** Light-absorbing dyes are added to some phosphors to control the spread of light. These dyes increase resolution but reduce speed.
5. **Crystal size.** The larger the individual phosphor crystals, the higher the light emission per x-ray interaction. The phosphor crystals of high-speed screens are approximately 8 μm. The crystals of fine-de-

tail screens are approximately half that size. The crystals of par-speed screens are of intermediate size.

6. **Concentration of phosphor crystals.** The higher the crystal concentration, the higher is the screen speed.

The following factors affect screen speed and are under the control of the radiologic technologist:

1. **Radiation quality.** As x-ray tube potential is increased, the intensification factor increases also (Fig. 15-4). Although this may seem contradictory to the discussion of x-ray absorption in Chapter 9, it is not. In Chapter 9, x-ray absorption was shown to decrease with increasing kVp. Remember, however, that the intensification factor is the ratio of the x-ray absorption in a screen-film combination to x-ray absorption in radiographic film alone. Screens have higher effective atomic numbers than x-ray films, and therefore, although true absorption in the screen decreases with increasing kVp, the relative absorption compared with that in film increases.
2. **Temperature.** X-ray intensifying screens emit more light per x-ray interaction at low temperatures than at high temperatures; the intensification factor decreases with temperature. This characteristic, though

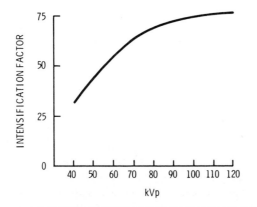

Fig. 15-4. Graph showing approximate variation of the intensification factor with kVp. At 70 kVp the intensification factor for a typical par-speed screen is 60.

relatively unimportant in a clinic with a controlled environment, can be significant in field work in hot or cold climates.

3. **Film development.** Only the superficial layers of the emulsion are affected when x-ray film is exposed to light. The emulsion is nearly uniformly affected, however, when the film is exposed to x rays. Therefore excessive developing time for screen films results in a lowering of the intensification factor because the emulsion nearest the base contains no latent image, yet it can be reduced to silver if the developer is allowed sufficient time to penetrate the emulsion to that depth. This, too, is relatively unimportant in modern radiology, since films manufactured for use with screens have thinner emulsion layers than those produced for direct exposure.

Resolution

The use of screens adds one more step to the process of imaging the human body with x rays. Although screens are widely used, they have the disadvantage of lower resolution compared with direct-exposure radiographs. Resolution is measured in a number of ways and can be given a numerical value. For our purposes a general description should be sufficient.

Resolution is the ability of a system to image an object faithfully. A photograph in focus shows good resolution; one out of focus shows poor resolution. Fig. 15-5 shows the differences in resolution between a direct-exposure film and a par-speed screen-film combination obtained when imaging an x-ray test pattern.

Such a test pattern is called a line-pair test pattern. It has a lead grid line separated by an equal-size interspace. As discussed more com-

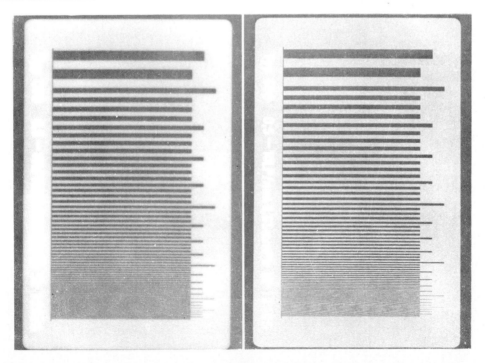

Fig. 15-5. Radiographs of an x-ray test pattern made with direct-exposure film *(right)* and a par-speed screen-film combination *(left)*. The difference in image clarity and resolution is obvious.

pletely in Chapter 22, when resolution is expressed by the number of line pairs per millimeter (lp/mm), the higher the number, the smaller the object that can be imaged and the better the resolution. Very fast screens can resolve 7 lp/mm, and fine-detail screens can resolve 15 lp/mm (Table 15-1). Direct-exposure film can resolve 50 to 100 lp/mm. The unaided eye can resolve about 10 lp/mm.

When x rays interact with the screen phosphor, a larger area of the film emulsion is activated by the emitted light than would be with direct x-ray exposure, and this results in reduced resolution. Generally, **those conditions that in-**

crease the intensification factor reduce resolution. Thus high-speed screens have low resolution and fine-detail screens high resolution. Resolution improves with smaller phosphor crystals and thinner phosphor layers. Fig. 15-6 shows how these factors affect image resolution. Unfortunately, these factors are not under the control of the technologist. Therefore screens should be selected with care.

SCREEN-FILM COMBINATIONS

Screens and films are manufactured for compatibility. Best results will be obtained if they are selected with this in mind. **Use only those**

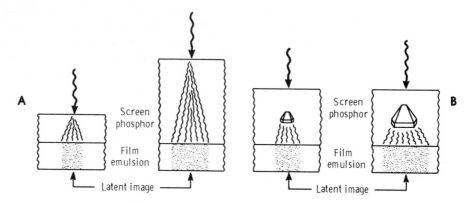

Fig. 15-6. **A,** Reduction in image resolution is greater when phosphor layers are thick. **B,** Reduction is also greater when crystal size is large. These same conditions increase screen speed by producing more light photons per incident x ray.

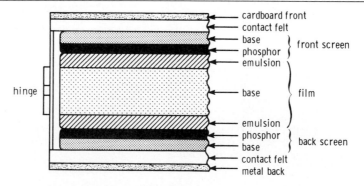

Fig. 15-7. Cross-sectional view of cassette containing front and back screens and loaded with double-emulsion film.

films for which the screens are designed. X-ray intensifying screens are nearly always used in pairs. Fig. 15-7 is a cross section of a properly loaded film cassette containing front and back screens with a double-emulsion film. Production of the latent image will be nearly evenly divided between front and back screen with less than 1% being contributed directly by x-ray interaction. Each screen exposes the emulsion with which it is in contact.

Cassette

The **cassette** is the rigid holder that contains the screens and film. Some of the important characteristics of a good cassette are indicated in Fig. 15-7. The front surface, the side facing the tube, should be made of material with a low atomic number, such as plastic or cardboard, and should be as thin as practicable yet sturdy. Attenuation of the x-ray beam by the front cover of the cassette is undesirable. Attached to the inside of the front cover is the front screen, and attached to the back cover is the back screen. The radiographic film is loaded between these two screens. Until recently, screens were supplied in pairs and identified for front and back. The back screen was thicker than the front screen so that each film emulsion layer would be exposed to the same quantity of light. Inadvertently interchanging these screens would result in a loss of contrast and resolution and might produce dull, pale films. It is now generally agreed that the advantage of specific front and back screens is far outweighed by the disadvantages arising from cost and confusion in handling. Today most cassettes are loaded with identical screens front and back.

Between each screen and the cassette cover will be some sort of **compression device,** such as felt or rubber, that maintains close film-screen contact when the cassette is closed and latched. The back cover is usually made of heavy metal to minimize backscatter. The x rays transmitted through the film-screen combination to the back cover will be absorbed photoelectrically more readily in a high-Z material than in a low-Z material. If the back plate were made of a low-Z material, x rays could be transmitted through the entire cassette, and some might be scattered back to the film by the cassette holding device or a nearby wall. This is called **backscatter** radiation and results in decreased image clarity. Sometimes the cassette hinges or hold-down clamps on the back cover are imaged. This is due to backscatter radiation and normally occurs only during high-kVp radiography when the x-ray beam is sufficiently penetrating.

Carbon fiber material

One of the materials the United States developed early in its space exploration program was **carbon fiber.** This material was developed for nose cone applications because of its exceeding strength and heat resistance. It consists principally of graphite fibers ($Z_C = 6$) in a plastic matrix that can be formed to any shape or thickness.

This material is now used widely in radiology in devices designed to reduce patient exposure. A cassette with a front consisting of carbon fiber material will only absorb approximately half the x rays that are absorbed in a conventional aluminum or cardboard cassette.

Carbon fiber is also being used as pallet material for fluoroscopic examination tables and computed tomography couches.

Use of carbon fiber not only reduces the patient exposure but may also result in longer x-ray tube life because of the lower radiographic techniques required.

Direct exposure vs. screen-film exposure

The principal advantage to the use of screens is that fewer x-ray photons are needed than in direct-exposure techniques to produce the same density on the radiographic film. Table 15-2 shows the relative number of x-ray photons and light photons at various stages for radiographs taken directly and with a par-speed screen-film

Table 15-2. Comparison of relative number of x-ray photons and light photons at various stages for direct and screen-film exposures*

Stage	Type of exposure	
	Direct	Screen-film
Incident x-ray photons	1000	20
X rays absorbed by film	10	<1
X rays absorbed by screens	—	5
Light photons produced	—	5000
Light photons incident on film	—	3000
Light photons absorbed by film	—	1000
Latent images formed	10	10

*Intensification factor = 1000/20 = 50.

combination. This table assumes an intensification factor of 50.

The steps where major differences occur are due to the interaction of x rays with the screen phosphor and to the large number of visible-light photons produced by each of these interactions. Unfortunately, the number of latent images formed is less than 1% of the number of visible photons produced.

Spectrum matching

One reason that calcium tungstate is a useful screen phosphor is that it emits visible light in the violet-to-blue region. A stimulated screen observed through a protective window will appear dark blue. The sensitivity of conventional radiographic film is greatest in the blue-violet region of the spectrum, and consequently the light emitted by calcium tungstate screens is readily absorbed in the radiographic film. If the screen phosphor emitted green or red light, its intensification factor would be greatly reduced because it would require more visible-light photons to produce a latent image.

Fig. 15-8 shows the relative emission spectra for calcium tungstate and zinc cadmium sulfide and the relative sensitivities of radiographic film and the human eye. Some phosphors luminesce in the yellow or even orange region. Formerly used conventional fluoroscopic screens made of **zinc cadmium sulfide,** for example, luminesce with yellow-green light. These screens were used because the wavelength of light they emit closely matches the sensitivity of the human eye. They would be less useful for x-ray intensifying screens because the color spectrum would be mismatched with conventional silver halide film. Conventional fluoroscopic screens have been replaced by image intensifiers and therefore are no longer used.

Rare earth screens

From its introduction in 1896 by Thomas Edison until recently, calcium tungstate ($CaWO_4$) had been employed almost exclusively as the phosphor of choice for radiogrpahic intensifying screens. However, such screens exhibit only 3% to 5% x-ray–to–light conversion efficiencies, which are relatively poor. Newer phosphor materials have been developed for such screens, and they have become the material of choice. Table 15-3 lists these newer phosphors and the general identification of the screens into which they have been incorporated. Except for barium fluorochloride, the other materials are identified as **rare earth substances,** and therefore all these screens have come to be known as **rare earth screens.** The term "rare earth" describes those elements of group III in the periodic table (see Fig. 3-3) having atomic numbers of 57 to 71. These elements are generally minerals found in low abundance in nature. Those used in newer screens are **gadolinium, lanthanum,** and **yttrium.** The compositions of the four principal rare earth phosphors are (1) terbium-activated gadolinium oxysulfide (Gd_2O_2S: Tb), (2) terbium-activated lanthanum oxysulfide (La_2O_2S: Tb), (3) terbium-activated yttrium oxysulfide (Y_2O_2S: Tb), and (4) lanthanum oxybromide (LaOBr).

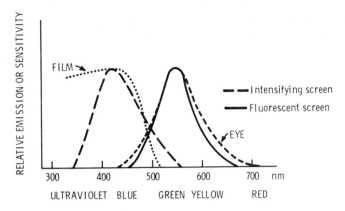

Fig. 15-8. Importance of spectral matching is demonstrated by this graph, which shows the relative emission spectra for intensifying and fluoroscopic screens and the relative sensitivities of radiograph film and the human eye.

Table 15-3. Composition and identification of new, fast intensifying screens

Supplier	Identification	Phosphor	Color
Agfa-Gevaert	NR series	Lanthanum oxybromide	Blue
DuPont	Quanta II	Barium fluorochloride	Blue
DuPont	Quanta III	Lanthanum oxybromide	Blue
Fuji	Greenex	Gadolinium oxysulfide	Green
Gafmed	Rarex	Gadolinium oxysulfide and yttrium oxysulfide	Blue-green
Ilford	Rapide	Lanthanum oxybromide	Blue
Kodak	Lanex	Gadolinium oxysulfide	Green
3M	Trimax	Gadolinium oxysulfide	Green

Rare earth screens have a single, principal advantage over earlier calcium tungstate screens: **speed.** Rare earth screens are manufactured to perform at several speed levels, but each is approximately twice as fast as the calcium tungstate screen counterpart. This increase in speed is obtained without loss of resolution; however, with the fastest rare earth screens the effects of quantum mottle (radiographic noise) are noticeable and can become bothersome.

The advantages of rare earth screens are obvious. Since they are faster, lower radiographic technique can be employed, and this results in lower patient dose. Rare earth screens provide a general reduction in the radiation environment and, when used exclusively, can influence the design of the radiographic facilities and reduce the need for protective lead shielding. The lower radiographic technique will also result in increased tube life, perhaps by as much as a factor of two.

Rare earth screens obtain their increased sensitivity through higher x-ray absorption and more efficient conversion of x-ray energy into light. The light emitted by these screens, however, differs from that for calcium tungstate, and therefore specially matched film is required when using rare earth screens.

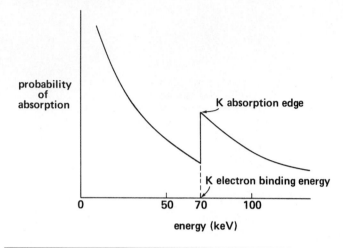

Fig. 15-9. Probability of x-ray absorption in a calcium tungstate screen as a function of the incident x-ray energy.

Higher x-ray absorption. When diagnostic x rays interact with a calcium tungstate screen, approximately 30% of the x rays are absorbed. The mechanism of absorption is almost entirely the photoelectric effect. Recall that photoelectric absorption occurs readily with the inner electrons of high atomic number atoms. In a calcium tungstate screen it is the tungsten atom that determines its absorption properties. Tungsten has an atomic number of 74 and a K-shell electron binding energy of 70 keV. In the diagnostic range, x-ray absorption in tungsten follows the relationship shown in Fig. 15-9.

At very low energies photoelectric absorption is very high. But as the x-ray energy increases, the probability of absorption decreases rapidly until the x-ray energy is equal to the binding energy of the K-shell electrons. At x-ray energies below this K-shell electron binding energy, the incident photon does not have sufficient energy to ionize K-shell electrons. When the x-ray energy equals the K-shell electron binding energy, the two K-shell electrons become available for photoelectric interaction. Consequently, at this energy there is an abrupt increase in the probability of photoelectric absorption. This abrupt increase is followed by another rapid reduction

Table 15-4. Atomic number and K-shell electron binding energy of high-Z elements in intensifying screen phosphors

Element	Chemical symbol	Atomic number (Z)	K-shell electron binding energy (keV)
Yttrium	Y	39	17
Barium	Ba	56	37
Lanthanum	La	57	39
Gadolinium	Gd	64	50
Tungsten	W	74	70

in photoelectric absorption with increasing x-ray energy.

The energy at which the incident x ray has energy equal to the K-shell electron binding energy is the energy at which photoelectric absorption is maximum for those electrons. The abrupt rise in the absorption characteristic is called the **K-shell absorption edge.**

The rare earth materials employed for radiographic intensifying screens all have atomic numbers less than that for tungsten. Consequently, they each have a lower K-shell electron binding energy. Table 15-4 lists the important

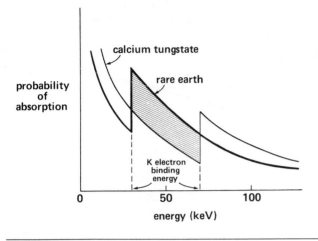

probability
of
absorption

calcium tungstate

rare earth

K electron
binding
energy

0　　　　50　　　　100

energy (keV)

Fig. 15-10. X-ray absorption probability in a representative rare earth screen compared with that for a calcium tungstate screen. In the energy interval between the rare earth K-shell electron binding energy and the tungsten K-shell electron binding energy, absorption in a rare earth screen is higher.

physical characteristics of the high atomic number elements in radiographic intensifying screens. Those elements with lower atomic numbers and lower K-shell electron binding energies result in lower x-ray absorption probabilities over most of the x-ray energy spectrum.

Fig. 15-10 shows that the probability for x-ray absorption in rare earth elements is lower than that for tungsten at all x-ray energies except those between the respective K-shell electron binding energies. Below the K-shell absorption edge for the rare earth elements, x-ray absorption is higher in tungsten. However, at an x-ray energy equal to the K-shell electron binding energy of the rare earth elements, the probability of photoelectric absorption is considerably higher than that for tungsten. The absorption probability of the rare earth materials decreases with increasing x-ray energy at approximately the same rate as that for tungsten. At x-ray energies above the K-shell absorption edge for tungsten, the rare earth elements again exhibit lower absorption than that for tungsten.

The result of this complex interaction process is that **in the x-ray energy range between the K-shell absorption edge for the rare earth element and for tungsten, rare earth screens absorb three to five times more x rays than a** **calcium tungstate screen.** Furthermore, for each x ray absorbed, more light is emitted by the rare earth screens.

Higher conversion efficiency. Rare earth screens exhibit better absorption properties than calcium tungstate screens only in the energy range between the respective K-shell absorption edges. This energy range extends from approximately 35 to 70 keV and corresponds to approximately half the useful x rays emitted during most examinations. However, outside this energy range conventional calcium tungstate screens absorb more x rays, and therefore an additional property of the rare earth phosphors contributes to their extraordinary speed. This additional property is called the **conversion efficiency** and is defined as the ratio of the x-ray energy absorbed to the visible-light energy emitted.

When an x-ray photon interacts photoelectrically with a phosphor and is absorbed, its energy reappears as either heat or light through a rearrangement of electrons in the crystal lattice of the phosphor. If all the energy reappeared as heat (electron and molecular motion), the phosphor would be worthless as an intensifying screen. In calcium tungstate approximately 4%

of the absorbed x-ray energy reappears as light. **The rare earth phosphors exhibit conversion efficiencies of 15% to 20%, four to five times that of calcium tungstate.**

Faster speed. It is the combination of improved conversion efficiency and higher x-ray absorption that results in the increased sensitivity, or speed, of rare earth screens.

Spectrum matching. Rare earth screens are available in many combinations with different films, resulting in varying relative speeds. When compared with par-speed calcium tungstate screens, rare earth screen-film combinations have relative speeds from 200 to 1200. Relative screen speeds of 200 to 800 provide image quality comparable to par-speed calcium tungstate screens. When using rare earth screen-film systems with relative speeds as high as 1200, image quality may be degraded somewhat by increased quantum mottle, but this may be acceptable for some types of examinations in view of the significantly reduced patient dose.

To be fully effective, rare earth screens must be used only in conjunction with film emulsions that have absorption characteristics matched to the emission of the screen. Calcium tungstate screens emit light in a rather broad continuous spectrum centered in the blue–to–blue-violet region with a maximum intensity at approximately 430 nm. This emission spectrum is shown in Fig. 15-11 along with that of a typical rare earth screen. The spectral emission of rare earth phosphors is more discrete, as indicated by the many peaks in the spectrum, and it is centered in the green region of the visible spectrum at approximately 540 nm. Terbium activation is responsible for the shape and intensity of this emission spectrum. The spectrum can be altered somewhat by varying the concentration of terbium atoms in the phosphor.

Conventional x-ray film is sensitive to blue and blue-violet light and rather insensitive to light of longer wavelengths. Such blue-sensitive films are used with calcium tungstate screens because their absorption spectrum matches the calcium tungstate emission spectrum. Fig. 15-12 shows this relationship graphically along with that for specially designed green-sensitive film

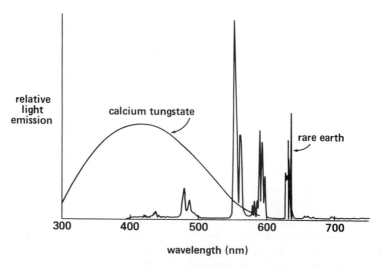

Fig. 15-11. Calcium tungstate emits a broad spectrum of light centered in the blue region, whereas rare earth screens have more discrete emissions centered near the green region of the spectrum.

for use with many rare earth screens. If a green-emitting screen were used with blue-sensitive film, the strong emissions in the green region would go undetected and system speed would be sharply reduced. To obtain maximum advantage and speed from rare earth screens, therefore, the film with which they are employed must be sensitized for the emission of the screen.

Use of a green-sensitive film creates problems in the darkroom. Safelight filters that are satisfactory for regular x-ray film will fog film manufactured for use with rare earth screens. Safelights that are colored even more to the red portion of the spectrum are required.

CARE OF SCREENS

Screens must be properly cared for if consistently high-quality radiographs are to be produced. When handling screens, one should take utmost care because even a small fingernail scratch can degrade the radiographic image. Screens should be handled only when they are new and being installed in cassettes and when they are being cleaned. When screens are

mounted in a cassette, the manufacturer's instructions must be followed carefully.

Screens must be periodically cleaned. The required frequency of cleaning is determined primarily by two factors: (1) the amount of use the screens receive and (2) the degree to which the air in which they are used is dust free. In a busy radiology service it may be necessary to clean screens once each month or even more often. Under other circumstances the cleaning frequency may safely be extended to 2 to 3 months.

There are special screen cleaning materials, and when they are used, the manufacturer's instructions should be followed carefully. One advantage to using these commercial preparations is that they often contain **antistatic** compounds, which can be quite helpful. Screens can also be cleaned with mild soap and water. They should be carefully rinsed and thoroughly dried. If the screen is damp, the film emulsion layer may stick to it, possibly causing permanent damage.

An equally important requirement in caring for screens is maintaining good screen-film contact. Screen-film contact can be checked by radiographing a wire mesh. Fig. 15-13, A, is a

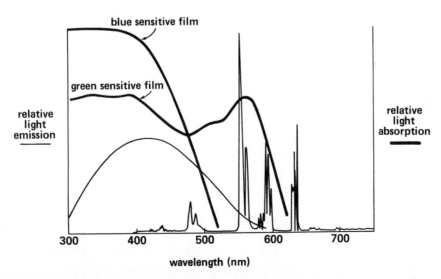

Fig. 15-12. It is essential that blue-sensitive film be used with blue-emitting screens and green-sensitive film with green-emitting screens.

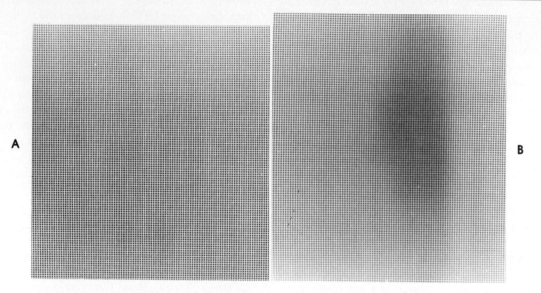

Fig. 15-13. Radiographs of wire mesh are used to check for screen-film contact. **A,** Good contact is evident. **B,** Region of poor contact is present because of a warped cover.

radiograph showing good screen-film contact. If there are any areas of blurring, as in Fig. 15-13, *B,* then poor screen-film contact exists and should be corrected. When new screens are installed in a cassette, this examination for screen-film contact should be made, and the radiograph should be retained as a baseline measurement. Additional wire mesh radiographs for screen-film contact should be made and compared with the baseline film at least once a year.

To test for screen-film contact, expose the cassette through the wire mesh at 50 kVp, 5 mAs and an SID of 100 cm. To view the result optimally, back away 2 to 3 m (6 to 10 ft) from the viewbox. Areas of poor screen-film contact will appear blurred and cloudy, indicating that the cassette should be repaired or replaced.

The following list summarizes the most common causes of poor screen-film contact. Observe that nearly all the causes listed can result from rough handling of cassettes, which is the principal cause of loss of good screen-film contact. Although the cassettes appear sturdy, they are precision pieces of equipment and should be treated accordingly.

Most common causes of poor screen-film contact

1. Worn contact felt
2. Loose, bent, or broken hinges
3. Loose, bent, or broken latches
4. Warped screens caused by excessive moisture
5. Warped cassette front
6. Sprung or cracked cassette frame
7. Foreign matter under the screen

Properly maintained x-ray intensifying screens will last indefinitely. X-ray interaction with the phosphor does not cause them to wear out. The only way they become useless and need replacement is through improper handling and maintenance.

FLUOROSCOPIC SCREENS

Screens that are used in conventional fluoroscopy and photofluorography behave much like x-ray intensifying screens and have many similar properties. These fluoroscopic screens convert the x-ray image into an image visible to the human eye. The phosphor employed in nearly all of them is **zinc cadmium sulfide** (ZnCdS). During conventional fluoroscopy, the fluoroscopic screen is backed by leaded glass to protect the fluoroscopist.

The light emitted from fluoroscopic screens is different from that emitted by x-ray intensifying screens in two major ways. The first is shown in Fig. 15-8. Fluoroscopic screens emit light in the yellow-green region of the visible-light spectrum. This is desirable because it closely matches the wavelength-dependent sensitivity of the human eye. The second difference is that fluoroscopic screens exhibit more **afterglow** than do x-ray intensifying screens.

This discussion of conventional fluoroscopic screens is brief and intended as a historical note rather than necessary instructional material. All fluoroscopy today is, or should be, image-intensified fluoroscopy. Early image intensifiers used zinc cadmium sulfide as the input phosphor, but newer image-intensifier tubes incorporate cesium iodide (CsI) because it is faster with higher resolution and less afterglow than ZnCdS. Image intensifiers and fluoroscopy are considered more completely in Chatper 18.

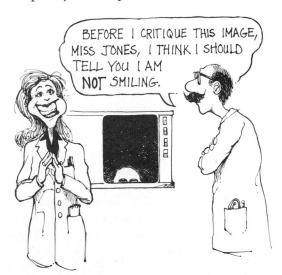

REVIEW QUESTIONS

1. Define or otherwise identify the following:
   a. Afterglow
   b. Isotropically
   c. Resolution
   d. Zinc cadmium sulfide
   e. Intensification factor
   f. Sensitivity spectrum
   g. Screen lag
   h. Phosphor
   i. Cassette compression
   j. Luminescence
2. Discuss the physical qualities that a material must possess to be used as a screen base material.
3. Describe the composition of a typical x-ray intensifying screen, including approximate layer thicknesses.
4. Discuss the two types of luminescence and how they are associated with intensifying screens and fluoroscopic screens.
5. What are the three main types of conventional intensifying screens and their approximate speeds? What accounts for the differences in screen speed?
6. The usual technique for an oblique radiograph of the foot employs direct-exposure film at 45 kVp, 150 mAs. If screens are used, the technique factors have to be changed to 45 kVp, 7.5 mAs to maintain the same average density. What is the approximate intensification factor for this screen-film combination?
7. Describe a technique designed to test for good screen-film contact.
8. What characteristics of phosphor materials make them especially suited for intensifying screens and fluoroscopic screens? What phosphor material is most often used for each?
9. Describe the construction of a film cassette, listing each layer from tube side to back.
10. Why do cassettes become worn with age? List the most common cassette malfunctions.

16

Radiographic quality

FILM FACTORS
GEOMETRIC FACTORS
SUBJECT FACTORS
CONSIDERATIONS FOR IMPROVED
RADIOGRAPHIC QUALITY

The term **radiographic quality** refers to the fidelity with which the anatomic structure under examination is imaged on the radiograph. A radiograph that faithfully reproduces structures and tissues is identified as a **high-quality radiograph.** A radiologist needs high-quality radiographs to make accurate diagnoses. Poor-quality radiographs contain images that are difficult for the human eye to interpret. They can lead to otherwise unnecessary reexaminations and, sometimes, missed diagnoses.

The quality of a radiograph is not easy to define, and it cannot be measured precisely. There are a number of factors that affect radiographic quality but no precise, universally accepted measures by which to judge it. Perhaps the two most important characteristics of radiographic quality are **resolution,** sometimes called sharpness, and **noise. Resolution is the ability to image two separate objects** and visually detect one from the other. **High-contrast resolution** refers

to objects having high subject contrast such as a bone–soft tissue interface. Conventional radiography is excellent for high-contrast resolution. **Low-contrast resolution** involves objects of very similar subject contrast such as the liver and pancreas. Computed tomography is excellent for low-contrast resolution. The actual size of objects that can be resolved will always be smaller under conditions of high contrast than under conditions of low contrast.

Noise is a term borrowed from electrical engineering. The hum, flutter, and whistle heard from a stereo system is **audio noise** that is inherent in the design of the system. The "snow" on television screens, especially in weak signal areas, is **video noise,** and it too is inherent in the system. **Radiographic noise is an undesirable fluctuation in the optical density of the image,** and it also is inherent in the imaging system. Fig. 16-1 shows an example of the appearance of noise on a radiograph. There are a

258

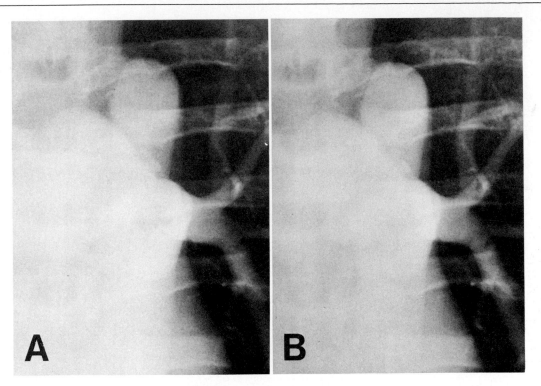

Fig. 16-1. This region of the aortic knob from a chest phantom radiograph illustrates radiographic noise. **A,** Radiograph with noise appears blotchy. **B,** Low-noise radiograph. (Courtesy Robert Waggener, University of Texas Health Science Center, San Antonio, Tex.)

number of contributing factors to radiographic noise, and some are under the control of the technologist. In general, the lower the noise, the better is the radiographic image.

Radiographic noise has three components: film graininess, structure mottle, and quantum mottle. **Film graininess** refers to the distribution in size and space of the silver halide grains in the emulsion. **Structure mottle** is similar to film graininess, but it refers to the construction of the phosphor of the radiographic intensifying screen. Film graininess and structure mottle are inherent in the image receptor. They are not under the control of the technologist, but they contribute very little to radiographic noise. **Quantum mottle** is somewhat under the control of the technologist, and it is the principal contributor to radiographic noise.

Quantum mottle refers to the random nature in which x rays interact with the image receptor. If an image is produced with just a few x-ray photons, the radiographic noise will be higher than if the image is formed from a large number of x rays. In general, **the use of high mAs, low kVp, and slower image receptors reduces radiographic noise.** The use of very fast intensifying screens results in increased quantum mottle.

These two characteristics of radiographic quality, resolution and noise, are intimately connected with a third characteristic—**speed.** Although the speed of the image receptor is not apparent on the radiographic image, it very much influences resolution and noise. In fact, a variation in any one of these characteristics will alter the other two, as illustrated in Fig. 16-2.

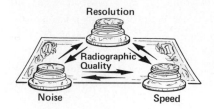

Fig. 16-2. Resolution, noise, and speed are interrelated characteristics of radiographic quality.

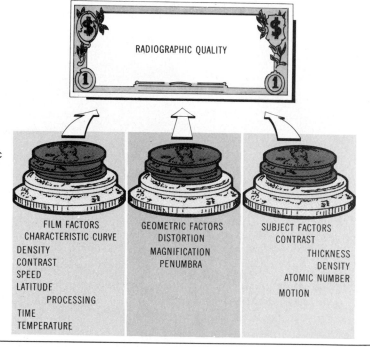

Fig. 16-3. Organizational chart of principal factors affecting radiographic quality.

As a general rule, the following statements apply:

1. **Fast image receptors have high noise and low resolution.**
2. **High resolution requires low noise and slow image receptors.**
3. **Low noise accompanies slow image receptors with high resolution.**

The radiologic technologist is provided with all the physical tools required to produce high-quality radiographs. The skillful technologist will properly manipulate these tools according to each specific clinical situation. Generally, the quality of a radiograph is directly related to the technologist's understanding of the basic principles of x-ray physics and of those factors affecting radiographic quality. Fig. 16-3 is an organizational chart of the principal factors affecting radiographic quality, most of which are under the control of the x-ray technologist. Each will be considered in detail.

FILM FACTORS

Unexposed x-ray film that has been processed appears quite **lucent,** like frosted window glass. It easily transmits light but not images. On the

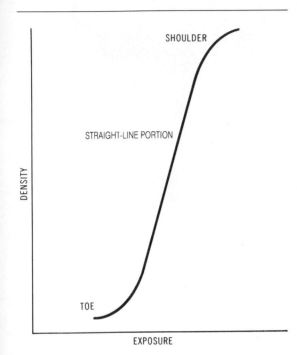

Fig. 16-4. Characteristic curve of radiographic film is the graphic relationship between density and exposure.

sometimes an H & D curve after Hurter and Driffield, who first described this relationship. A typical characteristic curve is shown in Fig. 16-4. At low and high exposure levels, large variations in exposure result in only a small change in density. These portions of the characteristic curve are called the **toe** and **shoulder,** respectively. At intermediate exposure levels, small changes in exposure result in large changes in density. This intermediate region, called the **straight-line portion** of the characteristic curve, is the area for proper exposure.

Two pieces of apparatus are needed to construct a characteristic curve: an aluminum step wedge, sometimes called a **penetrometer,** and a **densitometer.** The steps involved are outlined in Fig. 16-5. First, the film under investigation is exposed through the aluminum step wedge at some standard technique (for example, 70 kVp with 2.5 mm Al total filtration). When processed, the x-ray film will have areas of increasing density corresponding to sections of the step wedge with decreasing thickness. The step wedge is fabricated so that the intensity of exposure to the film under each step can be determined. The processed film is analyzed in the densitometer, a device that has a light source focused through a pinhole with a light-sensing device positioned on the opposite side of the film. The x-ray film is positioned between the pinhole and the light sensor, and the amount of light transmitted through each segment of the radiograph is measured. These data are recorded and analyzed and when plotted result in a characteristic curve.

Radiographic film is sensitive over a wide range of exposures. Screen film, for example, will respond to radiation intensities from under 5 to over 1000 mR. Consequently, the exposure values for a characteristic curve are presented in logarithmic fashion. Furthermore, it is not the absolute exposure that is of greatest interest but rather the change in density over each exposure interval. Therefore the log relative exposure is used as the scale along the x axis. Fig.

other hand, exposed, processed x-ray film can be quite **opaque.** Exposed film appears with various shades of gray, and heavily exposed film appears black. The study of the relationship between the intensity of exposure of the film and the blackness after processing is called **sensitometry.** The radiologic technologist will not normally be involved in sensitometric measurements, but knowledge of sensitometric aspects of radiographic film is essential.

Characteristic curve

The principal measurements involved in sensitometry are the exposure to the film and the percentage of light transmitted through the processed film. Such measurements are used to describe the relationship between **density,** the degree of blackness of the film, and exposure. This relationship is called a **characteristic curve,** or

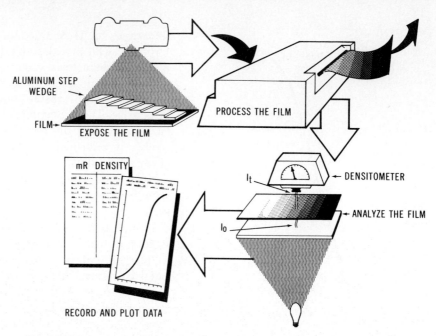

Fig. 16-5. Steps involved in construction of a characteristic curve.

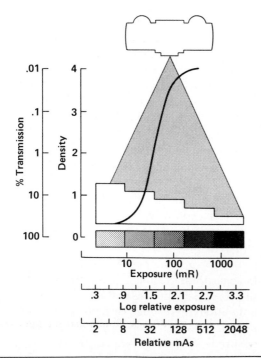

Fig. 16-6. Relationship among exposure, log relative exposure, and relative mAs for typical screen-film combination. Relationship between percent transmission and density is shown along the y axis.

16-6 shows exposure in mR and log relative exposure along the same scale for a representative screen-film combination. The log relative exposure scale is usually presented in increments of 0.3 because the log of 2 is 0.3. **An increase in log relative exposure of 0.3 results from doubling the exposure.** This can be accomplished by doubling the mAs as shown in Fig. 16-6.

Density. It is not enough to say that radiographic density is the degree of blackening of an x-ray film, or that a clear area of the radiograph represents low density, and a black area high density. Density has a precise numerical value that can be calculated if the level of light incident (I_0) on a processed film and the level of light transmitted through that film (I_t) can be measured. The **density** (D) is defined as follows:

(16-1)

$$D = log_{10} \frac{I_0}{I_t}$$

Density is short for optical density. It is a logarithmic function. Logarithms allow a wide range of values to be expressed by small numbers. Radiographic film contains densities ranging from near 0 to 4; these densities correspond to clear and black, respectively. A density of 4 actually means that only 1 in 10,000 light photons is capable of penetrating the x-ray film. Table 16-1 shows the range of light transmission corresponding to various levels of radiographic density.

High-quality glass has an optical density of 0, which means that all light incident on such glass is transmitted. Unexposed x-ray film allows no more than about 80% of incident light photons to be transmitted. Most unexposed and processed radiographic film has a density in the range of 0.1 to 0.15, corresponding to 79% and 71% transmission, respectively.

These undesirable densities are due to base density and fog density, the graphic interpretations of which are shown in Fig. 16-7. The base density is the density inherent in the base

Table 16-1. Relationship of density of radiographic film to light transmission through the film

Percent of light transmitted $(I_t/I_0 \times 100)$	Fraction of light transmitted (I_t/I_0)	Density $(log\ I_0/I_t)$
100	1	0
50	1/2	0.3
32	8/25	0.5
25	1/4	0.6
12.5	1/8	0.9
10	1/10	1
5	1/20	1.3
3.2	4/125	1.5
2.5	1/30	1.6
1.25	1/80	1.9
1	1/100	2
0.5	1/200	2.3
0.32	2/625	2.5
0.125	1/800	2.9
0.1	1/1000	3
0.05	1/2000	3.3
0.032	1/3125	3.5
0.01	1/10,000	4

of the film. It is due to the composition of the base and the tint added to the base to make the radiograph more pleasing to the eye. Base density usually has a value of approximately 0.05. Fog has been previously described as the development of silver grains that contain no useful information. Film fog results from inadvertent exposure of film during storage, undesirable chemical contamination, improper processing, and a number of other influences. Fog density on a processed radiograph should not exceed 0.05. Higher fog levels will drastically reduce the quality of the radiograph.

EXAMPLE: The light incident on the radiograph of a long bone has a relative value of 1500. If the light transmitted through the radiopaque bony structures has an intensity of 480, and the light trans-

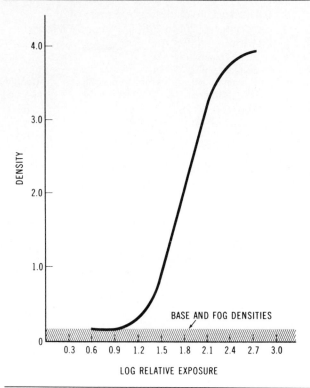

Fig. 16-7. Base and fog densities contribute no diagnostic information to the radiograph and should be as low as possible.

mitted through the radiolucent soft tissue has an intensity of 2, what are the approximate respective film densities? Refer to Table 16-1 if necessary.

ANSWER:
$$D = log_{10} \frac{I_0}{I_t}$$

a. For bone:
$$D = log_{10} \frac{1500}{480}$$
$$= 0.5$$

b. For soft tissue:
$$D = log_{10} \frac{1500}{2}$$
$$= 2.9$$

The useful range of radiographic densities is approximately 0.25 to 2.5. However, approximately 75% of all radiographs show image patterns in the range of 0.5 to 1.25 optical density. Attention to this part of the characteristic curve is essential.

Reciprocity law. One would think that the density on the photographic film would be strict-

ly dependent on the total exposure and independent of the time of exposure. This, in fact, is the reciprocity law. It states that **the density of a photographic film is proportional only to the energy imparted to the film.** Whether a film is exposed over a very short period of time (for example, 1 ms) or over hours or even days, the reciprocity law states that the optical density will be the same if the total energy imparted to the film is constant. The reciprocity law holds for direct exposure with x rays, but it does not hold for exposure of film by visible light. Consequently, **the reciprocity law fails for screen-film exposures** at exposure times less than approximately 10 ms or longer than approximately 10 s. Film density will be somewhat less at such short or long exposure times than exposure times within that range, even though the radiation exposure is the same. Consequently, reciprocity law failure is not of much importance in

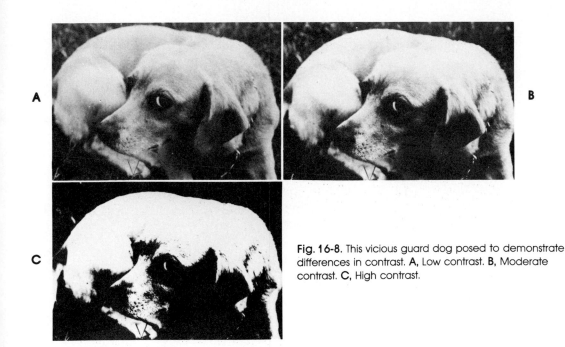

Fig. 16-8. This vicious guard dog posed to demonstrate differences in contrast. **A,** Low contrast. **B,** Moderate contrast. **C,** High contrast.

diagnostic radiology except for some special procedures that require millisecond timing. For these few situations a technique change of increasing mAs will be required.

Contrast. When a high-quality radiograph is placed in an illuminator, the differences in density it contains are obvious and result in the image. These density differences are called **radiographic contrast.** A radiograph that has sharp differences in density is called a high-contrast radiograph. On the other hand, if the density differences are small and not distinct, the radiograph is of low contrast. Fig. 16-8 illustrates the difference between high contrast and low contrast with a photographic scene.

Radiographic contrast is the product of two separate factors:

1. **Film contrast** is inherent in the film and influenced somewhat by the processing of the film.

2. **Subject contrast** is determined by the size, shape, and x-ray–attenuating characteristics of the subject being examined.

Radiographic contrast can be greatly affected by changes in either film contrast or subject contrast. In the clinical setting it is usually best to standardize the film contrast and alter the subject contrast according to the needs of the examination. Subject contrast will be dealt with in greater detail later.

Film contrast is inherent in the type of film being employed. It can, however, be influenced by two other factors, the film density and the film-processing technique. Film selection is generally limited and determined somewhat by the intensifying screen employed. Screen-film images always have higher contrast than direct-exposure images. All these factors require some judgment on the part of the radiologic technologist.

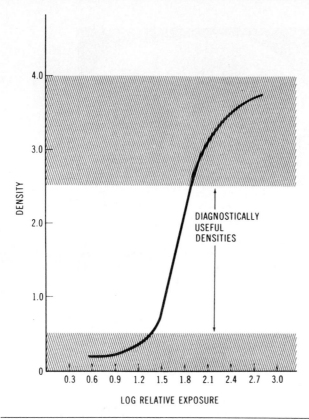

Fig. 16-9. If the exposure of the film results in densities that lie in the toe or shoulder regions, where the slope of the curve is less, contrast will be lost.

The best control the technologist can exercise is exposing the film properly so that the apparent densities lie within the diagnostically useful range: 0.5 to 2.5. When the exposure of the film results in densities outside this range, contrast is lost. Fig. 16-9 demonstrates this property. Put another way, if the exposure of the radiograph results in densities corresponding to the extreme toe or shoulder of the characteristic curve for that film, then film contrast will be lost. On the other hand, since most radiographic densities lie in the toe region, it is important to expose the x-ray film so that the range of densities observed will lie in the diagnostically useful range, particularly the region from 0.5 to 1.25 optical density.

Standardized film-processing techniques are absolutely necessary for consistent film contrast and good radiographic quality. Deviation from manufacturer recommendations will result in reduced contrast.

The characteristic curve of a film allows one to judge at a glance the relative degree of contrast for that particular film. Mathematically, **film contrast is equal to the slope of the straight-line portion of the characteristic curve.** If this slope had a value of 1, then the straight-line portion of the characteristic curve would be angled up to 45 degrees. An increase of 1 unit along the log relative exposure axis would result in an increase of 1 unit along the density axis. The contrast would be 1. Film that has a contrast of 1 is very low-contrast film. Film with a contrast higher than 1 in effect amplifies the relative differences in x-ray exposure to the film. Film with a contrast of 3, for instance, would show large

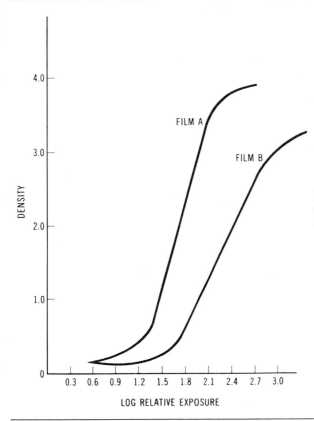

Fig. 16-10. Slope of the straight-line portion of the characteristic curve is greater for film A than for film B. Film A has higher contrast.

density differences over a small range of x-ray exposure.

Generally, it is not necessary for the radiologic technologist to have a precise knowledge of film contrast, but, from the appearance of the characteristic curve, the technologist should be able to distinguish high-contrast from low-contrast film. Fig. 16-10 shows the characteristic curves for two different types of x-ray film. Film A has higher contrast than film B, as shown by the fact that the slope of the straight-line portion of the characteristic curve is greater for A than for B.

Several methods are employed to numerically specify film contrast. The one most often employed is **average gradient.** The average gradient is the slope of a straight line drawn between the two points on the characteristic curve at density levels 0.25 and 2 above the combined base and fog densities. The equation for average gradient is

(16-2)

$$Average\ gradient = \frac{D_2 - D_1}{LRE_2 - LRE_1}$$

where D_2 is the optical density of 2 plus base and fog, D_1 is the optical density of 0.25 plus base and fog, and LRE_2 and LRE_1 are the log relative exposures associated with D_2 and D_1, respectively. This method is diagramed in Fig. 16-11 for a film having a combined base and fog density of 0.2.

Most radiographic films have an average gradient in the range of 2.5 to 3.5. Since the average gradient of x-ray film is usually much larger than 1, x-ray film acts as an amplifier of subject con-

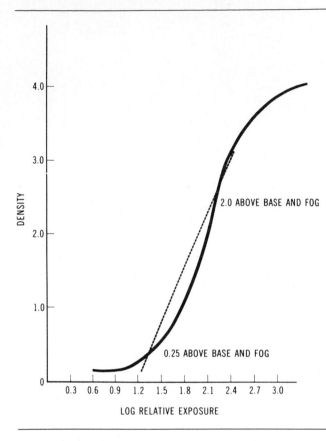

Fig. 16-11. Average gradient is the slope of the line drawn between the points on the characteristic curve that correspond to density levels 0.25 and 2.0 above the combined base and fog densities.

trast; that is, the range of the number of x-ray photons producing the latent image is effectively expanded, and the subject contrast is enhanced.

Film contrast may also be identified by **gradient.** The gradient is the slope of the tangent at any point on the characteristic curve. **Toe gradient** is probably more important than average gradient or midgradient, since most densities appear in the toe region of the characteristic curve.

EXAMPLE: A radiographic film has a base density of 0.06 and a fog density of 0.11. At what densities should one evaluate the characteristic curve to determine the film contrast?

ANSWER: The curve should be evaluated at densities 0.25 and 2 above base and fog densities, that is, at points corresponding to densities of 0.25 + 0.06 + 0.11 and 2 + 0.06 + 0.11, or 0.42 and 2.17.

EXAMPLE: If densities of 0.42 and 2.17 on the characteristic curve in the preceding example correspond to log relative exposures of 0.95 and 1.75, what is the average gradient?

ANSWER: *Average gradient* $= \dfrac{D_2 - D_1}{LRE_2 - LRE_1}$

$$= \frac{2.17 - 0.42}{1.75 - 0.95}$$

$$= \frac{1.75}{0.8}$$

$$= 2.19$$

Speed. The ability of an x-ray film to respond to a minimum quantity of x-ray exposure is a measure of its **sensitivity** or, more commonly, its **speed.** An exposure of less than 1 mR can be detected with a screen-film combination, whereas several mR are necessary to produce a measurable response with direct-exposure film.

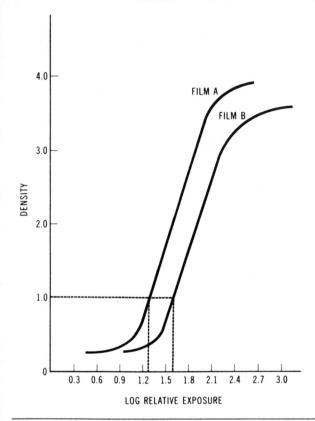

Fig. 16-12. Speed of a film is the reciprocal of the exposure, in roentgens, needed to produce a density of 1. Film *A* is faster than film *B*.

The characteristic curve of an x-ray film is also useful in identifying film speed. Fig. 16-12 shows the characteristic curves of two different x-ray films. Since film *A* requires less exposure than film *B* to produce any density, film *A* is said to be faster than film *B*. The characteristic curves of fast films are positioned to the left of those of slow films along the log relative exposure scale. X-ray films are identified as either fast or slow according to their relative sensitivity to exposure.

Usually the identification of a given film as so many times faster than another film is sufficient for the technologist. If film *A* were twice as fast as film *B*, film *A* would require only half the exposure required by film *B* to produce a specified density. Moreover, the image on film *A* might be of poor quality because of increased radiographic noise.

In sensitometry the density specified for determining film speed is 1, and the speed is measured in **reciprocal roentgens.** The following is the definition of film speed:

(16-3)

$$Speed = \frac{1}{\begin{array}{c} Number\ of\ roentgens \\ needed\ to\ produce\ a\ density\ of\ 1 \end{array}}$$

EXAMPLE: The characteristic curve of a given film shows that 25 mR are needed to produce a density of 1 on that film. What is the film speed?

ANSWER: $Speed = \dfrac{1}{25 \text{ mR}} = \dfrac{1}{0.025 \text{ R}} = 40$

Latitude. The fourth x-ray film characteristic easily obtained from the characteristic curve is the film **latitude.** Latitude refers to the range of exposures over which the x-ray film will respond

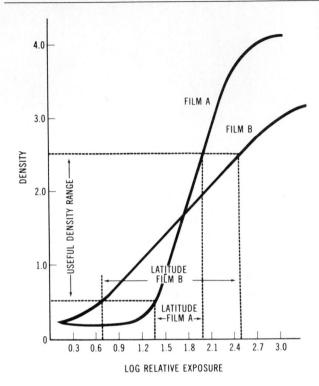

Fig. 16-13. Latitude of a film is the exposure range over which it responds with diagnostically useful densities.

with densities in the diagnostically useful range. Fig. 16-13 shows two films of comparable speeds but different latitudes. Film *B* responds to a much wider range of exposures than film *A* and is said to have wider latitude than film *A*. Films with wide latitude are said to have **long gray scale,** and those with narrow latitude have **short gray scale.** From Fig. 16-13 it should be clear that **latitude and contrast are inversely proportional:** high-contrast film has narrow latitude, and low-contrast film has wide latitude.

Film processing

Proper film processing is required for optimum film contrast primarily because the degree of development has a pronounced effect on the level of film fog and on the density resulting from a given exposure at a given film speed. The important factors affecting the degree of development are (1) the composition of processing chemicals, (2) the degree of film agitation during development, (3) the development time, and (4) the development temperature. The two factors particularly subject to control by the radiologic technologist are the time and temperature of development.

Development time. As development time is varied, the characteristic curve for any film will vary in shape and in position along the log relative exposure axis. These changes are represented in Fig. 16-14. If the characteristic curves were analyzed for contrast, speed, and fog level, each would be shown to vary as in Fig. 16-15. Speed and fog increase with lengthening development time. Contrast increases and then de-

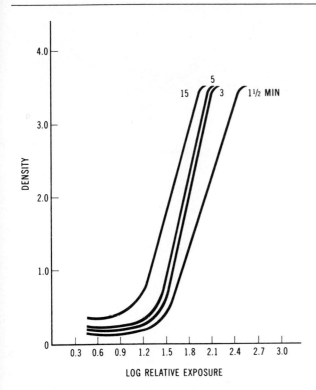

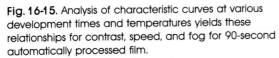

Fig. 16-14. As development time increases, changes occur in the shape and relative position of the characteristic curve.

Fig. 16-15. Analysis of characteristic curves at various development times and temperatures yields these relationships for contrast, speed, and fog for 90-second automatically processed film.

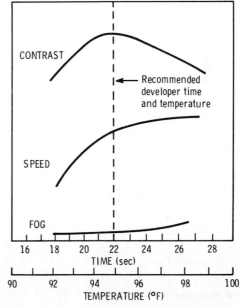

creases with development time. The development time recommended by the manufacturer is the time that will result in maximum contrast at relatively high levels of speed and low levels of fog. When development time extends much beyond the recommmended period, the film contrast decreases and the fog level increases.

Development temperature. The relationship just described for variations in development time applies equally well to variations in development temperature. If the average gradient, speed, and fog level for the characteristic curves representative of various temperatures were plotted as a function of development temperature, the results would appear as in Fig. 16-15. As with time of development, the maximum contrast is obtained at the recommended development temperature. The fog level increases with increasing temperature, as does x-ray film speed.

Most hand processed films require development at 68° F (20° C) for 5 minutes. Within a small range, a change in either time or temperature can be compensated for by a change in the other. It should be clear, however, that a small change in either time or temperature alone can result in a large change in the sensitometric characteristics of the x-ray film. With rapid processing, monitoring of time and temperature for film development is even more important than for hand processing. If the processing time of an automatic processor is optimized at 90 s, a variation of 5 s in development time can result in significant changes in radiographic qualtiy.

GEOMETRIC FACTORS

Making a radiograph is similar in many ways to taking a photograph. Proper exposure time and intensity are required for both. Images are recorded in both because the x rays and the visible-light photons travel in straight lines. In that regard, an x-ray image may be considered analogous to a shadowgraph. Fig. 16-16 shows the familiar shadowgraph that can be made to

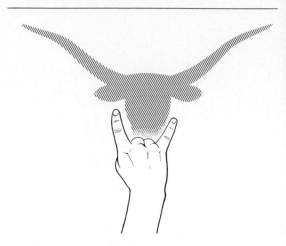

Fig. 16-16. A shadowgraph is analogous to a radiograph. (Dedicated to Xie Nan Zhu, Guangzhou, People's Republic of China.)

appear on a wall if light is shone on a properly contorted hand.

The sharpness of the shadow image on the wall is a function of a number of geometric factors. For example, the closer to the wall the hand is placed, the sharper the shadow will be. Similarly, the farther from the hand the light source is, the sharper the shadow will be. These geometric conditions also apply to radiology and the production of high-quality radiographs. There are three principal geometric factors that affect radiographic quality: (1) magnification, (2) distortion, and (3) characteristics of the x-ray tube. The latter cannot normally be controlled by the radiologic technologist.

Magnification

All images on the radiograph are larger than the object they represent, a condition called **magnification.** For most clinical examinations it is desirable to maintain as low a magnification as possible. During some situations, however, magnification is desirable and is carefully planned into the radiographic examination. This type of examination is called **magnification radiography.** It will be dealt with in Chapter 18.

Quantitatively, magnification is measured and expressed by the magnification factor *(MF)*, which is defined as follows:

(16-4)

$$MF = \frac{Image\ size}{Object\ size}$$

The magnification factor is dependent on the conditions of examination. For most radiographs taken at an SID of 100 cm, the magnification factor will be approximately 1.1; for radiographs taken at 180 cm SID, it would be approximately 1.05.

EXAMPLE: If a heart measures 12.5 cm from side to side at its widest point, and its image on a chest radiograph measures 14.7 cm, what is the magnification factor?

ANSWER: $MF = \dfrac{14.7\ cm}{12.5\ cm} = 1.176$

In the usual radiographic examination it is not possible to determine the object size. The image size may be measured directly from the radiograph. In such situations the magnification factor can be determined from the ratio of the SID to the source-to-object distance (SOD):

(16-5)

$$MF = \frac{SID}{SOD}$$

Fig. 16-17 shows that this method of calculating the magnification factor results from the basic geometric relationship between similar triangles. If two right triangles have a common hypotenuse, the ratio of the height of one to its base will be the same as the ratio of the height of the other to its base. In this representation the object size and the image size are both two times the size of the base of their respective triangles. This is the situation that generally is encountered in radiology. The SID is known and can be measured directly. The SOD can be estimated relatively accurately by a radiologic technologist who has a good foundation in human anatomy.

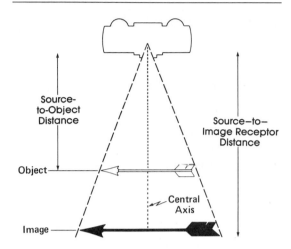

Fig. 16-17. Magnification can be measured by the ratio of image size to object size or SID to SOD.

EXAMPLE: A lateral film of the lumbar spine taken at 100 cm SID results in the image of a vertebral body with maximum and minimum dimensions of 6.4 cm and 4.2 cm. The width of the patient at that level is 40 cm, and the film-to-tabletop distance is 5 cm. What is the object size?

ANSWER: $MF = \dfrac{100}{100 - (40/2 + 5)} = \dfrac{100}{75} = 1.33$

Therefore the object size is

$$\frac{6.4}{1.33} \times \frac{4.2}{1.33} = 4.81\ cm \times 3.16\ cm$$

One might ask if these relationships hold for images off the central axis as shown in Fig. 16-18. The magnification factor will be the same for objects positioned off the central axis as for those lying on the central axis if the object–to–image receptor (OID) distance is the same and if the object is essentially flat. The two previous relationships for calculating the magnification factor are appropriate for use with the off-axis subject. In Fig. 16-18 the projection lines indicate that the two triangles of interest, although not right triangles, are still similar triangles; therefore the ratio of height to base is the same in both.

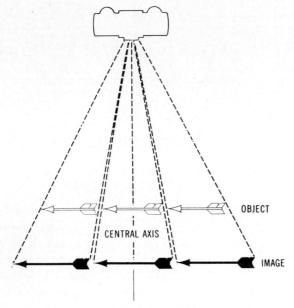

Fig. 16-18. Magnification of an object positioned off the central x-ray axis is the same as that for an object in the central axis if the objects are in the same plane.

Fig. 16-19. Graph showing value of magnification factor at 90, 100, and 180 cm SID for various object-to-film distances.

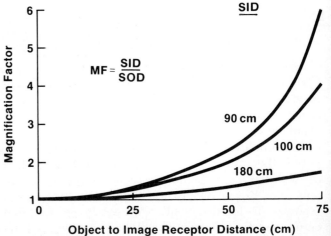

$$MF = \frac{SID}{SOD}$$

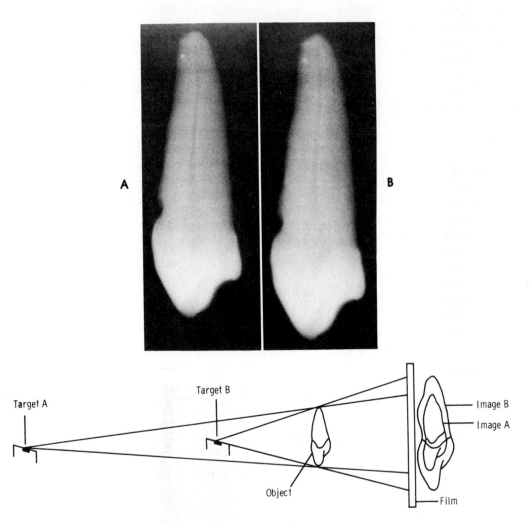

Fig. 16-20. Periapical radiographs of a bicuspid. **A,** 40 cm SID. **B,** 20 cm SID. The long-cone technique results in noticeably less magnification.

In summary, there are two factors that affect magnification, and, to maintain minimum magnification, one should observe the basic rules:

1. Large SID: use as large a source–to–image receptor distance as possible.
2. Small OID: place the object as close to the image receptor as possible.

The SID is standardized in most radiology departments to 180 cm for chest work, 100 cm for routine examinations, and 90 cm for some special studies such as portable films and skull films. Fig. 16-19 shows the value of the magnification factor for these three SIDs and for OIDs varying from 0 to 75 cm.

There are two familiar clinical situations in which minimum magnification is routinely obtained. Most chest radiographs are taken at 180 cm SID from the posterior-anterior projection. This projection results in a smaller heart–to–image receptor distance than an anterior-posterior projection. Magnification is reduced because of the large SID and the small OID. Many dentists now take bite-wing and periapical exposures at 40 cm SID rather than at 20 cm SID, the technique that prevailed for years. Using the 40 cm SID, known as **long-cone technique** dental radiography, has many advantages over the short-cone technique. One such advantage is less magnification. Fig. 16-20 shows periapical radiographs of the bicuspid taken at 20 and 40 cm SID. The difference in magnification is obvious even though the OID is small in each case.

Distortion

The previous discussion concerning magnification assumed a very simple object, an arrow, lying perpendicular to the central x-ray beam at a fixed OID. If any one of these conditions is changed, as they all are in most clinical examinations, the magnification will not be the same over the entire object. **Unequal magnification of different portions of the same object is called**

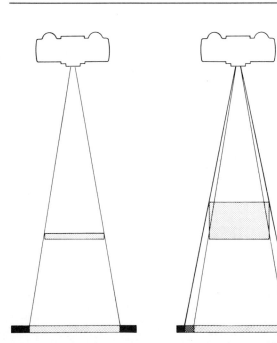

Fig. 16-21. Thick objects result in unequal magnification and therefore more distortion than thin objects.

distortion. Distortion can hinder proper interpretation of the radiograph. Two conditions contribute to image distortion: (1) the size and shape of the object and (2) the position of the object.

Object size and shape. Thick objects are distorted and thin objects are not. With a thick object the OID changes measurably across the object. Consider, for instance, two rectangular structures of different thicknesses, as shown in Fig. 16-21. Because of the change in OID across the thicker structure, the image of that structure will be more distorted than the image of the thinner structure.

Object shape also affects image distortion. The images produced by a disk and a sphere of the same diameter will be the same on the central axis. Lateral to the central axis, both images will be distorted. Fig. 16-22 demonstrates this property of image distortion. If the OID remains constant, both the disk and the sphere will appear elliptic in the image plane lateral to the central axis, but the sphere will be less distorted than the disk.

Object position. If the object plane and the image plane are parallel, the image will be undistorted, but if the object plane and image plane are not parallel, distortion will occur. Such distortion is a possibility in every radiographic examination if proper patient positioning is not maintained. Fig. 16-23, an example of gross distortion, shows that the image of an inclined arrow can be smaller than the object itself. In such a condition the image is said to be **foreshortened.** The amount of foreshortening (the amount of reduction in image size) increases as the angle of inclination increases.

If an inclined object is not located on the central x-ray beam, the degree of distortion will be affected by not only the object's angle of inclination but also its lateral position from the cen-

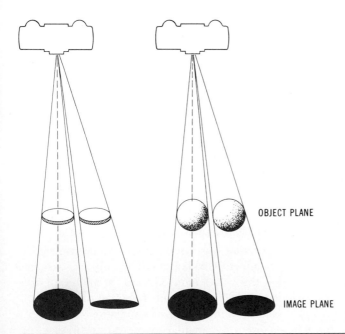

OBJECT PLANE

IMAGE PLANE

Fig. 16-22. Object shape influences distortion. Radiographs of a disk or sphere will appear as circles if the object is on the central axis. If they are lateral to the central axis, both will appear elliptic.

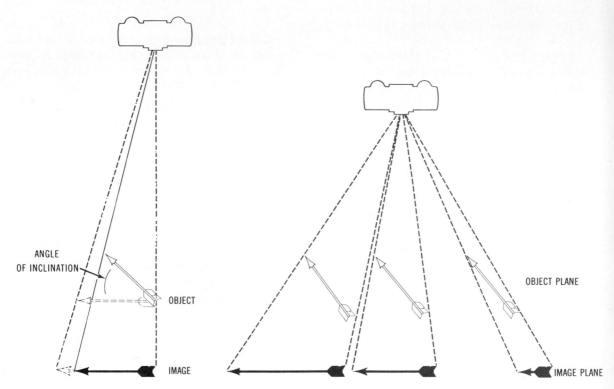

Fig. 16-23. Inclination of an object results in a foreshortened image.

Fig. 16-24. An inclined object positioned lateral to the central x-ray beam may be severely distorted by magnification or foreshortening.

tral x-ray beam. Fig. 16-24 illustrates this situation and shows that the image of an inclined object can be severely foreshortened or considerably magnified.

With multiple objects positioned at various OIDs, **spatial distortion** can occur. Spatial distortion is the misrepresentation in the image of the actual spatial relationships among the objects. Fig. 16-25 demonstrates this condition for two arrows of the same size, one of which lies on top of the other. Because of the position of the arrows, only one image should be seen, representing the superimposition of the arrows. However, unequal magnification of the two objects causes arrow *A* to appear larger than arrow *B* and to be positioned more laterally. This distortion is minimum for objects lying along the central x-ray beam. As object position is shifted laterally from the central axis, spatial distortion can become significant.

Geometric unsharpness

Thus far our discussion of the geometric factors affecting radiographic quality has assumed that the x rays emitted from the target all originate at the same point. In actual practice there is not a point source of x-radiation but rather a square or rectangular source varying in size from

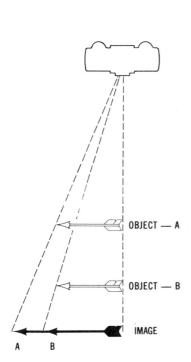

Fig. 16-25. When objects of the same size are positioned at different distances from the film, spatial distortion occurs.

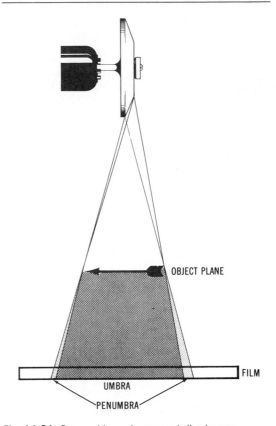

Fig. 16-26. Geometric unsharpness is the image blurring caused by the measurable size of the focal spot. Another name for geometric unsharpness is penumbra.

approximately 0.3 to 2 mm on a side, depending on the type of x-ray tube in use.

Fig. 16-26 illustrates the result of using x-ray tubes with measurable effective focal spots as imaging devices. The point of the object arrow in Fig. 16-26 will not appear as a point in the image plane because the x rays used to image the point originate in different locations in the target. A blurred region on the radiograph over which the radiologic technologist has little control will result because the effective focal spot size is not a point. This phenomenon is called **geometric unsharpness,** or **penumbra,** and as illustrated it is greater on the cathode side of

the image. Penumbra reduces resolution and is undesirable. Fig. 16-26 shows that for the same radiographic condition there will be a region in which the object is properly imaged, called the **umbra.**

Three conditions result in high penumbra:
1. Large effective focal spot
2. Short SID
3. Long OID

The geometric relationships governing magnification also influence penumbra. As the geometry of the source, object, and image are altered to produce greater magnification, they also produce increased penumbra blurring of the

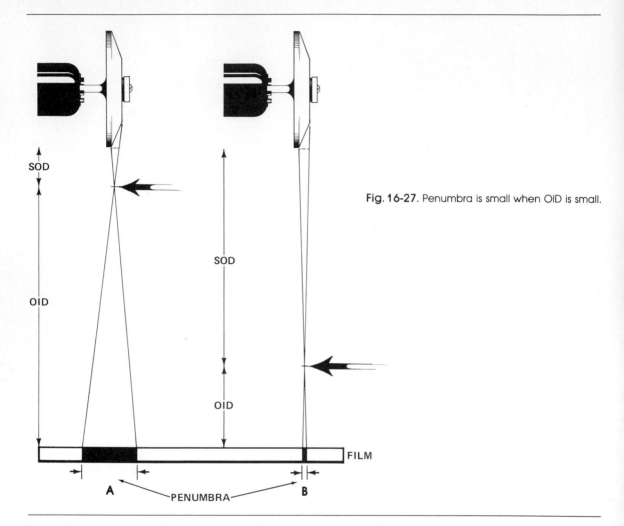

Fig. 16-27. Penumbra is small when OID is small.

radiograph. Consequently, these conditions should be avoided when possible.

The region of geometric unsharpness can be calculated using similar triangles. If an arrowhead were positioned near the tube target, as in Fig. 16-27, *A*, the size of the penumbra would be larger than that of the effective focal spot. Generally, the object is much closer to the film, as in Fig. 16-27, *B*, and therefore the penumbra is much smaller than the effective focal spot. From these drawings one can see that two similar triangles are described. Therefore the ratio of the source-to-object distance (SOD) to the object–to–image receptor distance (OID) is the same as the ratio of the sizes of the effective focal spot and the penumbra. Mathematically, this is rendered as follows:

(16-6)

$$Penumbra\ (P) = (Effective\ focal\ spot) \frac{OID}{SOD}$$

EXAMPLE: An x-ray tube target having a 1.6 mm effective focal spot is used to image an object in a chest cavity estimated to be 8 cm from anterior chest wall. If the radiograph is taken posterior-anterior at 180 cm SID, with a tabletop film separation of 5 cm, what will be the size of the penumbra?

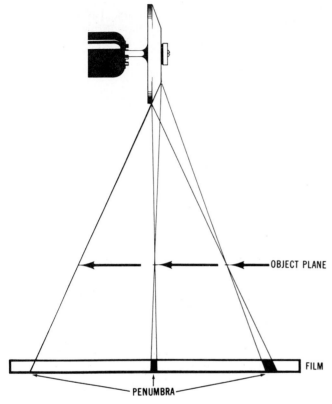

Fig. 16-28. Effective focal spot size is largest on the cathode side, and therefore the geometric unsharpness of a radiograph is greatest on the cathode side.

ANSWER: $P = (1.6 \text{ mm}) \dfrac{8 + 5}{180 - (8 + 5)}$

$= (1.6 \text{ mm}) \dfrac{13}{167}$

$= (1.6 \text{ mm})(0.078)$

$= 0.125 \text{ mm}$

To minimize penumbra, one uses small focal spots and positions the patient so that the part of the body under examination is close to the film. The SID is usually fixed.

Heel effect. The heel effect, introduced in Chapter 7, was described as a varying intensity across the x-ray field caused by attenuation of x rays in the heel of the anode. Another characteristic of the heel effect is unrelated to x-ray intensity but affects geometric unsharpness. The size of the effective focal spot is not constant across the radiograph. A tube said to have a 1 mm focal spot has a smaller effective focal spot on the anode side and a larger effective focal spot on the cathode side. This condition is diagramed in Fig. 16-28.

This variation in focal spot size results in a variation in penumbral size. **The penumbra is small on the anode side and large on the cathode side.** Consequently, images to the cathode side of a radiograph have higher geometric unsharpness and poorer resolution than those to the anode side. This situation is significant when x-ray tubes with low target angles are used at short SIDs.

SUBJECT FACTORS

The third general group of factors affecting radiographic quality concerns the patient. These factors are those associated not so much with the positioning of the patient as with the selection of a radiographic technique that properly compensates for the patient's size, shape, and composition. Patient positioning is basically a requirement associated with the geometric factors affecting radiographic quality.

Subject contrast

The contrast of a radiograph viewed in an illuminator is called **radiographic contrast.** As indicated previously, radiographic contrast is a function of the film contrast and the subject contrast. In fact, the radiographic contrast is simply the product of the film contrast and the subject contrast.

(16-7)
$$Radiographic\ contrast = \\ Film\ contrast \times subject\ contrast$$

EXAMPLE: Direct-exposure film having an average gradient of 3.1 is used to radiograph a long bone having a subject contrast of 4.5. What is the radiographic contrast?

ANSWER: *Radiographic contrast* = (3.1)(4.5)
= 13.95

In practice, subject contrast is difficult to determine quantitatively. The factors that affect subject contrast, on the other hand, can be readily described as follows:
1. Patient thickness
2. Tissue density
3. Effective atomic number
4. Object shape
5. Kilovoltage

Several of these factors were discussed in Chapter 9 in their relation to the effective attenuation of an x-ray beam. The effect of each on subject contrast is a direct result of differences in attenuation in body tissues.

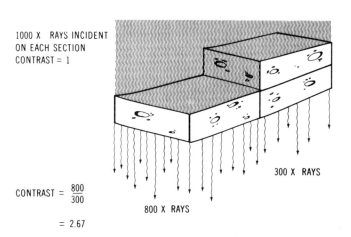

1000 X RAYS INCIDENT
ON EACH SECTION
CONTRAST = 1

300 X RAYS

CONTRAST = $\frac{800}{300}$

800 X RAYS

= 2.67

Fig. 16-29. Variation in thickness of body part contributes to subject contrast.

Patient thickness. Given a standard composition, a thick body section will attenuate more x rays than a thin body section. Fig. 16-29 demonstrates this difference in attenuation. The same number of x rays are incident on each section, and therefore the contrast of the incident x-ray beam is 1; there is no contrast at all. If the same number of x rays exited each section, the subject contrast would be 1. However, since more x rays are transmitted through thin body sections than through thick ones, subject contrast will be greater than 1. The degree of subject contrast is directly proportional to the relative number of x rays exiting adjoining sections of the body.

Tissue density. Adjoining sections of the body may have equal thicknesses yet greatly different densities. Tissue density is an important factor affecting subject contrast. Consider, for example, the radiograph of an ice cube in water. The materials have the same thickness and chemical composition. The ice, however, is not so dense as the water and therefore will be imaged. The

effect of density on subject contrast is demonstrated in Fig. 16-30.

Effective atomic number. Another important factor affecting subject contrast is the effective atomic number of the tissue being examined. In Chapter 9 it was shown that Compton interactions are independent of atomic number, but photoelectric interactions vary greatly with atomic number. The effective atomic numbers of tissues of interest were reported in Table 9-1. In the diagnostic range of x-ray energies, the photoelectric effect is of considerable importance; therefore the subject contrast is greatly influenced by the effective atomic number of the tissue being radiographed.

Shape. The shape of the anatomic structure under investigation influences the radiographic quality not only through its geometry but also through its contribution to subject contrast. Obviously, a structure having the form of a truncated wedge that would coincide with the x-ray beam would have maximum subject contrast, as

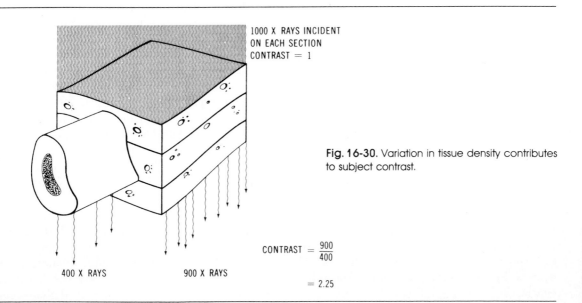

1000 X RAYS INCIDENT
ON EACH SECTION
CONTRAST = 1

400 X RAYS   900 X RAYS

$$CONTRAST = \frac{900}{400}$$

$$= 2.25$$

Fig. 16-30. Variation in tissue density contributes to subject contrast.

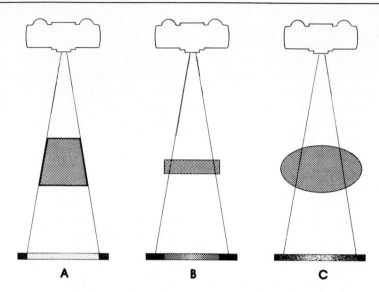

Fig. 16-31. Shape of the structure under investigation contributes to absorption unsharpness.

shown in Fig. 16-31, *A*. All other anatomic shapes have reduced subject contrast because of the change in thickness that they present to incident x-ray photons. Fig. 16-31, *B* and *C*, shows examples of two shapes that result in a reduced subject contrast.

This characteristic of the subject affecting subject contrast is sometimes termed **absorption unsharpness.** It reduces radiographic quality during imaging of any anatomic structure, but it is most troublesome during angiographic procedures where vessels with small diameters are under examination.

Kilovoltage. The radiologic technologist has no control over the four previous factors influencing subject contrast. The absolute magnitude of subject contrast, however, is greatly controlled by the kVp of operation. In fact, kVp is probably the most important influence on subject contrast. Kilovoltage also influences film contrast but not to the extent it controls subject contrast.

Fig. 16-32 shows a composite of a series of radiographs of an aluminum step wedge taken at kVp's ranging from 40 to 100. Low kVp results in high subject contrast, sometimes called **short-scale contrast,** since the radiographic image will appear either black or white with few shades of gray. On the other hand, high kVp results in low subject contrast, or **long-scale contrast.**

It would be easy to jump to the conclusion that low-kVp techniques are always more desirable than high-kVp techniques. However, there are two major disadvantages to low-kVp radiography. One is high patient dose; the other is loss of exposure latitude. A radiographic technique that produces low subject contrast allows for wide latitude in exposure factors. Optimization of radiographic technique is not so critical when using high kVp.

Subject contrast can be greatly enhanced by the use of contrast media. The high atomic numbers of iodine (Z = 53) and barium (Z = 56) result in extremely high subject contrast. Contrast media are effective because they accentuate subject contrast through increased photoelectric absorption.

Fig. 16-32. Radiographs of an aluminum step wedge demonstrating change in contrast with varying kVp. (Courtesy Eastman Kodak Co.)

Motion unsharpness

Movement of either the patient or the x-ray tube during the x-ray exposure will result in a blurring of the radiographic image. This loss of radiographic quality, called **motion unsharpness,** may result in reexamination.

Normally, motion of the x-ray tube head is not a problem. In tomography the tube head is deliberately moved in a precise geometric pattern during exposure to blur the images of structures on either side of the plane of interest. Tomog-

raphy is described in Chapter 18. Sometimes the table or another restraining device is caused to move by auxiliary equipment such as a moving grid mechanism.

Patient motion usually accounts for motion unsharpness. Motion unsharpness can be reduced by careful instruction of the patient by the radiologic technologist: "Take a deep breath and hold it. Don't move."

Motion unsharpness is primarily affected by

four factors. By observing the following guidelines, the radiologic technologist can reduce motion unsharpness:

1. Use the shortest possible exposure time.
2. Restrict patient motion by instruction or restraining device.
3. Use a large SID.
4. Use a small OID.

Note that the last two have the same relation to motion unsharpness as to geometric unsharpness. With the use of three-phase power and 400-speed receptors for Bucky technique, motion has essentially been removed as a clinical problem.

CONSIDERATIONS FOR IMPROVED RADIOGRAPHIC QUALITY

The radiologic technologist normally has the tools available to produce high-quality radiographs. The selection of proper radiographic technique, proper imaging devices, and proper patient preparation is not straightforward and cannot be simply stated in a general rule. These factors, all of which affect radiographic quality, are very much interrelated. For any given radiologic examination, a proper interpretation and application of each of these factors must be made. A small change in one may require a compensating change in another.

Patient positioning

The importance of patient positioning should now be clear. Proper patient positioning requires that the anatomic structure under investigation be placed as close to the image receptor as practical and that the axis of this structure lie in a plane parallel to the plane of the image receptor. The central x-ray beam should be incident on the center of the structure. Finally, the patient must be effectively restained to minimize motion unsharpness.

To be able to position patients properly, the radiologic technologist must have a good knowledge of human anatomy. If multiple structures are being radiographed and are to be imaged with uniform magnification, they must be equi-

distant from the film. The various techniques described in textbooks on radiographic positioning are designed to produce radiographs with minimum image distortion and maximum image resolution.

Imaging devices

Usually a standard type of screen-film combination is employed throughout a radiology department for a given examination. Generally, extremity and soft tissue radiographs are taken with the fine-detail screen-film combinations. Most other radiographs employ double-emulsion film with screens. The newer, structured grain x-ray films used with high-resolution intensifying screens produce exquisite images with very limited patient dose.

Several general principles regarding these imaging devices should be considered when selecting the proper combination for any particular examination:

1. Use of intensifying screens decreases patient dose by a factor of at least 20.
2. As the speed of the image receptor increases, image resolution is made worse and radiographic noise increases, resulting in reduced radiographic quality.
3. Direct exposure of x-ray film always results in lower contrast than exposure of a screen-film combination.
4. Low-contrast imaging procedures allow for a wider margin of error in producing an acceptable radiograph.

Selection of technique factors

Before each radiographic examination the radiologic technologist is required to exercise good judgment in selecting optimum radiographic technique factors: kVp, mA, and time of exposure. The considerations that determine the value of each of these factors are many and are complexly interrelated. Few generalizations are possible.

One generalization that can be made for all radiographic exposures is that the time of exposure should be as short as possible. Image quality is improved with short exposure times. One of the reasons three-phase radiographic equipment is better than single-phase equipment is that shorter exposure times are possible with three-phase equipment.

We can dispose of exposure time with a simple statement: **keep it as short as possible.** Similar simple statements cannot be made about the selection of kVp or mA. Since time is to remain a minimum, we may now consider the selection of kVp, mA, and the resulting mAs.

The kVp primarily influences the quality of the x-ray beam, but it also has an effect on quantity. As the kVp is increased, the penetrability of the x-ray beam and the total number of x rays emitted at any x-ray energy are also increased.

The mAs affects only the radiation quantity. As mAs is increased, the quantity of x-radiation is increased proportionately.

The radiologic technologist should strive for optimum radiographic contrast and density by exposing the patient to the proper quantity and quality of x-radiation. **The primary control of radiographic contrast is kVp.** As kVp is increased, both the quantity and and quality of x-radiation increases; more x rays are transmitted through the patient so that a higher portion of the primary beam reaches the film. Thus kVp also affects radiographic density. Of those x rays that interact with the patient, the relative number of Compton interactions increases with increasing kVp, resulting in less differential ab-

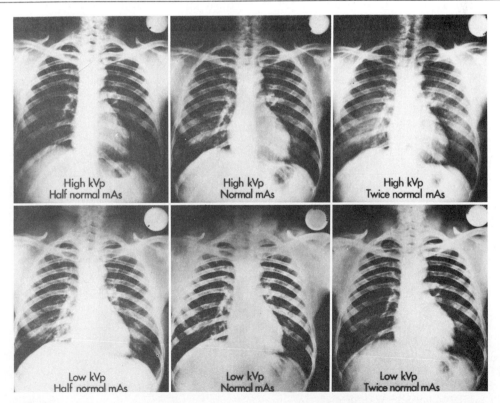

Fig. 16-33. Chest radiographs demonstrating one advantage of high-kVp technique—greater latitude and margin for error. (Courtesy Eastman Kodak Co.)

sorption and reduced subject contrast. Furthermore, with increased kVp there is increased scatter radiation and consequently higher fog density on the radiograph. The result of increased kVp is loss of contrast. When radiographic contrast is low, latitude is high, and there is greater margin for error. The principal advantages to the use of high kVp are the great reduction in patient dose and the wide latitude of exposures allowed in the production of a diagnostic radiograph. Fig. 16-33 shows a series of chest radiographs that demonstrate the increased latitude resulting from high-kVp technique; the relative technique factors are indicated on each radiograph. To some extent the use of grids can compensate for the loss of contrast accompanying high-kVp technique.

The primary control of radiographic density is mAs. As mAs is increased, the radiation quantity increases, and therefore the number of x rays arriving at the film increases, resulting in higher radiographic density and lower radiographic noise. In a secondary way the mAs also influences contrast. Recall that maximum contrast is obtained only when the film is exposed over a range that results in densities along the straight-line portion of the characteristic curve. Too low an mAs will result in insufficient density, which will reduce radiographic contrast. Excessive mAs will result in high radiographic density and an accompanying loss of radiographic contrast.

A number of other factors influence radiographic density and contrast and therefore radiographic quality. A change in SID results in a change in radiographic density because x-ray intensity varies with distance. Adding filtration to the x-ray tube head reduces the intensity but

Table 16-2. Principal factors affecting the making of a radiograph*

	Patient dose	Magnification	Geometric unsharpness	Motion unsharpness	Absorption unsharpness	Radiographic density	Radiographic contrast
Film speed	−	0	0	−	0	0	0
Screen speed	−	0	0	−	0	+	0
Grid ratio	+	0	0	0	0	−	+
Processing time and temperature	0	0	0	0	0	+	−
Patient thickness	+	+	+	+	+	−	−
Field size	+	0	0	0	0	+	−
Use of contrast media	0	0	0	0	0	−	+
Focal spot size	0	0	+	0	0	0	0
SID	0	−	−	−	0	−	0
OID	0	+	+	+	0	0	+
Screen-film contact	0	0	−	0	0	0	+
mAs	+	0	0	0	0	+	−
Time	+	0	0	+	0	+	−
kVp	+	0	0	0	0	+	−
Voltage waveform	+	0	0	0	0	+	−
Total filtration	−	0	0	0	0	−	−

*As the factors in the left-hand column are increased while all other factors remain fixed, the cross-referenced conditions are affected as shown: +, increase; −, decrease; 0, no change.

increases the quality. Table 16-2 summarizes the principal factors that influence the making of a radiograph.

The current trend in radiographic technique is to use high kVp with a compensating reduction in mAs to produce a radiograph of satisfactory quality while reducing patient exposure and the likelihood of reexamination because of an error in technique.

REVIEW QUESTIONS

1. Define or otherwise identify the following:
   a. Average gradient
   b. Density
   c. Foreshortening
   d. Penumbra
   e. Opaque, radiopaque
   f. Densitometer
   g. Motion unsharpness
   h. Spatial distortion
   i. Radiographic quality
   j. Latitude
2. Discuss the secondary factors that influence radiographic density and contrast.
3. Construct a characteristic curve for a typical screen-film combination and carefully label the axes.
4. The intensity of the light emitted by a view box is 1000, and the intensity of the light transmitted through the film is 1. What will be the density of the film, and will it appear light, gray, or black?
5. Base and fog densities for a given film are 0.35. At densities 0.25 and 2 above base and fog densities, the characteristic curve shows log relative exposure values of 1.3 and 2, respectively. What is the average gradient?
6. X-ray films A and B require 15 mR (3.9 μC/kg) and 45 mR (12 μC/kg), respectively, to produce a density of 1. Which is faster, and what is the speed of each?
7. An x-ray examination of the heart taken at 100 cm SID shows a cardiac silhouette measuring 13 cm in width. If the OID distance is estimated at 15 cm, what is the actual width of the heart?
8. A skull film is taken at 50 cm SID with a tube having a 0.4 mm focal spot. A vessel lying 8 cm from the film is imaged. What is the size of the penumbra?

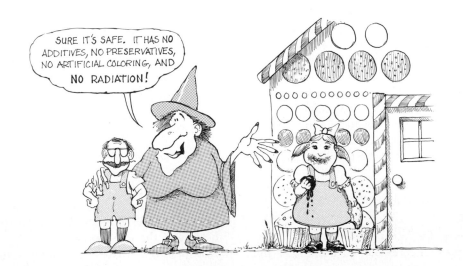

SURE IT'S SAFE. IT HAS NO ADDITIVES, NO PRESERVATIVES, NO ARTIFICIAL COLORING, AND NO RADIATION!

17

Radiographic technique

EXPOSURE TECHNIQUE FACTORS
IMAGE QUALITY FACTORS
RADIOGRAPHIC EXPOSURE GUIDES

Radiographic technique is generally described as the combination of settings selected on the control panel of the x-ray machine to produce a desired effect on the radiograph. The geometry and position of the x-ray tube, the patient, and the image receptor are included in this description.

Radiographic techniques may be described by identifying two groups of factors. The first group includes the **exposure technique factors:** kilovoltage, milliamperage, time, and distance (SID). These factors determine the basic characteristics of radiation exposure of the patient and image receptor. The second group includes the **image quality factors:** density, contrast, detail, and distortion. These factors provide the radiologic technologist with a specific and orderly means to produce, evaluate, and compare radiographs. Understanding how to use each of these factors is essential for the production of quality images.

EXPOSURE TECHNIQUE FACTORS
Kilovoltage

The effects of kVp on the x-ray beam have been described in previous chapters. For the purpose of understanding kVp as an exposure technique factor, one should assume that **kVp is the primary control of beam quality** and therefore beam penetrability. A higher-quality primary beam is one with higher energy and thus is more likely to penetrate the anatomy of interest. Kilovoltage has more effect than any other factor on image receptor exposure because it not only affects beam quality, but also secondarily influences beam quantity. With increasing kVp, x rays are more penetrating, more are present, and they produce more scatter radiation. Consequently the kVp selected will determine to a great degree the amount of x rays in the remnant beam and therefore the resulting density on the film. Finally, and perhaps most importantly, **kilovoltage controls the scale of contrast** on the finished radiograph.

Milliamperes and time

Milliamperes (mA) and time (seconds, s) are usually combined and used as one factor, mAs, in radiographic technique selection. The mAs determines the number of x rays in the primary beam and therefore **principally controls radiation quantity.** It has little influence over radiation quality. **The mAs is the key factor in the control of density** on the radiograph. One obtains mAs by multiplying the milliamperage by the time:

(17-1)

$$mA \times Time = mAs$$

EXAMPLE: A radiographic technique calls for 600 mA at 200 ms. What is the mAs?

ANSWER: 600 mA $\times$ 200 ms = 600 mA $\times$ 0.2 s
          = 120 mAs

Time and mA can be used to compensate for one another in an indirect fashion. This is described by the following:

(17-2)

$$\frac{Time \; (first \; exposure)}{Time \; (second \; exposure)} = \frac{mA \; (second \; exposure)}{mA \; (first \; exposure)}$$

EXAMPLE: A radiograph of the abdomen requires 300 mA and 500 ms. The patient was unable to hold his breath, resulting in unacceptable motion unsharpness. Therefore a second exposure was made with an exposure time of 200 ms. Calculate the new mA that was required.

ANSWER:
$$\frac{500 \; ms}{200 \; ms} = \frac{x}{300 \; mA}$$
$$(200 \; ms) \, x = (500 \; ms) \, (300 \; mA)$$
$$(200 \; ms) \, x = (0.5 \; s) \, (300 \; mA)$$
$$(200 \; ms) \, x = 150 \; mAs$$
$$x = \frac{150 \; mAs}{200 \; ms}$$
$$x = \frac{150 \; mAs}{0.2 \; s}$$
$$x = 750 \; mA$$

If the generator is properly calibrated, the same mAs and therefore the same radiographic density can be produced with various combinations of mA and time, as seen in Table 17-1.

Distance

Distance affects exposure of the image receptor according to the inverse square law, covered in Chapter 4. The source–to–image receptor distance (SID) selected to make an exposure largely determines the intensity of the x-ray beam at the image receptor. **Distance has no**

Table 17-1. Products of milliamperage (mA) and time (ms) for the same mAs

mA		ms (s)	Product in mAs
100	$\times$	100 ($\frac{1}{10}$)	10
200	$\times$	50 ($\frac{1}{20}$)	10
300	$\times$	33 ($\frac{1}{30}$)	10
400	$\times$	25 ($\frac{1}{40}$)	10
600	$\times$	17 ($\frac{1}{60}$)	10
800	$\times$	12 ($\frac{1}{80}$)	10
1000	$\times$	10 ($\frac{1}{100}$)	10

effect on radiation quality. The following relationship derived from the inverse square law relates a change in mAs with a change in SID to produce the same optical density:

(17-3)

$$\frac{mAs \; (first \; exposure)}{mAs \; (second \; exposure)} = \frac{(SID)^2 \; (first \; exposure)}{(SID)^2 \; (second \; exposure)}$$

EXAMPLE: An examination requires 100 mAs at 180 cm SID. If the distance is changed to 90 cm SID, what should be the new mAs?

ANSWER:
$$\frac{100}{x} = \frac{(180)^2}{(90)^2}$$
$$\frac{100}{x} = \frac{32,400}{8100}$$
$$32,400 \, x = 810,000$$
$$x = \frac{810,000}{32,400}$$
$$x = 25 \; mAs$$

Of course an easier solution method would be:

$$\frac{100}{x} = \frac{(180)^2}{(90)^2} = \frac{180^2}{90} = 2^2 = 4$$
$$4x = 100$$
$$x = 25 \; mAs$$

When ready to make a radiographic exposure, the radiologic technologist selects specific settings for each of the factors described: kilovoltage, mAs, and distance (SID). The control panel selections are based on an evaluation of the patient, the thickness of the part, and the type of accessories used.

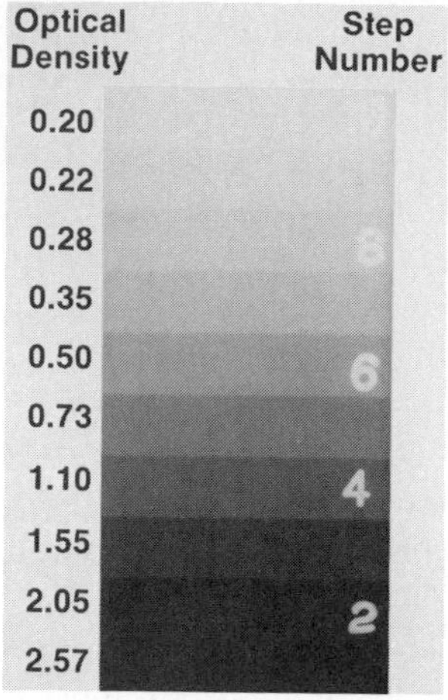

Optical Density	Step Number
0.20	9
0.22	
0.28	8
0.35	
0.50	6
0.73	
1.10	4
1.55	
2.05	2
2.57	

Fig. 17-1. Amount of light transmitted through a radiograph is determined by the density of a film. This step-wedge radiograph shows a representative range of densities.

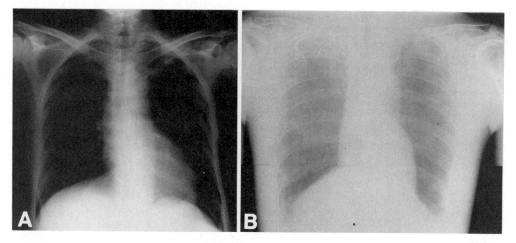

Fig. 17-2. A, Overexposed radiograph of the chest is too black to be diagnostic. **B,** Likewise, underexposed chest radiograph is unacceptable because there is no detail to the lung fields.

IMAGE QUALITY FACTORS

Image quality factors refer to the characteristics of the radiographic image and include density, contrast, definition, and distortion. These factors provide a means for the radiologic technologist to produce, review, and evaluate radiographs. Image quality factors are considered the "language" of radiography, and often it is difficult to separate one such factor from another.

Density

Optical density, sometimes called **radiographic density** or simply **density,** is described as the blackening of the finished radiograph. Density can be present in varying degrees, from complete black, where no light is transmitted, to almost clear. Black is numerically equivalent to an optical density of 3 or 4, whereas clear is less than 0.2. The blackening present on the film is a result of development of the silver bromide crystals in the film emulsion and directly relates to the amount of exposure received from x rays or from the visible light of intensifying screens.

Density was defined in Chapter 16 as:

(17-4)

$$D = log_{10} \frac{I_o}{I_t}$$

Density is the logarithm to the base 10 of the ratio of light incident on a film (I_o) to the light transmitted through the film (I_t), as illustrated in Fig. 17-1. Chapter 16 discussed this in more detail.

In medical radiography most problems relate to density by the film being "too dark" or "too light." A film that is too dark has a high optical density, resulting in **overexposure.** This situation is generally caused by too much radiation exposing the film. A film that is too light has been insufficiently exposed to radiation, resulting in **underexposure** and a low optical density. Either of these conditions can result in unacceptable image quality, which may require re-

peating. Fig. 17-2 shows clinical examples of the two extremes of overexposure and underexposure.

Density can be controlled in radiography by two major factors: **mAs and distance (SID).** A significant number of problems would arise if one continually changed the distance from the x-ray source to the image receptor. Therefore distance is usually standardized at either 90 cm for portable examinations, 100 cm for table studies, and 180 cm for upright chest examination. Fig. 17-3 illustrates the change in density at these SIDs when other exposure technique factors remain constant. Distance then becomes fixed instead of a variable. Consequently mAs becomes the primary variable technique factor that is used to control radiographic density.

Density increases directly with mAs, which means that if the density is to be increased on a radiograph, the mAs would be increased accordingly. **When the density of the film is the only characteristic to change, the appropriate factor to make this change would be the mAs.** Density can be affected by other factors, but mAs becomes the factor of choice for controlling density. If the radiologic technologist wants only to see a slight increase in density, then the mAs must be increased by approximately 30%. Less than that will not produce a detectble change.

Since an increase in density on the finished radiograph is accomplished with a proportionate increase in mAs, is the same true with kilovoltage? The answer is yes, but a qualified yes. As kVp is increased, the quality of the beam is increased and more x rays will be able to penetrate the anatomic part of interest. This results in more remnant radiation exposing the image receptor. Other qualitative factors change when kVp is used to adjust for density. This makes it much more difficult to optimize density with kVp. It takes the eye of an experienced radiologic technologist to determine if density is the

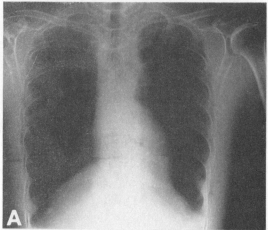

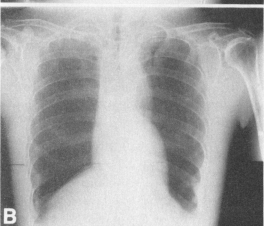

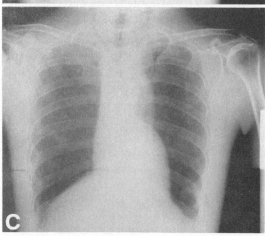

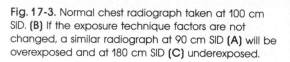

Fig. 17-3. Normal chest radiograph taken at 100 cm SID. **(B)** If the exposure technique factors are not changed, a similar radiograph at 90 cm SID **(A)** will be overexposed and at 180 cm SID **(C)** underexposed.

only factor to be changed or if contrast should also be changed to optimize the radiographic image.

Technique changes involving kVp become complicated. A change in kVp affects penetration, scatter, patient dose, and especially contrast. It is generally accepted that to increase the density on the radiograph using kVp, an increase in kVp by 15% would be equivalent to doubling the mAs. This is known as the **Fifteen percent rule.** Fig. 17-4 illustrates the density change when one applies the Fifteen percent rule.

The simplest method to increase or decrease the density on the radiograph is to increase or decrease the mAs. This reduces other possible factors that could affect the finished image. These various factors that affect film density are listed in Table 17-2.

Contrast

The function of contrast in the image is to make anatomic detail more visible. Therefore contrast is one of the most important factors in radiographic quality evaluation. The radiologic technologist should be able to examine the finished radiograph and determine that sufficient contrast is present to produce the best possible image detail.

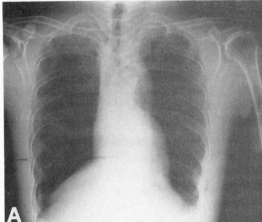

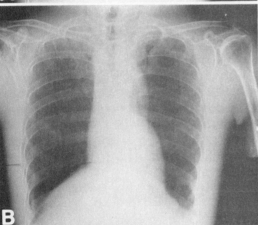

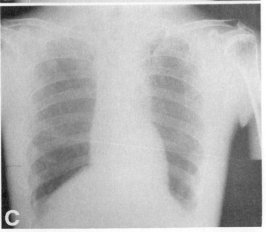

Fig. 17-4. Normal chest radiograph taken at 70 kVp **(B)**. If the kilovoltage is increased 15% to 80 kVp **(A)**, overexposure occurs. Similarly, at 15% less, 60 kVp **(C)**, the radiograph is underexposed.

Table 17-2. Technique factors affecting radiographic density

Factor increased	Effect on density
mAs	Increases
kVp	Increases
SID	Decreases
Thickness of part	Decreases
Mass density	Decreases
Development time	Increases
Image receptor	Increases
Beam restriction	Decreases
Grid ratio	Decreases

Contrast is defined as the difference in density on adjacent anatomic structures or the variation in density present on a radiograph. The difference in density of adjacent structures is the most important factor. Fig. 17-5 shows an image of the spinal column and pelvis, illustrating the difference in densities of adjacent structures. High contrast is visible at the bone–soft tissue interface along the spinal column. The soft tissues of the psoas muscle and kidneys exhibit much less contrast, although details of those structures are readily visible. The contrast of the

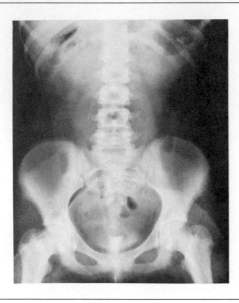

Fig. 17-5. Radiograph of the abdomen showing the vertebral column with its inherent high contrast. The kidneys, pelvis, and psoas muscle are low-contrast tissues that are better visualized with low kVp.

soft tissue, low-contrast resolution, can be enhanced with reduced kVp but only at the expense of higher patient dose.

Contrast on a radiograph is necessary or the outline or border of a structure may not be visible. Contrast is the result of differences in attenuation of the x-ray beam as it passes through various tissues in the body. The penetrating ability of the beam is important since relative penetrability among tissues determines the image contrast.

The penetratability of the primary x-ray beam is controlled by kilovoltage; thus **kVp becomes the major factor for control of radiographic contrast.** To obtain adequate contrast, the anatomic part must be adequately penetrated; therefore penetration becomes the key to understanding radiographic contrast. Compare the radiographs shown in Fig. 17-6. Fig. 17-6, *A*, represents high contrast or "short scale," whereas Fig. 17-6, *B*, represents a radiograph with low contrast or "long scale."

The terminology for describing radiographic contrast must be studied carefully. Consider the terms "short scale" and "long scale" of contrast.

Scale of contrast means the range of optical densities from the lightest to the blackest part of the radiograph. For example, think of using a scissors to cut a small patch representing each density on the radiograph, then arranging the patches in order from the lightest to darkest. The result would be a scale of densities. High-contrast radiographs produce shorter scales. They exhibit black to white in just a few apparent steps. Low-contrast radiographs produce longer scales and have the appearance of many shades of gray. Fig. 17-7 presents two radiographs of a step wedge. The one taken at 50 kVp shows that only five steps are visible. At 90 kVp all thirteen steps are visible because of the long scale of contrast.

Often the radiologic technologist is required to increase or decrease contrast because of an inadequate image. To increase contrast, one must make the range of optical densities more black and white with a greater difference in the optical density of adjacent structures. In other words, one is requested to produce a radiograph with a shorter contrast scale. Accomplishing this requires a reduction in kVp. To reduce contrast,

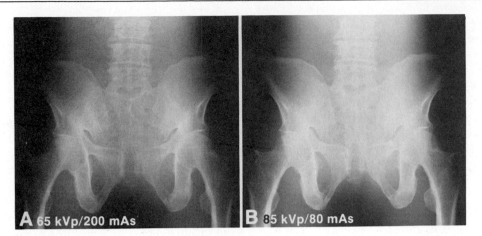

Fig. 17-6. Radiographs of a pelvis phantom demonstrate short scale of contrast **(A)** and long scale of contrast **(B)**.

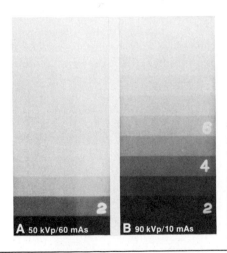

Fig. 17-7. Images of a step wedge exposed at low kVp **(A)** and high kVp **(B)** illustrate the meaning of short scale and long scale of contrast, respectively.

one must produce a radiograph with longer scale contrast and therefore with more grays. This is done by increasing kVp. Normally a 4 kVp change is required to visually affect the scale of contrast, although at higher kVp a greater change may be required.

High contrast, high degree of contrast, and the term "a lot of contrast" all define short scale of contrast and are obtained by the use of lower-

kVp exposure techniques. **Low contrast and low degree of contrast** are the same as long scale of contrast and result from higher kVp selections. These relationships in radiographic contrast can be summarized as follows:

High kilovoltage produces:	Lower kilovoltage produces:
Longer scale	Shorter scale
Low contrast	Higher contrast
Less contrast	More contrast

In addition to kilovoltage, many other factors influence radiographic contrast. The mAs will secondarily influence contrast. If the mAs is too high or too low, the predominant optical densities will fall on the shoulder or toe of the characteristic curve where contrast is low. Use of intensifying screens results in shorter contrast scale when compared with nonscreen exposures. Beam restriction removes scatter radiation from the radiograph, thereby producing a radiograph of shorter scale contrast. Grids also help reduce the amount of scatter reaching the film, thus producing radiographs of shorter scale contrast. Grids with high ratio will increase the contrast. The exposure technique factors that affect contrast are summarized in Table 17-3.

Detail

Radiographic detail describes the sharpness of small structures on the radiograph. With adequate detail, even the smallest parts of anatomy are visible and the radiologist can more readily detect tissue abnormalities. Radiographic detail must be evaluated by two means: (1) **sharpness of image detail** and (2) **visibility of image detail.**

Sharpness of image detail refers to the structural lines or borders of tissues in the image and the amount of clarity or unsharpness (penumbra) of the image. The factors that generally control the sharpness of detail are the geometric factors discussed in Chapter 16: focal spot size, SID, and object–to–image receptor distance (OID). Sharpness of image detail is also influenced by

Table 17-3. Exposure technique factors that affect radiographic contrast

Factor increased	Effect on contrast
kVp	Decreases
mAs	Decreases
Development time	Decreases
Screen-film use	Increases
Beam restriction	Increases
Grid ratio	Increases

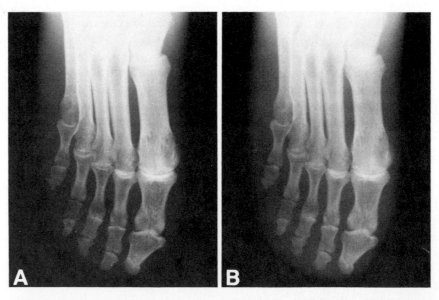

Fig. 17-8. Radiograph **A** was taken with a 1.0 mm focal spot and exhibits far greater detail than **B,** which was taken with a 2.0 mm focal spot x-ray tube.

the type of intensifying screens used and the presence of motion. **To produce the best sharpness of image detail, one should use the smallest appropriate focal spot and the longest standard SID and place the anatomic part as close to the image receptor as possible.** Fig. 17-8 shows two radiographs of a foot. One was taken under optimum conditions and the other with poor technique. The difference is obvious.

Visibility of image detail describes the ability to see the detail on the radiograph. It refers to any factor that would result in the deterioration or obscuring of the image detail. For example, fog will reduce the ability to see structural lines on the image. An attempt to produce the best defined image can be accomplished by using all the correct factors, but if the film is fogged by light or radiation, as in Fig. 17-9, the details present will not be fully visible. One might conclude that good detail would have been present but that the visibility of image detail was poor.

It is assumed that any factor that affects density and contrast will affect the visibility of detail in the image. Key factors that provide the best visibility are beam restriction, use of grids, and all other methods that result in reduced scatter radiation reaching the image receptor.

Distortion

The fourth image quality factor is distortion, the misrepresentation of object size and shape on the finished image. Because of the position of the tube, the anatomic part of interest, and the image receptor, the final image may poorly misrepresent the object.

Poor alignment of the image receptor or the x-ray tube can result in **elongation** of the image. Elongation means the object or part of interest appears longer than normal. Poor alignment of the anatomic part may also result in **foreshortening** of the image. Foreshortening occurs when the anatomic part appears smaller than normal. Fig. 17-10 provides examples of elongation and foreshortening.

Distortion can be minimized by proper alignment of the tube, the anatomic part of interest, and the image receptor. This is the fundamental importance to **patient positioning.** Chapter 16 presented a discussion of these principles.

Table 17-4 summarizes the principal radiographic image quality factors. The primary controlling technique factor for each image quality factor is given, as well as secondary technique factors that influence the image quality factor.

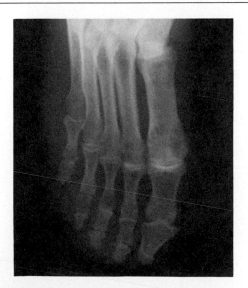

Fig. 17-9. Same radiograph in 17-8, *A,* except the visibility of image detail is reduced because of safelight fog.

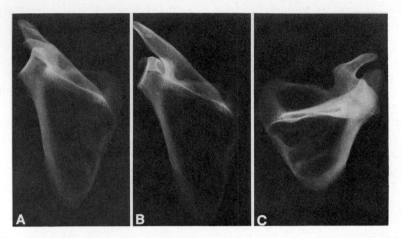

Fig. 17-10. A, Normal projection of the scapula. **B,** Elongation of the scapula. **C,** Foreshortening of the scapula.

Table 17-4. Principal radiographic image quality factors

Factor	Controlled by:	Influenced by:
Density	mAs	kVp
		Distance
		Thickness of part
		Mass density
		Development time
		Image receptor speed
		Beam restriction
		Grid ratio
Contrast	kVp	mAs
		Development time
		Screen-film combination
		Beam restriction
		Grid ratio
Detail	Focal spot size	SID
		OID
		Motion
		All factors related to density and contrast
Distortion	Patient positioning	Alignment of tube, anatomic part, and image receptor

RADIOGRAPHIC EXPOSURE GUIDES

Radiographic exposure guides are charts that provide a means for determining the specific technical factors to be used for a given radiographic examination. It is important for the radiologic technologist to know how to manipulate these technical factors to produce the desired density, contrast, definition, and detail on the finished radiograph. However, it is not necessary to become creative with each new patient. A guide or chart should be available for each radiographic unit that supports a standardized method for the radiologic technologist to produce high-quality images consistently.

In order for a **radiographic exposure chart** to meet with success, the radiologic technologist must understand its purpose, how it was constructed, how it is to be used, and most importantly, when to make adjustments for body habitus and pathologic processes. When used properly, the radiographic exposure chart allows for consistently good diagnostic images. The scale of contrast and density are more predictable than if no standard chart is used.

Radiographic exposure charts can be prepared to accommodate all types of facilities. The four principal types of charts are based on **variable kilovoltage, fixed kilovoltage, high kilovoltage,** and **automatic exposure.** Each of these charts provides the technologist with a guide in the selection of exposure factors for all patients and all examinations. Most facilities will select a particular type for use and then prepare similar charts for each radiographic examination room. The type of chart usually depends on the radiologist, the type of equipment available, the screen-film combination, and the accessories available.

Radiographic exposure charts and their use become an important issue in patient protection. Radiologic technologists are required to use their skill in producing the best possible image with a single exposure. Repeat examination serves only to increase the radiation dose to the patient. The preparation of these charts becomes an important and challenging task, and once in use, the charts must constantly be evaluated. This allows for the least radiation exposure to the patient as possible.

The preparation of a chart does not require one to create it completely from scratch. Many authors have made available guides that can be used in preparation of specific charts. **It is important that radiographic exposure charts from books and pamphlets not be used as printed.** Each radiographic unit is unique in its radiation characteristics. Therefore a specific chart should be prepared for each room and tested individually.

Before the preparation of the radiographic exposure chart begins, the x-ray equipment must be calibrated and the processing system thoroughly evaluated. The total filtration should be determined. Although 2.5 mm Al is the prescribed standard, one may find 4 or 5 mm Al total filtration as well. This significantly alters contrast and will make a considerable difference in any technique chart. The type of grid to be used should be selected and the collimator or beam restrictor checked for accurate light field, or x-ray beam coincidence. This is most important so that all variables are reduced to a minimum. When a radiographic exposure chart is found to be inadequate, these are the factors that should be tested first.

Variable-kVp chart

The variable-kVp radiographic exposure chart employs a fixed mAs and a kVp that varies according to the thickness of the anatomic part. **Kilovoltage varies with the thickness of the anatomic part by 2 kVp per centimeter.** The basic characteristic of the variable-kVp chart is the **short scale of contrast.** Generally, exposures made with this method provide radiographs of shorter contrast scale because of the use of lower kVp.

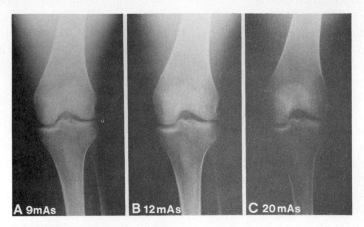

Fig. 17-11. Radiographs of a knee phantom taken at 58 kVp. Obtained at 12 mAs, **B** was selected to begin the variable-kVp chart.

Exposures directed by the variable-kVp chart usually result in higher patient dose and less exposure latitude. For success, the radiologic technologist must be accurate in measuring the anatomic part before selecting the exposure factors from the chart. Without such care and attention, anatomy may not be fully penetrated as a result of the lower kVp.

To begin preparation of a variable-kVp radiographic exposure chart, select the body part for examination. For example, if the knee is chosen, use a knee phantom for all test exposures. First, measure the thickness of the knee phantom accurately, using a caliper designed for that purpose. Multiply the part thickness by 2 and add 30; this will indicate a kVp with which to begin.

EXAMPLE: A phantom knee measures 14 cm thick. What kVp should be used to begin construction of a variable-kVp technique chart?

ANSWER: $14 \text{ cm} \times 2 = 28 + 30$
$= 58 \text{ kVp}$

The kilovoltage setting for examination of the knee will be 58 kVp. The next task is to select the optimum mAs at this kVp. This will depend on the image receptor characteristics and effectiveness of scatter radiation control. For example, when using 200-speed screens with an 8:1 grid, make test exposures at 58 kVp with 9 mAs, 12 mAs, and 20 mAs. Fig. 17-11 shows representative images taken at 9, 12, and 20 mAs. Select the radiograph that produces the best density, or make additional exposures at other mAs values if necessary. The result of this exercise is the first line of the variable-kVp technique chart. The kVp and mAs to be used when radiographing a knee measuring 14 cm have been established, as shown in Table 17-5.

At this point, the chart can be expanded to include knees with other thicknesses. To prepare a variable-kVp radiographic exposure chart for other anatomic parts, the same procedure is used. When completed and ready to use on patients, one must be ready for some minor adjustments and continuing refinement of each chart.

Fixed-kVp chart

The fixed-kVp radiographic exposure chart is the one used most often. It was developed by

---

Table 17-5. Variable-kVp chart for examination of the knee

Knee—AP/lat	Part thickness (cm)	Kilovoltage
mAs: 12	8	46
SID: 100 cm	9	48
Grid: 12:1	10	50
Collimation: to part	11	52
Image receptor	12	54
speed: 200		
	13	56
	14	**58**
	15	60
	16	62
	17	64
	18	66

---

the late Arthur Fuchs and is a method for selecting exposures that produce radiographs with a longer scale of contrast. The kVp is selected as the optimum required for penetration of the anatomic part. This usually results in somewhat higher values for most examinations than with the variable-kVp technique. Once selected, the kVp is fixed at that level for each type of examination and not varied according to differences in the thickness of the part. The mAs is changed according to the thickness of the anatomic part to provide the proper optical density. For example, all examinations of the knee might require 80 kVp with mAs adjusted to accommodate for differences in thickness.

The fixed-kVp method generally requires higher kVp. One benefit of this technique is that on average, the patient receives a lower radiation dose. There is greater latitude and more consistency with exposures of the same anatomic part. Measurement of the part is not as critical because part size is grouped as small, medium, and large. For most examinations of the trunk of the body, the optimum kVp is 80. For most distal extremities, the optimum would be approximately 60 kVp.

To prepare a fixed-kVp radiographic exposure chart, the first step is to separate anatomic part thickness into three groups—small, medium, and large—by identifying the range thickness that is to be included in each group. Using the abdomen as an example, small might be 14 to 20 cm, medium 21 to 25 cm, and large 26 to 31 cm. For test exposures, use an abdomen phantom as a member of the medium group and begin with 80 kVp. Produce radiographs at mAs increments of 40, 60, 80, and so on until the proper density is obtained. Again, the density selected will depend on the type of image receptor and available scatter radiation control devices. Fig. 17-12 demonstrates this process with radiographs of such an abdomen phantom.

Once the proper density has been established, the chart can then be expanded to include small and large anatomic parts. For small anatomy, one should reduce the mAs by 30%. For large anatomy, one should increase the mAs by 30%. For a part that is swollen as a result of trauma, a 50% change is required. Table 17-6 presents the hypothetic results of this procedure.

High-kVp chart

For high-kVp charts, the kVp selected would generally be greater than 100. For example,

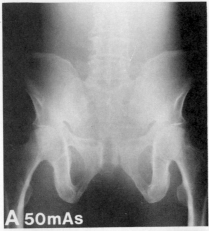

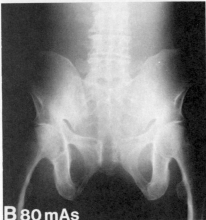

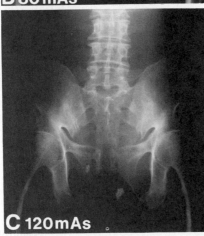

Fig. 17-12. Radiographs of an abdomen phantom used to construct a fixed-kVp chart. All exposures were taken at 80 kVp. From this series, 80 mAs **(B)** was selected to begin the chart.

overhead radiographs for procedures using barium sulfate would employ 120 kVp for each exposure. High-kilovoltage exposure techniques are ideal for barium work to ensure adequate penetration of the barium. This type of exposure technique could also be used for routine chest radiography to provide improved visualization of the various tissue densities present in the lung fields and mediastinum. Lower, or more conventional, kVp settings provide increased subject contrast between bone and soft tissue, whereas when 120 kVp is selected for chest radiography, all skeletal tissue will be penetrated and exhibit increased visualization of the different soft tissue densities present. To prepare a high-kVp chart, the procedure used is basically the same as for preparing the fixed-kVp chart. All exposures for a particular anatomic part would use the same kVp. Obviously the mAs would be much less. Test exposures would be made using a phantom to determine the appropriate mAs for adequate density. Fig. 17-13 shows a chest radiograph made at 120 kVp. Notice the improved visualization of the tissue markings of the bronchial tree and the mediastinal structures, compared with the low kVp radiographs of Fig. 17-4.

One additional advantage for using the high-kVp exposures is the reduced dose of radiation to the patient.

Automatic exposure systems

Automatic exposure systems are being employed more often in radiographic imaging, especially with the use of computer-assisted control units. These systems utilize an electronic exposure timer, such as described in Chapter 7,

Table 17-6. Fixed-kVp chart for examination of the abdomen

Abdomen—AP	Part thickness (cm)	Required mAs
kVp: 80	Small: 14-20	50
SID: 100 cm	Medium: 12-25	80
Grid: 12:1	Large: 26-31	110
Collimation: to part		
Image receptor speed: 200		

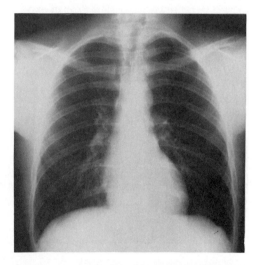

Fig. 17-13. High-kVp chest radiograph illustrating the improved visualization of mediastinal structures.

Table 17-7. Factors to consider when constructing a radiographic exposure chart for automatic systems

Factor for selection	Rationale for selection
Kilovoltage	To select for each anatomic part
Density control	To adjust according to the thickness of part
Beam restriction	To reduce patient dose and ensure proper response of automatic exposure control
Accessory selection	To optimize the radiation dose/image quality ratio

that terminates the exposure when the proper radiographic density is obtained. The density results from exposure to the film, which is measured by either a photocell or an ionization chamber. The principles associated with automatic exposure systems have already been described, but the importance in using radiographic exposure charts with these systems has not been covered.

These automatic control x-ray systems are not completely automatic. It is incorrect to assume that because the radiologic technologist does not have to select kVp, mA, and time for each examination, a less qualified or less skilled operator can use the system. Generally, the technologist must use a guide for the selection of kVp and optical density setting. Sometimes only optical density as a function of patient size must be selected. The kVp selection is more in keeping with that of the fixed-kVp method. Density selections are numerically scaled to allow for differences in the thickness of the part.

Patient positioning must be absolutely accurate because the specific body part must be placed over the phototiming device to ensure proper exposure. In addition to the accuracy in positioning, it is recommended that the anatomic part be measured before each examination for determining the appropriate density setting.

The factors shown in Table 17-7 must be considered when preparing the radiographic exposure chart for an automatic x-ray system. The kVp is selected according to the specific anatomic part being examined. The optical density control will be positioned according to the part thickness. The specific accessories to be used, such as film, screens, and grid, will determine to a great extent the previous selections. It is critical to ensure that beam restriction confines the x-ray field only to the anatomic part under investigation or to the image receptor, whichever is smaller. Excessive scatter radiation will affect the response of the automatic exposure control and reduce image contrast.

Many of the control panels of newer radiographic units, such as the one in Fig. 17-14, allow the radiologic technologist simply to select the anatomic part directly by name or symbol. Such systems are called **anatomic programmed radiography (APR).** These systems are under microprocessor control, but they require input from the technologist for proper programming.

The principle of APR is similar to automatic exposure with the radiographic exposure chart stored in the microprocessor of the control unit. The service engineer loads the controlling programs during installation and calibrates the exposure control circuit for the general conditions of the facility. The technologist needs only to select the part and the relative size before each exposure. However, the programmed instructions must be continuously adjusted by the technologist until the entire panel of examinations is optimized for best image quality.

REVIEW QUESTIONS

1. Define or otherwise identify the following:
   a. Fifteen percent rule
   b. Image detail
   c. Definition
   d. Image quality factors
   e. Scale of contrast
   f. APR
   g. Optical density
   h. Elongation
   i. Variable-kVp chart
   j. Distortion
2. List and discuss the four exposure technique factors. How does each affect radiographic density?

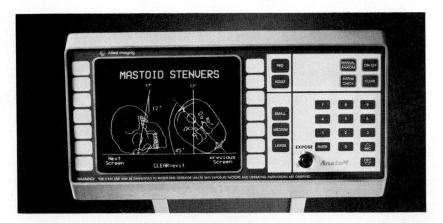

Fig. 17-14. Amount of light transmitted through a radiograph is determined by the optical density of a film. This step-wedge radiograph shows a representative range of optical densities. (Courtesy Allied Universal Imaging, Inc.)

3. Explain how kilovoltage influences the scale of contrast.

4. A radiographic technique calls for 82 kVp at 400 mA, 200 ms and an SID of 90 cm. What is the mAs?

5. A radiographic technique of 150 mA, 200 ms results in an acceptable radiograph except for patient motion. If the exposure time is reduced to 25 ms, what should the mA be?

6. An acceptable chest x ray was taken at 180 cm SID with 10 mAs. If the 400 mA station is used, what will be the new exposure time at 90 cm SID?

7. Identify the range of radiographic densities that are too light, too dark, and just right.

8. When a change in radiographic density is required, what exposure technique factor should be changed and why?

9. When a change in radiographic contrast is required, what exposure technique factor should be changed and why?

10. List and discuss the nature of the four types of radiographic exposure charts.

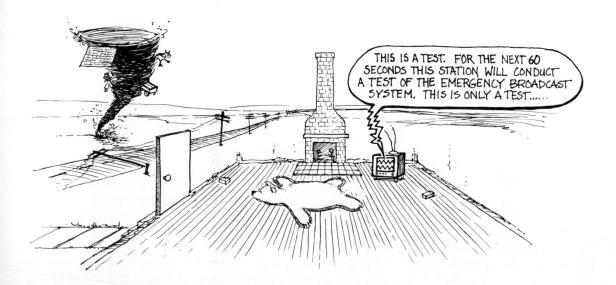

18

Special x-ray equipment and procedures

FLUOROSCOPY
TOMOGRAPHY
STEREORADIOGRAPHY
MAGNIFICATION RADIOGRAPHY

Many areas of x-ray diagnosis require special equipment and specialized techniques to obtain the required diagnostic information. Such procedures are designed to visualize more clearly a given anatomic structure, usually at the expense of nonvisualization of other structures.

The equipment and procedures discussed here include tomography, cinefluorography, stereoradiography, magnification radiography, and fluoroscopy. Fluoroscopy is actually a rather routine type of x-ray examination except for its application in the visualization of vessels, in which case it is called **angiography.** The two main areas of angiography are neuroradiology and vascular radiology, and, as with all fluoroscopic procedures, radiographs are obtained also. The recent introduction of computer technology into fluoroscopy and radiography is placing increasing demands on the training and performance of technologists. These subjects will only be lightly touched on here, with the intention of present-

ing their basic principles. Later chapters will explain more completely the emerging role of computer science in radiology.

FLUOROSCOPY

Ever since Thomas A. Edison invented the fluoroscope in 1896, it has been a valuable tool in the practice of medicine. The primary function of the fluoroscope is to perform dynamic studies; that is, **the fluoroscope is used to visualize the motion of internal structures and fluids.** During fluoroscopy, the radiologist views a continuous image of the motion of internal structures while the x-ray tube is energized. If something is observed that the radiologist would like to preserve for later study, a radiograph can be exposed with little interruption of the fluoroscopic examination. Such a radiograph is known as a **spot film.** The layout of a modern fluoroscopic system is shown in Fig. 18-1.

Conventional fluoroscoopy has been replaced

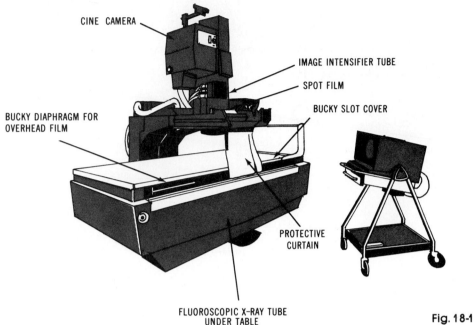

CINE CAMERA

IMAGE INTENSIFIER TUBE

SPOT FILM

BUCKY SLOT COVER

BUCKY DIAPHRAGM FOR
OVERHEAD FILM

PROTECTIVE
CURTAIN

FLUOROSCOPIC X-RAY TUBE
UNDER TABLE

Fig. 18-1. Modern fluoroscope.

by image-intensified fluoroscopy. During conventional fluoroscopy, the radiologist observes the image on a fluoroscopic screen (described in Chapter 15). During image-intensified fluoroscopy, the radiologic image usually is displayed on a television monitor. The image-intensifier tube and the television chain are described later.

For a radiographic examination, the x-ray tube current is measured in hundreds of mA. During fluoroscopy, the x-ray tube is operated at less than 5 mA. When image intensification was first introduced, it was anticipated that tube current could be reduced by at least a factor of ten and that as a result patient dose would be reduced by a factor of ten. For a variety of reasons this tube-current reduction has not materialized. During image-intensified fluoroscopy, tube currents of 1 to 3 mA are normal. Consequently, the patient dose during fluoroscopy remains high, considerably higher than doses resulting

from radiographic examinations. Representative patient doses are reported in Chapter 32.

The kVp of operation depends entirely on the section of the body being examined. Modern fluoroscopic equipment allows the radiologist to select an image brightness level that is subsequently maintained automatically by varying the kVp or the mA, or sometimes both. Such a feature of the fluoroscope is called **automatic brightness control (ABC), automatic brightness stabilization (ABS), automatic exposure control (AEC), or automatic gain control (AGC).**

Illumination

The principal advantage of image-intensified fluoroscopy over conventional fluoroscopy is the increased image brightness. Just as it is much more difficult to read a telephone book in dim illumination than in bright illumination, it is much harder to interpret a dim fluoroscopic image than a bright one. Illumination levels are

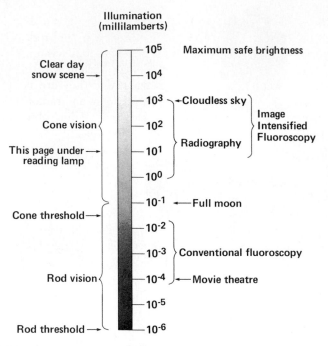

Fig. 18-2. Range of human vision is wide; it covers eleven orders of magnitude.

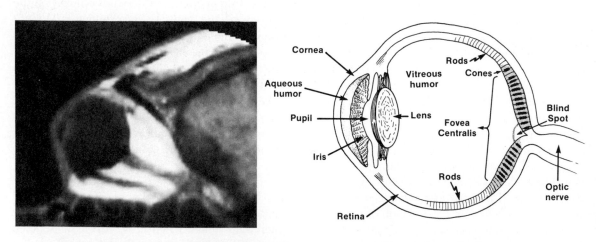

Fig. 18-3. The human eye's appearance on CT scan and the parts responsible for vision. (Courtesy Ed Hendricks, Ph.D., University of Colorado.)

measured in units of lamberts (L) and millilamberts (mL) (1 L = 1000 mL). It is not necessary to know the precise definition of a lambert; its importance lies in demonstrating the wide range of illumination levels over which the human eye is sensitive. Fig. 18-2 lists some approximate illumination levels for familiar objects. Radiographs are visualized under illumination levels of 10 to 1000 mL; fluoroscopy is performed at similar illumination levels.

Human vision

The structures in the eye responsible for the sensation of vision are called **rods** and **cones.** Fig. 18-3 is a cross section of the human eye, identifying its principal parts. Light incident on the eye must first pass through the **cornea,** a transparent protective covering, and then through the **lens,** where the light is focused onto the **retina.** Between the cornea and the lens is the **iris,** which behaves like the diaphragm of a photographic camera to control the amount of light admitted to the eye. In the presence of bright light the iris contracts and allows only a small amount of light to enter. During dark conditions, such as a darkened movie theater, the iris dilates, that is, opens up, and allows more light to enter. In digital fluoroscopy there is an iris between the image-intensifier tube and the TV camera tube that functions in a similar fashion.

When light arrives at the retina, it is detected by the rods and the cones. Rods and cones are small structures; there are more than 100,000 of them per square millimeter of retina. The cones are concentrated on the center of the retina in an area called the **fovea centralis.** Rods, on the other hand, are most numerous on the periphery of the retina. There are no rods at the fovea centralis.

The rods are very sensitive to light and are used during dim light situations. The threshold for rod vision is approximately 10^{-6} mL. Cones, on the other hand, are less sensitive to light; their threshold is only 5×10^{-3} mL, but they are capable of responding to intense light levels whereas rods cannot. Consequently, cones are used primarily for daylight vision, called **photopic vision,** and rods are used for night vision, called **scotopic vision.** This aspect of visual physiology explains why dim objects are more readily viewed if they are not looked at directly. Astronomers and radiologists are familiar with the fact that a dim object can be seen better if viewed peripherally, where rod vision dominates.

The ability of the rods to visualize small objects is much worse than that of the cones. This ability to perceive fine detail is called **visual acuity.** Cones are also much more able to detect differences in brightness levels than rods. This property of vision is termed **contrast perception.** Furthermore, cones are sensitive to a wide range of wavelengths of light. Cones perceive color, but rods are essentially color blind.

Practical fluoroscopic technique

The visual features distinguishing rods from cones emphasize that cone vision is preferred over rod vision. During fluoroscopy, maximum image detail is desired, and if this is to be achieved image brightness must be high. This is the principal reason for using the image intensifier. It raises the illumination from the low level of conventional fluoroscopy, about 10^{-3} mL, into the cone-vision region, where visual acuity is greatest.

Before image-intensified fluoroscopy was used, the radiologist's eyes had to become accustomed to dim illumination for at least 15 minutes. **Dark adaptation** was the process of wearing red goggles under normal illumination so that the amount of light entering the eye was reduced, allowing dilation of the iris and stimulation of rod vision for use during conventional fluoroscopy.

The brightness of the fluoroscopic image is dependent primarily on the anatomic structure under investigation, the kVp, and the mA. Patient anatomy cannot be controlled by the tech-

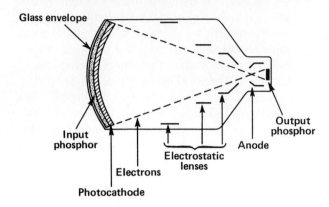

Fig. 18-4. Image-intensifier tube is a complex electronic vacuum tube that converts the pattern of the x-ray beam into a bright light image.

nologist. The influence of kVp and mA on fluoroscopic image qualtiy is similar to their influence on radiographic image quality. Generally, high kVp and low mA are preferred.

Image intensification

The image-intensifier tube is a complex electronic device that receives the remnant x-ray beam, converts it into light, and increases the light intensity. Fig. 18-4 is a rendition of an x-ray image-intensifier tube. The tube is usually contained in a glass envelope that provides some structural support but more importantly maintains a vacuum. When installed, the tube is mounted inside a metal container to protect it from rough handling and possible breakage.

X rays that exit the patient and are incident on the image-intensifier tube are transmitted through the glass envelope and interact with the **input phosphor,** which is cesium iodide. When an x ray interacts with the input phosphor, its energy is converted into a burst of visible-light photons as occurs with radiographic intensifying screens.

The next active element of the image-intensifier tube is the **photocathode,** which is bonded directly to the input phosphor with a thin, transparent, adhesive layer. The photocathode is a thin metal layer, usually composed of cesium and antimony compounds, that responds to stimulation by light with the emission of electrons, a process known as **photoemission.** Thus the photocathode is sometimes called a photoemissive surface. The terminology is similar to **thermionic emission,** which refers to electron emission following heat stimulation. Photoemission is electron emission following light stimulation. The number of electrons emitted by the photocathode is directly proportional to the intensity of light falling on it. Consequently, this number of electrons is proportional to the intensity of the incident x rays.

The image-intensifier tube is approximately 50 cm long. A potential difference of about 25,000 V is maintained across the tube between photocathode and anode so that the electrons of photoemission will be accelerated to the anode. Near the anode is the output phosphor, where the electrons interact and produce a burst of light. If there is to be an accurate image pattern, the electron path from photocathode to output phosphor must be precise. The engineering aspects of maintaining proper electron travel are called **electron optics** because the electrons emitted over the face of the image-intensifier tube must by focused just like visible light. The devices resopnsible for this control, called **electrostatic focusing lenses,** are located along the length of the image-intensifier tube. The electrons arrive at the output phosphor with high

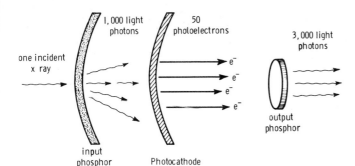

Fig. 18-5. In an image-intensifier tube each incident x ray that interacts with the input phosphor results in a large number of light photons at the output phosphor. The representative image intensifier shown here has a brightness gain of 3000.

kinetic energy and contain the image of the input phosphor in minified form.

When these high-energy electrons interact with the output phosphor, a considerable amount of light is produced. The **output phosphor** usually is made of zinc cadmium sulfide crystals. Each photoelectron that arrives at the output phosphor results in approximately fifty to seventy-five times as many light photons as were necessary to create it. The entire sequence of events from initial x-ray interaction to output image is summarized in Fig. 18-5.

The increased illumination of the image is due to the multiplication of the light photons at the output phosphor compared with those at the input phosphor and the image minification from input phosphor to output phosphor. The ability of the image-intensifier tube to increase the illumination level of the image is called its **brightness gain.** The brightness gain is simply the product of the **minification gain** and the ratio of the number of light photons at the output phosphor to the number at the input phosphor. This ratio is known as the **flux gain.**

(18-1)

> *Brightness gain =*
> *Minification gain × Flux gain*

The minification gain is simply the ratio of the square of the diameter of the input phosphor to the square of the diameter of the output phosphor. Output phosphor size is fairly standard at 2.5 or 5 cm. Input phosphor size varies from 10 to 35 cm and is used to identify image-intensifier tubes.

EXAMPLE: What is the brightness gain for a 17 cm image-intensifier tube having a flux gain of 120 and a 2.5 cm output phosphor?

ANSWER: *Brightness gain* $= \dfrac{17^2}{2.5^2} \times 120$

$$= 46 \times 120$$
$$= 5520$$

The brightness gain of most image intensifiers is 5000 to 20,000, and it decreases with tube age and use. The image-intensifier tube allows for great flexibility in manipulation of fluoroscopy information. Fig. 18-6 demonstrates some of the modes of operation that can be accommodated with the image-intensifier tube.

Multifield image intensification

Most of the newer image intensifiers are of the multifield type, sometimes called **dual-focus** or **trifocus** tubes. These multifield image intensifiers provide for considerably more flexibility for all fluoroscopic examinations, and they are standard components in digital fluoroscopy. Dual-focus tubes come in a varied range of sizes, but perhaps the most popular is the 25 cm−17

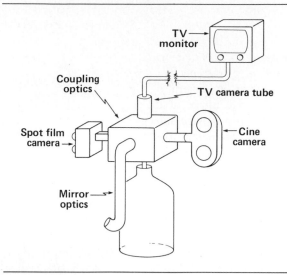

Fig. 18-6. Some possible modes of operation with an image-intensifier tube.

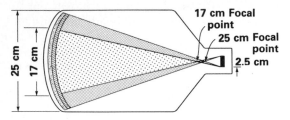

Fig. 18-7. A 25/17 image-intensifier tube produces a magnified image in the 17 cm mode.

cm (25/17) design. Trifocus tubes of 25/17/12 or 23/15/10 are also often employed.

These numeric dimensions refer to the diameter of the input phosphor of the image-intensifier tube. The operation of a typical multifield tube is illustrated by the 25/17 type shown in Fig. 18-7. In the 25 cm mode the photoelectrons from the entire input phosphor are accelerated to the output phosphor. When switched to the 17 cm mode, the voltage on the electrostatic focusing lenses is increased, and this causes the electron focal point to move further from the output phosphor. Consequently, only electrons from the center 17 cm diameter of the input phosphor are incident on the output phosphor. The principal result of this change in

focal point is to reduce the field of view and thereby magnify the image. Use of the smaller dimension of a multifield image-intensifier tube always results in a magnified image with a magnification factor in direct proportion to the ratio of the diameters. A 25/17 tube operated in the 17 cm mode will produce a magnified image 1.5 times larger than the image produced in the 25 cm mode.

This magnified image comes at a price. When operating in the magnified mode, the minification gain is reduced and there are fewer photoelectrons incident on the output phosphor. A dimmer image results.

To maintain the same level of brightness, the x-ray tube mA is automatically increased, and this increases the patient dose. The increase in dose is approximately equal to the ratio of the area of the input phosphor used or 2.2 times $(25^2 \div 17^2)$ the dose obtained in the wide field of view mode.

This increase in patient dose results in better image quality. The patient dose is higher because more x-ray photons per unit area are used to form the image. This results in lower noise and higher contrast. That portion of any image resulting from the periphery of the input phosphor is inherently unfocused and suffers from **vignetting,** a reduction in brightness at the periphery. Because only the central region of the input phosphor is used in the magnification mode, image resolution is better. In the 25 cm mode, a CsI image-intensifier tube can image approximately 0.125 mm objects (4 lp/mm); in the 10 cm mode, the resolution is approximately 0.08 mm (6 lp/mm). This compares with a resolution of 0.25 to 0.17 mm (2 to 3 lp/mm) available with the older image-intensifier tube having ZnCdS as the input phosphor. The concept of spatial frequency as measured in lp/mm was first introduced in Chapter 15 and will be discussed more completely in Chapter 22. At this stage it is sufficient to know that high spatial frequency is associated with increased lp/mm and smaller resolution.

Fluoroscopic image monitoring

Optical monitoring. Two methods for observing the image are preferred in image-intensified fluoroscopy. One is a system of optical lenses and mirrors that magnifies the image from the output phosphor onto a viewing glass. This is called a **mirror-optics system,** and, although adequate, it has several disadvantages. The field of view for a mirror-optics system is small, allowing only one person to observe the image at a time. Also, a significant amount of light photons is lost in this optical system, so that full advantage is not taken of the image-intensifier tube.

Television monitoring. A television monitoring system, although more expensive than a mirror-optics system, is preferred. When television is employed, the output phosphor of the image-intensifier tube is coupled directly to a TV camera tube. The **vidicon** is the TV camera tube most often used in television fluoroscopy. It has a sensitive input surface of the same size as the output phosphor of the image-intensifier tube. The TV camera tube converts the light image pattern into an electric signal and conveys this

signal to the television monitor, where it is reconstructed as an image on the television screen. A significant advantage to the use of television monitoring is that brightness level and contrast can be electronically controlled. With television monitoring, several observers can view the fluoroscopic image at the same time. It is even possible to place monitors outside the examination room for others to observe. Television monitoring also allows for storage of the image in its electronic form on a magnetic tape or disk for subsequent playback and image manipulation. Television monitoring is an essential part of the digital fluoroscopic equipment described in Chapter 21.

Television camera. The television camera consists of a cylindric housing, approximately 15 cm in diameter by 25 cm in length, that contains the heart of the camera, the TV camera tube. It also contains electromagnetic coils for properly steering the electron beam inside the tube. There are a number of such TV camera tubes available for television fluoroscopy, but the **plumbicon** and **vidicon** are most often used.

Fig. 18-8 shows a typical vidicon, a cylindric tube approximately 15 cm long by 3 cm in diameter. The **glass envelope** serves the same function that it does for the x-ray tube—to maintain a vacuum and provide mechanical support for the internal elements. The internal elements are the cathode and its **electron gun,** assorted **electrostatic grids,** and a **target assembly** that serves as an anode.

The electron gun is a heated filament that supplies a constant electron current by thermionic emission. These electrons are formed into an electron beam by the control grid, which also assists in accelerating the electrons to the anode. The electron beam is further accelerated by additional electrostatic grids. The size of the electron beam and its position is controlled by external electromagnetic coils known as deflection coils, focusing coils, and alignment coils.

At the anode end of the tube the electron beam passes through a wire mesh–like structure

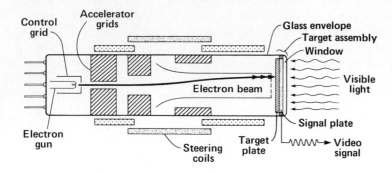

Fig. 18-8. A vidicon TV camera tube and its principal parts.

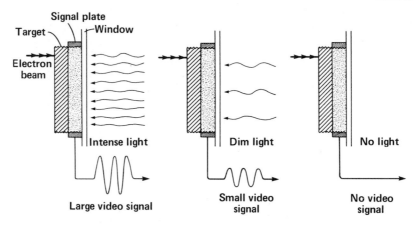

Fig. 18-9. The target of a TV camera tube conducts electrons, creating a video signal only when illuminated.

and interacts with the target assembly. The target assembly consists of three layers sandwiched together. The outside layer is the **face plate,** or **window,** a thin part of the glass envelope. Coated on the inside of the window is a thin layer of metal or graphite called the **signal plate.** The signal plate is thin enough to transmit light yet thick enough to be an efficient electrical conductor. Its name derives from the fact that it conducts the video signal out of the tube into the external video circuit. On the inside of the signal plate is applied a photoconductive layer of antimony trisulfide. This layer is called the **target,** or **photoconductive layer,** and it is this layer with which the electron beam interacts. Antimony trisulfide is photoconductive because,

when illuminated, it conducts electrons; when dark, it behaves as an insulator.

The mechanism of the target assembly is very involved but can be described simplistically as follows. When light from the output phosphor of the image-intensifier tube strikes the window, it will be transmitted through the signal plate to the target. If the electron beam is incident on the same part of the target at the same time, some of its electrons will be conducted through the target to the signal plate and conducted from there out of the tube as the video signal. If that area of the target is dark, there will be no video signal, The magnitude of the video signal is proportional to the intensity of light. This process is illustrated in Fig. 18-9.

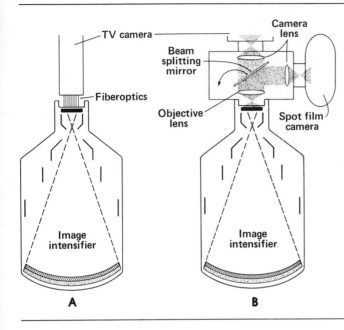

Fig. 18-10. TV camera tubes are coupled to an image-intensifier tube in two ways. **A,** Fiber optics. **B,** Lens system.

Coupling the television camera. Image intensifiers and TV camera tubes are manufactured so that the output phosphor of the image-intensifier tube is the same diameter as the window of the TV camera tube, usually 2.5 or 5 cm. Two methods are commonly used to attach, or **couple,** the TV camera tube to the image-intensifier tube, and these are shown in Fig. 18-10.

The simplest method is to use a bundle of **fiber optics.** The fiber-optics bundle is only a few millimeters thick and contains thousands of optic fibers per square millimeter of cross section. One advantage of this type of coupling is its small, compact assembly, making it easy to manipulate the image-intensifier tower. This coupling is also rugged and can withstand relatively rough handling. The principal disadvantage is that it cannot accommodate auxilliary imaging devices such as cine or spot film cameras. With this type of coupling, cassette-loaded spot films are necessary.

To accept a cine or spot film camera, a lens coupling, as shown in Fig. 18-10, *B,* is required. This type of coupling results in a much larger

assembly that should be handled with care. It is absolutely essential that the lenses and mirror remain precisely adjusted. Malposition will result in an unsharp image. The **objective lens** accepts the light from the output phosphor and converts it into a parallel beam. When recording an image on film, this beam is interrupted by a **beam-splitting mirror** so that only a portion, from 10% to 90%, is transmitted to the television camera, while the remainder is reflected to a film camera. The amount of reflectance is determined by the film and camera system employed. Such a system allows the fluoroscopist to view the image while it is being filmed. Usually the beam-splitting mirror is retracted from the beam when a film camera is not in use. Both the television camera and the film camera are coupled to lenses that focus the parallel light beam onto the film and target of the respective cameras. These **camera lenses** are the most critical elements in the optic chain in terms of alignment. Although the lenses are shown as simple convex lenses, it should be understood that each is a compound lens system consisting of several separate lens elements.

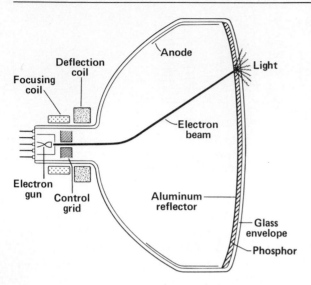

Fig. 18-11. A TV picture tube (CRT) and its principal parts.

Television monitor. The video signal is amplified and transmitted by cable to the television monitor, where it is transformed back into a visible image. The television monitor forms one end of a closed circuit television system. The other end is the television camera. There are two immediately obvious differences between closed circuit television fluoroscopy and a home television set—no audio and no channel selection. There are usually only two controls that the technologist will manipulate—contrast and brightness.

The heart of the television monitor is the **TV picture tube** or cathode-ray tube (CRT). Such a tube is illustrated in Fig. 18-11. It has many similarities to the camera tube—glass envelope, electron gun, and external coils for focusing and steering the electron beam. It is different from a camera tube in that it is very much larger and its anode assembly consists of a fluorescent screen and graphite lining.

The video signal received by the picture tube is **modulated;** that is, its magnitude is directly proportional to the optic signal received by the camera tube. Unlike the camera tube, the electron beam of the picture tube varies in intensity

according to the modulation of the video signal. The intensity of the electron beam is controlled by a **control grid,** which is attached to the electron gun. This electron beam is focused onto the output fluorescent screen by the external coils. Here the electrons interact with an output phosphor and produce a burst of light. The phosphor is composed of linear crystals aligned perpendicularly to the glass envelope to reduce **lateral dispersion.** It is usually backed by a thin layer of aluminum that transmits the electron beam but reflects the light.

Television image. The image on the television monitor is formed in a complex way that can be described rather simply. It involves transforming the visible-light image of the output phosphor of the image-intensifier tube into an electrical video signal that is created by a constant electron beam in the TV camera tube. The video signal then modulates, or varies, the electron beam of the TV picture tube and transforms that electron beam into a visible image at the fluorescent screen of the picture tube.

Both electron beams, the constant one of the camera tube and the modulated one of the picture tube, are finely focused pencil beams that

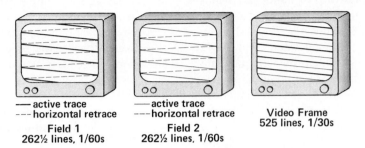

—— active trace
--- horizontal retrace
Field 1
262½ lines, 1/60s

—— active trace
--- horizontal retrace
Field 2
262½ lines, 1/60s

Video Frame
525 lines, 1/30s

Fig. 18-12. A video frame is formed from a raster pattern of two interlaced video fields.

are precisely and synchronously directed by the external electromagnetic coils of each tube. The beams are **synchronous** because they are both always at the same position at the same time and move in precisely the same fashion.

The movement of these electron beams produces a **raster** pattern as shown in Fig. 18-12, where the screen of a TV picture tube is illustrated. Although the following discussion relates to a picture tube, remember that the same electron-beam pattern is occurring in the camera tube. The electron beam begins in the upper-left corner of the screen and moves to the upper-right corner, creating a line of varying intensity of light as it moves. This is called an **active trace.** The electron beam then is **blanked,** or turned off, and it returns to the left side of the screen as shown. This is called the **horizontal retrace.** There follows a series of active traces followed by horizontal retraces until the electron beam is at the bottom of the screen. This is much like the action of a typist who types a line of information (the active trace), returns the carriage (the horizontal retrace), and continues this sequence to the bottom of the page. Whereas the typist completes a page, the electron beam completes a **television field.**

The similarity stops there, however, because the typist would continue on another page. The electron beam is blanked again and undergoes a **vertical retrace** to the top of the screen. It now describes a second television field, the same

as the first except that each active trace lies between two adjacent active traces of the first field. This movement of the electron beam is termed **interlace,** and two interlaced television fields form one **television frame.**

In the United States our power is supplied at 60 Hz and therefore there are 60 television fields per second and 30 television frames per second. This is fortuitous because the flickering of home movies shown at 16 frames per second or of old-time movies—the "flicks"—does not appear on the television image. Flickering is not detectable by the human eye at rates above about 25 frames per second. At a frame rate of 30 per second, each frame is 33 ms long.

In the camera tube, as the electron beam reads the optic signal, the signal is erased. In the picture tube, as the electron beam creates the optic signal, it immediately fades; hence the term "fluorescent screen." Therefore each new television frame represents 33 ms of new information.

Standard broadcast and closed circuit TV are called 525-line systems because they have 525 lines of active trace per frame. Actually there are only about 490 lines per frame because of the time required for retracing. Other special purpose systems have 875 or 1000 lines per frame and therefore have superior **vertical resolution.** These high-resolution systems are particularly important for digital fluoroscopy.

The **horizontal resolution** is determined by a

property called **bandwidth** or **bandpass.** Bandpass is expressed in frequency (Hz) and describes the number of times per second that the electron beam can be modulated. A 1 MHz bandpass would indicate that the electron beam intensity could be changed a million times each second. The higher the bandpass, the higher the horizontal resolution. The objective of television designers is to create a television frame having equal horizontal and vertical resolution. Commercial television systems have a bandpass of about 3.5 MHz; those used in fluoroscopy are about 4.5 MHz; 1000-line, high-resolution systems have a bandpass of about 20 MHz.

Even though these numbers may seem to indicate a relatively high resolution, **the television monitor remains the weakest link in image-intensified fluoroscopy.** A 525-line system can do no better than about 2 lp/mm, but the image intensifier is good to about 5 lp/mm. Therefore, to take advantage of the superior resolution of the image intensifier, the image must be recorded on film through an optically coupled photographic camera.

Cinefluorography. In cinefluorography the TV camera tube is replaced with a movie camera that records the image on film for later playback. Cinefluorography finds most application in certain angiographic procedures, especially those associated with **cardiac catheterization.** The patient dose is much higher than that required for recording of images electronically on magnetic tape or disk, but the image quality is also higher.

Both 16 and 35 mm film movie cameras are used for cinefluorography. The 35 mm film format requires more patient exposure than the 16 mm film format, but the image quality is also better. Cine cameras are driven by **synchronous motors** controlled by the line voltage, which is 60 Hz (1 Hz = 1 cycle per second). Therefore they have framing frequencies of 7.5, 15, 30, and 60 frames per second. Naturally, the higher the framing frequency, the higher the radiation dose. High framing frequencies are necessary

for cardiac studies, but 7.5 frames per second may be adequate for intestinal examinations.

All present cinefluorographic systems are **synchronized.** That is, the x-ray tube is energized only during the time when the cine film is in position for exposure. The tube is not energized during the time between frames when the film is advancing because this would result in considerably excessive and unnecessary patient exposure.

Spot filming. The conventional cassette-loaded spot film is used with image-intensified fluoroscopes. The spot film is positioned between the patient and the image intensifier. When a cassette spot film exposure is desired, the radiologist must actuate a control that properly positions the cassette and changes the operation of the x-ray tube from low fluoroscopic mA to high radiographic mA. Sometimes a second or two is required for the rotating anode to be energized to a higher speed. Exposures with cassette-loaded spot films require more patient dose, and the delay necessary before exposure can be made is sometimes a nuisance. Cassette-loaded spot films, however, do provide a familiar format for the radiologist and have high image quality.

Recent developments in large format spot film cameras are resulting in the slow disappearance of cassette-loaded spot films. The spot film camera is similar to a movie camera except that it exposes only one frame when activated. It receives its image from the output phosphor of the image-intensifier tube and therefore requires less patient exposure than the cassette-loaded spot film. It does not require significant interruption of the fluoroscopic examination, nor is there the additional heat load on the x-ray tube associated with cassette-loaded spot films. Current spot film cameras use film sizes of 70, 90, and 105 mm. As a general rule, **a larger film format results in better image quality but increased patient dose.** Even with 105 mm spot films, however, the patient dose is small compared to cassette-loaded spot films.

TOMOGRAPHY

A conventional film of the chest or abdomen images all structures contained in these portions of the body with approximately equal clarity. The structures, however, are superimposed on one another, and often this superimposition results in a masking of the structure of interest. When this occurs, a procedure called **tomography** may be necessary.

The tomographic examination is designed to bring into focus only those objects lying in a plane of interest while blurring structures on either side of the plane. Actually, the object is not focused in the normal sense, but rather its radiographic contrast is enhanced by the blurring of the adjacent structures. Since the introduction of computed tomography and magnetic resonance imaging, with their excellent low-contrast resolution, tomography has been employed with less frequency. Tomography is now applied principally to high-contrast anatomy.

During the tomographic examination, the ra-

diographic tube head is caused to move in a precise fashion while the film moves synchronously. There are five basic types of tomographic movements: linear, circular, elliptical, hypocycloidal, and trispiral.

Linear tomography

The simplest tomographic examination is linear tomography. During linear tomography (Fig. 18-13), the radiographic tube is mechanically attached to the image receptor and moves in one direction while the image receptor moves in the opposite direction. The capacity to perform tomography can be obtained inexpensively by altering a conventional radiographic table to accommodate tube and film motion. With this type of linear tomography, the tube and the film remain in the same plane during motion, as shown in Fig. 18-13, A. Apparatus specially designed for linear tomography is usually constructed so that the tube head and the image receptor move in concentric arcs during the ex-

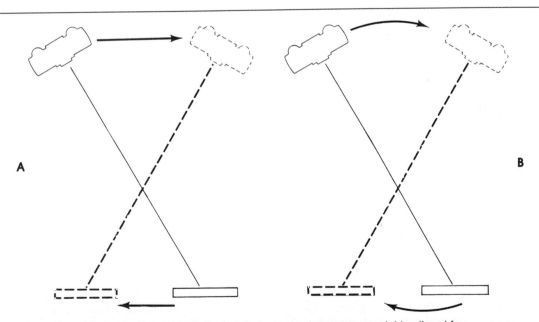

Fig. 18-13. A, Cassette tray and tube head of a general purpose x-ray table altered for tomography move in a plane. **B,** Those of a table designed specifically for tomography move in an arc.

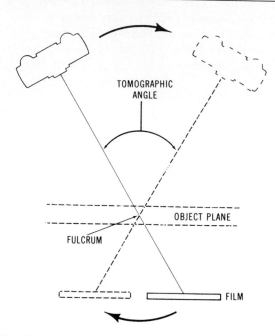

Fig. 18-14. Relationship of fulcrum, object plane, and tomographic angle.

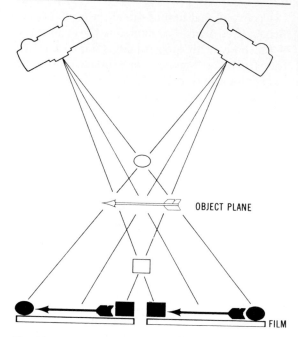

Fig. 18-15. Only objects lying in the object plane are properly imaged. Objects on either side of this plane are blurred because they are imaged across the film.

amination, as shown in Fig. 18-13, *B*. This latter method of linear tomography results in higher-quality tomographs, but it is more expensive.

Other aspects of the linear tomographic examination are shown in Fig. 18-14. The fulcrum is the imaginary pivot point about which the tube and the film move. The fulcrum lies in the **focal,** or **object, plane,** and only those anatomic objects lying in this plane will be imaged and focused. The farther from the object plane an anatomic structure is, the more blurred its image will be. The angle of movement is known as the **tomographic angle.** It determines the thickness of cut, the thickness that will be clearly imaged.

Fig. 18-15 illustrates how structures in the object plane are imaged while other structures are not. The examination begins with the tube head and the film positioned on opposite sides

of the fulcrum. The exposure begins as the tube and film move simultaneously in opposite directions. The image of a structure lying in the object plane, such as the arrow in Fig. 18-15, will have a fixed position on the radiograph throughout the tube travel. On the other hand, the images of structures lying outside the object plane, such as the ball and box in Fig. 18-15, will have varying positions on the film according to the position of the tomographic movement. Consequently, the ball and box will be blurred. The larger the tomographic angle, the more blurred the images of structures outside the object plane will be.

The blurring of objects lying outside the object plane is simply a example of **motion unsharpness** caused by the moving tube head. In theory, only objects lying precisely in the object plane, which is the plane of the fulcrum, will be properly

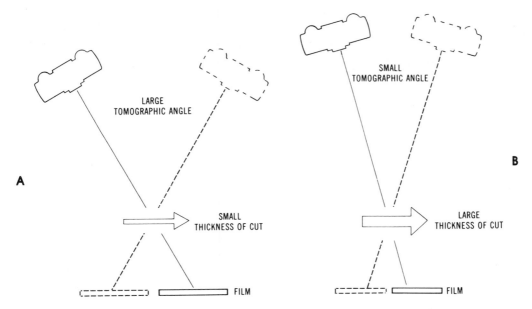

Fig. 18-16. Thickness of cut is determined by the tomographic angle. **A,** A large tomographic angle results in a small thickness of cut. **B,** A small tomographic angle results in a large thickness of cut.

imaged. Objects lying outside this plane will exhibit increasing motion unsharpness with increasing distance from the object plane. In practice, however, structures throughout a given volume of tissue described by two planes parallel to and equidistant from the object plane are in focus. This tissue volume is shown schematically in Fig. 18-16. The thickness of tissue that will be properly imaged is called the **tomographic layer,** and its width is described numerically by the **thickness of cut.**

The thickness of cut is controlled by the tomographic angle, **The larger the tomographic angle, the smaller the thickness of cut.** Table 18-1 shows the approximate relationship between tomographic angle and thickness of cut. When the tomographic angle is very small (for example, 0 degrees), the in-focus layer is the entire anatomic structure, and we have a con-

Table 18-1. Approximate values for thickness of cut during linear tomogrtaphy as a function of tomographic angle

Tomographic angle (degrees)	Thickness of cut (mm)
0	Infinity
2	31
4	16
6	11
10	6
20	3
35	2
50	1

ventional radiograph. When the tomographic angle is 10 degrees, the thickness of cut is approximately 6 mm; structures lying farther than 3 mm from the object plane will appear blurred.

Multidirectional tomography

Tomographs sometimes appear streaked. This occurs when linear structures such as long bones lie outside the object plane and are oriented in the direction of film movement. Another disadvantage of linear tomography is that the in-focus section is not very distinct, and the degree of blurring varies over the radiograph. This effect is primarily objectionable during wide-angle tomography. It occurs because the distance from tube to patient and the angulation of the x-ray beam change during exposure, resulting in nonuniform density across the radiograph. If sharper tomographs are to be obtained, a multidirectional motion is necessary.

Actually a tomograph can be produced if the x-ray tube and film move synchronously in any direction or pattern of directions. Because of engineering considerations, four multidirectional movements, shown in Fig. 18-17, are employed: circular, elliptical, hypocycloidal, and trispiral. For a given tomographic angle, the hypocycloidal and trispiral movements will result

in the sharpest tomographic image. The circular tomographic movement is the poorest of the four, but it is considerably better than linear tomography for the production of sharp, thin-sectioned tomographs. The major disadvantage of multidirectional tomography is cost. These units can be quite expensive.

Zonography

If the tomographic angle is less than about 10 degrees, the thickness of cut will be quite large, as shown in Table 18-1. This type of tomography is called **zonography** because a relatively large zone of tissue is brought into focus. Zonography is employed when the subject contrast is so low that thin-section tomography would result in a poor image. Zonography finds most application in chest examinations. Usually tomographic angles of 1 to 5 degrees are employed.

Practical considerations

The principal advantage to tomography is **improved radiographic contrast**. By blurring over-

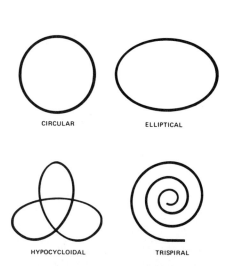

Fig. 18-17. Multidirectional tomography movements for tube head and film tray.

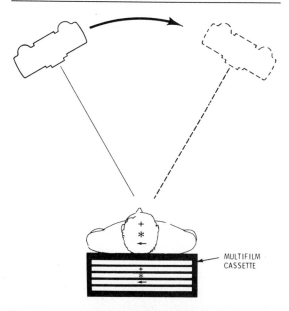

Fig. 18-18. Multifilm tomography provides simultaneous tomographic views of different object planes within the body.

lying and underlying tissues, the subject contrast of the tissues of the tomographic layer is enhanced. The more irregular the movement of the x-ray tube and image receptor, the greater will be the contrast enhancement. Irregular tube-receptor movement does not affect the thickness of the tomographic layer, only the tomographic angle.

The principal disadvantage of tomography is increased patient dose. The x-ray tube is energized during the entire tube travel, which can be several seconds long. A single nephrotomographic exposure, for example, can result in a patient dose of 1000 mrad (10 mGy). Furthermore, most tomographic examinations require several exposures to make certain that the plane of interest is brought into focus. A sixteen-film tomographic examination can result in a patient dose of several rad.

One attempt to reduce patient dose during tomography is a technique known as **simultaneous multifilm tomography.** During simultaneous multifilm tomography, a book cassette is

loaded with four to six films in booklike fashion and positioned as in Fig. 18-18. The screen-film combination of each page of the book must be adjusted so that radiographic density remains constant throughout. The separation of one film from another can be varied but is usually 0.5 to 1 cm. In effect, simultaneous multifilm tomography accomplishes with one exposure the same objective that conventional tomography does with four to six exposures.

The determination of the thickness of cut is made by selecting the proper tomographic angle. The plane of cut is determined by adjusting the height of the radiographic tube from the table or by repositioning the patient between exposures with an adjustable table.

Grids are employed during a tomographic examination for the same reason that they are employed during conventional radiography. **During tomography, linear grids must be used, and the grid lines must be oriented in the same direction as the tube movement.** For linear tomography this usually means that the grid will be positioned with its grid lines parallel with the length of the table. For multidirectional tomography the grid must change its orientation in accordance with movement of the tube head, as shown in Fig. 18-19, while the film remains in the fixed orientation., In effect, the grid rotates over the film during multidirectional tomography.

STEREORADIOGRAPHY

During the early part of this century, the stereoscope (Fig. 18-20) was a popular device. When two properly exposed photographs are inserted into it, the stereoscope provides three-dimensional images and photographic viewing with great depth perception. Today the use of stereoscopes is mostly limited to children's toys.

Similarly, in the early years of this century, stereoradiography was prominent, whereas today its use is limited. **Stereoradiography** involves making two radiographs of the same object and viewing them stereoscopically, usually with a specially constructed stereoscope. Ster-

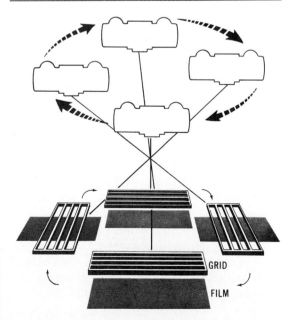

Fig. 18-19. Movement of x-ray tube, film, and grid during multidirectional tomography.

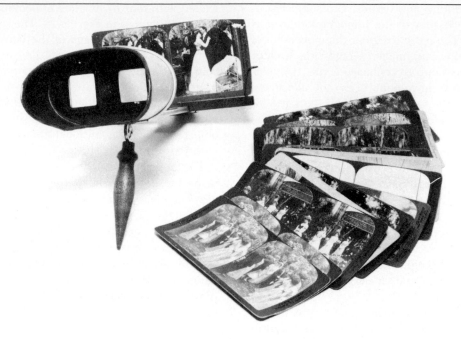

Fig. 18-20. Early twentieth century stereoscope. (Courtesy Sharon Briney-Glaze.)

eoradiography provides a three-dimensional image instead of the flat image obtained with conventional radiography.

Stereoradiography can be particularly helpful in locating foreign bodies and identifying calcified lesions in dense or thick body sections where interpretation of right-angle radiographs might be difficult. Stereoradiography also provides for superior interpretation of the relative location of internal structures. The interpretation of particularly confusing radiographs may be helped by stereoscopic radiography.

The principal disadvantage of stereoradiography is that it requires twice the patient exposure. Additionally, it takes practice to produce good stereoradiographs, and considerable patient cooperation is required.

Making stereoradiographs

Stereoradiographs involve the exposure of two films with the x-ray tube shifted in position between the two. The critical condition that the radiologic technologist must satisfy to produce a good stereoradiograph is the degree of tube shift. Stereoradiography should not be confused with tomography. In stereoradiography the film position does not change. The tube shift is dependent on a number of factors, principally the SID, the viewing distance, and the interpupillary distance. These factors are complexly interrelated. A good rule of thumb assumes an interpupillary distance of 65 mm and a viewing distance of approximately 65 cm. These values are in the ratio of 1:10, which is approximately what the ratio of the tube shift to SID should be. Fig. 18-21 illustrates this principle. Should the viewing distance change significantly, the ratio of tube shift to SID should be changed accordingly. For most situations, however, the following generalization is sufficient:

(18-2)

$$Tube\ shift = 0.1 \times SID$$

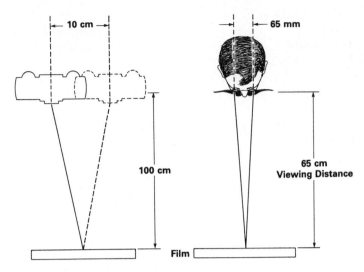

Fig. 18-21. Degree of tube shift required in making a stereoradiograph is dependent on the SID, the interpupillary distance, and the viewing distance.

EXAMPLE: Chest stereoradiographs are made at 180 cm SID. What should be the amount of tube shift on either side of the midline?

ANSWER: *Tube shift* = 0.1 × 180 cm
                          = 18 cm

Therefore the shift should be 9 cm to each side of the midline.

If the SID equals the viewing distance, the tube shift should equal the interpupillary distance.

When using grids while making stereoradiographs, one must take care that the tube shift is in the same direction as the grid lines. With low-ratio grids and large SIDs, a tube shift across the grid lines is usually acceptable. The tube shift should also be across any dominant linear structures such as long bones. If the direction of the tube shift is the same as the direction of the linear structure, the stereoscopic effect will be lessened. This rule is easy to remember, since it also applies to tomography. The stereoscopic

effect will be lost if there is any patient movement between exposures. This should be carefully explained to the patient to obtain maximum cooperation.

Stereoradiography takes practice and patience. The following steps are involved. They are simple but must be precisely followed to produce satisfactory results.

1. Properly position the patient and line up the film and x-ray tube as though a single radiograph were to be taken.
2. Determine the SID and the appropriate tube shift distance.
3. Shift the tube half the required distance from the midline and expose the film. The film should be marked to identify the direction of the tube shift.
4. Change films and mark the new film for identity.
5. Shift the tube an equal distance to the opposite side of the midline and expose the second radiograph.

6. Process both radiographs under identical conditions.
7. View them stereoscopically.

Viewing stereoradiographs

Stereoradiographs are normally viewed in stereoscopes specially designed for radiographs. These stereoscopes are optical devices incorporating lenses, prisms, mirrors, or combinations thereof. One such stereoscope is illustrated in Fig. 18-22. The important requirement for viewing stereoradiographs is the proper positioning of the film. Basically, the radiographs should be viewed in the same position in which they were made, as though the eyes were the x-ray tube. The tube side of the film should be toward the eyes. The radiographs should be positioned side by side along the direction of the tube shift, not perpendicular to it. The right eye should view the film made when the tube was shifted to the right of center, and the left eye should view the film made when the tube was shifted to the left of center.

Many radiologists are proficient at cross-eyed stereoscopy. This technique requires no special viewing equipment. The stereoradiographs are positioned in reverse order to their normal relationship and viewed by crossing the eyes.

MAGNIFICATION RADIOGRAPHY

Magnification radiography is a technique used principally by vascular radiologists and neuroradiologists. Many feel that it enhances the visualization of fine vessels and bony structures.

Magnification radiography uses the principles of magnification described in Chapter 16. To obtain a magnified radiograph, the object is placed at a distance from the film, as shown in Fig. 18-23. The degree of magnification is given by the

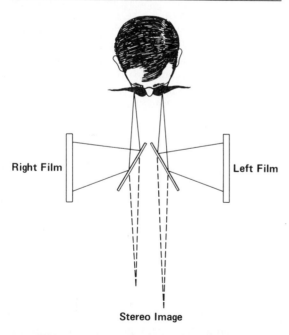

Fig. 18-22. Basic principle employed in viewing a stereoradiograph.

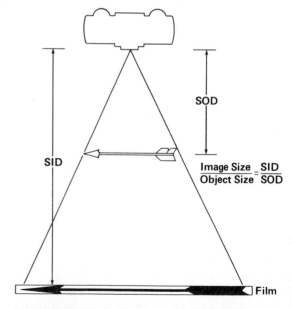

$$\frac{\text{Image Size}}{\text{Object Size}} = \frac{\text{SID}}{\text{SOD}}$$

Fig. 18-23. Principle of magnification radiography. The magnification factor is equal to the ratio of image size to object size.

magnification factor (MF), described in equation 16-5 as

$$MF = \frac{SID}{SOD}$$

where SID is the source–to–image receptor distance and SOD is the source–to–object distance.

EXAMPLE: A magnified radiograph of the sella turcica is taken at 100 cm SID with the object positioned 25 cm from the film. If the image of the sella turcica measures 16 mm, what is its actual size?

ANSWER: $MF = \dfrac{100}{(100 - 25)} = 1.33$

$$\frac{Image\ size}{Object\ size} = MF$$

$$Object\ size = \frac{Image\ size}{MF}$$

$$= \frac{16}{1.33}$$

$$= 12.0\ mm$$

A small focal spot must be used to make a magnified radiograph. The geometric unsharpness resulting from an unnecessarily large focal spot can destroy the diagnostic value of the radiograph. Usually grids are not needed for magnified radiography. The large object–to–image receptor distance (OID) results in a significant air gap so that scatter radiation is diverted away from the film. The larger the OID, the lower the amount of scatter radiation reaching the film.

The principal disadvantage of magnification radiography, like so many specialized techniques, is increased patient dose. To obtain a magnification factor of 2, one must position the patient halfway between the source and the film. Recall that radiation intensity is related to the square of the distance, which suggests a fourfold increase in patient dose. In reality, most magnification radiographs result in only two or three times the normal patient exposure because grids are not used.

REVIEW QUESTIONS

1. Define or otherwise identify the following:
   a. Photopic vision
   b. Tomographic angle
   c. Automatic brightness control
   d. Magnification factor
   e. Visual acuity
   f. Flux gain
   g. Hypocycloidal
   h. Angiography
   i. Vidicon
   j. Photoemission
2. Describe the operation of the fluoroscope and the advantages of image-intensified fluoroscopy over conventional fluoroscopy.
3. Discuss the anatomy of vision as it influences fluoroscopy.
4. Diagram the image-intensifier tube, label its principal parts, and discuss their functions.
5. A 23 cm image-intensifier tube has a flux gain of 52. What is its brightness gain?
6. When image intensification is employed, what modes of monitoring are possible?
7. Diagram hypocycloidal tomography and identify the fulcrum, tomographic angle, object plane, image plane, grid position, and film position.
8. Portable films taken at 76 cm SID are to be used stereoscopically. What degree of tube shift to either side of midline should be used?
9. What steps are necessary for making good stereographs?
10. L-4 is radiographed at an SID of 150 cm and an SOD of 50 cm. The width of L-4 on the radiograph measures 72 mm. What is its true width?

19

Mammography

BASIS FOR MAMMOGRAPHY
X-RAY APPARATUS
IMAGE RECEPTORS
XERORADIOGRAPHIC PROCESS
CONCLUSION

Radiographic examination of soft tissues, called **soft tissue radiography,** requires selected techniques that differ greatly from conventional radiography because of the substantial differences in the anatomic structures being radiographed. In conventional radiography the subject contrast is great because of the large differences in mass density and effective atomic number among bone, muscle, fat, and lung tissue. In soft tissue radiography, however, only muscle and fat structures are imaged, and these tissues have similar effective atomic numbers (Table 9-1) and similar effective densities (Table 9-2). Consequently, in soft tissue radiography the techniques employed are designed to enhance differential absorption in these very similar tissues.

A prime example of soft tissue radiography is **mammography**—radiographic examination of the breast. As a distinct type of radiographic examination, mammography was first attempted in the 1920s. However, the lack of adequate equipment precluded its development at that time. In the late 1950s, Dr. Robert Egan renewed interest in mammography with his demonstration of a successful technique using low kVp, high mAs, and direct film exposure. Since that time, mammography has undergone considerable development and now enjoys widespread application.

The principal motivation for continuing the development and improvement of mammography is the incidence of breast cancer. Breast cancer is the leading cause of cancer death in women and the leading cause of death from all causes for women in the 40 to 50 age group. Each year about 90,000 new cases of breast cancer are reported in the United States. One third of these result in death. Equally frightening is the knowledge that one out of every ten women will develop breast cancer during her life.

Most physicians believe that early detection of breast cancer should result in more effective treatment and fewer deaths. X-ray mammography has proved to be an accurate breast cancer detection method, the accuracy of which can be extended still further. With continuing development of dedicated mammographic x-ray apparatus and imaging systems, the image quality is being improved and the patient dose reduced. Patient dose in mammography is of primary importance when considering the overall efficacy, because it is known that radiation can cause breast cancer as well as detect it. Radiation carcinogenesis (the induction of cancer) is discussed in Chapter 29. The dose necessary to produce breast cancer is unknown; however, the dose experienced in mammography is well known and is covered in Chapter 32. This chapter concerns the technique, equipment, and procedures employed in mammography.

BASIS FOR MAMMOGRAPHY

Normal breasts consist of three principal types of tissue: fibrous, glandular, and adipose (fat). In a premenopausal woman the fibrous and glandular tissues are structured into various ducts, glands, and connective tissues. These are surrounded by a thin layer of fat. Postmenopausal breasts are characterized by a degeneration of this fibroglandular tissue and an increase in the adipose tissue. The tissue most sensitive to the induction of cancer by radiation is the glandular tissue. If a malignancy is present, it will be manifested by a distortion of the normal ductal and connective tissue patterns and may have associated deposits of microcalcifications. These are calcific deposits appearing as small grains of varying sizes. The sizes of interest for breast cancer detection are those microcalcifications less than approximately 500 μm.

Because mass density and effective atomic number for soft tissue components of the breast are so similar, conventional radiographic technique is useless. In the 70 to 100 kVp range, Compton scattering predominates with soft tissue; thus differential absorption among tissues

of similar composition is minimum. Low kVp must be employed to maximize the photoelectric effect and therefore enhance differential absorption.

Recall that x-ray absorption in tissue occurs principally by photoelectric effect and Compton effect. The degree of absorption is determined by the mass density and the effective atomic number. Absorption caused by differences in mass density by photoelectric and Compton effects is simply proportional to the mass density. Absorption caused by differences in the effective atomic number, however, is directly proportional for Compton interactions and **proportional to the cube of the effective atomic number for photoelectric interaction.** Furthermore, at low x-ray energy, photoelectric absorption becomes increasingly more frequent than Compton scattering.

Therefore x-ray mammography requires a low-kVp technique. However, as kVp is reduced, the penetrability of the x-ray beam is also reduced, which in turn requires an increase in the mAs. If the kVp is too low, an inordinately high mAs may be required, and this could be unacceptable because of the increased patient dose. **Patient dose, of course, is the principal disadvantage of x-ray mammography.** Technique factors between 25 and 50 kVp are usually employed as an effective compromise between the increasing dose at the low-kVp range and reduced image quality at the high-kVp range.

X-RAY APPARATUS

Acceptable radiographic results can rarely be obtained with conventional x-ray apparatus; therefore specially designed, dedicated x-ray machines should be used for mammography. Nearly all x-ray apparatus manufacturers now produce such units; Fig. 19-1 shows four popular models. Dedicated mammographic units are designed for flexibility in patient positioning with a compression device, low-ratio grid technique, automatic exposure control, and microfocus x-ray tubes for magnification radiography.

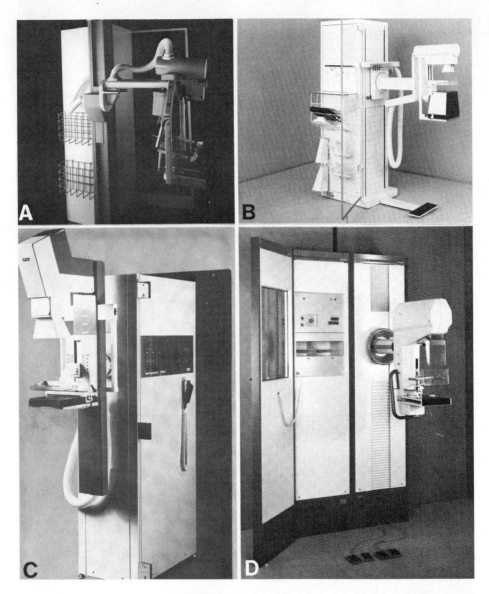

Fig. 19-1. Representative available dedicated mammography units. **A,** The Xerox 120 System. **B,** The Phillips Mammo Diagnost. **C,** The CGR Senographe 500 T. **D,** The Siemens Mammomat. (**A** courtesy The Xerox Corp.; **B** courtesy Phillips Medical Systems, Inc.; **C** courtesy Thompson-CGR; **D** courtesy Siemens Medical Systems.)

Target composition

Mammographic x-ray tubes are manufactured with either a tungsten target or a molybdenum target. Fig. 19-2 shows the x-ray emission spectrum from a tungsten-target tube operating at 30 and 50 kVp. Note that the bremsstrahlung spectrum predominates and that the only characteristic x rays present are those from *L*-shell transitions. **These *L*-characteristic x rays are of no value in mammographic imaging because their energy, approximately 12 keV, is too low to penetrate the breast.** These photons are all absorbed and serve only to contribute to patient dose. The x rays most useful for enhancing differential absorption in breast tissue and for maximizing radiographic contrast are those in the 20 to 30 keV range. The tungsten target supplies sufficient x rays in this energy range but also an abundance of x rays above and below this range.

Fig. 19-3 shows the emission spectrum from a molybdenum-target tube with its near absence of bremsstrahlung x rays. The most prominent x rays are characteristic, with energy of approximately 20 keV resulting from *K*-shell interactions. Molybdenum has an atomic number of 42, compared with 74 for that of tungsten, and this difference is responsible for the differences in emission spectra. Bremsstrahlung x rays are produced much more readily in high-Z target atoms. Molybdenum *K*-characteristic x rays have energy corresponding to the *K*-shell electron binding energy; this just happens to be within the range of energies that are most effective for mammographic imaging. The change in tube potential from 30 to 50 kVp results in a minor change in the shape of the emission spectrum from a molybdenum-target x-ray tube.

Filtration

At the low tube potentials employed for mammography it is important to have the proper type and thickness of filtration in the beam. **Under no circumstances should total beam filtration be less than 0.5 mm Al equivalent.** Most mammographic tubes have inherent filtration of approximately 0.1 mm Al equivalent. If it is a tungsten-target tube, it should have added filtration of aluminum. If it is a molybdenum-target tube, then molybdenum filtration of 30 μm is recommended. Regardless of the tube target or filtration, the half-value layer (HVL) is always very low.

Mammography tubes fabricated with a target of molybdenum-tungsten alloy are also employed. Such tubes emit a mixed radiation spec-

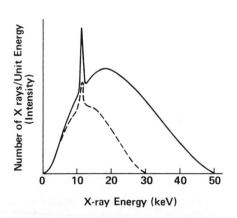

Fig. 19-2. X-ray emission spectrum for a tungsten-target x-ray tube operated at 30 and 50 kVp.

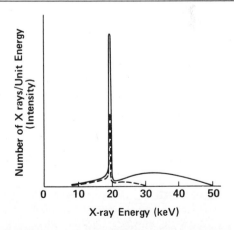

Fig. 19-3. X-ray emission spectrum for a molybdenum-target x-ray tube operated at 30 and 50 kVp.

trum having the characteristics of each of those target elements. By selecting either an aluminum or molybdenum filter, one can shape the x-ray emission spectrum to compatibility with the type of image receptor employed.

Heel effect

The heel effect is of considerable importance to mammography. The conic shape of breasts should require that the radiation intensity near the chest wall be higher than that to the nipple side so that near uniform exposure of the image receptor will occur. This could be accomplished by positioning the cathode to the chest wall, as shown in Fig. 19-4. In practice this is not necessary because vigorous compression ensures that a uniform thickness of tissue is imaged.

If such an arrangement is employed, however, the image of a structure near the chest wall will be degraded somewhat because of the increased geometric unsharpness created by the larger effective focal spot size. Therefore, if this were a primary consideration, the anode would be positioned toward the chest wall, as diagrammed in Fig. 19-5.

In summary, then, it can be said that (1) the cathode should be positioned to the chest wall for equal radiation intensity, and (2) the anode should be positioned toward the chest wall for best image sharpness. In fact, manufacturers of dedicated mammography equipment accommodate both these situations satisfactorily by employing a relatively long source–to–image receptor distance (SID), 50 to 70 cm, with the anode to the chest wall, as seen in Fig. 19-5. Target angles of approximately 20 degrees are employed.

Compression

Compression is important in many aspects of conventional radiology, but it is of particular importance in mammography. **Compression should always be employed in x-ray mammography.** Several advantages resulting from the use of compression are demonstrated in Fig. 19-6. A compressed breast is of more uniform thickness, and therefore the image pattern will be more uniform. Tissues near the chest wall are less apt to be underexposed and tissues near the nipple are less apt to be overexposed. Sec-

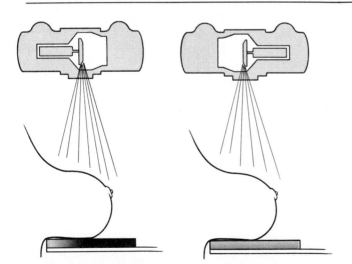

Fig. 19-4. Heel effect can be used to advantage in mammography by positioning the cathode toward the chest wall so that a more uniform image density will be produced.

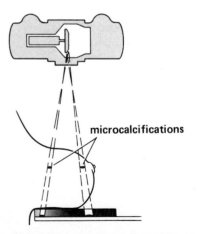

microcalcifications

Fig. 19-5. If the anode is positioned toward the chest wall, resolution of objects to that side will be enhanced because of the smaller effective focal spot size.

ond, by compression, all object structures are brought closer to the image plane, and geometric unsharpness is reduced. Finally, absorption unsharpness, radiation dose, and scatter radiation are all reduced.

All dedicated mammographic x-ray units have a built-in stiff compression device that is parallel with the surface of the image receptor. Vigorous compression of the breast is necessary for optimum image quality.

Grids

The use of fiber interspaced grids during screen-film mammography is increasing. Although mammographic image contrast is high because of the low kVp used, it is not high enough. Many now use moving grids with a ratio of 3:1 to 5:1 focused to the SID to enhance image contrast. Use of such grids does not compromise high-contrast spatial resolution, but it does increase patient dose. Use of a 4:1 ratio grid will almost double the patient dose when compared to nongrid screen-film mammography. The dose is acceptably low, however, and the improvement in visibility of image detail is significant.

Magnification mammography

Magnification techniques are now frequently used in mammography, producing images 1½ times normal size. Special equipment is required for magnification mammography, such as microfocus tubes, adequate compression, and patient positioning devices. Effective focal spot size should not exceed 0.3 mm. **Magnification mammography should not be used routinely** because:

1. Normal mammograms are adequate for most patients.
2. The entire breast may not be completely imaged.
3. Patient dose may be doubled.

IMAGE RECEPTORS

There are three types of image receptors employed in mammography: direct-exposure film, screen-film, and Xerox. The latter two are employed at the present time and both have distinctive characteristics. Direct-exposure mammography has the distinct disadvantage of excessively high patient dose; consequently, this modality has been replaced by the other two as the image receptor of choice.

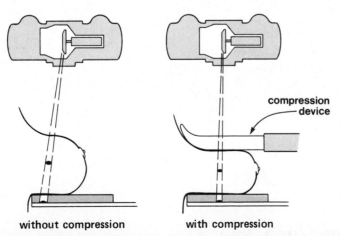

Fig. 19-6. Use of compression in mammography has three advantages: uniform image receptor exposure, reduced geometric unsharpness, and reduced absorption and scatter.

Direct-exposure film

Direct-exposure films were the first to be employed in mammography. Initially such films were those developed for industrial radiographic purposes, but, as the Egan technique became more widely accepted, film manufacturers produced similar films, specifically identified for mammography. Direct-exposure films are fine-grain, double-emulsion films with high contrast and extremely high resolution. These films are supplied in prepackaged sealed paper envelopes or in bulk for use with fiberboard or plastic cassettes. The high contrast has the undesirable correlate of narrow latitude. There is not much room for error in radiographic technique. Overexposure or underexposure occurs more frequently. The high-resolution properties of direct exposure are of limited benefit. Patient motion and the geometric unsharpness resulting from measurable focal spot size limit the overall system resolution to much less than that of the film.

Direct-exposure films are slow. They are five to fifty times slower than screen-film combinations, and consequently they require five to fifty times as much patient dose as the screen-film examination. This is the principal disadvantage of direct-exposure mammography, and it is the principal reason for its replacement by screen-film examination or xeroradiography. **No one should be doing direct-exposure mammography today.**

Screen-film combinations

Radiographic intensifying screens and films have been especially designed for x-ray mammography. The films are primarily single emulsion, although some special double-emulsion films are now available. Regardless of the type of film, it must have matched photosensitivity for the light emission of the associated intensifying screen. Special emulsions coupled with rare earth screen material are available. The screen-film combination is placed in a low-attenuating cassette, specially designed, to produce good screen-film contact. **The emulsion surface must always be adjacent to the screen, and the combination package must be positioned so that the emulsion surface is toward the x-ray tube.**

The use of the intensifying screen increases

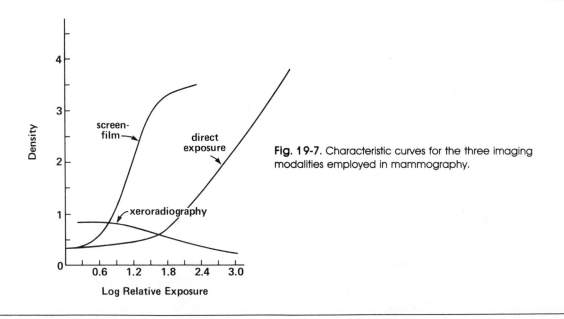

Fig. 19-7. Characteristic curves for the three imaging modalities employed in mammography.

the speed of this imaging system significantly, resulting in a patient dose much less than that experienced with direct-exposure examination. The use of screens also enhances the radiographic contrast compared with that from direct-exposure examination. The resolution of the screen-film combination is less than that of direct-exposure film but better than that of conventional screen-film radiograph.

Acceptable screen-film mammography requires that a molybdenum target x-ray tube be used. Because the breast tissue has such low subject contrast, a low-energy x-ray beam such as that from molybdenum is required to obtain maximum radiographic contrast. Furthermore, the x-ray tube should be operated at 28 kVp or less, and the x-ray beam should be shaped with molybdenum filtration, usually 30 μm, in order to accentuate the 20 keV characteristic x-ray emission.

Fig. 19-7 shows representative characteristic curves for direct-exposure film, screen film, and xeromammography. The curve for xeromammography is not derived in precisely the same manner as that for the films; nevertheless, it

does demonstrate a surprising lack of contrast. In view of this lack of contrast one might ask what is responsible for the success of xeromammography. The answer is a phenomenon characteristic of xeroradiography known as **edge enhancement.**

Xeromammography

Conventional radiography is based on the formation of a latent image by a photographic emulsion and wet chemistry processing to produce the visible image. Xeroradiography is quite different. It is based on the formation of an electrostatic latent image by a photoconductive material and a dry processing technique for the visible image. Its name, xeroradiography, comes from the Greek (*xeros:* dry; *graphin:* to write) and Latin (*radius:* ray).

Xeroradiography was invented in 1939 by Chester Carlson, a physicist, whose rights to the process were exploited around 1947 by the Hayloid Corporation. This company subsequently became the Xerox Corporation. Although many years were spent by Xerox in developing the process for medical imaging, it was not until

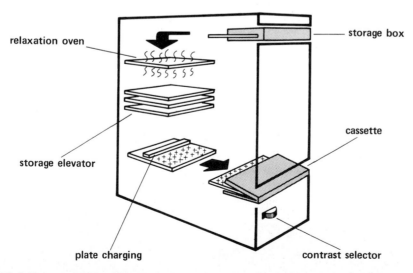

Fig. 19-8. Xerox conditioner, its principal parts, and their function. (Courtesy Xerox Corporation.)

1956 that the first commercially available system was produced.

Although both tungsten and molybdenum target x-ray tubes may be employed for xeromammography, tungsten is preferred. Xeromammograms do not rely so much on subject contrast as on soft tissue boundaries, which are greatly amplified by edge enhancement. Because edge enhancement does not depend heavily on beam quality, very good images can be obtained at higher kVp with more filtration than screen-film images. Techniques of 40 to 50 kVp with 1 to 3 mm Al filtration are typically employed. Use of a molybdenum target x-ray tube for xeromammography will result in acceptable images, but at higher patient radiation dose.

XERORADIOGRAPHIC PROCESS

The basic element of the xeroradiographic process is the **image receptor.** The image receptor is a plate of aluminuim 2 mm thick and measuring approximately 23 × 36 cm. This aluminum plate serves as the **base** for the x-ray–sensitive photoconductive material, selenium, which is deposited carefully with a controlled thickness of 150 μm. The selenium is a semiconductor; that is, it behaves not as an electrical insulator nor as an electrical conductor but somewhere in between. It is also **photoconductive; in the dark it behaves as an insulator, but, when exposed to light or x rays, it is a conductor of electrons.** A discussion of the xeroradiographic process will better describe the action of this unique type of image receptor.

There are two pieces of apparatus associated with xeroradiography. The first, the conditioner, prepares the image receptor for x-ray exposure. The second, the processor, converts the electrostatic latent image into a visible image through a dry processing technique.

Conditioner

Fig. 19-8 illustrates the various parts of the conditioner and the action of each on the image receptor plate. Xerox plates are stored in the dark in a multistage cassette or storage box. On command from the operator, the Xerox plate is removed from the storage box and transported to the **relaxation oven.** At this station the plate is heated so that any residual electrostatic charge on the surface will be removed. This step is necessary to prevent ghost images from the previous x-ray exposure from appearing on the new image.

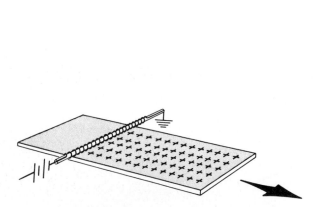

Fig. 19-9. Charging the Xerox plate by corona ionization of the air surrounding a high-voltage wire.

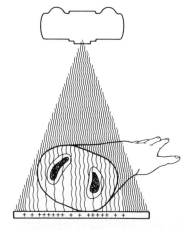

Fig. 19-10. Irradiation of the Xerox plate produces an electrostatic latent image.

After relaxation the plate has no residual surface charge. It is transported to a storage elevator where it is cooled to room temperature. This storage elevator holds sixteen plates and advances them sequentially.

The next station places a uniform positive charge on the surface of the Xerox plate. This is done by passing the plate very near to a wire that has a high (7000 to 10,000 V) positive voltage applied to it. Such a high electric potential will create ionization of air molecules in the vicinity of the wire, as shown in Fig. 19-9. This ionization pattern is called the **corona** and results in the negative electrons being attracted to the wire while the remaining positive ions are attracted to the surface of the Xerox plate as it passes nearby. The result of this station is formation of the uniform positive charge on the surface of the Xerox plate. Those familiar with the operation of the conditioner know that there are three contrast settings: B, C, and D. Position B results

in lowest contrast. Position D results in highest contrast. Position D is recommended for mammography. The differences in contrast are produced by the intensity of the positive charge deposited on the surface of the plate. Highest contrast, position D, results because the voltage on the wire is highest and causes more positive ions to be formed on the surface of the plate.

From the plate-charging station the image receptor is transferred to an exposure cassette. The cassette is sealed lighttight, as is the entire conditioning operation.

X-ray exposure

Once charged and ready for exposure, the image receptor must be used within approximately 30 minutes. If the charged plate is held longer than that before exposure, the surface charge will begin to leak, and a loss in sensitivity will result. During exposure, the cassette must be handled carefully so as not to disrupt the surface

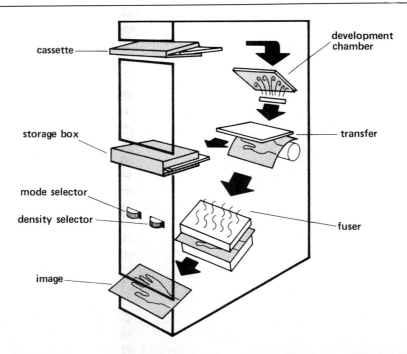

Fig. 19-11. Processor converts the electrostatic image into a visible image. (Courtesy Xerox Corporation.)

charge of the selenium plate. Rough handling of the cassette can result in artifacts from unintentional surface discharge.

When the selenium plate is x-irradiated (Fig. 19-10), the uniform electrostatic surface charge is reduced in proportion to the number of x rays that interact with the plate. After exposure the number of positive charges remaining under a thick part of the object will be greater than those remaining under a thin part of the object. The remaining electrostatic charges form a pattern representative of the distribution of x rays interacting with the plate and therefore representative of the object being radiographed. The result is an invisible electrostatic image, which is the xeroradiographic latent image. To make the latent image visible, the Xerox plate must be processed.

Processor

Image processing is accomplished in a unit known as the **processor** (Fig. 19-11). Following exposure, the technologist inserts the Xerox cassette into the processor, and the cassette is automatically opened. All processing stages take place in the dark. The Xerox plate advances to the **development chamber.** In the development chamber a fine cloud of charged, blue particles

is blown onto the plate. These particles form a powder called the **toner.** Because the particles are charged, they adhere to the plate in approximately the same distribution as the electrostatic charge pattern—the latent image. It is during this process that the mode of image display can be varied to either positive or negative. This is done by controlling the charge placed on the toner. In the development chamber the density of the final image can also be regulated by controlling the amount of toner applied to the plate. Satisfactory results may be obtained with either positive-mode or negative-mode xeromammography. However, patient dose is 30% to 50% lower in negative mode.

The Xerox plate, now containing a visible image of toner particles, is transferred from the development chamber to a station where the plate comes into contact with specially treated paper. This is the **transfer station,** and here the toner particles are removed from the Xerox plate and transferred to the paper. Now the visible image is on paper. The Xerox plate is transported from this station back to the storage box. When the storage box is full, it will be transferred from the processor to the conditioner and recycled.

At the same time the plate is returned to the

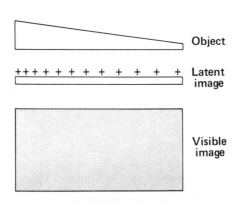

Fig. 19-12. Xeroradiograph of an inclined wedge results in a uniform image toner density that does not faithfully represent the object's thickness.

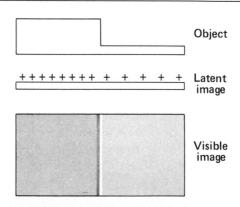

Fig. 19-13. Xeroradiograph of a step wedge images edge clearly. The toner density under each step is approximately the same.

storage box, the paper is transported to the **fuser,** the final station of the processor. In this station the Xerox paper is heated, which causes the toner particles to be melted into the thermoplastic layer of the paper. This is fusing and results in a permanent visible image. From the fusing station the Xerox paper with its image drops to the reception drawer.

Edge enhancement

The principal characteristic of the Xerox image is **edge enhancement.** Edge enhancement is the ability to amplify the contrast at the interface between two structures even when there is only minimum subject contrast. Xeroradiography has very low inherent contrast, as shown in the characteristic curve in Fig. 19-7. If an

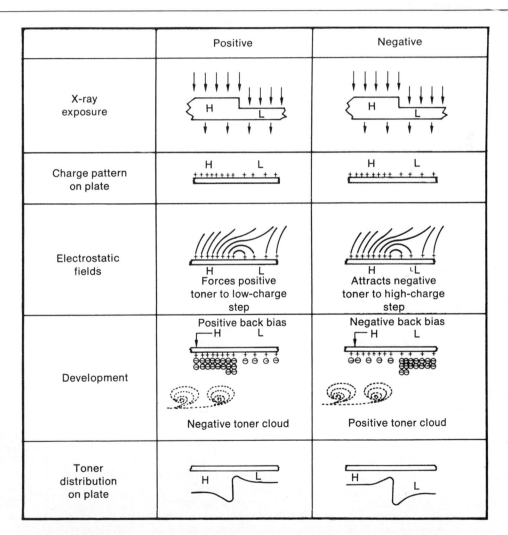

Fig. 19-14. Sequence of events that results in the edge enhancement of a xeroradiograph. (Courtesy Xerox Corporation.)

inclined wedge were imaged xeroradiographically (Fig. 19-12), the toner density on the image would be approximately uniform even though the thickness of the object varies. If the thickness of the object varied abruptly, as in the step wedge shown in Fig. 19-13, the toner distribution on the image would still be rather uniform except at the edge of the step. In Fig. 19-13 the toner density under the thin step appears much darker than under the thick step; this is to be expected for the step image with the conventional film. However, this is in fact something of an optical illusion. Lay your pencil across the edge of the image to obscure that edge, and you will notice that now the densities under both steps appear similar.

What has happened here is characteristic of the xeroradiographic process. Toner is robbed from one side of the edge and laid down more heavily on the other side, resulting in enhancement of the edge. Thus edge enhancement has amplified the contrast at the edge and has caused an apparent density difference on each side of the edge. It is this edge enhancement that is characteristic of xeroradiography and results in high-quality images, especially in mammography.

To understand precisely how edge enhancement works, follow the sequence of steps outlined in Fig. 19-14. Following an exposure of any object containing an edge, the electrostatic charge pattern associated with the edge will be irregular. The latent image contains more positive charges under the thick portion of the edge than under the thin. This latent image does not itself have an enhanced edge, but these charge differences cause edge enhancement during processing.

The latent image produces imaginary lines of electrostatic force that are relatively uniform above regions of uniform charge distribution. They are abrupt above regions with changing electrostatic charge patterns. The toner particles are attracted to the plate along these imaginary lines of force. Relatively fewer toner particles will be deposited where the latent image charge pattern is weak. At the edge, however, toner particles will be robbed from the low-charge side and deposited on the high-charge side. This uneven distribution of toner on the plate at each interface image produces a region of toner build-up with an adjacent **halo,** or absence of toner. The result is visible edge enhancement. The edge refers not only to that of a step wedge but also to any discontinuity.

Because of these physical characteristics, xeroradiography has several advantages over film radiography. **Since the system contrast is low, the exposure latitude is very wide.** It is difficult to produce a technically poor xeroradiograph. The resolution properties of xeroradiography are comparable to those of screen-film systems. The image receptor is reusable, although it can become damaged with rough handling. The final image is produced with a chalklike powder on paper that can be viewed with normal room

Table 19-1 Characteristics of the three types of image receptors employed for mammography

Receptor	Recommended x-ray tube target	Imaging properties	Mean glandular dose (mrad)
Screen-film (no grid)	Molybdenum	Good resolution; moderate latitude; images rounded structures well	60
Screen-film (grid)	Molybdenum	Improved contrast resolution	150
Xerox 125	Tungsten	Good resolution; wide latitude; images microcalcifications well; edge enhancement	400

light. Consequently, not only a darkroom but also a viewbox is unnecessary. These are dubious advantages, however, since all x-ray installations have these facilities.

As the price of precious metals, including silver, continues to escalate, radiographic film will follow suit. Xeroradiography does not require silver. On the other hand, xeroradiography does require special processing apparatus, and this can add considerable expense to an existing x-ray facility.

Good xeromammograms can be produced with either a tungsten-target tube or a molybdenum-target tube, whereas mammographic imaging with screen-film systems should be conducted only with a molybdenum-target tube. The kVp of operation is relatively unimportant; however, values from 40 to 55 kVp with total filtrations of 2 to 4 mm Al are recommended because patient dose will be considerably reduced with no significant sacrifice of image quality.

CONCLUSION

Of the three imaging systems just described, the latter two are recommended. Patient dose is too high with direct-exposure mammography. Patient doses are lower with screen-film mammography and with xeromammography. The subject of patient dose in mammography is treated in greater detail in Chapter 32. Table 19-1 summarizes some of the more important characteristics of each of these three types of mammographic image receptors.

Concern over radiation exposure or radiation effect should never be cause for a patient refusing mammography. In fact, radiation exposures in modern mammography are so low that regularly scheduled mammograms are recommended by advisory groups even for asymptomatic patients. The recommendations of the American Cancer Society and the American College of Radiology follow:

1. All women should have the first, or baseline, mammogram between ages 35 and 40.

2. Between age 40 and 50 mammographic examination should be repeated at 1- or 2-year intervals.
3. Beyond age 50 one should have an annual mammmogram.

Of course, symptomatic patients should be mammographed at any time and frequency as indicated.

REVIEW QUESTIONS

1. Define or otherwise identify the following:
   a. Minimum filtration for mammography
   b. SID
   c. Compression in mammography
   d. Adipose tissue
   e. Edge enhancement
   f. Photoconductive
   g. Relaxation
   h. Corona
   i. Toner
   j. Fuser
2. Describe the anatomy of the breast, including the types of tissue and structural sizes.
3. Discuss changes in image quality and patient dose in mammography as kVp is increased.
4. Graphically compare the x-ray emission of a tungsten-target tube with a molybdenum-target tube operated at 40 kVp.
5. The electron binding energies for molybdenum are K shell, 20 keV; L shell, 2.6 keV; M shell, 0.5 keV. What are the possible characteristic x-ray energies when operated at 30 kVp?
6. Discuss the influence of the heel effect on image quality in mammography.
7. If the operating potential of a mammographic x-ray machine is increased from 30 to 50 kVp, what will be the approximate increase in patient dose if the mAs remains constant?
8. Why must screen-film mammography be performed with a molybdenum target tube?

20

Introduction to computer science

A computer is an electronic data processing machine that can perform computations and word manipulations in very little time. Once a numeric or alphabetic operation has begun, the human operator can often leave the machine until the task is complete, since the instructions for carrying out the task can be stored in the computer's memory. Computers can also make choices in a limited fashion, which allows some operations to be essentially automatic.

At the present time computer applications are exploding at an incredibly fast rate. In addition to scientific, engineering, and business applications, the computer is becoming more familiar in everyday life. We know the computer is somehow involved in video games, automatic bank tellers, and highway toll booths. It may not be equally as obvious that computers now control such things as many supermarket checkouts, ticket reservation centers, industrial processes, traffic lights and even automobile ignition sys-

tems. The widespread availability of the personal computer promises to feed this explosion.

Computer applications in radiology are accelerating equally rapidly. The first large-scale computer application in radiology was computed tomographic (CT) scanning. Digital fluoroscopy and digital radiography are now routine in many clinics. Nuclear magnetic resonance imaging also applies computer technology in a fashion similar to computed tomography. Computers are now used to control x-ray generators for even more automation and precision in setting radiographic and fluoroscopic technique.

HISTORY OF COMPUTERS

The earliest calculating tool, the abacus (Fig. 20-1), was invented thousands of years ago in the Orient and is still used in some countries today. However, it was not until two seventeenth century mathematicians, Blaise Pascal and Gottfried Leibniz, built mechan-

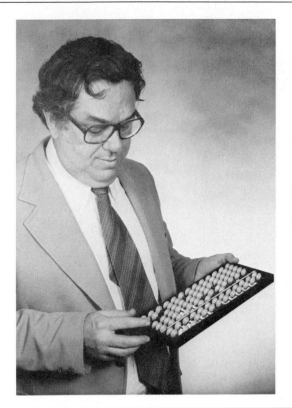

Fig. 20-1. The abacus is the earliest calculating tool. (Courtesy Robert J. Wilson, University of Tennessee Health Science Center.)

ical calculators using pegged wheels that one could automatically perform the four arithmetic functions—addition, subtraction, multiplication, and division. From the seventeenth century to World War II, little was done in the way of creating what we now recognize as the modern computer.

The first general purpose modern computer was developed in 1944 at Harvard University. It was originally called the Automatic Sequence Controlled Calculator (ASCC); now it is identified simply as the Mark I. It was an electromechanical device and was exceedingly slow and prone to malfunction. The first general purpose electronic computer was developed in 1946 at the University of Pennsylvania. It was called ENIAC (**e**lectronic **n**umerical **i**ntegrator **a**nd **c**alculator) and it contained over 18,000 vacuum tubes, which failed at an average of one every 7 minutes (Fig. 20-2). Neither the Mark I nor the ENIAC had their instructions stored in a memory device.

In 1948 scientists at the Bell Telephone Laboratories led by William Shockley developed the **transistor,** and that made possible the development of the "stored-program" computer and thus the continuing explosion in computer science. The transistor allowed the Sperry-Rand Corporation to develop UNIVAC (**univ**ersal **a**utomatic **c**omputer), which appeared in 1951, as the first commercially successful general purpose stored-program electronic digital computer.

The word **computer** today is used as an abbreviation for any general purpose stored-program electronic digital computer. **General**

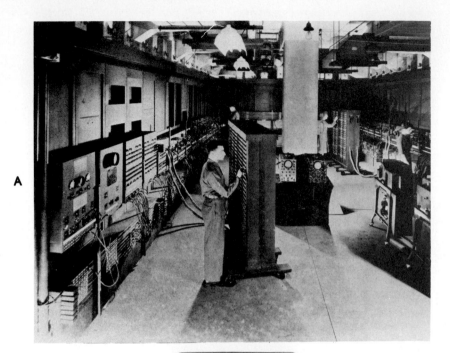

A

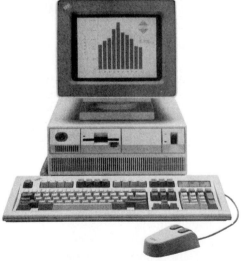

B

Fig. 20-2. A, The ENIAC computer occupied an entire room. It was completed in 1946 and is recognized as the first all-electronic general purpose digital computer. **B,** Today's microcomputer has more capacity and sits on a desk. (**A** courtesy Sperry-Rand Corporation; **B** courtesy IBM.)

purpose identifies a computer as able to solve any solvable problem. This is unlike a special purpose computer, which is designed for a particular singular task, such as control of an assembly-line robot or automobile ignition. All modern computers are **stored program** because they have their instructions (programs) and data stored in their memory. These stored-program computers are laid out so that the sequence of steps to be followed during any calculation is preestablished. **Electronic** implies that the computer is powered by electrical and electronic devices rather than by a mechanical device. Finally, **digital computers** have largely replaced analog computers. The difference between analog and digital is illustrated in Fig. 20-3, which shows an analog indicating meter and a digital meter. In a analog device the result, or display, is continuously variable in proportion to the intensity of a given electric signal. In a digital device the signal is first converted to digital form and then used in a display or computation. The meters shown both indicate 3.2 V, but the digital meter is more precise and easier to read.

Calculators can handle only arithmetic functions, whereas computers can handle arithmetic and **logic functions** such as "do," "if," "then," and "else." Logic functions require that the computer evaluate an intermediate computation and perform any of a number of subsequent computations depending on the result of the intermediate computation. A radiographic operating console controlled by a **microprocessor,** which

is a computer on a chip, will consider many characteristics of an examination—for example, body part, size, and image receptor—and logically select the proper technique.

Computers have undergone four generations of development, distinguished by the technology of their electronic devices. First-generation computers were vacuum-tube machines. Second-generation computers, which became generally available in the 1950s, were based on individually packaged transistors. Third-generation machines used integrated circuits (IC). **Integrated circuits** consist of many transistors and other electronic elements fused onto a **chip,** a tiny piece of semiconductor material, usually silicon. The fourth generation of computers, which first appeared in the early 1970s, was an extension of the third and incorporated **large-scale integration** (LSI). This is now being replaced by **very large-scale integration** (VLSI), which places hundreds of thousands of transistors and other circuit elements on a chip less than 1 cm in size (Fig 20-4).

Today's computers come in basically three sizes. The **microcomputer** is the smallest. It appears as a personal computer, a word processor, and a control for many industrial processes. The **minicomputer** is somewhat larger in capacity and flexibility. Most computer applications in radiology employ a minicomputer. The **mainframe computer** is used for very large applications by organizations such as the U.S. Census Bureau.

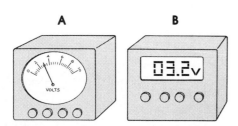

Fig. 20-3. A, An analog voltmeter. **B,** A digital voltmeter indicating 3.2 V.

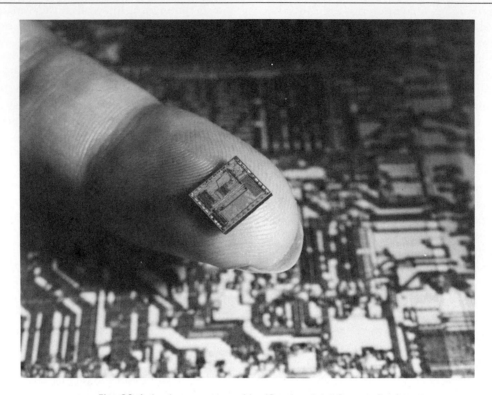

Fig. 20-4. A microprocessor chip. (Courtesy Intel Corporation.)

ANATOMY OF A COMPUTER

There are two principal parts to a computer—
hardware and software—each of which have several components. The **hardware** is everything
about the computer that is visible—the nuts,
bolts, and chips of the system that form the central processing unit and the various input/output
devices. The **software** is invisible. It consists of
the computer programs and languages and the
manner in which data are processed.

Central processing unit

The **c**entral **p**rocessing **u**nit (CPU) is built
around a **microprocessor.** In a small computer,
the microprocessor is a single large-scale integrated circuit on a silicon chip less than a centimeter on a side that contains thousands of individual circuit elements (Fig. 20-4). The CPU
is to the computer what the nucleus is to the

living cell—a primary control center. Fig. 20-5
is a photomicrograph of the 80286 16-bit microprocessor produced by the Intel Corporation. It
is an extremely powerful and fast microprocessor
designed for high-performance, large, multi-
user, multitask computer systems. The CPU on
this chip supervises all of the other components
of the computer, performs the mathematical manipulations, and even stores information. As illustrated in Fig. 20-6, the CPU consists of a
control unit, an arithmetic unit, and sometimes
memory. When memory is also included in the
CPU, the device is called a microcomputer instead of a microprocessor.

Control unit. When data are entered into the
computer through an input device such as the
keyboard or a diskette, the **control unit** identi-

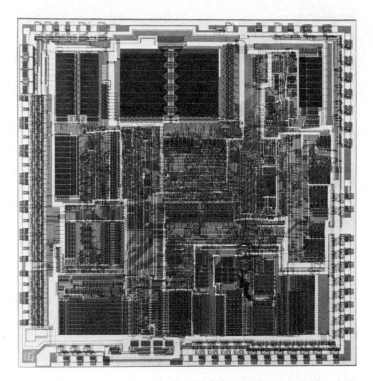

Fig. 20-5. This 16-bit microprocessor incorporates 128,000 transistors on a chip of silicon less than 1 cm on a side. The width of the conductive lines and spacings is 1.5 μ wide. (Courtesy Intel Corporation.)

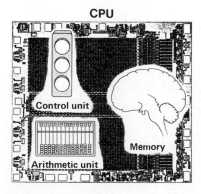

Fig. 20-6. The central processing unit contains a control unit, an arithmetic unit, and sometimes memory.

fies the route of entry and directs the data to the arithmetic unit or to memory. Similarly, when a computation is completed, the control unit will transfer the results to the output device selected.

The control unit is the computer's basic overseer in charge of interpreting the user's program instructions in the proper order. If a calculation is required, it passes data to the arithmetic unit. It also stores and retrieves data from memory or input/output devices as required. The speed at which these tasks are done is determined by the frequency of an external electronic clock that synchronizes CPU operation with the rest of the computer. Clock frequencies in excess of 10 MHz allow the computer to perform millions of simple operations per second. The fastest computer can perform a billion calculations a second, and machines ten and even a hundred times faster are being designed.

Arithmetic Unit. The arithmetic unit is that portion of the CPU that holds the numbers that are involved in the calculations, performs the logic and numeric calculations, and then temporarily holds the results until they can be transferred to memory. The speed of the arithmetic unit in performing these computations is also controlled by the external clock. In the arithmetic unit, the clock synchronizes a very high-speed calculator that performs the four basic arithmetic functions and the logic functions.

Memory unit. The CPU contains two types of memory. It has **registers,** in which it stores temporary information, and **main memory,** in which the programs and data are kept. **Direct memory access** (DMA) controllers are available for many computers. These devices speed up the transfer of bulk data between main memory and external devices bypassing the CPU itself. Generally, the control unit fetches instructions and data from the memory and, except for DMA operations, transfers data between the memory and various input and output devices.

A major change in computer technology in the mid-1970s was the change from magnetic-core memory to semiconductor memory. **A magnetic core** consists of small magnetic dipoles that exist in one of two states depending on the direction of an electric current passing through them. Compared with semiconductor memory, magnetic-core memory is expensive and slow. However, the word "core" still survives in computer terminology and is still sometimes used to refer to primary memory even though primary memory now is based on semiconductors and not magnetic loops.

Digital radiologic imaging owes its rapid development in part to semiconductor memory. **Semiconductor memory** consists of extremely small storage circuits etched on a silicon chip. The individual chips are arranged in groups to form a **memory module** complete with all interconnections to plug into the computer.

Semiconductor storage operates on the principle of a **flip-flop,** in which a switch is set in one of two states variously described as zero or one, A or B, "yes" or "no," "true" or "false," and "plus" or "minus." Each individual flip-flop stores one **bit** (**b**inary dig**it**) of information.

Primary memory is available as **read only memory** (ROM) and **random access memory** (RAM). ROM is wired in at the factory and cannot be changed. ROM usually contains the primary computer instructions called **system programs.** These instructions get the computer going when it is first turned on. ROM is also used extensively in such single-application chips as word processors, pocket calculators, and video games.

RAM is sometimes called **read-write memory.** RAM is used for storing computational instructions or data that might change from time to time.

All primary memory is **addressed;** that is, each memory location has a unique label identifying its position. This operates much like your home address, which allows you to receive mail that is uniquely yours. It allows the computer's

CPU access to the data at specific spots in memory without disturbing the rest of memory. A sequence of memory locations may contain steps of a computer program or a string of data. The CPU keeps track of what address in the program it is at so that it can hop to other memory locations to read or write data and then return to the proper place in the program.

All information to be processed by the computer must pass through primary memory, and therefore it is most efficient to have sufficient primary memory to retain all the necessary data and instructions for processing. Many applications, however, require additional **secondary memory,** usually in the form of disks or tape, which are described later in this chapter.

In CT scanning, for instance, when contiguous transverse images are reconstructed in a coronal or sagittal plane, the images are sequentially routed from secondary memory to primary memory to the arithmetic unit of the CPU.

Input/output devices

The process of transferring information into primary memory is known as an **input operation.** The process of transferring the results of a computation from primary memory to storage or the user is known as an **output operation.** Input/output devices, commonly referred to as **I/O devices,** allow the computer operator to communicate with the computer. In addition, I/O devices can provide secondary memory to handle information that is too large to be contained in primary memory at one time. Until recently, the most universal I/O device was the keypunched computer card. "Do not fold, spindle, or mutilate" were the famous instructions. Now "key to tape" and "key to disk" have largely replaced cards.

The I/O devices principally involved in computer applications in radiology are the keyboard, the video display terminal, the printer, the multiformat camera, and secondary memory devices. Fig. 20-7 illustrates how the control unit behaves as an interface between these various I/O devices and primary memory. Because VLSI computers have become cheaper and more powerful, some I/O devices have evolved into very powerful data processing units in themselves. Some operate nearly independently with only minimum interaction with the control unit.

Video display terminal. The I/O device most familiar to the radiologic technologist is the **video display terminal** (VDT) or, more simply, the terminal. Terminals are found on every CT scanner, digital x-ray imager, and MR imager. A terminal consists of a keyboard and a **cathode-ray tube** (CRT) display. We recognize the CRT display as a television set.

Terminal keyboards are nearly all electronic. Each key depression produces a code, and the computer responds with a character on the screen of the CRT display. This is the usual method of data entry to the computer. The keyboard resembles that of a conventional typewriter except that, in addition to the alphabetic key pad, there is usually a separate, calculator-type, ten-numeral key pad. There also are usually other key pads containing special-function keys, such as arrows left, right, up, and down, and function keys for use with a special operation, such as a radiologic examination. Digital fluoroscopy (Chapter 21), for instance, uses special-function keys for masking, reregistration, and time interval difference imaging.

Video display terminals may be designed for alphanumeric display only or for graphic display as well. Alphanumeric display is the display we normally encounter. It is a series of letters and numerals that conveys information. If graphic output is also available, one would be able to display the results of numeric computations graphically. Virtually all radiologic terminals provide for alphanumeric and graphic output.

The characters needed for the display of text are generated by patterns of dots from a special ROM called a **character generator.** A typical VDT will display 24 lines of 80 characters each. Each character is produced by a matrix that typ-

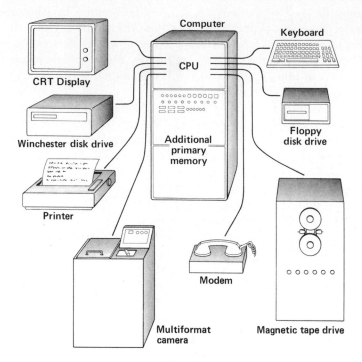

Fig. 20-7. The control unit is a part of the CPU and is directly connected with additional primary memory and various input/output devices.

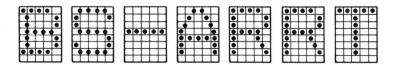

Fig. 20-8. Dot matrix characters produced in the OCR system.

ically consists of 63 dots (9 dots high by 7 dots wide), where only the dots required to form a character are displayed, such as those shown in Fig. 20-8. This system of characters from dots forms a larger computer-compatible system known as the **optical character recognition (OCR)** system. The characters on the CRT display and many printers are formed this way.

Video display terminals are either intelligent or nonintelligent—"smart" or "dumb"—devices. The smart terminal is also known as a **programmable,** or logic, terminal. This is the type employed for most radiologic applications. It consists of a small microprocessor with an associated small memory that contains a program in it to direct the operation of the terminal, validate input, and direct communications with a larger computer. The dumb terminal must be

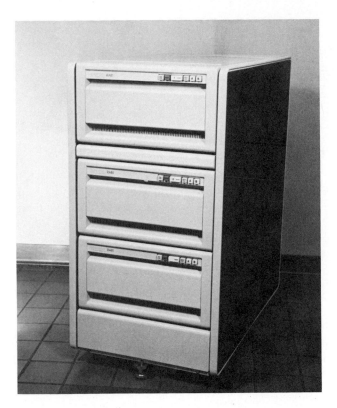

Fig. 20-9. A Winchester disk drive system. (Courtesy Digital Equipment Corporation.)

connected directly to a computer. It behaves strictly as a passbox for the operator's input. It does not edit, compute, or perform any logic on its own.

Magnetic disks. The principal medium for secondary memory is a magnetic disk. It is either rigid, like a phonographic record, or flexible. The former is usually called a hard disk; the latter is called a diskette or a floppy disk.

In 1973 IBM introduced a sealed hard disk that it called a 30-30 because its storage capacity was 30 Mbytes. The 30-30 was soon nicknamed a **Winchester disk** after the repeating rifle.

The Winchester disk is roughly equivalent in size and appearance to an LP phonograph record. Data are stored on the disk in a series of concentric magnetic tracks. If they could be

seen, the tracks would be similar in appearance to the grooves in a record. Most disks are rigid aluminum platters, coated on both sides with a recording material that can be magnetized. The data are recorded as binary digits and are accessible for reading or writing by positioning a read-write head on the disk. Both the top and bottom surfaces are used. For large amounts of data, a number of disks are stacked, as illustrated in Fig. 20-9. Winchester disks are random access in nature; that is, the data are grouped into fixed-length blocks, each of which is addressed. These blocks of data thus can each be separated, read, and written. Winchester disks are frequently employed in radiologic imaging procedures because of their large capacity and relative speed as secondary memory devices.

Floppy disks, either 3½, 5¼, or 8 inches in

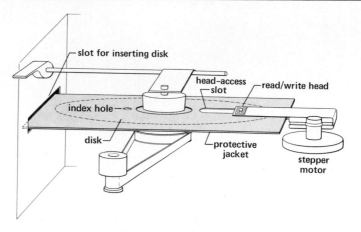

Fig. 20-10. The floppy disk has become standard equipment on many radiographic imaging systems. The basic mechanism of the floppy disk drive is shown here.

diameter, are in widespread use in radiologic imaging. These diskettes are very lightweight and made of a flexible plastic material. Floppy disks are small, inexpensive, and controlled by a relatively inexpensive disk drive, which is shown in a cutaway view in Fig. 20-10. However, they are much slower and of lower capacity than other media. They are primarily used in micro- and minicomputer systems. In radiology they are conveniently used to store patient images. Depending on the matrix size (Chapter 22) and the type of diskette, from two to twenty patient images can be stored on each disk.

Optical disks. The newest secondary memory device is the **laser disk** or **optical disk.** This device stores digital data on a mirrored surface by modulating the reflective properties of the surface to laser light. The principal advantage of the optical disk is storage capacity. Whereas a floppy disk can store 500 kbytes of data and a hard disk 500 Mbytes of data, current optical disks can store several Gbytes (1 gigabyte = 10^{12} bytes), and higher capacity is coming.

Systems are currently being developed that utilize many optical disks in jukebox fashion. It is envisioned that in the all-digital radiology de-

partment of the future the optical disk jukebox will replace the film file room. The compact disc (CD) recently introduced for audiophiles is an optical disk.

Magnetic tape. Magnetic tape is another secondary memory device. Since it is both the cheapest and slowest form of storage, it is used mainly for archiving patient images. The tapes come in various formats. The size of computer tape used most often in radiology is 1.25 cm (0.5 in) wide, 720 m (2400 ft) long, and has nine magnetic data tracks. It can accommodate the records of dozens of patients.

Magnetic tape has a polyester base. It is coated on one side with iron oxide, which when magnetized is the recording medium. The tape is fed across the read-write heads, The write head produces a small magnetic field when an electric current is passed through it. The magnetic field is reversed when the direction of the current is reversed. The two binary digits, 0 and 1, thus are easily represented by changes in the current. When the magnetic field produced by the head comes in contact with the magnetic coating on the tape, it magnetizes a small spot on the coating. When a tape is to be read, this series of tiny magnetic fields moves rapidly past the read head. As each field comes in contact with the read head, it produces an electric current. The direction of the current depends on the direction of the field, and therefore the information originally recorded is retrieved. This entire process is based on electromagnetic induction (Chapter 6). It is a little like the process that occurs in a transformer.

Multiformat camera. Perhaps the output device most often employed in computer applications in radiology is the multiformat camera. All computer-assisted images are ultimately displayed on a CRT, making them directly compatible with the multiformat camera.

Laser camera. Gaining in favor for producing hard-copy images from digital equipment is the laser camera. Instead of using the computer output to control CRT, it is used to modulate the intensity of a laser beam which is directed onto single-emulsion film. The images are sharper than multiformat camera images, and the contrast is more easily optimized. Digital image manipulation such as windowing, highlighting, and enhancing are possible. Laser camera images are characterized by a totally dark background, unlike the masked background of the multiformat camera image. The principal disadvantage of the laser camera is cost; it is up to twice as expensive as a multiformat camera.

Printers. Although in radiology the final result is an image, usually from a multiformat or laser camera, for most applications of computers the ultimate output is in printed form. Printers are often available with radiologic equipment, but they are seldom used. Nevertheless, it is important to know the different types of printers that one might encounter.

Large main-frame computers that generate exceedingly huge quantities of output will print results on a high-speed **line printer.** Such printers are capable of printing up to 1000 lines per minute, with 132 columns per line; even faster is the laser printer, which can print 14,000 lines per minute. These high-speed printers are rarely encountered in radiology.

Dot matrix printers are relatively inexpensive but moderately fast, They can print up to 350 characters per second. The dot matrix printer is the most popular type accompanying many micro- and minicomputers and is likely to be the printer a radiologic technologist would use. Many dot matrix printers are bidirectional; that is, they print one line from left to right and the next line from right to left. Dot matrix printers form the characters of the OCR system used in CRTs. Most use a carriage of nine pins although as many as twenty four have been employed. The pins punch an inked ribbon onto paper, as shown in Fig. 20-11. Some use specially treated paper and heated pins. Such printers are called **thermal printers.**

Daisy wheel printers are slower than dot matrix printers, only fifty characters per minute, but they produce typewriter-quality characters. Daisy wheel printers are most often employed with word processors.

Modem. Electronic data transmission over conventional telephone lines is increasingly used as a means of information transfer. Transmission of patient images from one hospital to another can assist in diagnosis in a very cost-effective way. A telephone handset acoustic coupler called a modem (**mo**dulater-**dem**odulator) is employed. One simply dials a number to which the image is to be transmitted, places the telephone handset on the modem cradle (Fig. 20-12), and, through the keyboard, initiates the data transmission. Directly connected modems are faster than the acoustic coupled modem.

The modem converts the computer output signal to a series of tones (acoustics) that are transmitted (coupled) to the modem at the receiving station. In this fashion an image can be transmitted in just a few minutes.

COMPUTER SOFTWARE

All that has been described thus far regarding the computer has been hardware. Hardware refers to the fixed visible components of the sys-

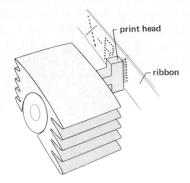

Fig. 20-11. The dot matrix printer is a relatively inexpensive computer-controlled printer that functions with nine pins striking a typewriter-like ribbon onto paper.

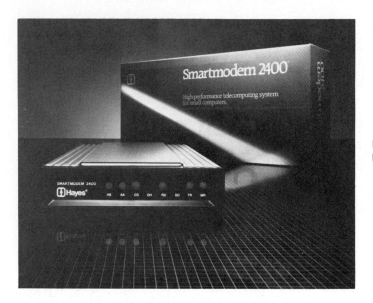

Fig. 20-12 A modem. (Courtsey Hayes Microcomputer Products, Inc.)

tem. The CPU, all I/O devices, and other auxiliary or peripheral devices are hardware. But these are only half of the computer. The other half is software. **Software** refers to the instructions written in a computer language that guide the computer through its designated operations.

Although the computer can accept and report alphabetic characters and numeric information

in the decimal system, it operates in the binary system. In the decimal system, the system we normally use, ten digits (0 to 9) are used. The word "digit" comes from the Latin for finger or toe.) The origin of the decimal system is undoubtedly rooted in the fact that we have ten fingers and ten toes that simplify counting.

The decimal system is a number system to the

Table 20-1. Organization of binary number system

Decimal number	Binary equivalent	Binary number
0	0	0
1	2^0	1
2	$2^1 + 0$	10
3	$2^1 + 2^0$	11
4	$2^2 + 0 + 0$	100
5	$2^2 + 0 + 2^0$	101
6	$2^2 + 2^1 + 0$	110
7	$2^2 + 2^1 + 2^0$	111
8	$2^3 + 0 + 0 + 0$	1000
9	$2^3 + 0 + 0 + 2^0$	1001
10	$2^3 + 0 + 2^1 + 0$	1010
11	$2^3 + 0 + 2^1 + 2^0$	1011
12	$2^3 + 2^2 + 0 + 0$	1100
13	$2^3 + 2^2 + 0 + 2^0$	1101
14	$2^3 + 2^2 + 2^1 + 0$	1110
15	$2^3 + 2^2 + 2^1 + 2^0$	1111
16	$2^4 + 0 + 0 + 0 + 0$	10000

base ten. Other number systems have been formulated to many other base values. The duodecimal system, for instance, has 12 digits. It is used to describe the months of the year and the hours in a day and night. Computers operate on the simplest number system of all, the binary number system. It has only two digits, 0 and 1.

Binary number system

When counting in the binary number system, as shown in Table 20-1, one counts 0 to 1 and then counts over again. There are only two digits, 0 and 1, and the computer performs all operations by converting alphabetic characters, decimal values, and logic functions to binary values. That way, although the binary numbers may become exceedingly long, computation can be handled by properly adjusting the thousands of flip-flop circuits in the computer.

In the binary system, 0 is 0 and 1 is 1, but there the direct relationship with the decimal system ends. In fact, it ends at 0 because the 1 in binary notation comes from 2^0. Recall that any number raised to the zero power is 1, therefore

2^0 equals 1. In binary notation, 2 is equal to 2^1 plus 0. This is expressed as 10. The decimal 3 is equal to 2^1 plus 2^0, or 11 in binary form; 4 is 2^2 plus no 2^1 plus no 2^0, or 100 in binary form. As shown in Table 20-1, each time it is necessary to raise 2 to an additional power to express a number, the number of binary digits increases by one.

Just as we know the meaning of the powers of ten, it is necessary to easily recognize the powers of two. Power-of-two notation is used in radiologic imaging to describe image size, image dynamic range (shades of gray), and image storage capacity. Table 20-2 is a review of these power notations. Note the following similarity: In both power notations the number of zeros to the right of 1 equals the value of the exponent.

EXAMPLE: Express the number 193 in binary form.

ANSWER: 193 falls between 2^7 and 2^8. Therefore it will be expressed as 1 followed by seven binary digits. Simply add the decimal equivalents of each binary digit from left to right:

$$
\begin{array}{lll}
\text{Yes } 2^7 = 1 = & 128 \\
\text{Yes } 2^6 = 1 = & 64 \\
\text{No } 2^5 = 0 = & \text{No } 32 \\
\text{No } 2^4 = 0 = & \text{No } 16 \\
\text{No } 2^3 = 0 = & \text{No } 8 \\
\text{No } 2^2 = 0 = & \text{No } 4 \\
\text{No } 2^1 = 0 = & \text{No } 2 \\
\text{Yes } 2^0 = 1 = & 1 \\
\hline
11000001 = & 193
\end{array}
$$

Digital radiologic images are made of discrete picture elements, **pixels,** arranged in a matrix (see Chapter 21). The size of the image is described in the binary system of numbers by power-of-two equivalents. Most images are either 256×256 (2^8), 512×512 (2^9), or 1024×1024 (2^{10}). The 256×256 and 512×512 image matrices are particularly applicable to CT and MRI. The 1024×1024 is used in digital fluoroscopy and digital radiography.

Bits, bytes, and words

In computer language, a single binary digit, 0 or 1, is called a **bit.** The computer will employ as many bits as necessary to express a decimal digit. The twenty-six characters of the alphabet

Table 20-2. Power-of-ten, power-of-two, and binary notation

Power of ten	Power of two	Binary notation
$10^0 = 1$	$2^0 = 1$	1
$10^1 = 10$	$2^1 = 2$	10
$10^2 = 100$	$2^2 = 4$	100
$10^3 = 1000$	$2^3 = 8$	1000
$10^4 = 10,000$	$2^4 = 16$	10000
$10^5 = 100,000$	$2^5 = 32$	100000
$10^6 = 1,000,000$	$2^6 = 64$	1000000
	$2^7 = 128$	10000000
	$2^8 = 256$	100000000
	$2^9 = 512$	1000000000
	$2^{10} = 1024$	10000000000

and other special characters are usually encoded by 8 bits. To **encode** is to translate from ordinary characters to computer-compatible characters—binary digits. Depending on the microprocessor, a string of 8, 16, or 32 bits will be manipulated simultaneously.

Bits are grouped into bunches of eight called **bytes.** Computer capacity is expressed by the number of bytes that can be accommodated by computer memory. The most popular personal computers employ 8- and 16-bit microprocessors with 64 to 512 kilobytes of memory. One kbyte is equal to 8×1024 bits. Note that kilo is not metric in computer use. Instead it represents 2^{10}. The minicomputers used in radiology have capacities measured in megabytes, where 1 Mbyte = 1 kbyte $\times$ 1 kbyte = $2^{10} \times 2^{10} = 2^{20} = 1,048,576$ bytes.

EXAMPLE: How many bits can be stored on a 64-kbyte chip whose byte size is 8 bits?

ANSWER: $\dfrac{1024 \text{ bits}}{\text{kbytes}} \times 64 \text{ kbytes} \times 8 \text{ bits} = 2^{10} \times 2^6 \times 2^3 = 2^{19} = 524,288$

Depending on the computer configuration, 2 bytes usually constitute a **word.** In the case of a 16-bit microprocessor, a word would be 16 consecutive bits of information that are interpreted and shuffled about the computer as a unit. Each word of data in memory has its own address.

Computer programs

The sequence of instructions developed by a software engineer or programer is called a computer program. **Computer programs are the software of the computer.** It is useful to distinguish two classifications of computer programs—systems software and application programs. Systems software consists of programs that make it easy for the user to operate a computer to its best advantage. Computer buffs describe good, efficient software as "user friendly." Application programs are those written in a higher-level language expressly to carry out some user function. Most computer programs as we know them are application programs.

System software. The computer program most closely related to the system hardware is the operating system. The **operating system** is that series of instructions that organizes the course of data through the computer to the solution of a particular problem. Commands such as "load file" to begin a sequence or "save file" to store some information in secondary memory are typical of operating-system commands. This type of program is usually developed by the computer manufacturer and some may be stored in ROM in the CPU. Since the CPU only recognizes instructions in binary or machine-language form, formulating the operating system is perhaps the most tedious of all computer programing.

Computers ultimately only understand zeros and ones. To save humans the tedious task of writing programs in this form, other programs, called assemblers, compilers, and interpreters, have been written. These types of software provide a computer language to communicate between the language of the operating system and our everyday language.

An **assembler** is a computer program that recognizes such symbolic instructions as "subtract (SUB)," "load (LD)," and "print (PT)" and trans-

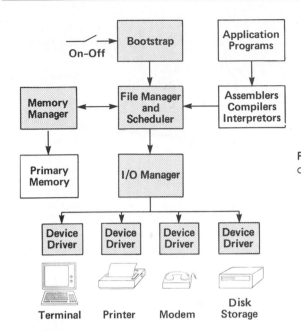

Fig. 20-13. The sequence of software manipulations to complete an operation.

lates them into the corresponding binary code. Assembly is the translation of a program written in symbolic, machine-oriented instructions into machine-language instructions.

Compilers and **interpreters** are computer programs that translate an application program from its high-level language such as Basic, Fortran, or Cobol into a form suitable for the assembler or into a form accepted directly by the CPU. Interpreters make program development easier because they are interactive. Compiled programs run faster.

Application programs. Computer programs that are written by the computer manufacturer, a software manufacturer, or the users themselves to permit the computer to perform a specific task are called **application** programs. Examples are Lotus 1-2-3, Displaywrite and D Base. Application programs allow the user to print a mailing list, complete an income tax form, evaluate a financial statement, or reconstruct an image from an x-ray transmission pattern. They are written in one of many high-level computer

languages and are then translated through an interpreter or compiler into a corresponding machine-language program that is subsequently executed by the computer.

The diagram in Fig. 20-13 illustrates the flow of the software instructions from turning the computer on to completing a computation. Initially, when the computer is first turned on, nothing is in its memory except a program called a **bootstrap.** This is frozen permanently in the primary memory. When the bootstrap program is started, it is capable of transferring the other necessary programs off the disk and into the computer memory.

The bootstrap program loads the operating system into primary memory, which in turn controls all subsequent operations. A machine-language application program can be input through one of several channels. It is loaded into primary memory where the prescribed operations occur. Following completion of the job, the results will be transferred from primary memory to an output device under the control of the operating system.

Table 20-3. Programing languages

Language	Date introduced	Description
FORTRAN	1956	Widely used; flexible; fast; mainly science and engineering applications
COBOL	1959	Mini- and main-frame computer applications in business
ALGOL	1960	Especially useful in high-level mathematics
BASIC	1964	Most frequently used with micro- and minicomputers; science, engineering, and business applications

FORTRAN Program

FORTRAN Statement	Type of Statement
Read (1,900) A,B,C 900 Format (3 F 10,2)	Input/Output
X = A+B+C Y = SQRT (X)	Arithmetic assignment
Write (3,900) X,Y	Input/Output
Stop	Control
End	Specification (to computer)

Fig. 20-14. A short FORTRAN program.

Computer languages

High-level programing languages allow the programer to write instructions in a form approaching human language, using words, symbols, and decimal numbers rather than the ones and zeros of machine language. An incomplete list of the more popular programing languages is given in Table 20-3. Using one of these high-level languages, one can write a set of instructions that will be understood by the system software and be executed by the computer through its operating system.

FORTRAN. The oldest language for scientific, engineering, and mathematic problems is **FORTRAN** (**for**mula **tran**slation). It is the most widely used algebraic language and is available for almost all computers. The algebraic languages are oriented toward the computational procedures for solving mathematic and statistic problems. Problems such as these, which can be expressed in terms of formulas and equations, are sometimes called **algorithms.** An algorithm is a step by step process used to solve a problem much like a recipe is to bake a cake except the algorithm is more detailed. It would include instructions to remove the shell from the egg. FORTRAN was developed in 1956 by IBM in

conjunction with some major computer users. It has changed substantially since that time but is defined by users according to a standard format.

The FORTRAN language consists of a vocabulary of symbols and words and rules for writing instructions. The nature of a FORTRAN program can best be illustrated by the short example shown in Fig. 20-14. This simple program directs the computer to read three values from an input device, to sum the three values, to take the square root of the sum, to print the sum and the square root, and then to stop.

BASIC. BASIC (**B**eginners **A**ll **P**urpose **S**ymbolic **I**nstruction **C**ode) is an algebraic programing language that was developed at Dartmouth College in 1964 as a first language for students. It is an easy-to-learn interpreter-based language whose simplicity leads to low-cost computer use. Major applications of BASIC are with micro- and minicomputer systems and particularly with the popular personal computer. It resembles other problem-oriented languages and can serve the engineer, student, or businessman equally well. BASIC contains a powerful arithmetic facility, several editing features, a library of common mathematic functions, and simple input and output procedures.

COBOL. One high-level procedure-oriented language designed for coding business data processing problems is COBOL (**Co**mmon **B**usiness **O**riented **L**anguage). A basic characteristic of business data processing is the existence of large files that are updated continuously. COBOL provides extensive file-handling, editing, and report-generating capabilities for the user.

Other program languages are variously identified. LOGO is a language designed for children. ADA is used principally for military applications. ALGOL and PASCAL are languages suited to the needs of mathematicians.

PROCESSING METHODS

Regardless of the operating software or the application programs in use, the essential modes of computer processing are time-sharing, online, and real-time systems. The modes often operate together as interactive systems when short response time between issuing a command and receiving a response is of major importance. Such processing methods are different from batch processing, which offers a relatively long turnaround time but aims at lowering computing costs. Many larger computer systems offer a choice of these several processing methods.

Batch processing

The most widely used mode of processing with main-frame computers uses a batch operating system. The users submit the complete job, which includes the program, the data, and the control statements. After a relatively long time, tens of minutes to hours, the results are available. Normally, the jobs in a batch are processed in sequence, one after the other. This method does not require the user to attend to the system once the batch has started. Batch processing can be handled by a remote job-entry, **RJE,** system in which users submit their batch jobs to a remote terminal connected to the computer by a cable or modem.

On-line systems

In an on-line system, certain transactions are processed immediately. In such a system, the users have multiple-access terminals, sometimes thousands of such terminals, from which they may introduce one or a few of the transactions exclusively. The response comes within seconds. Examples of on-line systems include airline reservation systems, automatic bank tellers, and supermarket checkout systems.

Time-sharing systems

The goal of time-sharing systems is to provide each user with the illusion of having the computer dedicated exclusively to himself. Several hundred users, the maximum number depending on the system, simultaneously interact with the computer. The time between the user's sign-on and sign-off is called a **session.** During a typical session, the user does the following:

1. Signs into the system by presenting a password
2. Enters a program under the control of a text editor
3. Usually saves this program under an assigned name
4. Has the program compiled
5. Runs the program

While the program is being run, the user may interact with it. For example, the user may request the result of a partial execution of a program, or the computer may make a request of the user and then proceed based on the result. This type of system is in use in most large research-and-development institutions where multiple-user groups must be accommodated.

Real-time systems

Real-time systems are most often designed as special purpose operating systems to provide for fast management of the system hardware. This is the case in most radiologic imaging. The processing of the incoming data (for example, from the detectors of a CT scanner) is completed in a matter of milliseconds or seconds at the most.

Real-time systems often use special purpose high-speed hardware to perform computationally intensive tasks like image reconstruction and filtering. **Pipeline processors** work like an assembly line. Different parts of the data are processed by different parts of the processor at the same time. The data move through the processor ("down the pipe") and are fully processed by the time they reach the output. **Array processors** perform the same computations in parallel on many items of data.

REVIEW QUESTIONS

1. Define or otherwise identify the following:
   a. Logic function
   b. Central processing unit
   c. Modem
   d. Character generator
   e. Winchester disk
   f. Byte
   g. Operating system
   h. Bootstrap
   i. Algorithm
   j. BASIC
2. What are the two principal parts of a computer and the distinguishing features of each?
3. Describe a CPU. Include its three principal parts and their functions.
4. What is the difference between a high-level and a low-level computer language? Name some high-level languages.
5. What input/output devices are commonly employed in radiology?
6. There are three general classes of computers. What are they? Which is normally employed in radiology?
7. List the applications of computer technology in diagnostic radiology.
8. A memory chip is said to have 256 Mbytes of capacity. If each byte is 16 bits deep, what is the total bit capacity?
9. Convert the following decimal numbers into binary form:
   a. 3
   b. 13
   c. 72
   d. 147
   e. 7342
10. Convert the following binary numbers into decimal form:
    a. 1011
    b. 10001
    c. 110001
    d. 1110010
    e. 10101011

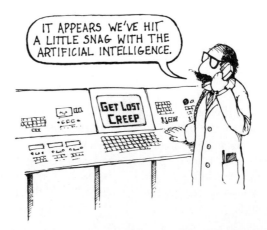

21

Digital x-ray imaging

DIGITAL IMAGING
DIGITAL FLUOROSCOPY
DIGITAL RADIOGRAPHY
PICTURE ARCHIVING AND
COMMUNICATION SYSTEM

Medical imaging is undergoing revolutionary change at this time. Since Roentgen's discovery of x rays, anatomic images have been obtained in basically the same fashion. Now that is changing and changing very rapidly.

A conventional static radiographic image is made like a shadowgraph, using a field of x rays that forms an image pattern after transmission through the patient. The image receptor, film or a screen-film combination, is a device that records this transmitted image directly. Fig. 21-1 diagrams the imaging chain for conventional radiography.

Conventional fluoroscopy likewise produces a shadowgraph-type image on a receptor that directly produces an image from the transmitted x-ray beam. Until the 1960s a fluoroscopic screen was the image receptor used for this type of dynamic examination. Currently, image-intensifier tubes serve as the image receptor. These are either optically coupled for direct viewing of the image or electronically coupled

to a television monitor for remote viewing, as described in Chapter 18. Fig. 21-2 diagrams the components employed in conventional fluoroscopy.

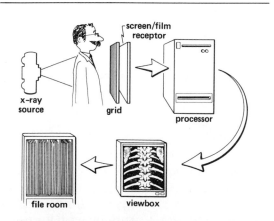

Fig. 21-1. The imaging chain in conventional radiography.

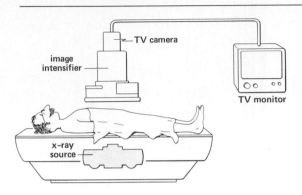

Fig. 21-2. The imaging chain in conventional fluoroscopy.

DIGITAL IMAGING

These conventional systems have served us well for many years, providing increasingly better diagnostic images. However, they both have several limitations. The static radiographic images require processing time that can delay the completion of the examination. This can be particularly bothersome in angiography and when film-subtraction techniques are employed. Once one has obtained such images, there is very little that can be done to enhance their information content. When the examination is complete, the images are in the form of hard-copy film that must be cataloged and stored for future review.

Another and perhaps more severe limitation is the noise inherent in these images. Radiography and fluoroscopy both employ area beams, that is, large rectangular beams of x rays. The Compton-scattered portion of the remnant x-ray beam increases with increasing field size. That increases the noise of the image and severely degrades low-contrast resolution. The use of grids is only marginally helpful in improving this situation.

These limitations can be overcome somewhat by the incorporation of computer technology into diagnostic x-ray imaging. This approach to imaging is based on transforming the conventional analog images into digital form, processing the digital data in helpful ways, and displaying it in a manner that makes it appear very much like a conventional image. Such data conversion and manipulation would not be possible if it were not for advanced computer technology.

Digital imaging techniques are being applied to computed tomography (CT), ultrasound, radioisotope studies, magnetic resonance imaging (MRI), digital fluoroscopy (DF), and digital radiography (DR). Digital fluoroscopy and radiography are currently under rapid development and clinical deployment. As our computer technology advances, so will digital x-ray imaging. Some predict that digital x-ray imaging will replace conventional x-ray imaging in the near future.

Standard nomenclature for identifying the methods of obtaining digital images has not yet been uniformly adopted. Terms such as **digital vascular imaging, digital subtraction angiography, computerized fluoroscopy, digital videoangiography, scan beam digital radiography,** and others appear frequently. In the following discussions we will use digital fluoroscopy (DF) to identify a digital x-ray imaging system that produces a series of dynamic images obtained with an **area x-ray beam** and an image intensifier. Digital radiography (DR) refers to the static images produced with a **fan x-ray beam** intercepted by a linear array of radiation detectors.

Development of the process

The development of digital radiologic imaging equipment was limited until sufficient computer technology was available to handle the large quantities of data generated. The microprocessor and semiconductor memory made this development possible. Initial activity began in the early 1970s, developed along two independent lines, and became a clinical reality by 1980.

The medical physics groups at the University of Wisconsin and the University of Arizona independently initiated studies of DF in the early 1970s. These studies were continued through the decade by the research-and-development groups of most x-ray equipment manufacturers. The approach in general was to utilize conventional fluoroscopic equipment and place a computer between the television camera and the television monitor. The video signal from the television camera was shunted through the computer, manipulated in various ways, and transmitted to the television monitor in a form ready for viewing.

The initial investigators of DF demonstrated that nearly instantaneous, high-contrast subtraction images could be obtained following intravenous injection. Although the intravenous route is still widely used, intraarterial injections are also used with DF. The two distinct advantages of DF over conventional fluoroscopy are the speed of image acquisition and the image-contrast enhancement.

Digital radiography has enjoyed a similar path of development by a number of different investigators. Although there are several approaches to DR, the approach developed in the late 1970s to complement computed tomography has enjoyed the widest application. This approach to DR is commonly referred to as **scanned projection radiography.** This modality employs a narrow fan beam of x rays that intercepts a linear array of radiation detectors. The signal from each detector is passed through a computer where it is used to reconstruct an image.

Although the image in digital x-ray techniques may appear as a conventional video or radiographic image, it is not. It is formed of individual image elements.

Image characteristics

The image obtained in digital x-ray procedures is unlike that obtained in conventional fluoroscopy or radiography. In those latter modalities, x rays form an image directly on the image receptor, the phosphor or film. With digital techniques, x rays form an electronic image on radiation detectors that is manipulated by a computer, temporarily stored in memory, and displayed as a **matrix** of intensities.

Image matrix. The term "image matrix" refers to a layout of rows and columns, usually of numbers, in boxes or cells. Fig. 21-3 shows a 10×10 matrix of cells, a 5×5 matrix of cells, and a 5×5 matrix of numbers in imaginary cells. Each digital image consists of a matrix of imaginary cells having various brightness levels on the video monitor. The brightness of a cell is determined by the computer-generated number in that cell.

Each imaginary cell of the image is called a **pixel** (picture element). In digital x-ray imaging the value of the pixel is unimportant. The value is relative and is used to provide subtraction images and to define the image contrast. In CT scanning the numeric information contained in each pixel is a CT number, also identified as a Hounsfield number or **Hounsfield unit.** The value of the Hounsfield unit can be used to judge the nature of the tissue represented by it. In MRI the value of the pixel also has a relationship to the composition and nature of the tissue imaged.

The size of the image matrix is determined by characteristics of the imaging equipment and by the capacity of the computer. Most digital x-ray imaging systems provide image sizes of 256×256, 512×512, and 1024×1024 ma-

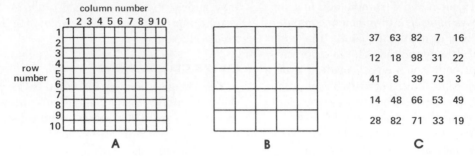

Fig. 21-3. Matrix refers to an arrangement of columns and rows. Three matrices are shown. **A,** 10 × 10 matrix of cells. **B,** 5 × 5 matrix of cells. **C,** 5 × 5 matrix of numbers in imaginary cells.

trices. Image resolution will be better with a larger image matrix.

EXAMPLE: How many pixels are contained in an image matrix described as 256 by 256?
ANSWER: $256 \times 256 = 65536$.

A 1024 by 1024 image matrix is sometimes described as a 1000-line system. In DF the image resolution is determined both by the image matrix and by the size of the image intensifier. A rough estimate of the theoretic limits of resolution can be obtained by dividing the size of the input phosphor of the image-intensifier tube by the matrix size.

EXAMPLE: What is the pixel size of a 1000-line imaging system operating in the 5-inch mode?
ANSWER: Five inches equals 127 mm. Therefore each pixel equals 127 divided by 1024, or 0.124 mm.

Fig. 21-4 illustrates the influence of matrix size on image quality. A 64 × 64 image matrix appears definitely "boxy," whereas a 512 × 512 image is a good represenation of the original analog image. A 1024 × 1024 image is indistinguishable from the original. Because of the rectangular shape of these images, only half of each image is shown.

Dynamic range. An imaging system that could display only black or white would have a dynamic range of 2^1, or 2. Such an image would be very high contrast but would display very little information. Although the value of each pixel is unimportant, the range of values is extremely important in determining the final image. This is especially true for subtraction techniques. The range of values over which a system can respond is called its **dynamic range.** Dynamic range in a digital system corresponds to the numeric range of each pixel. Visually, dynamic range refers to the shades of gray that can be represented.

The dynamic range of the human eye is approximately 2^5, or 32 shades of gray stretching from white to black. The dynamic range of the x-ray beam as it exits the patient is in excess of 2^{10}. Although we cannot visualize such a dynamic range, a computer with sufficient capacity can. The higher the dynamic range, the more gradual will be the gray scale representing the range from maximum x-ray intensity to minimum x-ray intensity. The greater the dynamic range, therefore, the better the image. This is particularly true of images from subtraction techniques.

Digital x-ray imaging systems are characterized by their dynamic range, which is determined by the capacity of the computer employed. Most use an 8-, 10-, or 12-bit dynamic range, meaning a 2^8, 2^{10}, or 2^{12} range. The elec-

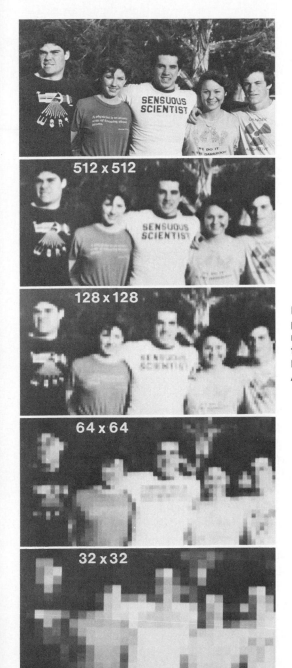

Fig. 21-4. These Wisconsin radiologic technology students posed to illustrate the loss of image resolution with decreasing matrix size. The 512 × 512 matrix is an acceptable rendition of the original. At a 32 × 32 matrix, the students became true blockheads. (Digitization courtesy Dennis Johnson, M.D., Anderson Hospital and Tumor Institute, Houston, Tex.)

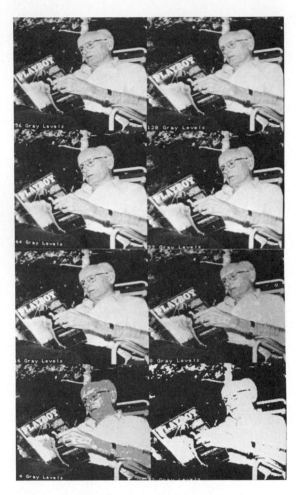

Fig. 21-5. This 34-year-old radiologist suffering from radiation-induced premature aging illustrates the meaning of dynamic range. The human eye can barely perceive the difference between sixteen and thirty-two gray levels. The computer can accurately distinguish 256 gray levels and more. (Digitization courtesy B. Wendt, Baylor College of Medicine, and R. Pennington, Rice University, Houston, Tex.)

tric signal that characterizes the x-ray intensity of the image is converted into digital form. The digital information is displayed as an image matrix, each pixel of which is capable of a range of 2^8 (0 to 256), 2^{10} (0 to 1024), or 2^{12} (0 to 4096).

Fig. 21-5 illustrates the effect of dynamic range on the image. Clearly a system with low dynamic range is high contrast but only over a limited portion of the image. High dynamic range allows for wide image latitude. The contrast of a **region of interest (ROI)** of the image can be electronically enhanced if the computer system has sufficient dynamic range. When a subtraction examination is undertaken, the information contained in the final image is far greater for a system with high dynamic range.

DIGITAL FLUOROSCOPY

A DF examination is conducted in much the same manner as a conventional study. To the casual observer the equipment employed is the same, but such is not the case. Fig. 21-6 shows the components necessary for DF. A computer has been added, as well as two video monitors and a more complex operating console.

Fig. 21-7 is representative of the operating console of a dedicated digital system. It contains typewriter and special function key pads in the left module for entering patient data and communicating with the computer. The right portion of the console contains additional special-function computer keys for data acquisition and image display. The module on the right also contains computer-interactive video controls and a pad for cursor and region of interest (ROI) manipulation. Other systems use a **trackball, joystick or mouse** instead of the pad. Two video screens are employed. The left screen is used to edit patient and examination data and to annotate final images. The right monitor will display subtracted images.

Generator

During DF, the undertable x-ray tube actually operates in the radiographic mode. The tube

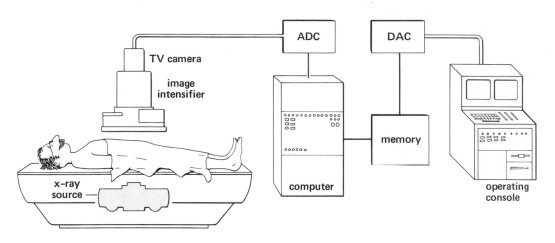

Fig. 21-6. The components of a digital fluoroscopic system.

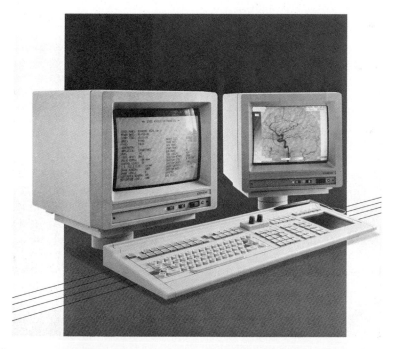

Fig. 21-7. A typical operating console for a digital fluoroscopic system. (Courtesy Siemens Medical Systems.)

current is measured in hundreds of mA instead of less than 5 mA as in conventional fluoroscopy. This is not a particular problem, however. Of course, if the tube were energized continuously, it would fail because of thermal overloading and the patient dose would be exceedingly high. DF images are obtained in much the same fashion that rapid-changer images are obtained in angiography.

Image acquisition rates of one per second to ten per second are common in most examinations. Since it requires 33 ms to read one video frame, x-ray exposures longer than that can result in unnecessary patient dose. However, that is a theoretic limit, and longer exposures may be necessary to ensure low noise and good image quality. Consequently, the x-ray generator must be capable of switching on and off very rapidly. The time required for the x-ray tube to be switched on and reach the selected level of kVp and mA is called the **interrogation time.** The time required for the x-ray tube to be switched off is the **extinction time.** DF systems must incorporate three-phase generators with interrogation and extinction times of less than 5 ms.

Video system

The video system employed in conventional fluoroscopy is usually a 525-line system. Such a system is adequate for DF, although higher resolution can be obtained with 1000-line systems. Conventional video, however, has two limitations that restrict its application in digital techniques. First, the interlaced mode of reading the target of the television camera can significantly degrade a digital image. Second, conventional TV camera tubes are relatively noisy. They have a signal-to-noise ratio of about 200:1, whereas a signal-to-noise ratio of 1000:1 is necessary for DF.

Interlace vs. progressive mode. In Chapter 18 we described the method by which a conventional TV camera tube reads off its target assembly. This was described as an interlace

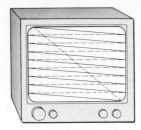

Fig. 21-8. The progressive mode of reading a video signal.

mode where two fields of 262½ lines each were read in ⅟₆₀ s (17 ms) to form a 525-line video frame in ⅟₃₀ s (33 ms). Reading the video signal in the progressive mode is illustrated in Fig. 21-8. Here the electron beam of the TV camera tube sweeps the target assembly continuously from top to bottom in 33 ms and then returns to the top for a second sweep in the same fashion. The video image is similarly formed on the television monitor. There is no interlace of one field with another, and this produces a sharper image.

Signal-to-noise ratio. All electronic devices are inherently noisy. Because of heated filaments and voltage differences, there is always a very small electric current flowing in any circuit. This is called background electricity or **noise.** It is similar to the noise on a radiograph in that it conveys no information and serves only to obscure **the signal,** the electric current that does convey information.

Conventional TV camera tubes have a signal-to-noise ratio of about 200:1. The maximum output signal will be 200 times greater than the background electrical noise. This is not sufficient for DF because the video signal is rarely at maximum and lower signals become even more lost in the noise. Especially when subtraction techniques are employed, image quality will be severely degraded by a system with a low signal-

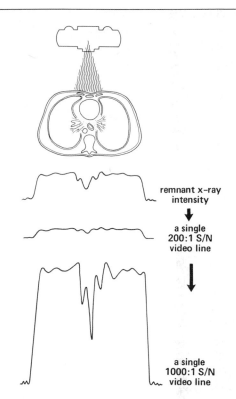

Fig. 21-9. The information content of a video system with a high signal-to-noise ratio is greatly enhanced. Shown here are a single video line through an object and the resulting signal at 200:1 and 1000:1 signal-to-noise ratios.

to-noise ratio and information will be lost. Fig. 21-9 illustrates the difference between the output of a 200:1 signal-to-noise TV camera tube and a 1000:1 tube. At 200:1 the dynamic range is less than 2^8, and at 1000:1 it is about 2^{10}. The tube with a 1000:1 signal-to-noise ratio contains five times the useful information and is more compatible with computer-assisted image enhancement.

Computer

DF employs minicomputers. The capacity of the computer is the most important factor in determining not only image quality but also the manner and speed of image acquisition. Important characteristics of a DF system that are computer controlled are the **image matrix size,** the **system dynamic range,** or bit depth, and the **image acquisition rate.** The output signal from the TV camera tube is transmitted by cable to an **analog-to-digital converter (ADC).** The ADC accepts the continuously varying television camera output signal, the analog signal, and digitizes it.

To be compatible with the computer, the ADC must have the same dynamic range as the computer. An 8-bit ADC would convert the analog signal into values between 0 and 256. A 10-bit ADC would be more precise in that the analog-to-digital conversion would range from 0 to 2^{10}, or 0 to 1024.

The output of the ADC is then transferred to main memory and manipulated so that a digital image in matrix form is stored. The dynamic range of each pixel, the number of pixels, and the method of storage will determine the speed that the image can be acquired, subtracted, and transferred to an output device.

If image storage is in primary memory, which is usually the case, then data acquisition and transfer can be as rapid as thirty images per second. However, if each video image must be transferred to a secondary memory such as a Winchester disk and recalled from secondary memory to primary memory for each subtraction event, then the time required for these transfers will limit the image acquisition rate. In general, if the image matrix is halved (for example, from 512 to 256), the image acquisition rate will be increased by a factor of four. A representative system might be capable of acquiring eight images per second in the 256 × 256 matrix mode; however, if a higher-resolution image is required and the 512 × 512 mode is employed, then only two images per second could be acquired. Even though the conducting path is very short, this limitation is imposed by the time required to transfer such enormous quantities of data by wire from one segment of memory to another.

Table 21-1. Comparison of temporal
and energy subtraction

Temporal subtraction	Energy subtraction
A single kVp is used.	Rapid kVp switching is required.
Normal x-ray beam filtration is adequate.	X-ray beam filter switching is preferred.
Contrast resolution of 1 mm at 1% is achieved.	Higher x-ray intensity is required for comparable contrast resolution.
Simple arithmetic image subtraction is necessary.	Complex image subtraction is necessary.
Motion artifacts are problem.	Motion artifacts are greatly reduced.
Total subtraction of common structures is achieved.	Some residual bone may survive subtraction.
Subtraction possibilities are limited by number of images.	Many more types of subtraction images are possible.

Image formation

The principal advantages of DF examination are the image subtraction techniques that are possible and the ability to visualize vasculature with a venous injection of contrast material. Unfortunately, an area beam must be employed. The associated scatter radiation reduces image contrast. However, image contrast can be enhanced electronically. Image contrast is obtained by subtraction techniques that provide for instantaneous viewing of the subtracted image, effectively in real time, during the passage of a bolus of contrast medium.

Temporal subtraction and energy subtraction are the two methods that receive the most attention in DF. Each has advantages and disadvantages, and these are described in Table 21-1. Temporal subtraction techniques are most frequently employed because of high-voltage generator limitations in the energy subtraction mode. When the two techniques are combined,

the process is called **hybrid subtraction.** Image contrast is enhanced still further by hybrid subtraction because of reduced patient motion between subtracted images.

Temporal subtraction. Temporal subtraction refers to a number of computer-assisted techniques whereby an image obtained at one time is subtracted from an image obtained at a later time. If, during the intervening period, contrast material was introduced into the vasculature, the subtracted image will contain only the vessels filled with the contrast material. Two methods are commonly employed—mask mode and time interval difference mode.

Mask mode. A typical **mask mode** procedure is diagramed in Fig. 21-10. The patient is positioned under normal fluoroscopic control to ensure that the region of anatomy under investigation is within the field of view of the image intensifier. A power injector is armed and readied to deliver 30 to 50 ml of contrast material at the rate of approximately 15 to 20 ml/s through a venous entry. If an arterial entry is chosen, 10 to 25 ml of diluted contrast material at 10 to 12 ml/s may be used. The imaging apparatus is changed from the conventional fluoroscopic mode to the DF mode. This requires an increase in x-ray tube current of twenty to one hundred times the conventional fluoroscopic mode and the activation of a program of pulse image acquisition.

The injector is fired and, following a delay of 4 to 10 s, before the bolus of contrast medium reaches the anatomic site, an initial x-ray pulse exposure is made. The image obtained is stored in primary memory and displayed on video monitor A. This is the **mask image.**

This mask image is followed by a series of additional images that are stored in adjacent memory locations. While these subsequent images are being acquired, the mask image is subtracted from each and the result is either stored in primary memory, if the capacity is sufficient, or dumped to a secondary memory, usually a

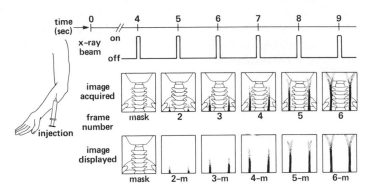

Fig. 21-10. A schematic representation of mask made fluoroscopy.

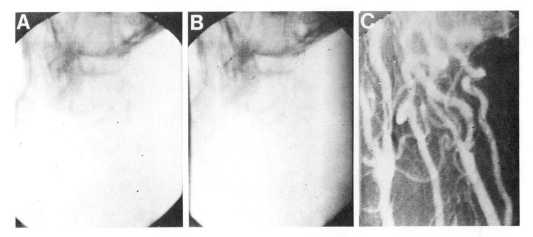

Fig. 21-11. A, The preinjection mask. **B,** The postinjection unenhanced image. **C,** An enhanced subtraction image produced when preinjection mask is subtracted from postinjection unchanged image. (Courtesy Charles Mistretta, Ph.D., University of Wisconsin, Madison.)

Winchester disk. At the same time the subtracted image is displayed on video monitor B. Fig. 21-11 shows a preinjection mask, an unenhanced image following a venous injection, and an enhanced image obtained by subtracting the first from the second.

The subtracted images appear in real time and are then stored on a Winchester disk. After the examination, each subtracted image can be recalled for closer examination.

As described here, each image was obtained from a 33 ms x-ray pulse. The time required for one video frame is 33 ms. Because the video system is relatively slow to respond and the video noise may be high, several video frames (usually four or eight) may be summed in memory to make each image. This process is called **image integration.** Although the process enhances image quality, it also increases patient dose.

In mask mode DF the imaging sequence following acquisition of the mask can be manually controlled or preprogramed. If preprogramed, the computer controls the data acquisition in accordance with the demands of the examination. For example, to evaluate carotid flow following a brachial vein injection, one could inject contrast material and, 2 s after injection, acquire a mask image. There then could follow another 2 s delay, followed by images obtained at the rate of two per second for 3 s, one per second for 5 s, and one every other second for 14 s. If the computer capacity for acquiring images is sufficient, any combination of multiple delays and varying image acquisition rates is possible.

Remasking. If, on subsequent examination, the initial mask image is inadequate because of patient motion, improper technique, or any other reason, later images may be used as the mask image. A typical examination may require a total of thirty images in addition to the mask image. If the intended mask image is technically inadequate and maximum contrast appears during the fifteenth image, one may obtain a better

subtraction image by using image number five as the mask rather than image number one. One can even integrate several images (for example, numbers four through eight) and use that composite image as the mask. Unacceptable mask images can be caused by noise, motion, and technique.

Time interval difference mode. Some examinations call for each subtracted image to be made from a different mask and follow-up frame. This is called **time interval difference** (TID) mode. Fig. 21-12 illustrates the sequence of image acquisition in a TID examination. TID imaging requires that a constant image acquisition rate be employed. In a cardiac study, for example, image acquisition begins 5 s after injection at the rate of fifteen images per second for 4 s. A total of sixty images will be obtained in such a study. These images are identified as frame numbers one through thirty. Each image is stored in a separate memory address as it is acquired. If a time interval difference of four images (268 ms) is selected, the first image to appear will be that obtained when frame one is subtracted from frame five. The second image will contain the subtraction of frame two from frame six, the third will contain the subtraction of frame three from frame seven, and so on.

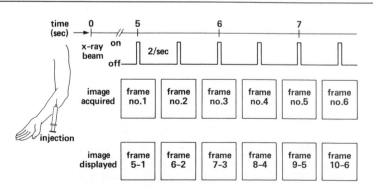

Fig. 21-12. The manner in which sequentially obtained images are subtracted in a time interval difference study.

In real time the images observed convey the flow of the contrast medium dynamically. Subsequent closer examination of each TID image shows it to be relatively free of motion artifacts but with less contrast than mask mode imaging. TID imaging is principally applied in cardiac monitoring, as shown in Fig. 21-13. These TID images of a dog heart show dyskinetic motion. In *h* the apex is expanding (white), while the rest of the left ventricular border is contrasting (black). In a normal heart the whole border is either white or black.

Misregistration. If patient motion occurs between the mask image and a subsequent image, the subtracted image will contain **misregistration artifacts,** as shown in Fig. 21-14. The same anatomy is not registered in the same pixel of the image matrix. This type of artifact can frequently be eliminated by reregistration of the mask, that is, by shifting the mask by one or more pixels so that **superimposition** of images is again obtained. Reregistration can be a tedious process. Often, when one area of an image is reregistered, another area will become misre-

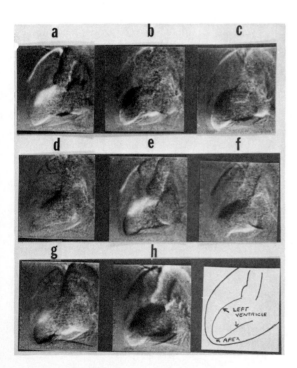

Fig. 21-13. TID images showing dyskinesia in a dog heart. (Courtesy Charles Mistretta, University of Wisconsin, Madison.)

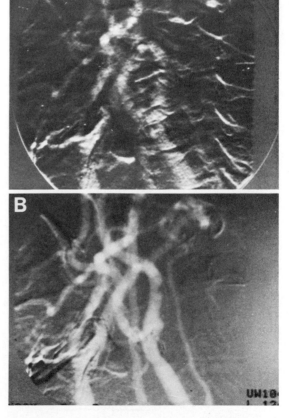

Fig. 21-14. Misregistration artifacts. (Courtesy Ben Arnold, South Bay Hospital, Redondo Beach, Calif.)

gistered. This can be controlled on some systems by ROI reregistration. Most systems can reregister not only in increments of pixel widths but also down to one tenth of a pixel width.

Energy subtraction. Temporal subtraction techniques take advantage of changing contrast media during the time of the examination and require no special demands on the high-voltage generator. Energy subtraction uses two different x-ray beams alternately to provide a subtraction image resulting from differences in photoelectric interaction. The basis for this technique is similar to that described in Chapter 15 for rare earth screens. It is based on the abrupt change in photoelectric absorption at the K edge of the contrast media compared with that for soft tissue and bone.

Fig. 21-15 shows the probability of x-ray interaction with iodine, bone, and muscle as a function of x-ray energy. The probability of photoelectric absorption in all three decreases with increasing x-ray energy. At an energy of 33 keV, there is an abrupt increase in absorption in iodine and a modest decrease in soft tissue and bone. This energy corresponds to the binding energy of the two K-shell electrons of iodine. When the incident x-ray energy is sufficient to overcome the K-shell electron binding energy of iodine, there is an abrupt and large increase

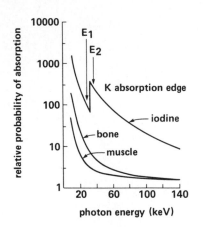

Fig. 21-15. Photoelectric absorption in iodine, bone, and muscle.

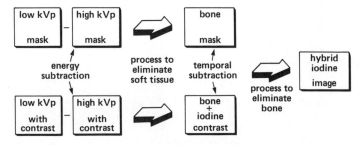

Fig. 21-16. Hybrid subtraction involves temporal and energy subtraction techniques.

in absorption. Graphically, this increase is known as the **K absorption edge.**

If one could employ monoenergetic x-ray beams of 32 and 34 keV alternately, the difference in absorption in iodine would be enormous and the resulting subtraction images would have very high contrast. Such is not the case, however, since every x-ray beam contains a wide spectrum of energies.

Energy subtraction has the decided disadvantage of requiring some method for providing an alternating x-ray beam of two different emission spectra. Two methods have been devised: (1) alternately pulsing the x-ray beam at 70 kVp and then 90 kVp and (2) introducing dissimilar metal filters into the x-ray beam alternately on a flywheel. The types of filters that have been employed in this alternating fashion are 4 mm Al and 2 mm Cu. The result of both approaches is an alternating x-ray spectra of two different energies.

Hybrid subtraction. Some DF systems are capable of combining temporal and energy subtraction techniques into what is called **hybrid subtraction.** This is illustrated in Fig. 21-16. Image acquisition follows the mask mode procedure as previously described. Here, however, the mask and each subsequent image are formed by an energy subtraction technique. If patient motion can be controlled, hybrid imaging can theoretically produce the highest-quality DF images.

DIGITAL RADIOGRAPHY

Digital radiography (DR) is advancing along several approaches simultaneously. It differs from conventional radiography in that film is not the image receptor. Other types of radiation detectors whose electrical output is proportional to the radiation intensity are used. Initially, this output signal may be in analog form, but it is converted to digital form. The image is displayed on a video monitor after computer processing.

Scanned projection radiography

Perhaps the first clinically useful application of DR was a complement to CT developed by the General Electric Company. This has come to be known as **scanned projection radiography** (**SPR**). Basically, SPR involves the use of the existing CT gantry and computer to generate an

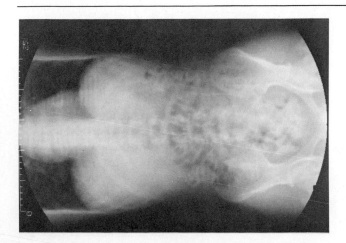

Fig. 21-17. This computed radiograph is typical of scan projection radiographs obtained with CT scanners. (Courtesy Larry Rothenberg, Ph.D., Memorial Hospital, New York City.)

image that looks surprisingly like a conventional radiograph. Fig. 21-17 is an example of such an image.

This image is similar to a conventional radiographic image in that there is superposition of tissues through the body. It differs from a conventional image in that it is virtually free of scatter radiation and is digital in form. The reduced scatter radiation results in enhanced radiographic contrast. The digital form of the image permits subtraction techniques as described for DF and provides for other types of numeric image manipulation.

Another way to view the production of the high-contrast image in DR is to consider that the rejection of scattered x-ray photons reduces the noise in the image. Remember that Compton-scattered photons carry no useful information but simply contribute to the background noise of an image. In any imaging system, **noise is the principal limitation to the detection of low-contrast objects.** Consequently, in DR the radiographic contrast is high and the detection of low-contrast objects is enhanced.

The principal disadvantage with DR is its poor high-contrast resolution. Whereas a conventional screen-film system can image 100 μm objects with ease, DR can do no better than about

500 μm. Of course, this degree of resolution is adequate for most examinations. In DR resolution is controlled principally by the design of the detector array and the speed with which the patient or x-ray beam is translated.

The more detectors there are per degree of fan x-ray beam, the better will be the high-contrast resolution. Since gas-filled detectors can be more tightly produced, such a system will usually exhibit better resolution.

As the speed of translation is reduced, fewer x rays will be detected in either the translation of the patient through the x-ray beam or the translation of the beam across the patient. This will restrict the resulting image quality by reducing both high- and low-contrast resolution.

The basic components of an SPR system are identified in Fig. 21-18. An x-ray beam is shaped into a fan by collimators that confine the beam to 5 to 10 mm thickness through an arc of 30 to 45 degrees. There are two collimators. The prepatient collimators shape the beam, reduce scatter radiation, and control patient dose. The postpatient collimators further reduce scatter radiation. On passing through the patient, the remnant x rays are intercepted by a detector array. Each detector responds with a signal that is related to the body part through which the x-

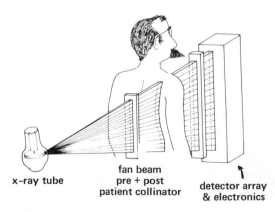

x-ray tube   fan beam
pre + post
patient collinator   detector array
& electronics

Fig. 21-18. The components of a digital radiographic system. (Courtesy Gary Barnes, Ph.D., University of Alabama, Birmingham.)

ray beam passed. The response of the total detector array therefore represents an attenuation profile of that body section.

To obtain enough profiles for a complete image, the source-detector assembly remains stationary and the patient is translated through the x-ray beam. Alternatively, the patient may remain stationary while the source-detector assembly translates. During translation, either the x-ray beam is pulsed or the interrogation of the detector array is intermittent. The sequential profiles obtained during translation are computer processed to form an image resembling a radiograph.

SPR designs with patient translation are incorporated into most CT scanners. By proper positioning of the x-ray tube–detector array, one can obtain AP, PA, lateral, and oblique views. Dedicated DR systems employ translation of the source-detector assembly across a stationary patient. A dedicated DR chest unit is illustrated in Fig. 21-19.

X-ray tube-detector assembly

An x-ray tube employed for DR must have a high heat capacity. A heat capacity in excess of 500 kHU is usually required, and some tubes have greater than 1 MHU capacity. The requirement for a high heat capacity occurs because of two characteristics of the system—imaging time and detector efficiency. One usually images 20 to 50 cm of the patient at a translation speed of 1 to 2 cm/s. The detectors may not be intrinsically as efficient as a screen-film receptor and, because of the precise beam collimation, few scattered photons reach the detectors. Consequently, techniques of 500 to 2000 mAs are required.

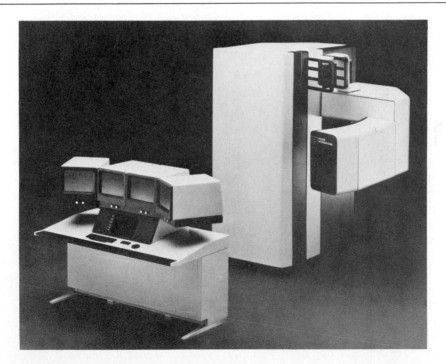

Fig. 21-19. A dedicated digital radiographic chest unit. (Courtesy Picker International.)

There are presently two basic designs employed in the detector array—a gas-filled detector assembly and scintillation detectors coupled to solid-state photodiodes. Similar designs were described earlier in relation to CT (see also Chapter 22). The gas-filled detector array usually contains xenon under high pressure in many small chambers. Xenon is used because its high Z, 53, results in high photoelectric absorption. The individual detector chamber can be made as small as 0.5 mm with an even smaller interspace.

The solid-state scintillation detector array incorporates individual crystal-photodiode assemblies. Such an array usually presents an active area to the x-ray beam of 5×20 mm. The interspace between detectors will vary from 1 mm to 5 mm. This results in a limit to the number of detectors that can be employed. The scintillation crystal usually employed is cadmium tungstate ($CdWO_4$), although bismuth germanate (BGO), cesium iodide (CsI), and sodium iodide (NaI) are also employed. The photodiode is a semiconductor material, usually silicon or germanium, whose response is proportional to the intensity of light incident on it.

Area beam

A principal limitation to the SPR mode of DR is the time required to obtain an image. In conventional radiography a latent image is produced in a matter of milliseconds. When a fan beam is used in digital radiography, several seconds may be required and this will increase image blur because of patient motion.

The image acquisition time in DR can be improved by increasing the translation time in SPR or by employing an area beam with an area image receptor as in conventional radiography. There is nothing special to providing an area beam. It is difficult, however, to fabricate an area image receptor that will retain the rapid response time required.

Two approaches are available. An assembly of solid-state detectors formed in matrix fashion can be used. The electronics associated with the enormous number of detectors required is quite large, and therefore the expense can be excessive. An electrostatic image receptor such as that employed in xeroradiography can be used, and the latent image read in point-by-point fashion to produce a digital image. Regardless of the type of area receptor employed, contrast resolution will be reduced.

Computed radiography

On the horizon are directly acquired digital radiographic images employing a **photostimulable phosphor.** This process is shown schematically in Fig. 21-20 and has been labeled **computed radiography (CR).** It is similar to xeroradiography in that a solid-state image receptor in plate form is used.

The image receptor resembles a conventional radiographic intensifying screen and is exposed in a cassette with conventional x-ray equipment. It is composed of barium fluorohalide compounds, which are energized when exposed to radiation. The sensitivity is approximately equal to a 200-speed screen-film combination or much greater when contrast resolution is sacrificed. The latent image consists of valence electrons stored in high-energy traps.

The latent image is made manifest by exposure to a pencil beam from a high-intensity laser. The laser beam causes the trapped electrons to return to the valence band with the emission of blue light. This is **light-stimulated phosphorescence,** as described in Chapter 15. The blue emission is viewed by an ultrasensitive photomultiplier tube. The electric signal, which is the output of the photomultiplier tube, is digitized and stored for subsequent display on a CRT or hard copy from a laser printer.

The spatial resolution of CR is not quite as good as conventional radiography, but the contrast resolution is superior because of available image-processing modes. The latitude of the system is exceptional, and for many examinations patient dose is considerably less. CR is still in development but promises to be of considerable importance to future radiology because of its digital nature.

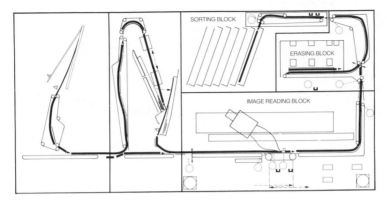

Fig. 21-20. Process of computed radiography using photostimulable phosphors. (Courtesy Fuji Photo Co.)

PICTURE ARCHIVING AND COMMUNICATION SYSTEM

Radiology is slowly evolving into totally digital imaging. Estimates of the present level of digitally acquired images range up to 35%. These images come from nuclear medicine, digital ultrasound, DSA, CT, and MRI. Analog images, such as conventional radiographs, can be digitized by a device such as that shown in Fig. 21-21. Such film digitizers are based on laser beam technology.

Essentially all these digital images are converted to film for interpretation and storage. A picture archiving and communication system (PACS), when fully implemented, will allow not only the acquisition but also the interpretation and storage of each medical image in digital form without resorting to film. The projected efficiencies of time and money are enormous. The three principle components to a PACS are the display system, the network, and the storage system.

Display system

The heart of a PACS display system is a CRT monitor. Some call it a video workstation, and Fig. 21-22 is an example of such a station. In order to truly replace film viewing, the CRTs must be high resolution, at least 2048 × 2048. Present image matrices used with digitally acquired images range from 128 × 128 to 512 × 512, which is considerably less than that required to equal the spatial resolution of film. However, PACS are equipped with a keyboard control for the various image-processing modes.

Some relaxation of the spatial resolution requirements of the workstation are allowed because of the electronic image-processing modes that are available. Image processing is possible because of the digital nature of the image and the interactive nature of the workstation. **Subtraction** of one image from another emphasizes vascular structures. **Edge enhancement** is effective for fractures and small, high-contrast objects. **Windowing** is useful for amplifying soft tissue differences. **Highlighting** can be effective in identifying diffuse nonfocal disease. **Pan, scroll,** and **zoom** allow for careful visualization of precise regions of an image. To be truly effective, each of these image-processing modes must be quick, not more than a few seconds. This requires that each workstation be microprocessor controlled and interactive with each imaging device and the central computer. To provide for such interaction, a network is required.

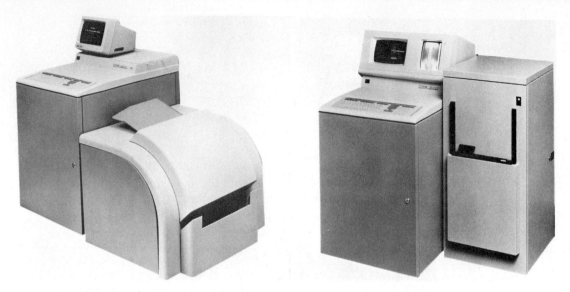

Fig. 21-21. This device called a digital teleradiography system uses a laser beam to convert an analog radiograph into a digital image. (Courtesy duPont Company.)

Network

Computer scientists use the term "network" to describe the manner in which many computers can be connected to interact with one another. In a business office, for instance, each secretary might have a microprocessor-based workstation, which is interfaced with a central office computer, so that information can be transferred from one workstation to another or to and from the main computer memory.

In radiology, as shown in Fig. 21-23, in addition to secretarial workstations, the network may consist of various types of imagers, PACS workstations, remote PACS workstations, a departmental mainframe, and a hospital mainframe. Each of these devices is called a **node** of the network. Nodes are interconnected, usually by cable within a building, by telephone or CATV line among buildings, and by microwave or satellite transmission to remote facilities. The name **teleradiology** has been given to the process of remote transmission and viewing of images. In order to be adaptable to any radiologic equipment, The American College of Radiology (ACR), in cooperation with the National Electrical Manufacturers Association (NEMA), has produced a standard imaging and interface format.

The network begins operation at the imager, where data are acquired in digital form. The images reconstructed from the data are then processed at the console of the imager or transmitted to a PACS workstation for processing. At any time, such images can be transferred to other nodes within or outside the hospital. Instead of running films up to surgery for viewing on a lightbox, one simply transfers the image electronically to the PACS workstation in surgery. When a radiologist is not immediately available for image interpretation, the image can be transferred to a PACS workstation in the radiologist's home. Essentially everywhere that film is required now, electronic images can be substituted. Time is essential when considering image manipulation, and therefore very large and fast computers are required for this task.

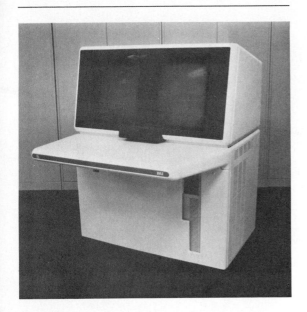

Fig. 21-22. This Diagnostic Review Station is a PACS workstation having two video monitors to network with the various digital imagers in radiology. (Courtesy J. Ed Barnes, Ph.D., General Electric Medical Systems.)

These requirements are relaxed for the information management and database portion of PACS. Such lower-priority functions of PACS include message and mail utilities, calendar reporting, text data, and financial accounting and planning.

From the PACS workstation, any number of coded diagnostic reports can be initiated and transferred to a secretarial workstation for report generation. The secretarial workstation in turn can interact with the main hospital computer for patient identification, billing, accounting, and interaction with other departments. Similarly, a secretarial workstation at the departmental reception desk can interact with a departmental computer for scheduling of patients, technologists, and radiologists and for analysis of departmental statistics. Finally, at the completion of an examination, PACS allows for more efficient image archiving.

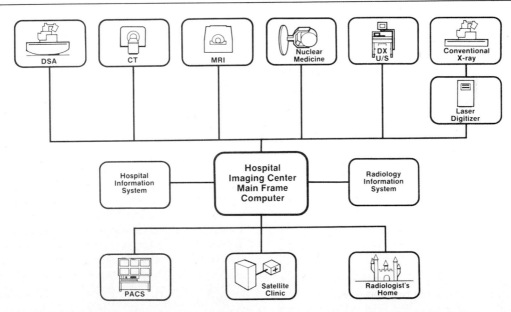

Fig. 21-23. The PACS network allows interaction among the various nodes of data acquisition, image processing, and image archiving.

Storage system

The principal motivation for PACS is archiving. How often are films checked out from the file room and never returned? How many films disappear from jackets? How many jackets disappear? How much effort is expended duplicating films for clinicians? Just the cost of the hospital space to accommodate a film file is sufficient to justify PACS.

With PACS, a film file room is replaced by a magnetic or optical memory device. Magnetic devices, such as high-capacity Winchester disks, are acceptable. The future of PACS, however, depends on the continuing development of the optical disk. Magnetic disk packs are available in configurations up to approximately 1000 megabytes or one gigabyte. Optical disks can accommodate one gigabyte on each side, and when positioned in a jukebox, as in Fig. 21-24, will accommodate 100 gigabytes. An entire hospital file room is thereby accommodated by a storage device the size of a desk. Electronically, images can be recalled from this archival system to any workstation in seconds.

The acceptance of PACS in general radiology is slow in coming. Although image quality is equal to that of film in most instances, the cost is still high and the acceptance by radiologists and clinicians is slow. Even though diagnosis in many instances is presently made from a CRT, a radiologist still feels more secure with hard copy. Undoubtedly, that will change with time.

REVIEW QUESTIONS

1. Define or otherwise identify the following:
   a. Digital subtraction angiography
   b. Matrix
   c. Pixel
   d. Voxel
   e. Registration
   f. Trackball
   g. Dynamic range
   h. Interrogation time
   i. ADC
   j. Hybrid subtraction
2. What are the principal advantages of digital fluoroscopy over conventional fluoroscopy?

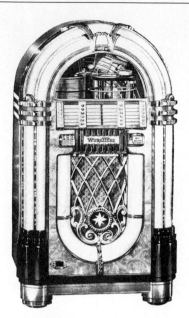

Fig. 21-24. This 1946 Wurlitzer jukebox with its 78 rpm platters serves as a model for the optical disc jukebox of PACS. (Courtesy Raymond Wilenzek, Ph.D., Ochsner Clinic, New Orleans.)

3. Describe the differences between a video system operating in the interlace mode and one operating in the progressive mode.
4. Describe the sequence of image acquisition in mask mode fluoroscopy.
5. What are the components of a scanned projection radiography system, and how is the image produced?
6. How does image resolution change with image matrix size and image-intensifier size?
7. Describe the difference between high-contrast resolution and low-contrast resolution.
8. How many pixels are contained in an image whose matrix size is described as 320 × 320?
9. A DF system is operated in a 512 × 512 image made with a 12 cm image intensifier. What is the size of each pixel?
10. The dynamic range of certain DF systems is described as being 8 bits deep. What does this mean?

22

Computed tomography

PRINCIPLES OF OPERATION
OPERATIONAL MODES
SYSTEM COMPONENTS
IMAGE CHARACTERISTICS
IMAGE QUALITY
QUALITY ASSURANCE

The components necessary to construct a computed tomographic (CT) scanner were available to physicists and engineers 20 years before Godfrey Hounsfield first demonstrated the process in 1970. Hounsfield was an engineer with EMI, Ltd., the British company most famous for recording the Beatles, and both he and his company have received justifiably high acclaim.

The CT scanner has already established itself as an invaluable radiologic diagnostic tool. Its development and introduction into radiologic practice will, without doubt, assume an importance as significant as the Snook interrupterless transformer, the Coolidge hot cathode x-ray tube, the Potter-Bucky diaphragm, and the image-intensifier tube. No other development in x-ray apparatus in the past 25 years is as significant. One could argue correctly that magnetic resonance imaging (MRI) is equally as significant. However, MRI is not an x-ray procedure.

Computed tomographic scanning has been variously identified as computerized axial to-mography (CAT), computerized transaxial tomography (CTAT), computerized reconstruction tomography (CRT), and digital axial tomography (DAT). **Computed tomography (CT)** is the nomenclature that has been substantially accepted to identify this diagnostic tool.

The CT scanner is revolutionary in that it does not record an image in the conventional way. There is no image receptor, such as film, an image-intensifier tube, or a Xerox plate, in a CT scanner. A collimated x-ray beam is directed on the patient, and the attenuated remnant radiation is measured by a detector whose response is transmitted to a computer. The computer considers the location of the patient and the spatial relationship of the x-ray beam to the region of interest. It analyzes the signal from the detector so that a visual image can be reconstructed and displayed on a television monitor. The image can then be photographed for later evaluation and file. The computer reconstruction of the cross-sectional anatomy is accomplished with mathematic equations adapted for computer processing called **algorithms.**

At one count there were over twenty manufacturers of CT scanners. Now there are less than ten. The cost of these systems varies from approximately $400,000 to over $1 million. The difference in operating characteristics and image quality is far greater over the range of CT scanners than for a comparable top-to-bottom range of conventional radiographic equipment. It is particularly important to perform a careful evaluation before purchasing a CT unit and to maintain the system continuously during use. Improper CT monitoring and maintenance produce poor images that may result in missed diagnoses and reirradiation of the patient.

PRINCIPLES OF OPERATION

When one images the abdomen with conventional radiographic technique, the image is created directly on the film image receptor and is relatively low in contrast. The image is not as clear as one might expect because of superposition of all the anatomic structures within the abdomen. The consequences of scatter radiation further degrade the visibility of image detail. To visualize and abdominal structure such as the kidneys better, conventional tomography can be employed. In a nephrotomogram the renal outline is much more distinct because the overlying and underlying tissues are blurred. In addition, the contrast of the in-focus structures has been enhanced. Yet, the image is still rather dull and unsharp. Fig. 22-1 depicts the arrangement for obtaining a radiograph of the abdomen and a nephrotomogram.

Conventional tomography is **axial tomography,** since the plane of the image is parallel with the long axis of the body and results in sagittal and coronal images. CT scanning results in a **transaxial tomogram.** The image is perpendicular to the long axis of the body (Fig. 22-2).

The precise methodology by which a CT scanner produces a cross-sectional image is extremely complicated and requires a good knowledge of physics, engineering, and computer science. However, the basic principles can be demonstrated if one considers the simplest of CT systems, consisting of finely collimated x-ray beam and single detector (Fig. 22-3). The x-ray source and detector are connected so that they move synchronously.

When the source-detector assembly makes one sweep, or **translation,** across the patient, the internal structures of the body attenuate the x-ray beam according to their density and effective atomic number, as discussed in Chapter 9. The intensity of radiation detected varies according to this attenuation pattern and forms a **projection** (Fig. 22-4). At the end of this translation the source-detector assembly will return to its starting position, and the entire assembly will **rotate** and begin a second translation. During the second translation, the detector signal

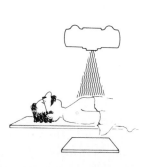
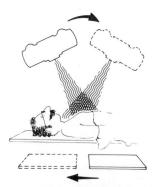

Fig. 22-1. Equipment arrangement for obtaining a radiograph and a conventional tomograph.

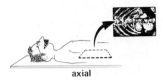

axial

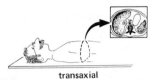

transaxial

Fig. 22-2. Conventional tomography results in an image that is parallel to the long axis of the body. CT scanning produces a transaxial image.

Fig. 22-3. In its simplest form a CT scanner consists of an x-ray source emitting a finely collimated x-ray beam and a single detector, both moving synchronously in a translate or rotate mode or a combination of both.

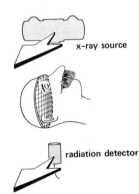

x–ray source

radiation detector

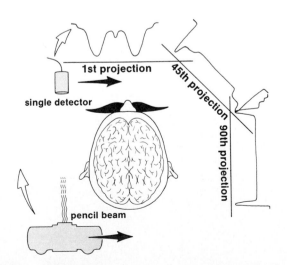

1st projection

45th projection

90th projection

single detector

pencil beam

Fig. 22-4. Each sweep of the source-detector assembly results in an electric signal that represents the attentuation pattern of the patient profile.

will again be proportional to the beam attenuation of anatomic structures, and a second detected intensity pattern will be described. If this process is repeated several times, a large number of intensity profiles will be generated. These intensity profiles are not displayed visually but are stored in numeric form in the computer. The computer processing of these data involves the effective superposition of each intensity profile to reconstruct the anatomic structures.

The superposition of the detector outputs does not occur as one might imagine. The detector signal during each translation is divided into multiple values in increments from about 80 to as high as 500. The value for each increment is related to the attenuation coefficient of the total tissue path. Through the use of simultaneous equations, a matrix of values is obtained that represents the cross-sectional anatomy.

OPERATIONAL MODES
First-generation scanners

The previous description of a finely collimated x-ray beam–single detector assembly translating across the patient and rotating between successive translations is characteristic of the early CT designs. These are now called **first-generation CT scanners.** The original EMI scanner required 180 translations, each separated by a 1-degree rotation (Fig. 22-5). It incorporated two detectors and split the finely collimated x-ray beam so that two contiguous slices or images could be generated during each scan. A third detector sampled the unattenuated beam as a reference. The principal drawback to these units was the time required to complete one scan. Scan time for first-generation units was almost 5 minutes.

These early scanners required a water-filled bag for patient positioning and detector normalization during scanning. The water was necessary to moderate the abrupt change in x-ray attenuation that would occur between air and skull bone.

Second-generation scanners

First-generation CT scanners can be considered a demonstration project. They demonstrated the feasibility of the functional marriage of the detector-source assembly, the mechanical

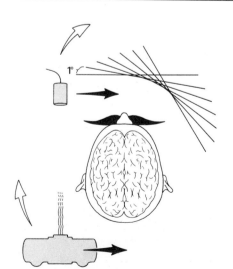

Fig. 22-5. First-generation CT scanners use a pencil x-ray beam and a single detector moving in the translate-rotate mode. A single slice image is generated following many such motions.

gantry motion, and the computer to produce an image. **Second-generation scanners** are also of the translate-rotate type, and these units continue to be produced. These units incorporate the natural extension of the single detector to a multiple detector assembly intercepting a fan-shaped rather than a pencil beam. Fig. 22-6 illustrates the difference between a pencil beam and a fan-shaped beam. A disadvantage to the fan beam is the increased scatter radiation. This affects the final image in much the same way as in conventional radiography. The characteristic features of a second-generation CT scanner are shown in Fig. 22-7.

The principal advantage to the second-generation CT scanner is speed. These scanners have five to thirty detectors in the detector assembly, and therefore shorter scan times are possible. Because of the multiple detector array, a single translation results in the same number of data points as several translations with a first-generation CT scanner. Consequently, each translation is separated by rotation increments of 5 degrees or more. With a 10-degree rotation increment, only eighteen translations would be required for a 180-degree scan. The simultaneous detection format of multiple detector channels also enhances image quality. Naturally the cost of second-generation scanners is considerably more than first-generation scanners because of the additional electronics and computer capacity required to accommodate multiple simultaneous information channels.

There are several advantages to the translation motion over later scanner designs that incorporate rotate-only modes. First, the inherent spatial resolution of a translation scanner is not limited by detector size. Second, each detector samples the entire cross-sectional anatomy, which can considerably reduce image artifacts. Finally, since all detectors translate across the patient into the raw, unattenuated beam, each one can be calibrated and normalized during each translation. This enhances image contrast and stabilizes CT numbers or Houndsfield units (HU).

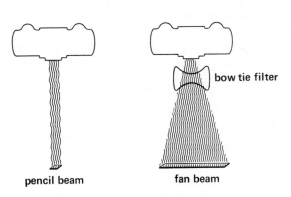

Fig. 22-6. The two x-ray beam profiles employed in CT scanning. With the fan beam a bow-tie filter is sometimes employed to equalize the radiation intensity reaching the detector array.

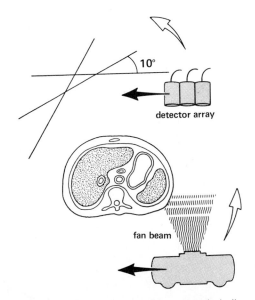

Fig. 22-7. Second-generation scanners operate in the translate-rotate mode with a multiple detector array intercepting a fan-shaped x-ray beam.

Third-generation scanners

The principal limitation to second-generation CT scanners is examination time. Because of the complex mechanical motion of translate-rotate and the enormous mass involved in the scan gantry, most units are designed for scan times of 20 s or more. To overcome this limitation, **third-generation scanners** evolved in which the x-ray tube and detector array were rotated concentrically about the patient (Fig. 22-8). As rotate-only units third-generation scanners currently accommodate scan times as low as 1 s.

The third-generation scanner employs a curvilinear detector array containing at least thirty elements and a fan beam. The number of detectors and the width of the fan beam, between 30 and 60 degrees, are both substantially larger than for second-generation scanners. In third-generation CT scanners the fan beam and detector array view the entire patient at all times. In the second-generation unit equipped with a linear detector array the x-ray path length is shortest for the central detector and increases in length as one moves to the periphery of the detector array. The curvilinear detector array results in a constant source-to-detector path length, which is an advantage for good image reconstruction. This feature of the third-generation detector assembly also allows for better x-ray beam collimation to reduce the effect of scatter radiation. This type of collimation is called **predetector** or **postpatient collimation,** and it functions much as a radiographic grid does in conventional radiographic examinations. There is also **prepatient collimation** to restrict patient dose. Prepatient collimation also determines the thickness of the tissue slice that is imaged. **Slice thickness** is also called **sensitivity profile.** Fig. 22-9 compares the detector assembly functions for second- and third-generation scanners.

One of the principal disadvantages of third-generation CT scanners is the occasional appearance of ring or circular artifacts. These can occur for several reasons. Each detector views a single anulus of anatomy (Fig. 22-10). Should any single detector or bank of detectors malfunction, the resulting errant or absent signal

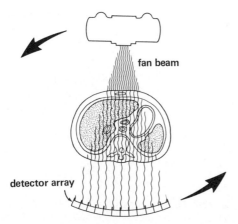

Fig. 22-8. Third-generation CT scanners operate in the rotate-only mode with a fan x-ray beam—multiple detector array revolving concentrically around the patient.

will result in a ring on the reconstructed image. Properly formulated image reconstruction algorithms will minimize such artifacts.

Fourth-generation scanners

The **fourth-generation** design for CT scanners is, as for those of the third generation, a rotate-only motion. However, with fourth-generation machines the x-ray source rotates but the detector assembly does not. Radiation detection is accomplished through a fixed circular array of detectors (Fig. 22-11), which contains as many as 1000 individual elements. The x-ray beam is fan shaped with characteristics similar to those of third-generation fan beams. These units are capable of scanning times as fast as 1 s, can ac-

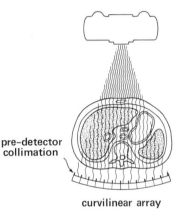 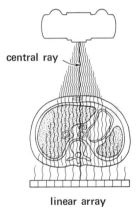

Fig. 22-9. The linear detector array is characteristic of first- and second-generation CT scanners; the curvilinear array is used in third- and fourth-generation units.

central ray

pre-detector collimation

curvilinear array

linear array

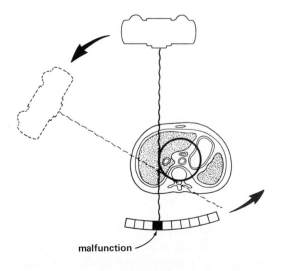

malfunction

Fig. 22-10. Ring artifacts can occur in third-generation scanners because each detector views an anulus of anatomy during each scan.

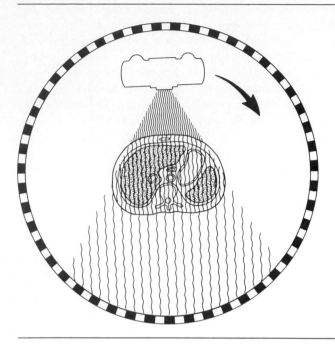

Fig. 22-11. Fourth-generation CT scanners operate in the rotate mode, but only the source rotates; the detector array is fixed.

commodate variable slice thickness through automatic prepatient collimation, and can provide the image manipulation capabilities of earlier scanners.

The fixed circular detector array of fourth-generation CT scanners does not result in a constant beam path from the source to all detectors, but it does allow each detector to be calibrated and its signal normalized during each scan, as is possible with second-generation scanners. Fourth-generation scanners are generally free of circular artifacts.

The principal disadvantage of fourth-generation machines appears to be patient dose, which is somewhat higher than that with other types of scanners. The cost of these units may be somewhat higher also because of the large number of detectors and their associated electronics. If scan time is important, then a third- or fourth-generation scanner is necessary.

Although many attempts at image quality comparison have been conducted, no general-

izations are possible, and a clear decision regarding the best image is not likely. Much of the final image quality is dependent on the mathematics of image reconstruction, and these techniques are continually being refined.

Future designs

There are continuing developments in CT scanner design that promise still further improvements in image quality at less patient dose. Some incorporate novel motions of either the x-ray tube or the detector array or both. Some involve patient motion as well. Faster scanners have been developed, making cine CT possible. There is continuing development of reconstuction algorithms so that the operator can select one of several for a particular examination.

SYSTEM COMPONENTS

Just as it was convenient to classify the components of a conventional x-ray unit according to three major systems—the operating console,

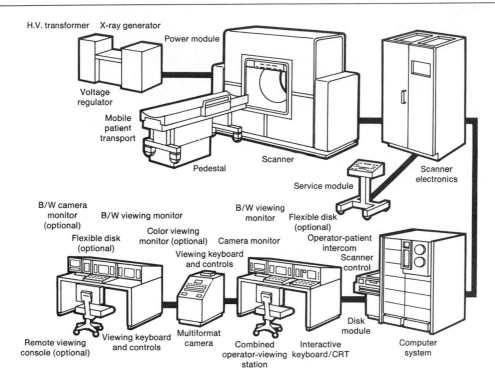

Fig. 22-12. Components of a complete CT scanner system. (Courtesy Picker International.)

the generator, and the x-ray tube—so it is convenient to identify the three major system components of a CT scanner: the gantry, the computer, and the operating console. Each of these major components has several subsystems involved in their operation. Fig. 22-12 shows the various components to a rather complete CT scanner.

Gantry assembly

The gantry assembly includes the x-ray tube, the detector array, the high-voltage generator, the patient support and positioning couch, and the mechanical support for each. These subsystems receive electronic commands from the operating console and transmit data to the computer for image production and analysis.

X-ray tube. X-ray tubes employed in CT scanning have special requirements. Although some operate at relatively low tube current (less than 100 mA), for many the instantaneous power capacity must be high. The anode heating capacity must be at least 500,000 HU, and some tubes designed specifically for CT have 1.5 million HU capacity. High-speed rotors are employed in most for best heat dissipation. Experience to date has shown that x-ray tube failure is a principal cause of scanner malfunction and the principal limitation on sequential scanning frequency.

Focal spot size is relatively unimportant in most designs, since the scanner is not based on principles of direct geometric imaging. Nevertheless, CT scanners designed for high spatial resolution imaging incorporate x-ray tubes with a small focal spot.

X-ray tubes are energized differently depending on the scanner design. For translate-rotate units the x-ray beam is "on" only during the translate portion. Tube currents up to 50 mA are employed in this mode. Rotate-only scanners operate with either a continuous or a pulsed beam. Continuous x-ray beams at tube currents up to 100 mA are produced during the entire rotation. Pulsed units produce x-ray beams at tube currents approaching 1000 mA with pulse widths from 1 to 5 ms at pulse repetition rates of 60 Hz.

Detector assembly. Early CT scanners employed one detector. Contemporary scanners use multiple detectors in an array from 10 to 2000 in two general classifications—scintillation and gas detectors.

Scintillation detectors. Early scintillation detector arrays contained crystal–photomultiplier tube assemblies, as described in Chapter 30. These detectors could not be packed very tightly together, and they required a power supply for each photomultiplier tube. Consequently, they have been replaced by crystal-photodiode assemblies. Photodiodes are smaller, cheaper, do not require a power supply, and are equally efficient as a CT radiation detector.

Sodium iodide (NaI) was the crystal used in the earliest scanners. This was quickly replaced by bismuth germanate ($Bi_4Ge_3O_{12}$ or BGO). Cesium iodide (CsI) and cadmium tungstate ($CdWO_4$) are the current crystals of choice.

The spacing of these detectors varies from one design to another, but generally one to four detectors per centimeter or one to three detectors per degree are available. The concentration of scintillation detectors is an important characteristic of a CT scanner that affects the spatial resolution of the system.

Scintillation detectors have relatively high intrinsic detection efficiency. Approximately 90% of the x rays incident on the detector will be absorbed and contribute to the output signal. Unfortunately, it is not possible to pack the detectors so that the space between them is small enough. The detector interspace may occupy 50% of the total area intercepting the x-ray beam. Consequently, the overall detection efficiency is only about 45%. Approximately 55% of the remnant x-rays exiting on the patient will contribute to patient dose without contributing to the image. This is diagramed in Fig. 22-13, which shows a comparison between the scintillation detector array and the gas detector array.

Gas detectors. Gas-filled detectors are also used in CT scanners (Fig. 22-14). They are constructed of a large metallic chamber with baffles spaced only at approximately 1 mm intervals. The baffles are like grid strips and divide the large chamber into many small chambers. Each small chamber functions as a separate radiation detector. The entire detector array is hermetically sealed and filled under pressure with a high atomic number inert gas such as xenon or a xenon-krypton mixture. Ionization of the gas in each chamber is proportional to the radiation incident on the chamber and is detected in much the the same way as the **ideal gas-filled detector** described in Chapter 30.

The intrinsic detection efficiency in such an assembly is only about 45%; however, the detector interspace can be reduced so small that very little of the face area of the detector assembly is not used. Consequently, the overall total detection efficiency is approximately 45%, similar to that for the scintillation detector array. All other characteristics being equal, therefore, patient dose is about the same for both types of detector arrays.

Cost. The crystal detector assembly is considerably more costly than the gas detector because of the associated electronics. However, the output signal is much higher from the crystal detector than from the gas-filled detector and therefore requires less amplification before processing.

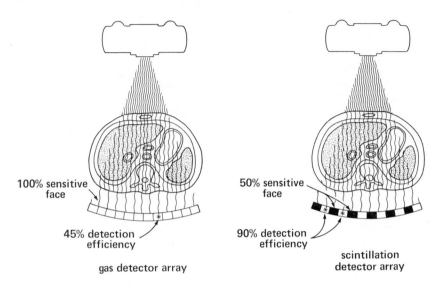

Fig. 22-13. Overall detection efficiency of a scintillation detector array is approximately equal to that of the gas detector array.

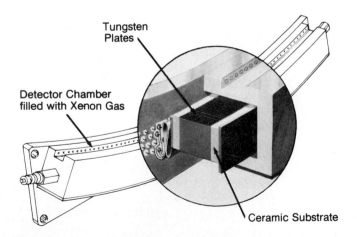

Fig. 22-14. Gas-filled detector array features small detectors in high concentration with little interdetector dead space. (Courtesy General Electric Co.)

The gas-filled detector array can be made with concentrations up to nine detectors per centimeter or seventeen detectors per degree.

Collimation

Collimation is required during CT scanning for precisely the same reasons that it is required in conventional radiography. Proper collimation reduces patient dose by restricting the volume of tissue irradiated. It also enhances image quality by limiting the volume of tissue available to generate scatter radiation. In conventional radiography there is only one collimator, that which is mounted on the tube housing. In CT scanning there are two collimators (Fig. 22-15). One is mounted on the tube housing or adjacent to it. This collimator limits the area of the patient that intercepts the useful beam and thereby determines the slice thickness and patient dose. This **prepatient collimator** usually consists of several sections so that a nearly parallel x-ray beam results. **Improperly adjusted prepatient collimators result in most of the unnecessary radiation dose during a CT scan.**

The **postpatient** or **predetector collimator** restricts the x-ray field viewed by the detector array. This collimator reduces the scatter radiation incident on the detector and, when properly coupled with the prepatient collimator, helps define the slice thickness.

High-voltage generator. All CT scanners operate on three-phase power. This accommodates the higher x-ray tube rotor speeds and the instantaneous power surges characteristic of pulsed systems. In other ways the generator is rather conventional. Some manufacturers conserve space by building the generator into the gantry or even by mounting the generator on the rotating wheel of the gantry so that winding and unwinding a power cable is unnecessary.

Patient positioning and support couch. The patient couch is one of the more important components of the CT scanner. In addition to supporting the patient comfortably, it must be constructed of low-Z material so that it does not interfere with x-ray beam transmission and patient imaging. Newer couches are fabricated from carbon fiber material that is low Z, very thin, yet adequately strong. It should be smoothly and accurately motor driven so that precise patient positioning is possible. It should be capable of automatic indexing so that the operator does not have to enter the room between each scan. Such a feature reduces the examination time required for each patient. Some units have been designed with fixed patient support couches. With these units the gantry indexes between scans.

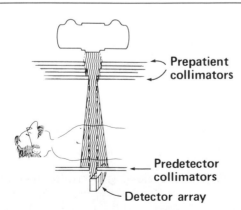

Fig. 22-15. CT scanners incorporate both prepatient collimators and predetector collimators.

Prepatient collimators

Predetector collimators

Detector array

Computer

The computer is a unique subsystem of the CT scanner. All other components are basically conventional in design and application. CT scanning would not be possible were it not for the high-speed digital computer. Depending on the image format, as many as 30,000 equations must be solved simultaneously; thus a rather large-capacity computer is required. Computer costs can easily run to one third the cost of the entire CT scan system, although such costs continue to be reduced substantially because of improving computer technology.

Computers require a special and controlled environment; consequently, each CT scan facility must have an adjacent room dedicated to the computer. In the computer room, humidity must be maintained at less than 30% relative, and temperatures must be maintained below 20° C. Higher temperatures and humidity can contribute to computer failure.

At the heart of the computer used in CT are the microprocessor and primary memory. These determine the time between the end of a scan and the appearance of an image, the **reconstruction time.** Reconstruction times up to 30 s are encountered in CT scanning. The efficiency of an examination is greatly influenced by reconstruction time, especially when a large number of slices are involved.

A few CT scanners use an **array processor** instead of a microprocessor for image reconstruction. The array processor has the reconstruction algorithm permanently wired in its memory and does many calculations simultaneously. It is significantly faster than the microprocessor, and an image is reconstructed in less than 1 s. However, any change in the algorithm requires a hardware change rather than simply reading in another program.

Control console

Many CT scanners are equipped with two consoles, one for the technologist to operate the unit and one for the physician to view the image and manipulate its contrast, size, and general visual appearance. The operator's console contains meters and controls for selecting proper radiographic technique factors, for proper mechanical movement of the gantry and patient couch, and for computer commands allowing image reconstruction and transfer. The physician's viewing console accepts the reconstructed image from the operator's console and displays it for viewing and diagnosis.

Operator's console. A typical operator's console is shown in Fig. 22-16. Controls and monitors for kVp and mA are provided. Operation is generally in excess of 100 kVp. The usual mA station will be 20 to 50 mA if the x-ray beam is continuous and several hundred mA if it is a pulsed beam. The length of time required per scan (**scan time**) is often selectable and varies from 1 to 10 s with the fastest scanners.

The thickness of the tissue slice to be imaged can also often be adjusted. Nominal thicknesses are 5 to 10 mm, but some units provide slice thicknesses as small as 1 mm for high-resolution scanning. Selection of slice thickness from the console is accomplished by automatic collimator adjustment. Controls will also be provided for automatic movement and indexing of the patient support couch. This allows the operator to program for contiguous slices or for intermittent slice images.

The operating console will have one and sometimes two television monitors. One is provided for the operator to indicate patient data on the scan (hospital identification, name, patient number, age, sex, etc.) and to provide identification for each scan (scan number, technique, couch position, etc.). A second monitor may be provided for the operator to view the resulting image before transferring it either to hard copy or to the physician's viewing console.

Physician's viewing console. Smaller, less expensive CT systems may not have a physician's viewing console. However, if the work

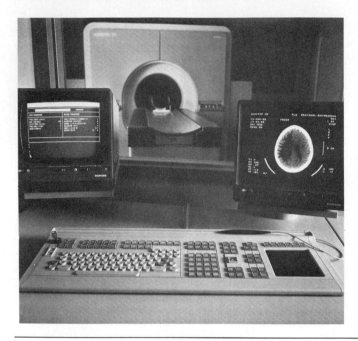

Fig. 22-16. Operator's console for a CT scanner showing the various control functions. (Courtesy Siemens Medical Systems, Inc.)

load is high and the system fully utilized, a physician's viewing console is absolutely essential so that patient scans can be reviewed and reported without interfering with scanner operations. For maximum effectiveness the physician's viewing console should be supported by an independent computer. If it requires the main computer for image manipulation, viewing can be slowed considerably when attempted during scanning, since the scan mode has precedence.

This console allows the physician to call any previous image and manipulate that image for maximum information. The manipulative controls provide for contrast and brightness adjustments, magnification techniques, region of interest viewing, and use of on-line computer software packages. This software may include computer programs to generate CT number histograms along any preselected axis, computation of mean and standard deviation of CT values within a region of interest, subtraction techniques, and planar and volumetric analysis. Reconstruction of images along coronal, sagittal, and oblique planes is also possible.

Image format. There are a number of useful image formats. Current scanners store image data on either **floppy disks** or **magnetic tapes.** If the floppy disk format is used, data from a single patient are transferred to a single disk that can be stored in a jacket with other patient reports and films. If magnetic tape storage is employed, data from many patients can be transferred to a single tape. Each tape will generally accommodate 150 scans or five to ten patients.

CT scan images are usually recorded on film in a multiformat or laser camera for later viewing and filing. Typical cameras employ 8 × 10 inch films and can provide one, two, four, or six images to a film. Naturally, the more images per film, the smaller the image. Some cameras use 14 × 17 inch film and therefore provide a larger image format.

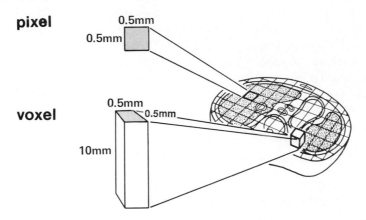

Fig. 22-17. Each cell in a CT image matrix is a two-dimensional representation (pixel) of a volume of tissue (voxel).

The weakest link in image storage using a multiformat camera can be the video monitor from which the image is photographed. For quality images a high-resolution monitor should be used.

IMAGE CHARACTERISTICS

The image obtained in CT scanning is unlike that obtained in conventional radiography. In radiography, x rays form an image directly on the radiation detector—the film. With CT scanners the x rays form a stored electronic image that is displayed as a matrix of intensities.

Image matrix

The CT scan image format consists of imaginary cells, each assigned a number and displayed as a density or brightness level on the video monitor. The original EMI format consisted of an 80×80 matrix, for a total of 6400 individual cells of information. Fourth-generation scanners provide matrices up to 512×512, resulting in 262,144 cells of information.

Each imaginary cell of information is a **pixel,** and the numeric information contained in each pixel is a CT number, or **Hounsfield unit.** The pixel is a two-dimensional representation of a corresponding tissue volume (Fig. 22-17). The tissue volume is known as a **voxel** (volume element), and it is determined by the product of the pixel size and the thickness of the CT scan slice. The larger the scan diameter, the larger will be each pixel for a given matrix size. On the other hand, the larger the reconstruction matrix, the smaller will be each pixel.

EXAMPLE: Compute the pixel size for the following characteristics of a CT scanner used for brain scans:
a. Scan and reconstruction diameter 20 cm, 120×120 matrix
b. Scan and reconstruction diameter 20 cm, 512×512 matrix
c. Scan and reconstruction diameter 36 cm, 512×512 matrix

ANSWER:

a. $\dfrac{120}{20} = 6$ pixels/cm or 1.7 mm/pixel

b. $\dfrac{512}{20} = 25.6$ pixels/cm or 0.4 mm/pixel

c. $\dfrac{512}{36} = 14.2$ pixels/cm or 0.7 mm/pixel

CT numbers

Each pixel will be displayed on the video monitor as a level of brightness and on the photographic image as a level of optical density. These levels correspond to a range of numbers from −1000 to +1000 for each pixel. A CT number of −1000 corresponds to air; a CT number of +1000 corresponds to dense bone. A pixel value of zero indicates water. Table 22-1 shows the CT values for various tissues of importance along with respective linear attenuation coefficients.

The precise CT number of any given pixel is related to the x-ray attenuation coefficient of the tissue contained in the voxel. As discussed in Chapter 9, the degree of x-ray attenuation is determined by the average energy of the x-ray beam and the effective atomic number of the absorber and is expressed by the attenuation coefficient.

The equation for determining the value of a CT number is

(22-1)

$$CT\ number = k\ \frac{\mu_o - \mu_w}{\mu_w}$$

where μ_o is the attenuation coefficient of the pixel under analysis, μ_w is the attenuation coefficient of water, and k is a constant that determines the scale factor for the range of CT numbers. This equation shows that the CT number for water is always zero. For the scanner to operate with precision, detector response must continuously be calibrated so that water is always represented by zero.

Obviously there is an enormous amount of information that is wasted when the actual dynamic range of the image is 2000 but is displayed on a video screen or film at no more than thirty-two shades of gray.

IMAGE QUALITY

The image quality of conventional radiographs is expressed in terms of resolution, noise, and speed. These characteristics are relatively easy to describe but somewhat difficult to measure and express quantitatively. Since CT images are composed of discrete pixel values that are then converted to film format, image quality is somewhat easier to characterize and to quantitate. There are a number of methods available for measuring CT image quality and four principal characteristics that are numerically assigned. These are spatial resolution, contrast resolution, linearity, and noise.

Table 22-1. CT number for various tissues and x-ray attenuation coefficients (cm⁻¹) at three operating kVp's

Tissue	CT number	Linear attenuation coefficient (cm⁻¹)		
		60 keV	84 keV	122 keV
Air	−1000	0.0004	0.0003	0.0002
Fat	−100	0.185	0.162	0.144
Water	0	0.206	0.180	0.160
Cerebrospinal fluid	15	0.207	0.181	0.160
White matter	46	0.213	0.187	0.166
Gray matter	43	0.212	0.184	0.163
Blood	40	0.208	0.182	0.163
Dense bone	1000	0.528	0.460	0.410

Spatial resolution

If one scans a regular geometric structure that has a sharp interface, as in Fig. 22-18, the image at the interface will be somewhat blurred. The degree of blurring is a measure of the spatial or high-contrast resolution of the system and is controlled by a number of factors. Since the image of the interface is a visual rendition of pixel values, one could analyze these values across the interface to arrive at a measure of spatial resolution.

Suppose the object organ in Fig. 22-18 were composed of material of a relatively high CT value (for examaple, 100) and that it was immersed in water, which has a CT number of zero. This would be a relatively high-contrast interface. The CT numbers across the interface might have actual values such as those shown in the object graph in Fig. 22-18. However, since the image is somewhat unsharp because of limitations of the CT scanner, the expected sharp edge of CT values is replaced with a smoothed range of CT values across the interface. This smoothing represents poor spatial resolution and results from several features of the CT scanner. The larger the pixel size and the lower the subject contrast, the poorer will be the spatial resolution. The design of the prepatient and predetector collimation will affect the level of scatter radiation and influence spatial resolution by affecting the contrast of the system.

The ability of the CT system to reproduce with accuracy a high-contrast edge is expressed mathematically as the **edge response function (ERF)**. The measured edge response function can be transformed into another mathematic expression called the **modulation transfer function (MTF)**. The MTF and its graphic representation are most often cited to express the spatial resolution of a CT system.

Although the MTF is a rather complicated mathematic formulation, its meaning is not too

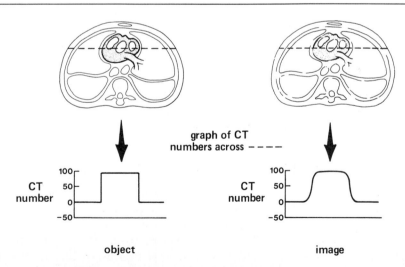

Fig. 22-18. A CT scan of an object organ with distinct borders such as the heart will result in an image with somewhat blurred borders. The actual CT number profile of the object would be abrupt, whereas that of the image would be smoothed.

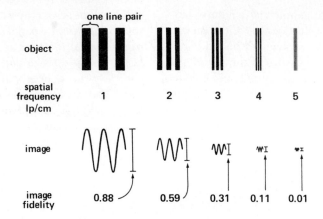

Fig. 22-19. As one images a bar pattern of increasing spatial frequency, the fidelity of the image decreases. The tracing of density across the image reveals the loss of fidelity.

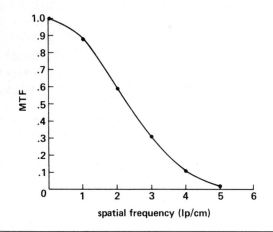

Fig. 22-20. Modulation transfer function is a plot of the image fidelity vs. spatial frequency. The six data points plotted here are from the analysis of Fig. 22-19.

difficult to represent. Consider, for instance, a series of bar patterns (Fig. 22-19) that are imaged by a CT scanner. One bar and its equal width interspace are called a **line pair (lp)**. The number of line pairs per unit length is called the **spatial frequency,** and for CT scanners it is expressed in line pairs per centimeter. A low spatial frequency represents large objects and a high spatial frequency small objects.

The image obtained from the low-frequency bar pattern will appear more like the object than the image from the high-frequency pattern. The loss in faithful reproduction with increasing spatial frequency occurs because of a number of deficiencies in the imaging system. CT scanner characteristics that contribute to such image degradation are collimation, detector size and concentration, mechanical-electrical gantry control, and the reconstruction algorithm. In simplistic terms the MTF is the ratio of the image to the object. If the image faithfully reproduced the object, the MTF of the system would have

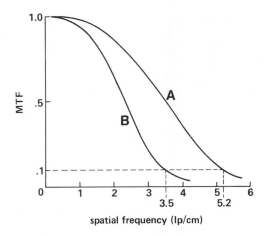

Fig. 22-21. MTF curves for two representative CT scanners are shown. Scanner *A* will produce higher resolution images than scanner *B*.

a value of 1. If the image were simply blank and contained no information whatsoever about the object, the system MTF would be equal to zero. Intermediate levels of fidelity result in intermediate MTF values. In Fig. 22-19 image fidelity is measured by the optical density along the axis of the image. At a spatial frequency of 1 lp/cm, for instance, the variation in optical density of the image is 0.88 that of the object. At 4 lp/cm it is only 0.1, or 10% that of the image. A graph of this ratio of image to object at each spatial frequency results in an MTF curve as shown in Fig. 22-20.

Fig. 22-21 shows the MTF for two different CT scanners and illustrates how one should interpret such a curve. An MTF curve that extends farther to the right indicates higher spatial resolution, which means the imaging system is better able to reproduce very small objects. Obviously this is a complex relationship, since it relates the imaging capacity of the system for various sized objects. Most CT scanners are judged by the spatial frequency at an MTF equal to 0.1, sometimes called the **limiting resolution.** As shown in Fig. 22-21, scanner A has a 0.1 MTF at 5.2 lp/cm, whereas B can only manage 3.5 lp/cm. Therefore A has higher spatial resolution

than *B*. The absolute object size that can be resolved by a scanner is equal to the reciprocal of the spatial frequency.

EXAMPLE: A CT scanner is said to be capable of resolution 5 lp/cm. What size object does this represent?

ANSWER: The reciprocal of 5 lp/cm $= (5 \text{ lp/cm})^{-1}$

$$= \frac{1}{5 \text{ lp/cm}}$$

$$= \frac{1 \text{ cm}}{5 \text{ lp}}$$

$$\frac{1 \text{ cm}}{5 \text{ lp}} = \frac{2 \text{ mm}}{\text{lp}}$$

Since a line pair consists of a strip and interspace of equal width, 2 mm/lp represents objects separated by a 1 mm interspace. The system resolution is therefore 1 mm.

Although CT scan resolution is most often expressed by the spatial frequency of the limiting resolution, it is easier to think in terms of the object size that can be reproduced. Fig. 22-22 illustrates the relationship between spatial frequency and object size. Currently, the best CT scanners have a limiting resolution of approximately 15 lp/cm, which corresponds to an object size of 0.3 mm.

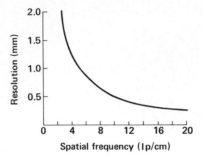

Fig. 22-22. Increasing spatial frequency means better resolution of smaller objects.

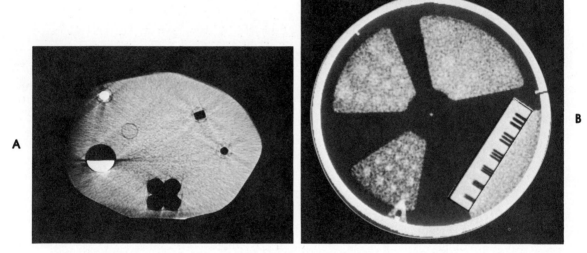

Fig. 22-23. A, This anthropomorphic phantom for evaluating CT scan image quality contains objects simulating a barium-filled stomach, intestinal folds, a rib, and airways. **B,** This phantom is designed to measure both low-contrast resolution and high-contrast resolution. (Courtesy Edwin C. McCullough, Ph.D., Mayo Clinic, Rochester, Minn.)

Specially designed phantoms are necessary for evaluating CT scanner performance. Such phantoms are usually fabricated from different density plastic in various shapes and configurations. The important measures of scanner performance that can be evaluated with phantoms are artifact generation, low-contrast resolution, and high-contrast resolution. Fig. 22-23, *A*, shows an anthropomorphic phantom designed to test the body mode of a CT scanner for generation of artifacts. Fig. 22-23, *B*, shows a specially designed phantom containing an array of low-contrast holes and high-contrast bars to test both low- and high-contrast resolution with a single scan.

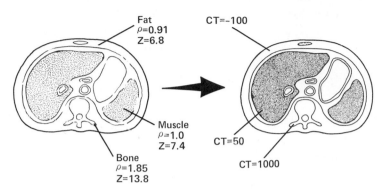

Fig. 22-24. There are not many differences in density and effective atomic number among tissues, but the differences are greatly amplified by the CT scanner. This results in exceptional low-contrast resolution.

Low-contrast resolution

The ability to distinguish material of one composition from another without regard for size or shape is called **low-contrast resolution.** This is an area in which the CT scanner excels. The absorption of x rays in tissue is characterized by the linear attenuation coefficient. This coefficient, as we have seen, is a function of photon energy and the atomic number of the irradiated tissue. In CT scanning the amount of radiation penetrating the patient is determined also by the density of the body part.

Consider the situation outlined in Fig. 22-24, a fat-muscle-bone structure. Not only are the atomic numbers somewhat different (Z = 6.8, 7.4, and 13.8, respectively), but the mass densities also are different (ρ = 0.91, 1.0, and 1.85). These differences are measurable but displayed minimally in conventional radiography. The CT scanner is able to amplify these differences in subject contrast so that the image contrast is high. On computer reconstruction the range of CT numbers will be approximately − 100, 50, and 1000, respectively. This amplified contrast scale allows the CT scanner to better resolve adjacent structures that are similar in composition.

The low-contrast resolution provided by CT scanners is considerably better than that available in conventional radiography. The ability to image low-contrast objects with a CT scanner is limited by the size and uniformity of the object and by the **noise of the system.**

System noise

If a homogenous medium such as water is scanned, each pixel should have a value of zero. Of course, this never occurs because the low-contrast resolution of the system is not perfect; therefore the CT numbers may average zero, but a range of values greater than or less than zero will exist. This variation in CT number about an average value is the **noise** of the system. If all pixel values were the same, system noise would be zero. The greater the variation of pixel values, the higher will be the system noise.

Noise is defined as percent standard deviation of a large number of pixels obtained from a water bath scan. It should be clearly understood that system noise depends on many factors of operations: (1) kVp and filtration, (2) pixel size, (3) slice thickness, (4) detector efficiency, and (5) patient dose. Ultimately it is patient dose, the number of x rays used by the detector to produce the image, that controls noise. System noise is defined as

(22-2)

$$Noise = \sqrt{\frac{\Sigma(x_i - \bar{x})^2}{n - 1}}$$

where x_i is each CT value, $\bar{x}$ is the average of at least twenty-five values, and n is the number of CT values averaged. In statistics noise is called a **standard deviation.**

Noise is manifested on the final image by apparent graininess. Low-noise systems appear very smooth in optical density rendition, and high-noise systems appear spotty or blotchy. **The resolution of low-contrast objects is limited by the noise of a CT scanner.**

System noise should be evaluated daily. This is done by scanning a 20 cm diameter water bath for a head scanner or a 40 cm diameter water bath for a body scanner. Most scanners have the ability to identify a region of interest and compute the mean and standard deviation of CT numbers in that region. When the technologist is monitoring for noise, the region of noise must encompass at least 100 pixels. Such noise measurements should include five determinations—four on the periphery and one in the center to monitor the spatial uniformity.

Linearity

The CT scanner must be frequently calibrated so that water is consistently represented by CT number zero and other tissues by their appropriate CT value. A check calibration that can be made daily requires scanning material of known CT numbers such as the American Association of Physicists in Medicine (AAPM) five-pin performance phantom shown in photograph and image form in Fig. 22-25. The five pins are each made of a different plastic material with known physical and x-ray absorption properties, as shown in Table 22-2. Following a scan of this phantom, the CT number for each pin would be recorded and its mean value and standard deviation would be plotted (Fig. 22-26). The plot of CT number vs. linear attenuation coefficient should be a straight line passing through CT number zero for water. A deviation from **linearity** is an indication of misalignment or malfunction of the scanner. A minor deviation would result in in-

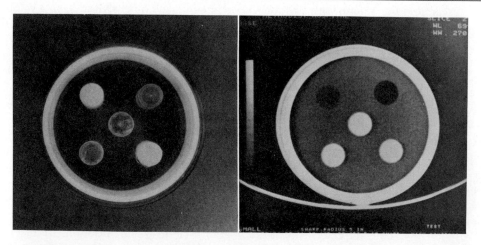

Fig. 22-25. Photograph *(left)* and CT image *(right)* of the five-pin test phantom designed by the American Association of Physicists in Medicine. The attenuation coefficient for each pin is known precisely and the CT number computed.

accurate CT number generation but would prob-ably not significantly affect the visual image.

Spatial uniformity

When one images a uniform object such as a water bath with a CT scanner, each pixel should have the same value, since each pixel represents precisely the same object composition. Fur-thermore, if the CT scanner is properly adjust-ed, that value should be zero. However, since the CT scanner is an extremely complicated electronic-mechanical device, such precision is not consistently possible. CT values for water may drift from day to day, even from hour to hour. At any time a water bath is scanned, the pixel values should be constant in all regions of the reconstructed image. Such a characteristic is called **spatial uniformity.** Testing for spatial uniformity can be done easily with those scan-ners equipped with a software package that al-lows the plotting of CT numbers along any axis of the scan as a histogram or as a line graph. If all the values of the histogram or line graph are within two standard deviations of the mean value

Table 22-2. Characteristics of the five-pin AAPM phantom

Material		Density (g/cm³)	Linear attenuation coefficient (cm⁻¹) at 60 keV	Approximate CT number
Polyethylene	C_2H_4	0.94	0.185	− 85
Polystyrene	C_8H_8	1.05	0.196	− 10
Nylon	$C_6H_{11}NO$	1.15	0.222	100
Lexan	$C_{16}H_{14}O$	1.20	0.223	115
Plexiglas	$C_5H_8O_2$	1.19	0.229	130
Water	H_2O	1.00	0.206	0

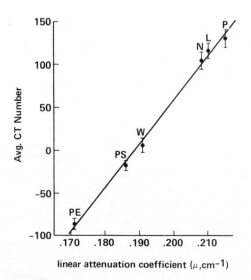

Fig. 22-26. Contrast linearity is acceptable if a graph of average CT number vs. the linear attenuation coefficient is a straight line.

Table 22-3. Frequency of quality-assurance measurements for CT scanners

Device	Measurements	Measurement interval
Water bath	Noise; spatial uniformity	Daily
Five-pin insert	Linearity	Monthly
Edge, wire, or hole array	Spatial resolution	Monthly
Ramp	Slice thickness	Monthly
Dosimeter	Dose	Monthly
Miscellaneous	Table incrementing; light localizer; collimation	Monthly

$(\pm 2\sigma)$, the system is said to exhibit acceptable spatial uniformity. Because of x-ray beam hardening or reconstruction inadequacies, there may be either cupping of CT numbers in the middle of the scan field or a falloff at the periphery.

QUALITY ASSURANCE

CT scanners are subject to all the misalignment, miscalibration, and malfunctioning difficulties of a conventional x-ray unit, and more. They have the additional complexities of the multimotional gantry, the interactive console, and the associated computer. Each of these subsystems allows more possibilities for drift and instability, resulting in degradation of image quality. For that reason a dedicated quality-assurance program is essential for each CT scanner. Such a program includes daily, weekly, monthly, and annual measurements and observations in addition to the ongoing preventive maintenance program.

Table 22-3 identifies the measurements and their required frequency for an adequate CT scanner quality-assurance program. The measurements specified for annual performance measurements should also be conducted on all new equipment and on all existing equipment following replacement or repair of a major component. In addition to the items identified in Table 22-3, an accurate log should be maintained showing the workload (number of patients, number of scans), maintenance activity, down time, and sample data from the daily quality-assurance measurements.

REVIEW QUESTIONS

1. Define or otherwise identify the following:
   a. Algorithm
   b. Transaxial
   c. Bismuth germanate
   d. Intrinsic detection efficiency
   e. Prepatient collimation
   f. Spatial frequency
   g. Hounsfield unit
   h. Image matrix
   i. MTF
   j. Noise
2. A second-generation CT scanner makes eight rotate-translate motions totaling 180 degrees in 16 s. How many degrees rotation between translations is this?
3. Discuss the characteristic design features of the four generations of CT scanners.
4. A fourth-generation CT scanner has 720 detectors and a 30-degree fan beam. How many detectors will be in the beam at any given time?
5. What is the voxel size of a CT head scanner with a 320 × 320 matrix size, a 20 cm reconstruction diameter, and a 0.5 cm slice thickness?
6. A bar- or grid-type test pattern has a spatial frequency of 8 lp/cm. What is the width of one bar?
7. A CT scanner is said to be capable of imaging 12 lp/cm. What is the size of such an object?

23

Physical principles of magnetic resonance imaging

WHY MRI?
FUNDAMENTAL CONCEPTS
NMR PARAMETERS
IMAGING PRINCIPLES

In the early 1970s, when computed tomography (CT) was beginning to make a significant impact in diagnostic radiology, another imaging modality based on **nuclear magnetic resonance (NMR)** spectroscopy was being investigated. **Magnetic resonance imaging (MRI),** as it is now called, is frequently employed in the clinical arena, and its potential impact on medicine apparently may be even greater than that of CT or ultrasound.

MRI is an extension of NMR techniques long employed in chemistry and physics that do not involve imaging. In the mid-1940s two different research groups under Felix Bloch and Edward Purcell were simultaneously investigating how the nuclei of materials behave in a magnetic field. They discovered that these nuclei will absorb radio waves at certain distinct frequencies. An analysis of the peaks in such a frequency spectrum yields information on the structure and motion of the individual molecules. Indeed,

NMR spectroscopy is widely used today in chemistry to obtain detailed information about complex molecules and in physics to study molecular motion. In 1952 Bloch and Purcell shared the Nobel Prize in physics for their investigations.

As it became apparent that NMR techniques were sensitive to the dynamics of chemical change, various investigators became increasingly interested in making measurements in living tissues. This interest was further spurred by investigations on excised rat tissue by Raymond Damadian. In 1971 he reported that there were significant differences in NMR parameters between normal rat tissues and several types of tumors. In 1973 Paul Lauterbur published a cross-sectional NMR image of two water-filled capillary tubes obtained with a modified NMR spectrometer. That was the first NMR image. Damadian obtained the first animal images in 1975. Many other imaging schemes using NMR were also investigated by Peter Mansfield, Waldo Henshaw, and others.

By the late 1970s MRI was progressing rapidly. The first human head scans were obtained in 1978, followed shortly thereafter by the first human body scans. Today, clinical MRI is established as an exceedingly excellent imaging modality.

Because the terms and quantities of MRI are so new to radiology, the following brief glossary (with the units of measure in boldface following each term) can be referred to while progressing through this and the following chapter:

Glossary of terms and quantities in MRI

Free induction decay (FID): The signal emitted by tissue after an RF pulse has excited the nuclear spins of that tissue at resonance. (**MHz**)

Gradient magnetic field: A change in the intensity of a magnetic field in space. If the change is smooth and proportional, it is called a linear gradient magnetic field. (**mT/cm**)

Gyromagnetic ratio: A constant, specific ratio for each nucleus, relating the precessional frequency in a magnetic field. (**MHz/T**)

Larmor frequency: The frequency at which a nucleus precesses in a magnetic field. (**MHz**)

Magnetic moment: A force created when a magnetic dipole is in a magnetic field. (**T**)

Magnetization: The large-scale macroscopic magnetic moment resulting from many nuclear magnetic moments. (**T**)

Precession: The wobble of the rotational axis of a spinning body about a stationary axis that describes a cone.

Radio frequency (RF): Electromagnetic radiation having frequencies from 0.3 kHz to 300 GHz. MRI employs RF in the range of approximately 1 to 100 MHz.

Resonance: Transfer of vibrating energy from one system to another. (**MHz**)

Specific absorption rate (SAR): The power absorbed by tissue during RF irradiation. (**W/kg**)

Spin density (SD): The concentration of nuclei in tissue precessing at the Larmor frequency and contributing to the MRI signal.

T_1 relaxation time: The time required for the interactions between nuclear spins and the tissue lattice to return to normal following RF excitation. Also called spin-lattice or longitudinal relaxation time. (**ms**)

T_2 relaxation time: The time required for the interaction between nuclear spins and adjacent nuclear spins to return to normal following RF excitation. Also called spin-spin or transverse relaxation time. (**ms**)

Tesla (T): The SI unit of magnetic field strength. The classic unit is gauss (G). 1 T = 10,000 G.

Why MRI?

MRI has several significant advantages over other diagnostic imaging modalities:

Best low-contrast resolution

No ionizing radiation

Direct multiplanar imaging

No bone or air artifacts

Direct flow measurements

Totally noninvasive

Contrast media not required

The MR image depends not on just a single parameter such as the x-ray attenuation coefficient, but on three principal independent parameters—T_1, T_2, and spin density (SD)—plus several secondary parameters. As shown in Fig. 23-1, these MRI parameters have a considerable range of values from one tissue to another. Whereas the x-ray attenuation coefficient of soft tissues differs by no more than 1%, spin density and T_1 relaxation time of the same tissues differ by 20% to 30%. T_2 relaxation time differs by as much as 40% among the same tissues. These intrinsic differences in MRI parameters result in **superior low-contrast resolution,** which is the main advantage to MRI. This advantage is vividly illustrated in Fig. 23-2, which shows both a CT and an MR image.

MRI uses on ionizing radiation. The images are obtained using magnetic fields and radio waves, thus avoiding even the slight risk that accompanies the low radiation doses of CT and conventional x-ray examination.

The region of the body imaged in MRI is not limited by the physical geometry of the gantry as in CT; it can be controlled electronically. This

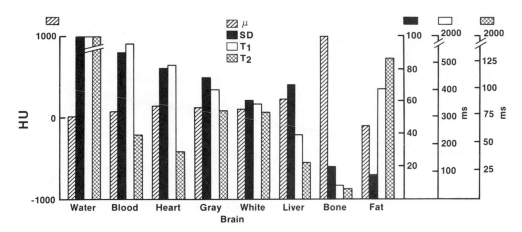

Fig. 23-1. This histogram demonstrates the very wide range of MRI parameters for soft tissues compared to the x-ray linear attenuation coefficient. The result is very good low-contrast resolution.

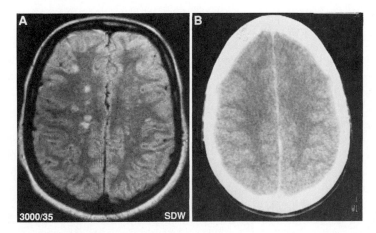

Fig. 23-2. The MR image **(A)** exhibits far superior low-contrast resolution than the CT image **(B)**.

allows direct imaging not only in axial planes, but also in true sagittal, coronal, and oblique planes. Even images of a volume of tissue can be produced without reorienting the patient. Such direct **multiplanar** imaging is a distinct advantage to MRI.

Many other less significant advantages to MRI exist. There are no bone or air artifacts as in CT. Blood flow can be imaged and quantitated. MRI is totally noninvasive. Because the low-contrast resolution is so superior, contrast media are not required.

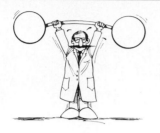

Fig. 23-3. Classic mechanics describes the motion of large objects, and quantum mechanics describes the motion of atoms and their constituents.

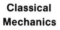

**Classical
Mechanics**

**Quantum
Mechanics**

FUNDAMENTAL CONCEPTS

In Chapter 3 it was pointed out that all fundamental particles possess certain inherent characteristics. A simple example of such a characteristic is "charge." For example, protons are positively charged and neutrons have no charge. Another less commonly known characteristic is **spin**. In simple terms, many particles can be visualized as being tiny spinning tops. Protons, neutrons, electrons, and all subatomic particles possess this property called spin. Spin is a consequence of the description of nature from the branch of physics called **quantum mechanics.** As shown in Fig. 23-3, classic mechanics describes the motion of large objects, whereas quantum mechanics describes the motion of atoms and their constituents.

Just as the sum of the charges of individual protons in a nucleus equals the total charge of the nucleus, so the individual spins of protons and neutrons also can be summed to yield the net total spin on the nucleus. Thus nuclei can also be thought of as small, positively charged spinning tops.

Magnetic moments

As was stated in the discussion of electromagnetism in Chapter 6, moving charges give rise to magnetic fields. Consequently, we might expect that something that is charged and spinning would also possess a magnetic field. This is indeed true. Consider the simplest nucleus, that of hydrogen, shown in Fig. 23-4. The charge and spin of the nucleus of hydrogen give rise to a magnetic field. Thus we must add another factor to our simple picture of the nucleus. The nucleus is a tiny spinning top with a north and south pole, just like a magnet. The nucleus is said to be a **magnetic dipole,** and the name for its inherent magnetism is **magnetic moment.**

In most materials, such as soft tissue, these little spinning magnetic nuclei are all oriented randomly. That is, if one nucleus has its spin and therefore its magnetic moment pointed up, there will be another nearby nucleus with its spin pointed down, as shown in Fig. 23-5. Other magnetic moments will be oriented in various directions. This random orientation causes all the spins and magnetic moments to cancel, so that the **net magnetization** in the patient of Fig. 23-5 is zero.

However, if the patient is placed in a strong magnetic field, as in Fig. 23-6, the magnetic dipoles will align themselves much as a compass needle aligns itself with the earth's magnetic field. Although all the magnetic dipoles are illustrated as being aligned in the same direction with the external magnetic field, they are not. This is simplification. Only about one in a million is so aligned, and nearly as many align against the field as with it. This situation can only be explained by quantum mechanics.

The atoms in any material are in constant thermal motion, and thus the nuclei are being con-

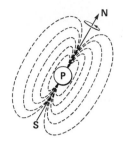

Fig. 23-4. The spinning proton of a hydrogen nucleus creates a magnetic field with a magnetic moment.

Fig. 23-5. In most materials and in all patients magnetic moments are randomly oriented. Consequently, the net magnetization is zero.

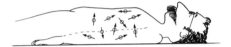

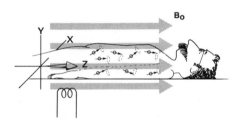

Fig. 23-6. Individual magnetic moments become aligned in the presence of an external magnetic field, creating net magnetization. By convention, the Z axis of an MR imager is horizontal.

tinually banged out of alignment. However, at any particular moment, slightly more of the nuclei will align with the field than against it, creating net magnetization of the patient. **The patient becomes a magnet.**

The strong external magnetic field is indicated by B_0. By convention, the B_0 field in most imagers is assigned the Z axis in space. This allows the B_0 field, the Z axis, and the long axis of the patient to be aligned.

Precession

In addition to charge, spin, and magnetic moment, each nucleus in the presence of an external magnetic field acts as a toy top or gyroscope.

Anyone who has observed a toy top spinning on a flat surface notices that the top does not just simply spin in an upright position. Rather, the axis of spin wobbles in a tiny circle. This wobble is called **precession.**

The precession of the spinning top occurs because it is influenced by the earth's gravitational field, as shown in Fig. 23-7, *A*. This is the principle of the gyroscope. If the gravitational field were increased, the frequency of precession would increase. If the top were taken aboard a space shuttle, no precession would occur.

Precession also occurs at the nuclear level, as shown in Fig. 23-7, *B*. The magnetic moment of the hydrogen nucleus does not simply align

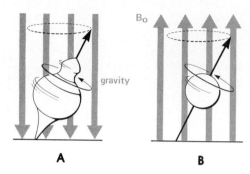

Fig. 23-7. A, A toy top precesses because of the earth's gravitational field. **B,** The hydrogen nucleus precesses in the presence of an external magnetic field, B_0.

itself with the external magnetic field, B_0, but it also wobbles about the direction of the external magnetic field lines. This magnetic precession is caused by an interaction between the external and the nuclear magnetic field.

How fast the magnetic moment precesses, that is, the **frequency of precession,** is determined solely by the strength of the external magnetic field and the type of nucleus involved. The relationship is

(23-1)

$$\omega = \gamma B_0$$

where ω is the frequency of precession in megahertz (MHz) and B_0 is the strength of the external magnetic field in tesla (T). Gamma, γ, is a constant value, called the **gyromagnetic ratio,** that is characteristic of each particular nucleus. It is to MRI as half-life is to radioactivity and has units of megahertz per tesla (MHz/T). This fundamental equation of MRI is called the **Larmor equation,** and the frequency of precession is called the **Larmor frequency.**

In summary, then, we have a simple picture of material such as a patient in a magnetic field. The magnetic moments of individual hydrogen nuclei tend to align themselves with the external

magnetic field and add together to produce a **net magnetization,** as illustrated in Fig. 23-6. The large arrow symbolizes the net magnetization of all the individual nuclear magnetic moments in the tissue. Although the individual hydrogen nuclei precess at a frequency determined by the Larmor relationship, they are **out of phase.** Therefore the net magnetic moment does not precess in such a situation and is represented by a large arrow on the $+Z$ axis.

We can now see how this property of nuclear magnetism could be useful in analyzing samples. Suppose we place a sample of unknown material in a magnet of known field strength. If we could somehow determine the frequencies of precession, then by the Larmor relationship we could calculate the gyromagnetic ratio for the nuclei in the sample. Since each type of nucleus has its own unique gyromagnetic ratio, this would then tell us which nuclei were present. The strength of each signal would indicate the relative abundance of each nuclear species.

If, in addition, we could somehow make this determination at various points in the sample, we could produce an image of the interior of the sample. This entire process hinges on our being able to somehow measure the frequencies of precession.

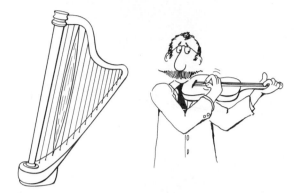

Fig. 23-8. Resonance occurs when one harmonically vibrating system interacts with another system of equal preferred frequency.

Resonance

The determination of the Larmor frequency of precession is carried out by making use of a process called **resonance.** Every physical system can be made to vibrate, and each system has a preferred frequency of vibration. This preferred frequency is the **resonant frequency.** The most efficient energy transfer between systems occurs at resonance. Fig. 23-8 shows a harp and a fiddle player. Each string of the harp is tuned by its **length and tension** to a different musical note or frequency. If the fiddler plucks a string that vibrates at the precise frequency of one of the harp strings, that harp string and no other will begin to vibrate and emit sound. **This is resonance.** Other everyday examples of resonance include radio and television transmission and reception, a child's swing, and the Tacoma Narrows Bridge (Fig. 23-9). Resonance brought the bridge down during a 1940 storm.

It turns out that, for reasonably strong magnetic fields, the frequency of precession of most nuclei of interest lies within the **radio band** of the electromagnetic spectrum. If we irradiate a patient containing precessing nuclei with a **radio frequency (RF) wave** of no specific frequency, then the chances are good that the wave will have little effect. However, if the frequency of

the RF wave exactly matches the Larmor frequency of the precessing hydrogen nuclei, then resonance will occur and, according to our simple model, the hydrogen nuclei will turn upside down, or "flip." By absorbing energy from the RF waves, the nuclei are energized and are now aligned against the external magnetic field, as shown in Fig. 23-10.

In addition to flipping the hydrogen nuclei into a higher energy state aligned against the B_0 field, another result occurs. The nuclei are caused to precess **in phase.** That is, they all precess not only at the same Larmor frequency, but also with the same orientation in space. Symbolically, the net magnetization vector is now seen to precess.

Before RF transmission the nuclei are said to be at **equilibrium** with the external magnetic field. Following RF exposure, they are **energized or excited.** The amplitude of the net magnetization vector at equilibrium is indicated as M_0. Therefore, M_0 is the **equilibrium magnetization vector,** and its amplitude is determined by several factors, including the number of nuclei present, called the **spin density (SD);** the gyromagnetic ratio, γ; and the strength of the external magnetic field, B_0. **The larger the M_0,**

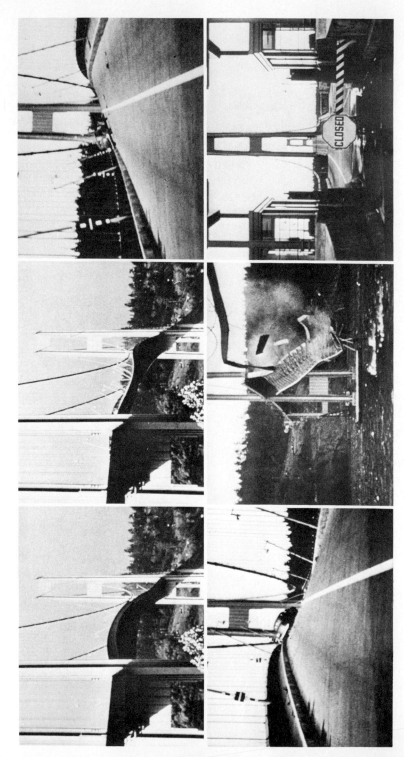

Fig. 23-9. The Tacoma Narrows Bridge was destroyed in high winds because of a resonance phenomenon. (Courtesy Civil Engineering Department, Rice University, Houston, Tex.)

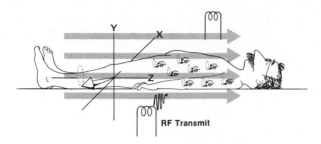

Fig. 23-10. Nuclei will absorb RF energy and flip when the RF is transmitted at the Larmor frequency.

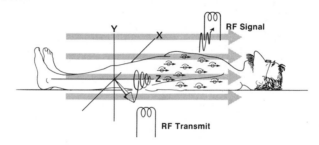

Fig. 23-11. Relaxation occurs when the nuclei return to their normal state of equilibrium after the RF is turned off.

the more intense will be the MRI signal and the brighter the MR image.

Following RF transmission, the nuclei are aligned against B_0 in an excited state, as in Fig. 23-10. If the RF was transmitted into the patient as a pulse, nuclear excitation exists only momentarily. One by one the nuclei flip and return to alignment with B_0. At the same time the **phase coherence** that was produced by the RF pulse fades. This complex manner of returning to equilibrium is called **relaxation,** and the time required for return is the **relaxation time.** During relaxation, an RF signal is emitted, as shown in Fig. 23-11, and this action is related to the MRI signal used to make an MR image.

NMR spectroscopy

Before proceeding to MRI, it is first necessary to include an introduction to its forerunner, NMR spectroscopy. The MRI signal emitted by the patient during relaxation is called a **free induction decay (FID),** as shown in Fig. 23-12. The FID relates signal intensity with time. If one takes this relationship and performs a rigorous mathematic exercise called a **Fourier transform,** the result is an NMR spectrum, as seen in Fig. 23-13. Fourier transformation converts the relationship of signal intensity vs. time to signal intensity vs. inverse time or frequency (Hz).

The NMR spectrum of a very simple molecule such as water (H_2O) is shown in Fig. 23-14. The

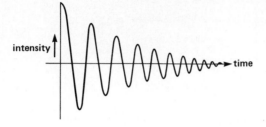

Fig. 23-12. Free induction decay (FID)
signal from hydrogen.

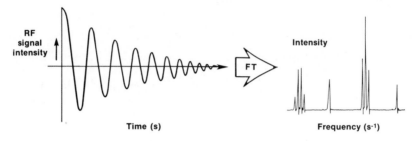

Fig. 23-13. Fourier transformation of an FID results in an NMR spectrum.

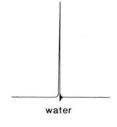

Fig. 23-14. NMR spectrum of hydrogen in water shows
a single resonance peak.

Fig. 23-15. NMR spectrum of hydrogen in methanol is
complex.

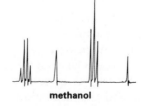

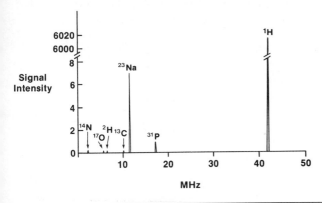

Fig. 23-16. The theoretic NMR spectrum of the body would contain resonance peaks representing various nuclei.

vertical axis is signal strength, and the horizontal axis is frequency. The single sharp peak is called a **resonance peak,** and it is centered at the Larmor frequency of precession of the hydrogen nuclei in a water molecule.

However, if we analyze hydrogen in a more complex molecule such as methanol (CH_3OH), we do not see just a single peak but several peaks, as shown in Fig. 23-15. This is because each hydrogen atom is bonded differently in the molecule. The magnetic field that each precessing hydrogen nucleus feels is mainly determined by the external magnetic field, B_0. However, this external field is minutely altered, or **perturbed,** for each nucleus by the presence of the slight magnetic fields of other nearby nuclei. This causes the resonant frequency of each nucleus to be slightly shifted with respect to that of other nuclei because of its position in the molecule. Thus, by carefully analyzing the positions of the resonant peaks in an NMR spectrum, one can deduce information about the structure of complex molecules. This field of science is termed **NMR spectroscopy,** and it is the first of many complicated steps to an MR image.

Nuclear magnetic resonance

If one takes the FID and applies a Fourier transform to it, one obtains an NMR spectrum. The details of performing Fourier transforms are not important. It is enough to know that one can

Table 23-1. Nuclear magnetic resonance properties of biologic nuclei

Nucleus	Relative abundance (%)	Relative MR imaging sensitivity	Gyromagnetic ratio (MHz/T)
^1H	99.9	1	43
^2H	0.015	91.7×10^{-3}	6.5
^{13}C	1.11	0.016	11
^{19}F	100	0.83	40
^{23}Na	100	0.093	11
^{31}P	100	6.6×10^{-2}	17
^{39}K	93.1	5.1×10^{-4}	2

produce an NMR spectrum from the analysis of the FID. Theoretically, one could sweep the patient with a broad band of RF, as in tuning a radio, and produce an NMR spectrum of many different nuclei, as shown in Fig. 23-16. Because hydrogen is so abundant and its gyromagnetic ratio so high, it has the highest sensitivity to NMR. Therefore pulsed RF at the hydrogen Larmor frequency is used for MRI.

In summary, **precessing nuclei in an external magnetic field are detected by resonance with applied radio frequency waves.** The term **nuclear magnetic resonance** thus is a good capsule description of the entire process.

A number of biologically important nuclei exhibit nuclear magnetic resonance, and they are shown in Table 23-1. For all except hydrogen, the nuclear abundance is too low or the MRI signal is too weak for imaging. Hydrogen is the most abundant element in the body; approximately 60% of all atoms are hydrogen, and most of them are in the water molecule. Although it is possible that the future may bring images with other nuclei, nearly all present attention is directed to hydrogen nuclei.

NMR PARAMETERS

The MRI signal contains information about not just a single parameter, but about three independent parameters. These are spin density, T_1, and T_2.

Spin density

Perhaps the simplest of these parameters to understand is **spin density (SD)**. As one might imagine, the strength of the signal received from the precessing nuclei is proportional to the number of nuclei within the detection volume of the MR imager. That is, if exactly the same experiment is performed on two samples, one of which has twice the number of hydrogen nuclei as the other, the signal received from this second sample is twice as large. In other words, one sample has twice the density of spinning protons as the other sample, meaning twice the number of detectable spins. **Spin density therefore is an indication of hydrogen concentration.**

T_1 relaxation time

To understand the other two parameters, T_1 and T_2, we must first take a closer look at the details of what happens to the nuclear spins when they abosrb energy from an RF pulse. When a patient is placed in a strong magnetic field, the spinning hydrogen nuclei attempt to align themselves with this field. However, thermal agitation prevents alignment of many of the nuclei. The constant bouncing of one molecule off another knocks some nuclei out of alignment. This is a continual process. As one disturbed nucleus is coming back into alignment, another somewhere nearby is being bounced out of alignment.

Thus at room temperature there is an **equilibrium** situation, and at any moment some of the nuclei are aligned and some are misaligned. It is useful to represent this equilibrium situation graphically by a large arrow pointing in the direction of the magnetic field. Since mathematicians always represent the Z axis as up, we must change our coordinate reference system and illustrate this condition, as in Fig. 23-17. Remember that the external magnetic field,

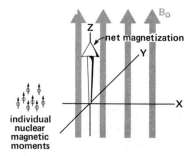

Fig. 23-17. Net magnetization of a tissue is the sum of all the nuclear magnetic moments in that tissue.

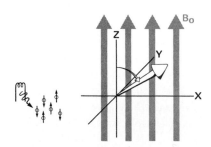

Fig. 23-18. When irradiated with an RF pulse at the Larmor frequency, the net magnetization is rotated away from the +Z axis.

B_0, is actually in a horizontal plane with the patient. The large arrow represents the **net magnetization** of the hydrogen nuclei, that is, the sum of all the scrambled up and down spins within the sample. The individual nuclei being shown in the same direction as the net magnetization is a simplification. At equilibrium this net magnetization is designated M_0.

When the sample is irradiated with a RF pulse at the Larmor frequency, some of the spins aligned with the magnetic field absorb energy from the RF wave and flip over to align against the field. This is represented by a rotation of the net magnetization away from the vertical direction, as shown in Fig. 23-18. The longer and/or stronger the RF pulse, the more spins get flipped, and therefore, the further away from vertical the net magnetization is rotated.

Indeed, it is possible to shape the pulse properly so that it rotates the net magnetization through a known angle, for example, 90 degrees onto the XY plane or even 180 degrees onto the $-Z$ axis. It is customary to name such an RF pulse after the angle through which the net magnetization is rotated. The two pulses just mentioned would be called a 90-degree pulse and a 180-degree pulse, as shown in Fig. 23-19.

What happens to the nuclear spins after ex-posure to a 90-degree RF pulse? In this case more spins than usual are misaligned and directed against the field since some have absorbed energy from the RF wave. The number that remain aligned with the field equal the number aligned against the field, so that the net magnetization along the Z axis, M_z, is zero. The spins aligned against the field will flip back into alignment with the field after the RF pulse is off, and the sample as a whole will gradually return to its normal state of equilibrium. This return to the normal state is not immediate, but occurs **exponentially with time** and is termed **relaxation.**

Another way of viewing this is illustrated in Fig. 23-20. A 90-degree pulse causes the net magnetization to be flipped down onto the XY plane. The gradual return of the nuclear spins to the normal state is represented by the rotation of the net magnetization back to its equilibrium position.

It is a property of these spinning nuclei that we receive no signal from them when they are in their equilibrium state. We only receive a signal when the net magnetization has some component lying in the xy plane. For example, consider again the net magnetization following the application of a 90-degree RF pulse. The

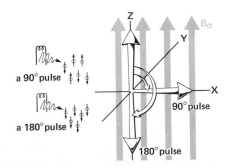

Fig. 23-19. The emitted RF pulse is usually shaped to rotate the net magnetization arrow through 90 degrees or 180 degrees.

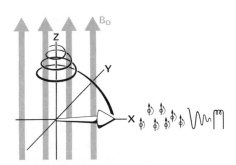

Fig. 23-20. When the RF pulse is removed, the nuclear moments gradually return to their normal equilibrium state with the emission of an RF signal.

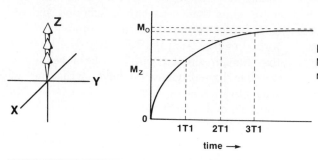

Fig. 23-21. Following an RF pulse the regrowth of M_z to M_0 is exponential in time. The time constant is the T_1 relaxation time.

strongest signal is received when it is totally in the XY plane. As the net magnetization rotates upward, the component of the net magnetization, M_{xy}, in the XY plane gets smaller, and therefore the amount of signal received becomes correspondingly less. Long before the M_z return to M_0, the MRI signal drops to zero because M_{xy} has shrunk to zero.

During return to equilibrium, two distinct, independent interactions are occurring among the hydrogen nuclei. The first is the manner in which the individual spins flip, one at a time, back to align with the B_0 field. The effect of this flipping is the regrowth of magnetization along the Z axis, M_z, to M_0, as shown in Fig. 23-21. This regrowth is exponential in time with a time constant, the T_1 relaxation time. Since T_1 relaxation is along the Z axis and B_0 field, it is sometimes called the **longitudinal relaxation time.**

The flipping of nuclear spins in a tissue is accomplished through the absorption of energy from an RF pulse. As the nuclear spins flip back to their normal position, they give up this energy to the sample as a whole. The nuclear spins are said to interact with the lattice of the tissue. T_1 thus is also called the **spin-lattice relaxation time.** T_1 is a characteristic of the tissue itself, much as half-life is unique for each radioisotope and the attenuation coefficient is unique for each x-ray absorber.

T_2 relaxation time

As one might guess, T_2 represents another type of relaxation. This type of relaxation refers to the second, independent interaction occurring among hydrogen nuclei after excitation by the RF pulse. The RF pulse causes the randomly oriented hydrogen nuclear spins to precess in phase, that is, they become **phase coherent.** Following a 90-degree RF pulse, the net magnetization is rotating at the Larmor frequency in the XY plane, as seen in Fig. 23-22. When the net magnetization is first tipped onto the XY plane, the net magnetization in each part of the tissue is pointed in precisely the same direction, namely, along the X axis. All regions of the tissue are said to be **in phase.** Within the tissue, however, individual nuclei are continually in motion. As they pass near each other, their magnetic moments interact, altering their rate of precession. With time the interactions of the slight magnetic field of one spinning nucleus alters the magnetic field of a neighbor, causing the neighbor to precess slightly faster or slower. The nuclear spins rapidly **dephase,** which causes M_{xy} to shrink while still precessing at the Larmor frequency.

This means that their sum is no longer as large as it was originally, and therefore the signal is no longer quite as strong. Indeed, if we waited a long enough time, the individual nuclear magnetic moments would gradually spread apart and

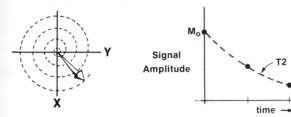

Fig. 23-22. Dephasing of spins in the XY plane results in harmonic reduction in the MRI signal to zero. This loss of M_{xy} is caused by T_2 relaxation.

be totally randomly oriented in the XY plane. The sum of all these randomly oriented arrows is zero, and thus the signal at this point is also zero. This decay of a signal because of **dephasing** of the net magnetization in the XY plane is exponential and is characterized by a decay time called the **T_2 relaxation time.** Since the decay results from passage of individual nuclear spins near each other, it is also referred to as the **spin-spin relaxation time.** It is also called the **transverse relaxation time** since it is in a plane perpendicular to B_0.

Although independent, T_1 and T_2 relaxation have an important boundary condition given by the following expression:

(23-2)

$$T_2 \leq T_1$$

T_2 relaxation times for body tissues are always less than or equal to T_1 relaxation times. T_2 relaxation times are measured in terms of tens of milliseconds, whereas T_1 relaxation times are hundreds of milliseconds. Table 23-2 presents approximate tissue relaxation times and spin densities.

MRI vs. CT

In summary, we may characterize tissue in an MR image by three NMR parameters. SD is the number of hydrogen nuclei available within the tissue voxel to contribute to the MRI signal. T_1

Table 23-2. Approximate spin density (SD) and relaxation times (T_1, T_2) for various tissues

Tissue	SD	T_1 (ms)	T_2 (ms)
Water	100	2700	2700
Skeletal muscle	79	720	55
Cardiac muscle	80	725	60
Liver	71	290	50
Fat	—	360	30
Bone	<12	<100	<10
Spleen	79	570	
Kidney	81	505	50
Gray matter	84	405	105
White matter	70	345	65

and T_2 relate to the response of the tissue after the spins have been excited by RF energy. The T_1 relaxation time characterizes the return of net magnetization along the Z axis to its normal equilibrium state and results from **spin-lattice interactions.** The T_2 relaxation time characterizes the exponential loss of signal caused by dephasing in the XY plane because of **spin-spin interactions.**

The MR image is usually the result of a mixture of these three quantities. By varying the imaging technique, we may choose to emphasize any one of these parameters in the image over the other two. Thus we may produce what are called **T_1-weighted images (T_1W)**, where the brightness of each pixel is caused primarily, but not solely, by variations in T_1. Similarly, **T_2-weighted (T_2W)** and **SD-weighted (SDW)** images may be obtained using different imaging techniques.

An MR image is determined by these three different properties of tissue. A CT image is characterized by just one, the x-ray attenuation coefficient. Therefore the MR image has better contrast for most tissues than the CT image. Furthermore, the NMR spectrum, which can be obtained during imaging, provides additional information about the biochemistry of the tissue.

The T_1 and T_2 values listed in Table 22-2 show that a fairly wide range in values exists between the various tissue types. There is also a considerable difference in values between pathologic and normal tissues. These values are only approximate since they vary from one MR imager to another.

IMAGING PRINCIPLES

Thus far we have dealt with MRI in general terms. The techniques of MR imaging are an extension of those of classic NMR spectroscopy and CT scanning. In NMR spectroscopy much effort is expended to obtain the most uniform primary magnetic field possible. The fields are typically uniform to 1 part in 10^5. The effect of any nonuniformity in the magnetic field is to broaden the lines of the NMR spectrum. If the nonuniformity is severe, the spectral lines will be broad enough to overlap one another and information may be lost.

Consider, for example, the simple situation illustrated in Fig. 23-23. This cross section of anatomy contains two voxels that are water filled. If the phantom is in a perfectly uniform magnetic field, then the resonant frequency of the water in each voxel will be precisely the same and a single sharp resonant peak will be observed.

If the magnetic field is nonuniform, however, one voxel senses a different field from that of the other voxel. The Larmor equation states that the resonant frequency of water in each voxel

will be slightly different. The total resultant signal then may appear as two close or overlapping peaks. NMR spectroscopists strive for the most uniform magnetic fields possible so as to obtain the most distinct peaks and the most detail in their spectra.

In MRI, however, we are not so much interested in obtaining spectral information as in determining from where in the sample the MRI signals are coming. Suppose we take our uniform magnetic field and on top of it superimpose a small second field, B_1, a **gradient magnetic field.** The term "gradient" refers to the uniformly changing nature of the field.

If we now image this anatomic section in this field, the spectrum will contain two distinct peaks, as shown in Fig. 23-24. This is once again due to each voxel feeling a distinctly different magnetic field and therefore possessing different resonant frequencies. Note, however, that if we know how the magnetic field varies, we can use the Larmor equation to predict how the frequency will shift, and vice versa. This means that by measuring the spacing between the peaks on our spectrum, we can calculate how far apart the two voxels are. We will have obtained information about the relative spatial positions of the water-filled voxels.

Thus, in a sense, MRI employs a technique opposite to that of classic NMR spectroscopy. In MR imaging the magnetic field is purposely made nonuniform by adding a second smaller gradient magnetic field. The NMR spectrum obtained while using a gradient field is just a projection of the spins onto a line along the direction of the gradient field.

Many techniques are possible for constructing an MR image from NMR signals. The earliest and easiest to understand is **back projection reconstruction.** First, the sample is irradiated with a shaped RF pulse designed to excite the spins in a uniform cross section of the sample. Then a gradient magnetic field is applied, and the sample is irradiated with one or more 90- or 180-degree RF pulses. The resulting FID is Fourier transformed to yield a spectrum. Since the FID

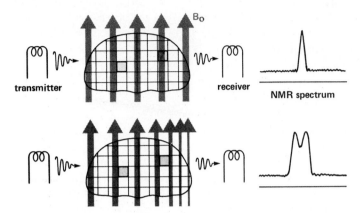

Fig. 23-23. A uniform primary magnetic field, B_0, produces a sharp NMR spectrum. A nonuniform magnetic field results in NMR spectral shifts.

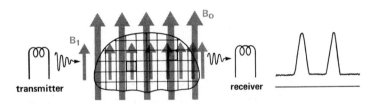

Fig. 23-24. By superimposing a gradient magnetic field, B_1, on the primary magnetic field, B_0, the position of each voxel will be indicated by the NMR spectrum.

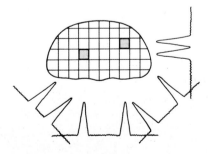

Fig. 23-25. By rotating the gradient magnetic field, multiple spectra are obtained that can be back projected to form an image.

was collected in a gradient magnetic field, the spectrum does not contain biochemical information, but rather represents a projection through the sample.

This projection is very similar to the projection data obtained in a CT scanner. Indeed, by controlling the direction of the gradient magnetic field, a series of projections at sequential angles through the patient can be collected, as seen in Fig. 23-25. We then perform a reconstruction by **back projection.**

At present, no manufacturer reconstructs images by back projection. A technique involving **two-dimensional Fourier transformation (2DFT)** is used. This requires a rigorous mathematic development that is not covered here. One may consider 2DFT to be a black box within the computer that decodes the MRI signals into images.

An MR imaging system thus is somewhat more complicated than a standard classic NMR spectrometer or a CT scanner. In addition to the large external magnet and RF transmitter and receiver used in spectroscopy, there must also be additional coils with their own separate power supplies to provide gradient magnetic fields. Additionally, a very large computer capable of reconstructing the image, as well as an image display system similar to the console screens available on CT scanners, is necessary. The basic difference between an NMR spectrometer and an MR imager is the **gradient magnetic field.**

REVIEW QUESTIONS

1. Define or otherwise identify the following:
   a. Longitudinal relaxation
   b. Larmor frequency
   c. FID
   d. Precession
   e. Spin density
   f. Tesla
   g. Felix Bloch
   h. Induction
   i. SAR
   j. Gyromagnetic ratio
2. What is the principal advantage to MR imaging? Can you name other advantages?
3. Describe what is meant by polarizing a patient; that is, creating net magnetization within the patient.
4. What is the Larmor frequency of an MR imager operated at 0.25 T? At 1.5 T?
5. What is a gradient magnetic field and why is it important to MRI?
6. What determines the brightness of a pixel in an MR image?
7. Describe the basic difference between an NMR spectrometer and an MR imager.
8. What determines the strength of the net magnetization, M_0?
9. List five nuclear species that have possible application for MRI.
10. Identify some representative values for T_1 and T_2 of several tissues.

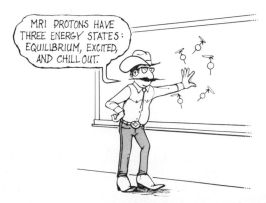

MRI PROTONS HAVE THREE ENERGY STATES: EQUILIBRIUM, EXCITED, AND CHILL OUT.

24

Magnetic resonance equipment and images

IMAGING MAGNETS
SECONDARY COILS
MR IMAGES
BIOLOGIC HAZARDS

Physically, a clinical magnetic resonance imaging (MRI) suite resembles a computed tomography (CT) scan facility. There is a large gantry-type assembly with an attached movable patient couch to transport and position the patient in the aperture of the gantry, as shown in Fig. 24-1. The MRI console, associated computer, and power supplies are usually located in separate rooms.

This resemblance to CT, however, is purely superficial. What appears to be an x-ray gantry contains not an x-ray tube and detectors but an enormous magnet, shim coils, gradient coils, and radio frequency (RF) transceiver coils. The power supply is not a high-voltage generator like that for an x-ray tube but a high-current power supply for the magnet and a precision power supply for the secondary coils.

IMAGING MAGNETS

In a clinical MR imager the patient is placed in a uniform magnetic field in the aperture of the gantry. Designing precision magnets of this size is not easy. At present the types of magnets suitable for MR imaging can be classified into three groups: permanent, resistive and superconducting. However, more than 95% of all imagers are of the superconducting variety, so this section concentrates on them.

Permanent magnets

One of the spinoffs of the large commercial ventures in home audio has been the development of relatively powerful permanent magnets. The newer materials, particularly ceramics, are inexpensive, easy to magnetize, lightweight, and capable of magnetic fields to about 0.3 tesla (T). Bricklike ceramics are assembled for use in MRI, but producing a uniform magnetic field in this fashion is difficult. However, the capital cost is much less that of the other magnets, and the operating cost is near zero.

Resistive magnet

In our discussions of electromagnetism in Chapter 6, we noted that a simple current-

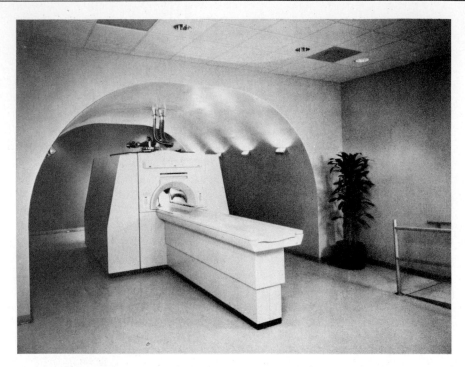

Fig. 24-1. Typical MR imager and patient positioning couch. (Courtesy Philips Medical Systems.)

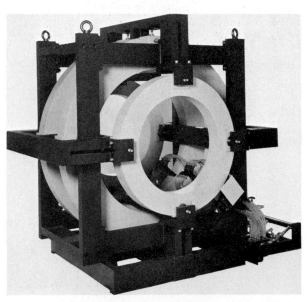

Fig. 24-2. Resistive magnet for MR imaging. (Courtesy Bruker Medical Instruments.)

carrying wire loop produces a magnetic field. By using several (usually four) large coils of roughly 1.5 m diameter, it is possible to arrange them concentrically so that the magnetic field within the coils is sufficiently uniform for MRI. Such an imaging magnet is shown in Fig. 24-2.

The design of such a multiple coil system is not as simple as it may appear. First, the coils must be both precisely manufactured and carefully positioned to meet the required field homogeneity. Second, MRI requires fairly large magnetic fields. The magnetic fields of the coils push strongly against one another, requiring that the coils be mounted in a rigid framework to minimize mechanical distortion. Third, continuous electric power on the order of tens of kilowatts (kW) is required to energize these resistive coils. The power consumption of such a magnet is equivalent to that of a large office building.

The wire used in such coils is a good conductor, but it is not a perfect conductor. Consequently these magnets have some small but finite resistance, and they are called **resistive magnets.** Even though the resistance of the wire is slight, a significant amount of heat is still produced because of the large electric current being passed through the coils. Such a magnet must be water cooled.

Superconducting magnets

Obviously it would be advantageous if one could make the coils out of some material that had no electrical resistance. Surprisingly, such a material exists. In the 1950s it was discovered that certain types of metal alloys will become perfect conductors; that is, they will have no resistance to the passage of an electric current when their temperature is dropped to approximately 10 Kelvin (K) (room temperature is 293 K). At room temperature these materials behave like other normal conductors, but at very cold, **cryogenic** temperatures they become **superconductors.**

A superconducting magnet is a magnet containing coils made from a superconducting metal alloy. An illustration of one manufactured for imaging is shown in Fig. 24-3. The superconducting magnet has certain distinct advantages over the resistive magnet. First, there is no problem of heat dissipation. Since the superconducting material possesses no resistance, none of the electrical energy is dissipated as heat. Second, since the loops of wire have no resistance, none of the energy of the electric current is ever lost. Once an electric current is started flowing in the coil, it will continue to flow indefinitely without the need for any exterior power source. Thus superconducting magnets do not require the water-cooling system or the large high-current power supply needed by resistive magnets.

The superconducting system can produce magnetic field strengths for imaging to 2 T, whereas resistive and permanent magnet systems can produce fields of only 0.3 T.

The disadvantage of a superconducting magnet lies in the difficulty of maintaining the magnet coils at near absolute zero. First, the entire coil assembly must be housed inside a giant, highly insulated bottle. This container has a smooth, shiny exterior and is much like a thermos bottle. It is called a **dewar.** Inside the dewar are two chambers. The outermost chamber is filled with liquid nitrogen, that is, nitrogen that has been cooled so much that it has condensed into a liquid. Liquid nitrogen has a temperature of 77 K, which is still not near enough to absolute zero. The liquid nitrogen layer simply acts as an intermediate buffer between the room temperature on the ouside and the interior chamber. This interior container is filled with liquid helium, which exists at 4.2 K. The superconducting coils are suspended in this bath of liquid helium. Separating these cryogenic chambers from each other and from the environment are vacuum chambers. This arrangement is shown in cross section in Fig. 24-4.

The expense associated with the maintenance of a superconducting magnet system comes from

RADIOLOGIC SCIENCE FOR
TECHNOLOGISTS: PHYSICS, BIOLOGY,
AND PROTECTION

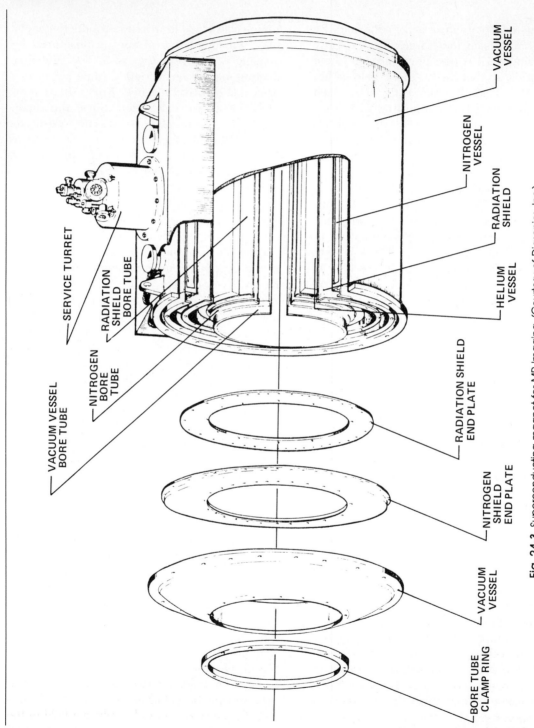

Fig. 24-3. Superconducting magnet for MR Imaging. (Courtesy of Diasonics, Inc.)

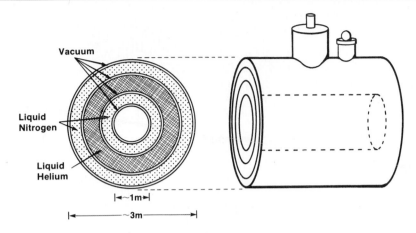

Fig. 24-4. Cross-sectional view of a superconducting magnet for imaging showing the successive insulating chambers.

Table 24-1. Advantages and disadvantages of the three main types of MRI magnets

Magnet type	Advantages	Disadvantages
Permanent	Low capital cost	Limited field strength
	Low operating cost	Fixed field strength
	Negligible fringe field	Very heavy
Resistive	Low capital cost	High power consumption
	Easy coil maintenance	Water cooling required
	Negligible fringe field	Significant fringe field
Superconductive	High field strength	High capital cost
	High field homogeneity	High cryogen cost
	Low power consumption	Intense fringe field

replenishment of the liquid nitrogen and liquid helium chambers. Despite the use of the best insulations available, the liquid helium and liquid nitrogen gradually evaporate and must be replaced periodically. Also, the handling of these **cryogenic liquids** and the filling of the chambers require some care and expertise. The recent discoveries of superconductivity at temperatures near 100 K could make the helium chamber unnecessary, greatly reducing cost.

In summary, each type of magnet system has advantages and disadvantages, as listed in Table 24-1. The permanent magnet is simplest in design and the least expensive to operate. The resistive magnet can be turned off but requires continuous power and water cooling. The superconducting system requires no continuous power source after it is up to field but may be more difficult to maintain.

SECONDARY COILS
Shim coils

A principal requirement of the imaging magnet is magnetic field homogeneity. A 1 T magnet, for instance, should produce a field in the imaging volume varying by not more than ± 50

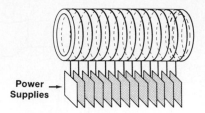

Fig. 24-5. Shim coils for improving the homogeneity of the main magnetic field.

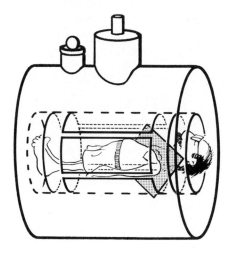

Fig. 24-6. Position of the three pairs of gradient coils is shown in relation to the patient.

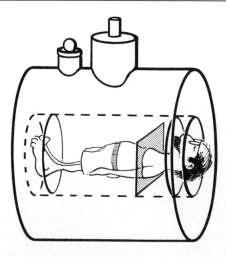

Fig. 24-7. Transaxial slice is selected for imaging by energizing the Z gradient coils.

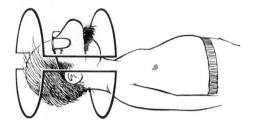

Fig. 24-8. The saddle coil is most often used with imagers having a horizontal external magnetic field.

µT or 50 ppm. If the homogeneity is worse than this, such as 100 ppm, then image quality will be degraded.

Just inside the aperture of the main magnet is positioned a drum with up to thirty individual windings, called **shim coils,** each with its own power supply, as shown in Fig. 24-5. After the main magnet has been brought up to field, the current and polarity of each shim coil will be adjusted to produce maximum homogeneity in the external magnetic field, B_0. This process is called **shimming the magnet.**

Gradient coils

As mentioned earlier, to obtain spatial information about the tissue from which the MRI signal is emitted, it is necessary that the primary magnetic field be slightly varied by using a **gradient magnetic field.** The gradient magnetic field is produced by electric coils called **gradient coils.** To obtain projections from a variety of directions, one must be able to orient the gradient magnetic field along either the X, Y or Z axes, or along any oblique plane. Three pairs of coils exist, as shown in Fig. 24-6, and they are identified as the X, Y and Z gradient coils, respectively.

Normally the Z gradient coils are used for selection of a transaxial slice. When the Z gradient magnetic field is on, the RF pulse can be precisely tuned so that only the hydrogen nuclei in a given slice of the patient are energized, as shown in Fig. 24-7. The strength of the gradient magnetic field and the shape of the RF pulse determine the width of the slice selected.

If a coronal slice is desired, the X gradient coils will be energized. Energizing the Y gradient coils will produce a sagittal slice, and energizing all three pairs of coils simultaneously will result in an oblique slice, as seen in Fig. 24-6.

For two-dimensional Fourier transformation (2DFT) imaging of transaxial anatomy, the Z gradient is on during the excitation RF pulse to select the appropriate slice. While receiving the MRI signals, the X and Y gradient coils will be sequenced on. The X gradient conventionally is termed the **frequency-encoding gradient** and the Y gradient the **phase-encoding gradient.**

Therefore, unlike CT, the plane of the scan can be determined totally electronically. The MRI system contains no moving parts and can produce not only transverse images but also sagittal, coronal, and indeed any oblique image of the volume of tissue lying within the gradient coils. Physically, the gradient coils are usually embedded in a ring fitting snugly inside the shim coils within the patient aperture.

RF probe

Usually the same antenna coil that transmits the RF pulse into the patient is also used to detect the MRI signal. Although engineers have certain general principles they can follow in designing RF antennas, the fabrication of an efficient antenna system for MRI remains something of an art. The shape of the antenna itself can range from a simple coil of wire to complex, three-dimensional, figure-eight shapes. The most popular coil configuration is the saddle-shaped coil shown in Fig. 24-8.

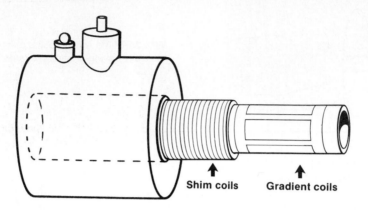

Fig. 24-9. Relative position of the secondary coils inside the main magnet.

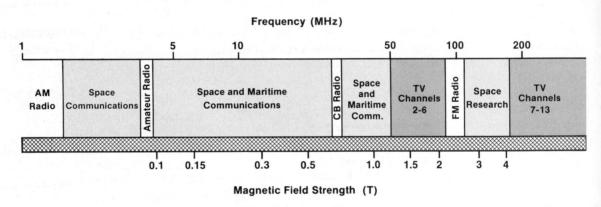

Fig. 24-10. The region of the FCC frequency allocation chart occupied by MRI is also crowded with commercial, industrial, and government broadcasts that can mask the NMR signals from a patient.

To maintain the coil in its intended shape and to protect it from damage, it is usually embedded in plastic, fiberglass, or some other insulator. This rigid unit, consisting of the antenna coil and its support material, is referred to as the **RF probe** or **probe assembly.** The RF probe is located inside the gradient coils and is closest to the patient. Fig. 24-9 shows the relative positions of the secondary coils.

Facility design

Because MRI involves no ionizing radiation, it is not necessary to shield the room with lead or other x-ray attenuating material. Depending on the design of the imager and the location of the room, however, it may be necessary to have the room shielded against radio interference and fringe magnetic fields. Also, great care must be taken to ensure that only nonmagnetic materials

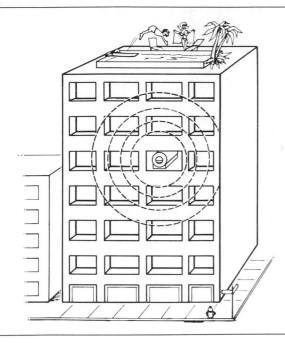

Fig. 24-11. The B_0 field of an imager consists of closed imaginary lines of the magnetic field. The magnetic field that extends outside of the patient aperture is the fringe magnetic field, and it is three dimensional.

are used for the structure and finish of the examination room.

Polyvinyl chloride (PVC) reinforcing rods should be substituted for iron reinforcing bars in any structural concrete slab or walls. All electrical penetrations into the room must have electric filters to remove interfering frequencies. Plumbing should not be iron but PVC or copper. Lighting should be direct current.

Electromagnetic shielding. The range of radio frequencies used in MRI imaging is very crowded with commercial and amateur radio broadcasts and other interference generated by power transmission and electronic systems. This RF interference can easily be strong enough to mask the faint MRI signals from the patient. Fig. 24-10 is a rendition of the FCC frequency allocation chart in the RF region of MRI. The potential sources of interference are many.

A carefully constructed wire-mesh shield enclosing the MR imager is necessary to attenuate these extraneous sources of RF. Such a shield is called a **Faraday cage** or an **RF shield.** This shielding, like x-ray lead shielding, need not be visible but can be covered by gypsum board or wood paneling. It is important to remember that this shielding exists solely to screen outside sources of RF interference. No radiation shielding is required either as a primary or secondary barrier for the protection of personnel, patients, or the general population as in x-ray imaging. Indeed, it is completely safe for attending personnel such as technologists and radiologists to remain in the room with the patient when necessary.

Magnetic shielding. The external magnetic field, B_0, of an MR imager is very intense and, as described in Chapter 5, consists of closed loops of lines of the magnetic field, as shown in Fig. 24-11. The magnetic field outside of the patient aperture is called a **fringe magnetic field** and must be considered in the design of an MRI

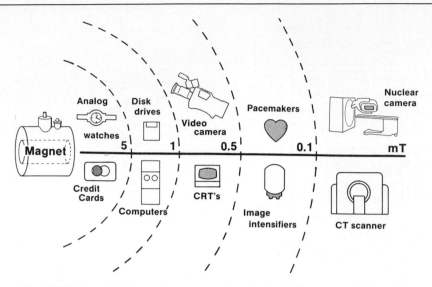

Fig. 24-12. Items to be excluded from various levels of the fringe magnetic field.

facility. This is especially important if the facility is to house a superconducting magnet with high field strength.

The problem with the fringe field is twofold. First, it can interfere with the proper operation of mechanical and electronic equipment. Electronic equipment is most sensitive. Any device such as a CRT, image-intensifier tube, or photomultiplier tube that operates on the principle of electron flow in a vacuum can be affected. The fringe magnetic field will cause the electron flow to be diverted. Electron microscopes are most easily influenced. Recommended exclusion areas for such equipment are shown Fig. 24-12.

Second, any large mass of ferromagnetic material, especially moving masses, can distort the homogeneity of the imaging volume by interacting with the fringe magnetic field. A distortion of the fringe magnetic field results in a compensating distortion in the imaging volume and degrades or destroys the image. Fig. 24-13 schematically shows how the addition of an iron wall

to reduce the intensity of the fringe magnetic field degrades the homogeneity of the imaging field.

MR IMAGES

MR imaging has many characteristics in common with other digital imaging modalities. Such characteristics as spatial resolution, low-contrast resolution, and noise are important criteria for judging an MR image.

Spatial resolution

At present the spatial resolution of MRI is equal to that of CT. When imaging high-contrast objects, structures less than 1 mm can be visualized routinely. Still higher spatial resolution can be obtained by reducing slice thickness or by increasing the amount of data collected. To increase data collection one must increase MRI signal acquisition, but this may require an unacceptably long examination time.

Another way to improve spatial resolution is by raising the MRI signal strength. Signal

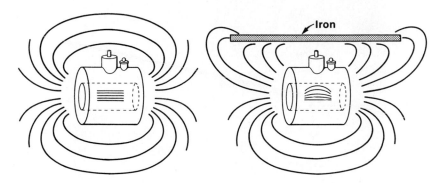

Fig. 24-13. Distortion of the fringe magnetic field by a ferromagnetic object will cause a compensating distortion in the imaging volume.

strength increases with the magnetic field strength. However, there are practical limitations to how strong a magnet can be used for MRI. Higher magnetic fields require more intense and higher-frequency RF pulses which is often an unacceptable solution.

Contrast resolution

One of the fundamental advantages of MRI is its potential for resolution of low-contrast structures. This, you will recall, is where CT scanning excels over conventional radiography. MRI does even better. A determining factor in the contrast between two tissues in a radiographic image is the difference in their x-ray attenuation coefficients. For most tissues these differences amount to less than 1%. In a conventional radiographic image, this 1% contrast is degraded by scatter radiation. In CT, scatter radiation is largely rejected so that 0.5% contrast can be imaged.

The difference in the MRI parameters among biologic tissues is frequently 30% or more, as seen in Fig. 23-1. For example, the difference in the x-ray attenuation coefficient between gray and white matter of the brain is roughly 0.5%, which is on the edge of detectability by CT scanning. However, the difference in MR parameters between gray and white matter is 30% to 40% and can be exploited to give dramatic differentiation of these two tissues.

We must remember that any MR image is a mixture of all three NMR parameters: spin density (SD), T_1, and T_2. By adjusting the RF pulse sequence used to excite the nuclear spins, one can alter the relative contribution of these three factors and significantly change the appearance of the image. For example, Fig. 24-14 shows four MR images of the brain. By using different RF pulse sequences, image contrast reversal can be produced, ranging from one in which the cerebrospinal fluid (CSF) space is lighter than the surrounding brain tissue, to one in which the CSF space is darker. Improper RF pulse selection can lead to total loss of contrast at what are termed **null regions.**

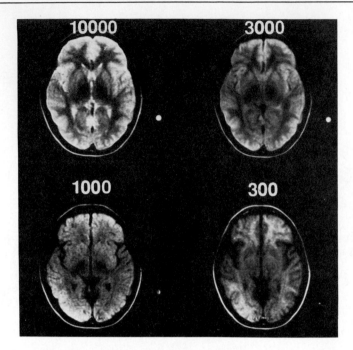

Fig. 24-14. Unlike x-ray imaging, MR images can be produced with contrast reversals simply by altering the RF pulse. This series of partial saturation images obtained at the indicated repetition times demonstrates contrast reversal due to changes in spin density and T_1 relaxation.

Thus the relative contrast between tissues as they appear on the image can be varied drastically by the RF pulse sequence chosen. It is important to remember that tissue containing no signal-producing hydrogen nuclei, such as air or cortical bone, will always appear dark on the image. Furthermore, fat and skin will usually appear bright because they have an abundance of hydrogen. The general relationship between the appearance of various tissues and their relative values of SD, T_1, and T_2 are shown in Table 24-2. These relationships are altered with tissue in a diseased state.

Examination time

When imaging the human anatomy, it is important to keep imaging times as short as prac-
tical to minimize the unsharpness caused by both voluntary and involuntary patient motion. As one might imagine, the best-quality images are usually obtained of extremities or the head, which can easily be restrained and exhibit little natural motion. This allows long data-acquisition times and a correspondingly high image quality. Indeed, this was one of the reasons why the first CT scanners with scan times of 4 minutes were dedicated head units. Reasonable-quality CT body images were not achievable until scan times could be reduced to below 30 s.

A similar time constraint applies to MRI. For example, during the production of each data acquisition, we excite the spins in the slice. For the next data acquisition, if we want the spins to start from the equilibrium state, we must wait

Table 24-2. The relative values of SD, T_1, and T_2 among normal tissues and the appearance of each in an MR image (value/appearance)

Tissue	Spin density	T_1	T_2
Fat and skin	High/white	Short/white	Long/white
Bone	Low/black	Very long/black	Very long/black
White matter	High/white	Short/white	Long/gray
Gray matter	High/white	Long/gray	Long/gray
CSF	Very high/white	Very long/gray	Very long/black

for these excited spins to return to equilibrium. This return, you will recall, is controlled by the parameter T_1, which in tissues is roughly 100 to 500 ms. Thus, in this instance, we must delay approximately 1 s between each projection. If a 256×256 image matrix is required, then at least 256 projections will be needed. Consequently, the minimum total scan time is 256 s, or more than 4 min. Some increased efficiency of data handling can be achieved by exciting and collecting data from other slices while waiting for previous slices to return to equilibrium. Thus one may, for example, collect data from twenty slices simultaneously over the span of approximately 10 minutes. However, each slice still represents data averaged over a considerable length of time. This is called **multislice imaging.** Much research is currently being devoted to reducing MR imaging times.

BIOLOGIC HAZARDS

Although we have very little information regarding the biologic response of humans to the fields of MRI, there is a large volume of research literature concerning the biologic responses to magnetic fields and to radio frequencies combined individually. It can be said with reasonable certainty at this time that **there are no harmful effects from MRI.** Furthermore, as research investigations in this area are accelerated, it can confidently be said that no long-term harmful effects are expected. There is simply no

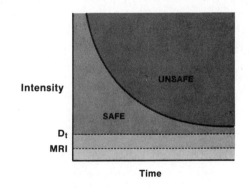

Fig. 24-15. The fields used in MRI exhibit threshold dose-response relationships.

underlying mechanism of action such as ionization to account for harmful effects.

Research investigations on laboratory animals, chromosomes, plant seeds, and molecular species have shown that biologic responses can be produced following extremely high intensities of MRI fields. In each case, however, **the dose-response relationship is threshold** in nature, as illustrated in Fig. 24-15, and the threshold is exceedingly high.

Three physical fields are associated with MRI that one might suspect of producing a biologic response. These are the strong static magnetic field (B_0), the time-varying gradient magnetic field (B_1), and the RF emission. In x-ray physics

Table 24-3. Units of dose associated with MRI

MRI field	Unit
Static magnetic field	Tesla (T)
Time-varying magnetic field	Tesla/second (T/s)
Radio frequency	Watts/kilogram (W/kg)

the dose of the physical agent is measured in rad (gray [Gy]). Since the radiation involved in MRI is nonionizing, different types of dose specifications are used. These specifications are summarized in Table 24-3. The static magnetic field strength is measured in tesla (T), varying magnetic fields in tesla per second (T/s), and radio frequencies (RF) in watts per kilogram (W/kg).

Static magnetic fields

Electric charges are not distributed uniformly throughout the body. Some molecules and membranes of the body have polarized electric charge distributions and therefore, in a sense, exhibit magnetic dipole characteristics. Other molecules, such as those constituting the nervous tissue, serve as conductors of electric current. In the presence of a very strong magnetic field, several electrochemical changes in tissue have been postulated.

Membrane permeability. Cellular and tissue membranes perform several important biologic functions, among them the passage of specific molecules. The ability of a molecule to penetrate a membrane and be transported to the other side is **the permeability of the membrane.** Because of the electric charge distribution on some membranes, changes in membrane permeability may occur in high magnetic fields. Such changes have not been observed in magnetic field strengths less than about 10 T.

Enzyme kinetics. Enzymes are rather large protein molecules with irregular charge distributions on their surfaces. In the presence of magnetic fields greater than approximately 10 T, the electric nature of these molecules changes. The effect of this change on the action of enzymes is unknown.

Nerve conduction. Nerve cells are electric conductors, much like a length of insulated copper wire. When electrons flow in a conductor in the presence of a magnetic field, a force is exerted on the electrons that tends to deviate their direction of flow and thereby forces the conductor aside. It is possible that such forces would interfere with the normal conduction of nerve cells and impair nervous function.

Biopotentials. Various tissues of the body, particularly muscle, experience changing electric potential during contraction. The electrocardiogram measures changing biopotentials in the heart having amplitudes of up to 10 mV. In the presence of a magnetic field, these biopotentials can be altered, thus possibly interfering with normal muscle function.

Gradient magnetic fields

Superimposed on the strong primary magnetic field are time-varying gradient magnetic fields. When a time-varying magnetic field interacts with the stationary electrons of certain tissues, an **electric current density** measured in microamperes per square centimeter ($\mu A/cm^2$) can be induced. There are three known responses to such induced current density, all of which occur at magnetic field intensities several orders of magnitude above those employed in MRI.

Visual phosphenes. If one passes a small electric current through the head with the eyes closed, a flash will appear on the retina. This flash is due to the activation of the molecule phosphene.

Bone healing. The passage of small electric currents through segments of fractured bone assists in healing. The current density used is about 10 $\mu A/cm^2$. Although the precise mechanism of action is unknown, it is employed effectively in many cases.

Cardiac fibrillation. When the heart loses its normal beat and begins to flutter uncontrollably, it is said to **fibrillate.** Cardiac fibrillation can lead to cardiac arrest and death. To stabilize a fibrillating heart, a large electric current can be passed through the cardiac muscle. Such **electric shock defibrillation** is commonplace in hospital coronary care units.

Likewise, an electric current can cause a normal heart to fibrillate. Experiments with dogs and humans have shown the minimum current densities for induction of fibrillation to be 300 mA/cm^2. Such currents are six orders of magnitude greater than those induced during MRI.

Radio frequency exposure

The principal result of the interaction between an RF field and tissue is heat. RF heating can easily be demonstrated, but the degree of heating is a complex function of the frequency and power density of the emitted RF. Heating is expressed as the **specific absorption rate (SAR)** measured in watts per kilogram (W/kg). The normal resting state is approximately 1.5 W/kg. During vigorous exercise, metabolic activity will equal perhaps 15 W/kg. In terms of temperature rise, a 1 K rise in tissue temperature requires an SAR of 5 W/kg.

Maximum permissible dose

The use of **maximum permissible dose (MPD)** is probably not correct for MRI, but standard nomenclature has not yet been adopted. Exposure guidelines have been suggested by the U.S. National Center for Devices and Radiological Health and the U.K. National Radiological Protection Board. These guidelines are shown in Table 24-4. They are set at such a low level that there is no likelihood of injury to patients or personnel from any biologic interaction.

Table 24-4. Suggested maximum exposure levels during MRI

Exposure condition	Maximum exposure	
	United States	United Kingdom
Static magnetic field	2 T	2.5 T
Time-varying magnetic field	3 T/s	20 T/s
Pulsed RF field	0.4 W/kg (whole body) 2 W/kg (maximum)	70 W

As we gain more imaging experience, develop more sophisticated equipment, and better identify the dose-response relationships involved, these suggested exposure levels are likely to rise.

Physical hazards

Although MRI is biologically safe, certain physical precautions must be taken near the magnet. Personnel must remember that the magnetic fields involved are strong and are capable of exerting significant forces on magnetic materials such as utensils made out of iron or steel. Care must be exercised with small miscellaneous objects such as pins and paper clips, since these may be easily sucked into the magnet. Special care is necessary when using larger objects such as wrenches, screwdrivers, and other hand tools. When such objects are brought near the magnet, the magnetic field is strong enough to pull these from your grasp with sufficient force to cause either injury to yourself, other personnel, or the patient or damage to the imager. These precautions also apply to the patient, who should be free of any metallic objects, even internally. Warning signs such as that in Fig. 24-16 are necessary.

MRI magnetic fields are also strong enough to affect such other personal items as bank cards and mechanical watches. Many credit cards con-

WARNING
MAGNETIC FIELD

THE FIELD OF THIS MAGNET ATTRACTS OBJECTS
CONTAINING IRON, STEEL, NICKEL OR COBALT.
SUCH OBJECTS MUST <u>NOT</u> BE BROUGHT INTO THIS
AREA. <u>LARGE</u> OBJECTS CANNOT BE RESTRAINED.

PERSONS WITH IMPLANTS OR PROSTHETIC
DEVICES SHOULD <u>NOT</u> ENTER THIS AREA.
PACEMAKERS MAY BE DISABLED.

DATA ON CREDIT CARDS AND MAGNETIC STORAGE
MEDIA CAN BE ERASED. WATCHES, CAMERAS, AND
INSTRUMENTS CAN BE DAMAGED.

Fig. 24-16. Representative warning sign for an MRI facility.

tain magnetic strips encoded with identification
information. Carrying such cards near the magnetic field can scramble the magnetically coded
information and invalidate the card. Also, the
tiny moving parts in a mechanical watch can
become magnetized, causing the watch to malfunction. It is possible, however, to take such a
damaged watch to a repairman to be demag-
netized. In general, solid-state watches are not
damaged by the magnetic field.

REVIEW QUESTIONS

1. Define or otherwise identify the following:
   a. Superconducting magnet
   b. Cryogenic
   c. Dewar
   d. Shim coils
   e. Faraday cage
   f. Null region
   g. Multislice imaging
   h. Phosphene
   i. SAR
   j. Degrees K

2. In what way does the MR image of the brain differ from CT?
3. What is the maximum static magnetic field to which a patient should be exposed?
4. List five potential hazards associated with MRI.
5. Discuss the relative advantages and disadvantages of a superconducting magnet for MRI.
6. What is the meaning of "shimming the magnet"?
7. Diagram the most popular shape for an RF probe assembly.
8. List ten items that should not be brought into an MRI examination room.
9. What are the relative values of the MRI parameters for bone, soft tissue, fat, and air?
10. How should each of those tissues appear on a T_2-weighted image?

25

Design of radiologic imaging facilities

DESIGNING TEAM
DEPARTMENTAL ACTIVITY
LOCATION OF X-RAY DEPARTMENT
PLAN LAYOUT
CONSTRUCTION CONSIDERATIONS

The success of a radiology service depends in great measure on the design of the quarters it occupies. The design of a new facility should begin years before construction if the facility is to meet its principal objective—providing good patient care, economically and with a minimum of motion by patients and employees.

The design of a radiologic facility will depend on the previous training and experience of persons consulted during the planning stage. For a design to be effective, it must be tempered by an analysis of flow patterns, equipment, use, and available resources.

X-ray departments are composed of many different types of rooms, each of which requires attention to interroom and intraroom design. Table 23-1 lists these various rooms and the type of facility for which they are required. For the purpose of this discussion, three types of facilities are identified, according to their size. First is the radiologic facility located in a private office or small hospital; next is the moderate-size com-munity hospital; and last is the large general hospital located in a medical center complex that serves teaching and research functions in addition to caring for patients. Some types of rooms are common to all radiologic facilities, regardless of the size of the institution housing them.

The backbone of any radiologic facility is, of course, the general purpose **radiographic-fluoroscopic (R-F)** examination room. Each such room must have an adjacent toilet. A darkroom, a film-viewing area, a film-file room, and space for necessary clerical support are also required for every radiologic facility. When planning large x-ray departments, consideration must be given to adequate space for patient waiting and dressing rooms, holding areas for stretcher patients, office and lounge space for radiologists and technologists, and special procedures x-ray rooms.

The design of radiologic facilities should account for nuclear medicine, ultrasound, MRI, and radiation therapy if these medical services are to be offered under the administrative con-

Table 25-1. Minimum room requirements for radiologic facilities according to type of institution*

Room	Private office	Community hospital	General hospital
Examination rooms			
R-F	X	X	X
Chest		X	X
Mammography			X
Special procedures			X
Patient rooms			
Waiting area	X	X	X
Dressing	X	X	X
Toilets	X	X	X
Film rooms			
Darkroom	X	X	X
Cassette loading			X
Automatic processor		X	X
Film conveyors			X
File	X	X	X
Technologist rooms			
Office		X	X
Lounge			X
Radiologist rooms			
Office	X	X	X
Viewing		X	X
Conference			X
Library			X

*An X indicates the room is necessary.

trol of radiology. Design of these types of facilities will not be considered here except in a general manner. Protective shielding of the examination room is not required for nuclear medicine and ultrasound as it is for x ray and MRI. Location of these facilities is not critical, except that the nuclear medicine laboratory should not be positioned so that its imaging apparatus could be in direct line with the useful beam of an adjacent radiographic room or in proximity to the MRI.

Radiotherapy facilities require considerably more shielding than diagnostic radiologic facilities and therefore are usually located on the lowest level of a hospital. The treatment rooms are most often positioned along an outer wall so that if the basement level is involved, advantage can be taken of the surrounding earth as shielding material.

Radiotherapy is a specialized part of radiology requiring special equipment and techniques. Cnsequently, its service is usually limited to large general hospitals. On the other hand, ultrasound and nuclear medicine are becoming more available to the small hospital and clinic and even to the private office.

DESIGNING TEAM

Unfortunately, too many radiologic facilities are designed by one person, usually either the radiologist in charge or the consultant architect, neither of whom has sufficient background to assume the required responsibility for the total design of the facility. The proper design of a radiologic facility requires the skills and experience of several persons. The designing team should have a minimum of six members, as outlined in Fig. 25-1. This team should be formally organized at the earliest possible stage of planning. It should meet in formal session as frequently as necessary and **record its deliberations** so that subsequent misunderstandings and errors will be minimized.

The principal member of the design team should be the **hospital administrator.** Only this person has an overview of the relationship of the radiology service to the rest of the hospital and knows the funds available and how they are allocated among the various hospital services. It is not uncommon to have a department superbly planned only to find that the resources are not available to acquire the required equipment after construction.

The **architect** is responsible primarily for construction details, including the structural engineering, the working drawings, and the decorating.

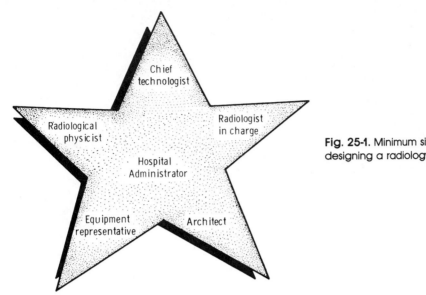

Fig. 25-1. Minimum six members of team designing a radiology department.

The **radiologist** and **chief technologist** provide the necessary information on facility work load, flow patterns, and anticipated future requirements. Their practical experience in departmental administration and patient services is invaluable to the design team.

The **radiologic physicist** is responsible for the specification of adequate protective barriers. The location of radiation rooms and the placement of equipment in those rooms must be planned to minimize radiation exposure to patients and employees. By careful computation the physicist can prescribe safe protective barriers using cost-saving materials and techniques.

The **equipment manufacturer** provides the necessary specifications of power requirements, space requirements, and radiation characteristics and can assist in locating equipment to maximally use available space.

The advice of all persons involved in the operation of the radiology department should be sought. Additional consultants should be retained as necessary.

DEPARTMENTAL ACTIVITY

One of the first considerations in properly designing an x-ray department is an estimation of future activity. Departmental activity can be measured in many ways, including number of patients per year, number of examinations per year, number of hospital beds, outpatient-to-inpatient ratio, and x-ray machine work load.

The United States Public Health Service has conducted several studies and found that 65% of the population of the United States receives a diagnostic x-ray examination each year. Nearly half the medical radiographic examinations are of the chest, as shown by Fig. 25-2. Fig. 25-3 shows that nearly two thirds of all x-ray examinations are conducted in hospitals. Private offices of radiologists and other physicians rank second in x-ray examinations. Radiologists supervise 70% of all x-ray procedures, and an examination averages 2.5 films.

Various authors and designers have developed rules of thumb for estimating required department size based on anticipated departmental ac-

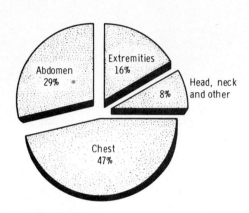

Fig. 25-2. Estimated frequency of radiographic examination by body site.

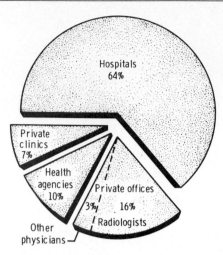

Fig. 25-3. Estimated frequency of x-ray examination by type of facility.

tivity. The more prominent of these are as follows:

$$\frac{\text{Number of examinations per year}}{5000} =$$
$$\text{Required number of x-ray rooms}$$

$$\frac{\text{Number of hospital beds}}{50} =$$
$$\text{Required number of x-ray rooms}$$

$$\text{Number of x-ray rooms} \times 1500 \text{ square feet} =$$
$$\text{Total space necessary}$$

$$\frac{\text{Number of examinations per year}}{4.5} =$$
$$\text{Total space necessary}$$

$$\text{Total space} \times 10\% = \text{Estimated growth per year}$$

The rule that there should be one diagnostic x-ray room for every 5000 annual x-ray examination is quite general. To be realistic, the determination of the number of x-ray examining rooms should be influenced by characteristics such as age, race, population density, and average income of the community to be served. If the area served is of low income and high population density, then outpatient examinations will represent the bulk of the radiology effort. Should this be the case, estimates of the percentage of outpatients referred for x-ray examination and the number of examinations per patient will be necessary. Knowing this, one can compute the number of outpatient examinations per day. If this number is divided by **twenty, the number of examinations per day a general purpose room can easily accommodate,** an estimate of the number of x-ray examining rooms needed for outpatient care can be made.

EXAMPLE: An average of 250 patients visit a medical clinic each day. If 20% of the patients are referred for x-ray examination and 5% of those referred are reexamined, how many x-ray rooms are required?
ANSWER:
$$250 \times 20\% = 50 \text{ x-ray patients by initial referral per day}$$
$$50 \times 5\% = 3 \text{ x-ray patients for reexamination per day}$$
$$50 + 3 = 53 \text{ total examinations per day}$$
$$53 \div 20 = 3 \text{ x-ray rooms required}$$

On the other hand, if the radiologic facility is housed in a specialty hospital, such as obstetrics and gynecology, surgical, or orthopedic, then inpatient examinations may represent the bulk of the radiology service. Should this be the case, perhaps the most important information necessary for proper design is the number of hospital beds. Depending on the nature of the hospital service, **somewhere between one and three x-ray rooms will be required for each 100 hospital beds.** In addition to the number of hospital beds, the anticipated occupancy rate, the approximate length of stay per patient, and the number of examinations per patient should be known to assist in planning for inpatient examinations. From this information the number of inpatient examinations per bed-day can be computed. If one again assumes the factor of twenty examinations per x-ray room per day, the number of x-ray rooms required for inpatient care can be estimated.

EXAMPLE: A 400-bed hospital has an 85% occupancy rate. On the average, 40% of the inpatients receive an x-ray examination during their 4-day stay. How many x-ray rooms are needed for inpatient care?

ANSWER:

$$\frac{400 \text{ beds} \times 85\% \text{ occupied} \times 0.4 \text{ exams/patient}}{4 \text{ days}} =$$

$$34 \text{ exams/day}$$

$$\frac{34 \text{ exams/day}}{20} =$$

$$2 \text{ x-ray rooms required for inpatient load}$$

The sum of the inpatient requirements, outpatient requirements, and considerations for future expansion will provide an estimate of the total number of examining rooms needed. In general, private offices have one or two rooms. Community hospitals with 200 beds or less have two to four rooms. Large general hospitals and teaching hospitals have ten to fifteen rooms or more.

Every x-ray examining room needs space, a requirement that should not be minimized. It is well known that, as the size of the x-ray examining room increases, the average radiation dose to employees decreases. Furthermore, the efficiency and morale of all employees are high when corridors are sufficiently wide, rooms are sufficiently large, and the interior of all spaces is brightly decorated, lighted, and properly ventilated.

The minimum size for any general purpose R-F x-ray room is 16 × 18 feet. Special procedures rooms must be at least 20 × 25 feet to accommodate the increased equipment load and the higher number of personnel required to operate the equipment. A room designed only for chest radiography may be proportionately smaller.

The total area assigned to the radiology department should be no less than 1500 square feet for each x-ray examining room. A larger ratio of total area to number of examining rooms is usually necessary in smaller facilities and special purpose facilities.

LOCATION OF X-RAY DEPARTMENT

Hospitals designed before about 1950 nearly always had the radiology department on the ground floor. The reasons for this were many, but the one most often quoted was the floor loading requirements resulting from the protective shielding of the x-ray rooms. In general, x-ray departments are still located on ground floors, but not for the same reason. The principal requirements for the location of the x-ray department prescribe that it be near the outpatient clinic, the emergency area, and surgery. For the convenience of patients, it is also helpful to locate the x-ray department near the clinical laboratories. In larger hospitals, separate radiologic facilities will be planned as an integral part of the emergency area, the admitting area, and special medical services. Locational restraints on the main x-ray department thus are minimum.

Modern structural engineering designs allow x-ray departments to be located on any floor of the hospital. In fact, when the departments are located on upper levels, the shielding requirements can be reduced by positioning the x-ray examining rooms along outside walls (nobody walks outside the twenty-third floor!). On ground level the x-ray examining rooms are generally located to the inside.

PLAN LAYOUT

The plan layout of the radiologic facility must take into account the various **traffic patterns,** some of which are diagramed in Fig. 25-4. Although patient flow is perhaps least important, it must be considered for its effect on the overall efficiency of the radiology service provided. **The traffic patterns produced by technologists and radiologists are of primary importance.** Both must be minimized to obtain maximum efficiency.

The radiologic technologists spend most of their time in the examining room but also must have ready access to the patient preparation area, the radiographic supply storeroom, the darkroom, and the professional staff. Departments that have more than four examining rooms should provide a lounge for technologists. The lounge must be located in the radiology area for the comfort and convenience of the technologists and also to discourage trips to the cafeteria or elsewhere for coffee breaks.

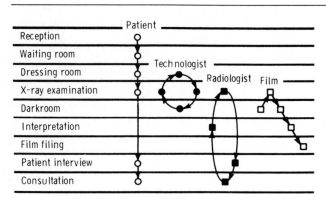

Fig. 25-4. Flowchart showing approximate movement of patient, technologist, radiologist, and film during an examination.

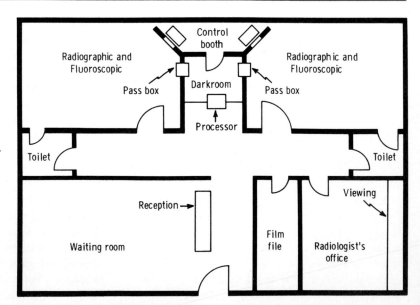

Fig. 25-5. Typical layout for two-room radiology service.

The plan layout of the radiologic facility should consider traffic pattern created by the radiologist. Radiologists spend most of their clinical time in the examining room, the reading room, or the consultation area. Often the reading room and consultation area are combined. Office space must be provided for the radiolo-

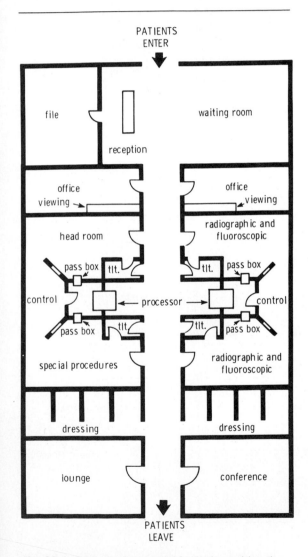

Fig. 25-6. Example of acceptable single-corridor plan, where patients enter at one end and exit at other.

gist. If the radiologist's activities are strictly clinical, an office should be located within the radiology area so that technologists and other physicians have easy access to it. On the other hand, if the radiologist is involved in teaching and research, then the office should be located in another part of the hospital so that the radiologist will be free of interruptions when not on clinical assignment.

The traffic pattern created by patient records is also of considerable importance. There are three principal types of patient records—the radiograph, the floppy disk, and the reported interpretation. These records create the worst traffic problem of all, and if not properly considered they can result in delays and lost records, causing inconvenience to patients and referring physicians. Lost or unobtainable films and reports often result in repeat examinations that otherwise would be unnecessary.

For private offices and small community hospitals the layout of the radiology department is fairly simple. An example of such a layout is shown in Fig. 25-5. For larger radiologic facilities a self-enclosed square or rectangular arrangement is usually best.

A typical **single-corridor plan** is shown in Fig. 25-6. Usually this type of design should be avoided because it results in counterflow among patients, technologists, and radiologists. If the corridor is not dead-ended, then it is probably continuous with other traffic patterns of the hospital. This, too, should be avoided. The only single-corridor plan with reasonable merit is one designed so that patients enter at one end and exit at the other.

A design incorporating a **central core** in a roughly square or rectangular area is usually most desirable. Such a design should locate the x-ray department in a way that future expansion can be accommodated. One such central-core design is shown in Fig. 25-7, where the x-ray examining rooms are positioned to the center with a central processing area. A second central-core design, shown in Fig. 25-8, has the x-ray examining rooms located along the outside walls

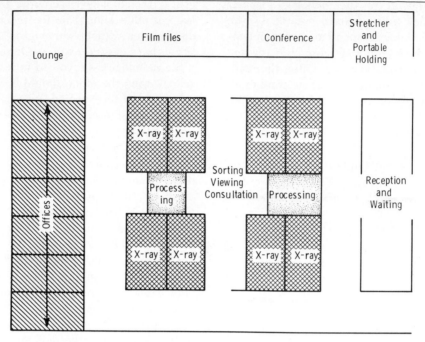

Fig. 25-7. Central-core design with x-ray rooms located in center of area.

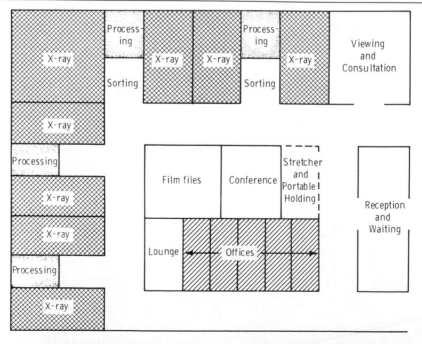

Fig. 25-8. Central-core design with x-ray rooms along outside walls.

with the administrative areas located to the interior.

Corridors used for outpatients should be 8 feet wide. Those accommodating inpatients with their wheelchairs and stretchers should be 12 feet wide.

CONSTRUCTION CONSIDERATIONS

Just like every other area of our exploding technology, the design and construction of medical facilities and the manufacture of radiologic equipment are rapidly changing some of their basic aspects. Items from shielding barriers to toilet fixtures are changing and forcing changes in the design and construction of radiographic facilities. Perhaps the most important requirement for the design of a modern radiologic facility is flexibility for future use and expansion.

Track-mounted movable partitions are a good method to prepare for the future. The average life of modern radiologic equipment is between 5 and 10 years. Replacement equipment may be larger or heavier or may require more power than the original equipment. The design of the radiologic facility should anticipate these changes.

X-ray examination room

Space and freedom from obstruction are key requirements in the design of an x-ray examination room. A large examining room has many advantages in addition to being comfortable for patients and radiologic personnel. Large rooms are easily altered and adapted for other uses. They result in lower personnel exposures because of the decrease in scatter radiation.

Fig. 25-9 shows the layout of a typical combination R-F room. The computation of the required protective barrier thickness is covered in Chapter 31. The protective barrier enclosing the operating console should be positioned relative to the radiographic tube head so that it is seldom in line with the useful beam. The viewing window should be as large as possible but not less than 24 × 36 inches. Too many console barriers incorporate 12-inch-square viewing windows, which necessitate a stepping stool for short technologists and require tall technologists to stoop to view the patients during examination. Unfortunately, this sometimes results in the technologist peering around the protective barrier during exposure. The control area should be roomy enough to accommodate several persons and ad-

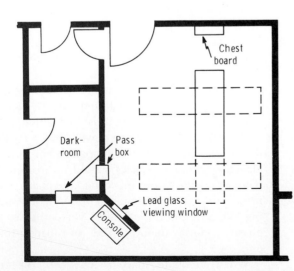

Fig. 25-9. Typical modern design of combination radiographic-fluoroscopic x-ray examining room.

equately store film. The minimum requirement is 25 square feet.

The location of the chest board is important. If an outside wall is available, it should be used for positioning the chest board, especially if the examining room is located above ground level. If the chest board must be positioned along an inside wall, additional lead shielding may have to be placed directly behind it.

Too often, electric cables for control of the fluoroscopic and radiographic tubes are strung along the floor or hung from the ceiling in such a manner that they become easily tangled. This results in loss of usable space behind the fluoroscope and interference with technologist movement in the room. An easy remedy is to use floor, wall, and ceiling troughs to convey the control cables. Should cable troughs be planned, the design must account for the loss of protective shielding and compensate accordingly.

In nearly every x-ray room the generator is located out of the way in the corner. New medical buildings often have interfloor distances of 12 to 15 feet with 8- or 9-foot drop ceilings in the x-ray examining rooms. This leaves 3 to 7 feet available in the false ceiling for the storage of x-ray apparatus, in particular, the generator. Use of a pulldown stairway and supporting struts in the false ceiling to position the x-ray generator will free an additional 10 to 30 square feet of floor space.

Darkroom

Many radiology experts believe the conventional darkroom is on its way out. Some predict that within a few years new construction will not even include a darkroom. These changes may come about because of improvements in automatic processors, daylight loaders, and cassetteless automatic film conveyers. Also contributing to the possible demise of the darkroom are new imaging techniques, such as xeroradiography, ionography, and photo imaging materials that do not incorporate silver halide as the principal ingredient. Also, the continuing development and application of digital image acquisition and stor-

age will hasten the obsolescence of the darkroom. Nevertheless, radiologic facilities currently under construction require adequate darkroom space. In large departments the darkroom facility can be either centrally located or dispersed throughout the department.

Central processing saves capital expenditures on the plumbing and electrical requirements and on the number of processors required. Central processing also can save on operating expenses, since it generally requires fewer darkroom personnel and less service and maintenance of processing equipment. The great advantage to central processing is the better quality control afforded by having all films processed under identical conditions. The size of the central processing area will depend on the overall size and activity of the radiology service.

If it is decided to have darkrooms distributed throughout the department, they can be smaller but should not be less than 8 feet along any wall. Generally, in such a situation one darkroom will be designed to service every two examining rooms. There are advantages to this arrangement. The traffic pattern of the technologist covers less distance, and communication with darkroom personnel is better. This results in less cassette wear and provides for immediate check of the radiograph by the technologist so that fewer patient recalls are necessary. With such a system, loss of film and loss of film identification are also less frequent.

The layout of a typical darkroom serving two examining rooms with an automatic processor is shown in Fig. 25-10. Care must be taken in providing adequate water and power service for the darkroom, with some anticipation for future changes. Storage space should be carefully planned. Ventilation must be adequate, and proper illumination should be provided. Warning lights should be installed over entrances to guard against unauthorized or inadvertent entry.

When adequate space is available, the entrance to the darkroom can be a maze arrange-

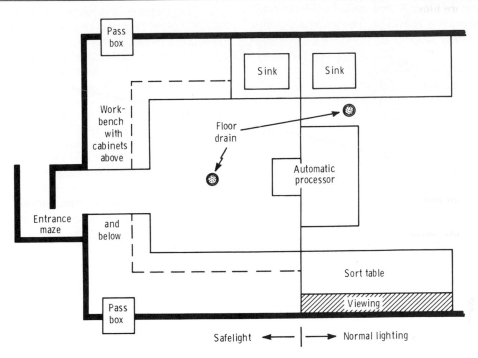

Fig. 25-10. This darkroom plan is sufficiently large for future use. It has adequate storage and work space and is designed to service two x-ray examining rooms.

ment, as shown in Fig. 25-10, although this arrangement is less necessary with automatically processed cut film than with roll film. When space is at a premium, conventional door entry may be necessary. In recent years some facilities have successfully used cleverly designed revolving doors.

The location, care, and intensity of safelights in the darkroom is important. Films are somewhat faster, averaging a relative speed of at least 200, and they are either blue or green sensitive. On average, they are handled open in the darkroom less than 1 minute. Tests should be performed regularly to ensure that safelights will not produce an optical density increase of greater than 0.05.

Painting the darkroom walls is no problem. Dark walls are not necessary; in fact, light walls are recommended. If the illumination from safe-lights is safe, that reflected from any surface will also be safe.

File room

The amount of space needed to file film will vary according to departmental activity. A minimum of 5-years storage is generally accepted, and this will require 7% to 10% of the available departmental space. Half of this space will have to be in the main section of the department, where the most recent films should be filed for easy access. On average, a 3-foot shelf space will hold 200 patient envelopes.

One must be sure to consider the weight requirements of film filing. Stored film weighs about 100 pounds per linear foot of shelf space. Most storage racks are 5 tiers high, so a total of 1500 pounds should be considered for each 3 feet of such stacked shelving.

The use of magnetic and optical media to store digital images is reducing the demand for film storage space.

REVIEW QUESTIONS

1. Who should be included in the designing team of a radiologic imaging facility? What would be their individual responsibilities?

2. Discuss the factors that should be considered when planning a routine radiographic-fluoroscopic (R-F) room. What effect would hospital size have?

3. A general hospital sees an average of 430 outpatients each day. Normally, 30% of the patients require x-ray examination, with 7% of those examined requiring reexamination. How many x-ray rooms would be needed to handle the outpatients in this hospital?

4. An obstetric and gynecologic hospital contains 250 beds and runs at a 75% occupancy rate. Forty percent of the inpatients are referred for x-ray examination. The normal period of hospitalization for these patients is 5 days. How many x-ray rooms would be needed for inpatient care?

5. A new chest clinic anticipates 10,000 patients each year with 90% requiring an x-ray examination. Of these patients, 20% require reexamination. How many x-ray rooms would be needed to handle the patient load in this clinic?

6. Plans for a new private radiology suite propose 5209 square feet to accommodate three radiographic-fluoroscopic rooms. Will this space be adequate initially? After 5 years of growth in this practice?

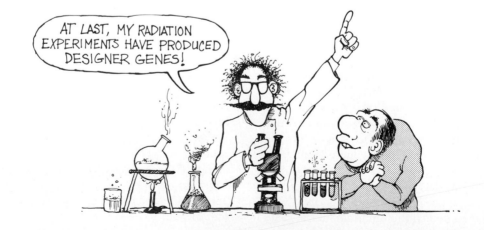

AT LAST, MY RADIATION EXPERIMENTS HAVE PRODUCED DESIGNER GENES!

26

Fundamental principles of radiobiology

FROM MOLECULES TO HUMANS

HUMAN BIOLOGY

LAW OF BERGONIÉ AND TRIBONDEAU

PHYSICAL FACTORS AFFECTING RADIOSENSITIVITY

BIOLOGIC FACTORS AFFECTING RADIOSENSITIVITY

RADIATION DOSE-RESPONSE RELATIONSHIPS

FROM MOLECULES TO HUMANS

It is known beyond a shadow of a doubt that x rays are harmful. If sufficiently intense, x rays can cause cancer, leukemia, and genetic damage. What is not known for certain is the degree of effect following diagnostic levels of x-radiation. We do know that the benefits derived from the diagnostic application of x rays in medicine are enormous. It is the job of the technologist, along with the radiologist, physicist, and maintenance engineer, to produce high-quality x-ray studies with a minimum of radiation exposure. This approach can result in the highest benefit and the smallest risk.

The effects of x rays on humans are the result of interactions at atomic levels (Chapter 9). These atomic interactions take the form of ionization or excitation of orbital electrons and result in the deposition of energy in tissue. The deposited energy can result in a molecular change, the consequences of which can be di-

sastrous if the molecule involved is critical. Fig. 26-1 summarizes the steps between radiation exposure and latent whole body injury.

When an atom is ionized, its chemical binding properties change. If the atom is a constituent of a large molecule, the ionization may result in breakage of the molecule or relocation of the atom within the molecule. The abnormal molecule may in time function improperly or cease to function, which can result in serious impairment or death of the cell.

This process is not irreversible. **At each stage in the sequence it is possible to recover from radiation damage.** Ionized atoms can become neutral again by attracting a free electron. Molecules can be mended by repair enzymes. Cells and tissues can regenerate and recover from the radiation injury.

If the radiation response occurs within minutes or days after radiation exposure, it is classified as an immediate or **early effect of radia-**

455

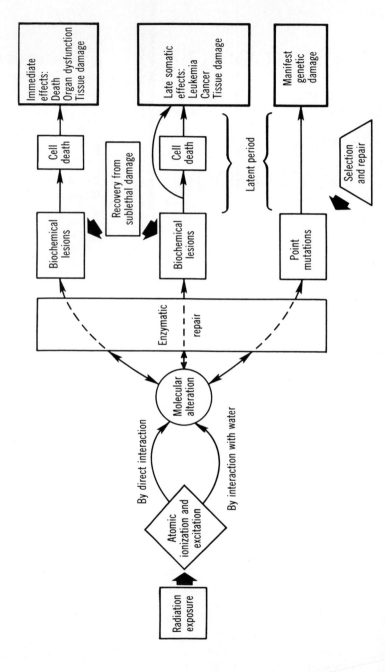

Fig. 26-1. Sequence of events following radiation exposure of humans can lead to several radiation responses. At nearly every step, mechanisms for recovery and repair are available.

tion. On the other hand, if the human injury is not observable for many months or years, it is termed a delayed or **late effect of radiation.**

The following outline summarizes the possible early and late human responses to radiation exposure. In addition, many other radiation responses have been experimentally observed in animals. Most of the human responses have been observed following rather large radiation doses. But we are cautious and assume that even small doses are harmful.

Human responses to ionizing radiation

A. Early effects of radiation on humans
1. Acute radiation syndrome
   a. Hematologic syndrome
   b. Gastrointestinal syndrome
   c. Central nervous system syndrome
2. Local tissue damage
   a. Skin
   b. Gonads
   c. Extremities
3. Hematologic depression
4. Cytogenetic damage
B. Late effects of radiation on humans
1. Leukemia
2. Other malignant disease
   a. Bone cancer
   b. Lung cancer
   c. Thyroid cancer
   d. Breast cancer
3. Local tissue damage
   a. Skin
   b. Gonads
   c. Eyes
4. Life span shortening
5. Genetic damage
   a. Cytogenetic damage
   b. Doubling dose
   c. Genetically significant dose
C. Effects of fetal irradiation
1. Prenatal death
2. Neonatal death
3. Congenital malformation
4. Childhood malignancy
5. Diminished growth and development

The following list gives some of the human population groups in which many of these radiation responses have been detected.

Human populations in which radiation effects have been observed

1. American radiologists
2. Atomic bomb survivors
3. Radiation accident victims
4. Marshall Islanders
5. Residents of areas of high environmental radiation
6. Uranium miners
7. Radium watch-dial painters
8. ^{131}I patients
9. Children treated for enlarged thymus
10. Ankylosing spondylitis patients
11. Thorotrast patients
12. Fetuses irradiated in utero
13. Volunteer convicts
14. Cyclotron workers

Radiobiology is the study of the effects of ionizing radiation on biologic tissue. The ultimate goal of radiobiologic research is the accurate description of the effects of radiation on humans so that radiation can be used more safely in diagnosis and more effectively in therapy.

HUMAN BIOLOGY

The composition of the human body has its ultimate basis in atoms, and that is the level at which radiation interacts. It is the atomic composition of the body that determines the character and degree of the radiation interaction. It is the molecular and tissue composition that defines the nature of the radiation injury. The following list summarizes the atomic composition of the body and shows that over 85% of the body is hydrogen and oxygen:

60.0% hydrogen
25.7% oxygen
10.7% carbon
2.4% nitrogen
0.2% calcium
0.1% phosphorus
0.1% sulfur
0.8% trace elements

Radiation interaction at the atomic level results in molecular change, and this in turn can produce a cell deficient in its normal growth and metabolism. Robert Hooke, the English schoolmaster, first named the **cell** as the basic biologic building block in 1665. Shortly thereafter, in 1673, Anton van Leeuwenhoek accurately described a living cell based on his microscopic observations. However, it was more than 100 years later, in 1838, that Schneider and Schwann showed conclusively that all plants and animals contain cells as their basic functional unit. This is the **cell theory.** The most significant milestone in recent studies of the living cell was the Watson and Crick description in 1953 of the molecular structure of deoxyribonucleic acid (DNA), the genetic substance of the cell.

Molecular composition

There are five principal types of molecules in the body:

80% water
15% protein
2% lipids
1% carbohydrates
1% nucleic acid
1% other

Four of these molecules—proteins, lipids (fats), carbohydrates (sugars and starches), and nucleic acids—are **macromolecules,** very large molecules sometimes consisting of hundreds of thousands of atoms. Proteins, lipids, and carbohydrates are the principal classes of **organic molecules.** An organic molecule is life supporting and contains carbon. One of the rarest molecules, a nucleic acid concentrated in the nucleus of a cell, is deoxyribonucleic acid (DNA), considered to be the most critical and radiosensitive target molecule.

Water is the most abundant molecule in the body and also the simplest. Water, however, plays a particularly important role in delivering energy to the target molecule, thereby contributing to radiation effects. In addition to water and the macromolecules, there are some trace elements and inorganic salts that are essential to proper metabolism.

Water. The most abundant molecular constituent of the body is water. It consists of two atoms of hydrogen and one atom of oxygen (H_2O) and constitutes approximately 80% of human substance. Humans are basically a structured aqueous suspension. The water molecules exist both in the free, or dissociated, state and in the bound state, that is, bound to other molecules. They provide some form and shape, assist in maintaining body temperature, and enter into some biochemical reactions. During vigorous exercise, body water is lost through perspiration to stabilize temperature and respiration, and it must be replaced to maintain **homeostasis** (the concept of the relative constancy of the internal environment of the human body). Water and carbon dioxide are end products in the **catabolism** (breaking down into smaller units) of macromolecules. **Anabolism,** the production of large molecules from small, and catabolism are collectively termed **metabolism.**

Proteins. Approximately 15% of the molecular composition of the body is protein. Proteins are long-chain macromolecules consisting of a linear sequence of **amino acids** connected by **peptide bonds.** There are twenty-two amino acids used in protein production, or **protein synthesis.** The linear sequence, or arrangement, of these amino acids determines the precise function of the protein molecule. Fig. 26-2 shows the general chemical form of a protein molecule. The generalized formula for a protein is $C_nH_nO_nN_nT_n$, where the subscript n refers to the number of atoms of each element in the molecule. T represents trace elements. In general, 50% of the mass of a protein molecule is carbon, 20% oxygen, 17% nitrogen, 7% hydrogen, and 6% other elements.

Proteins have a variety of uses in the body. They provide structure and support. Muscles are very high in protein content. Proteins also

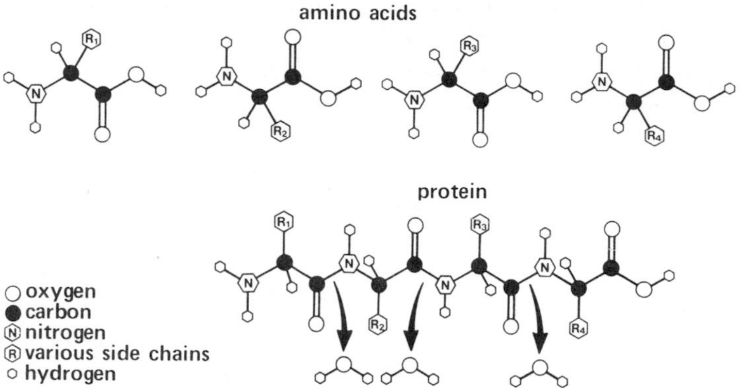

amino acids

protein

○ oxygen
● carbon
Ⓝ nitrogen
Ⓡ various side chains
○ hydrogen

Fig. 26-2. Proteins consist of amino acids linked by peptide bonds. To create the peptide bond, a molecule of water must be removed, as shown.

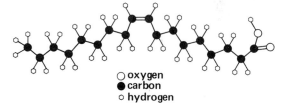

○ oxygen
● carbon
○ hydrogen

Fig. 26-3. Structural configuration of a lipid is represented by the following, a molecule of oleic acid: $CH_3(CH_2)_7CH = CH(CH_2)_7COOH$.

function as enzymes, hormones, and antibodies. **Enzymes** are molecules that are necessary in small quantities to allow a biochemical reaction to continue, even though they do not directly enter into the reaction. **Hormones** are molecules that exercise regulatory control over some body functions such as growth and development. Hormones are produced and secreted by the **endocrine glands**—the pituitary, adrenal, thyroid, parathyroid, pancreas, and gonads. **Antibodies** constitute a primary defense mechanism of the body against infection and disease. The molecular configuration of an antibody may be precise for attacking a particular type of invasive or infectious agent, the **antigen.**

Lipids. Lipids are organic macromolecules composed solely of carbon, hydrogen, and oxygen. They have the general formulation $C_nH_nO_n$. Structurally, lipids have the form shown in Fig. 26-3, and it is this structure that distinguishes them from carbohydrates. In general, lipids are composed of two kinds of smaller molecules, **glycerol** and **fatty acid.** Each lipid molecule is composed of one molecule of glycerol and three molecules of fatty acid.

Lipids are present in all tissues of the body and are the structural components of cell membranes. Lipids often are concentrated just under the skin and serve as a thermal insulator from the environment. Polar mammals, for instance, have a particularly thick layer of subcutaneous fat (blubber) as a means of protection from the cold. Lipids also serve as fuel for the body by providing energy stores. It is more difficult, however, to extract energy from lipids than from the other major fuel source, carbohydrates; this relationship, of course, is associated with the major dilemma in modern nutrition—obesity.

Carbohydrates. Carbohydrates are also called **saccharides. Monosaccharides** and **disaccharides** are sugars. The chemical formula for glucose, a simple sugar, is $C_6H_{12}O_6$. These molecules are relatively small. **Polysaccharides** are large and include plant **starches** and animal **glycogen.** The chemical formula for a polysaccharide is $(C_6H_{10}O_5)_n$, where n is the number of simple sugar molecules in the macromolecule.

Carbohydrates, like lipids, are composed solely of carbon, hydrogen, and oxygen, but their structure is different (Fig. 26-4). This structural difference determines the contribution of the carbohydrate molecule to body biochemistry. The ratio of the number of hydrogen atoms to oxygen atoms in a carbohydrate molecule is 2:1, as in water, and a large fraction of this molecule consists of these atoms. Consequently, carbohydrates were early considered to be watered, or **hydrated,** carbon; hence their name.

The chief function of carbohydrates in the body is to provide fuel for cell metabolism. To a lesser extent, some carbohydrates are incorporated into the structure of cells and tissues to provide shape and stability. The human polysaccharide, glycogen, is stored in the tissues of the body and used as fuel only when the simple sugar, glucose, is not present in adequate quantities. Glucose is the ultimate molecule that fuels the body. Lipids can be catabolized into glucose for energy but only with great difficulty. Polysaccharides are much more readily transformed into glucose. This explains why a chocolate bar, which is high in glucose, can provide a quick burst of energy for an athlete.

Nucleic acids. There are two principal nucleic acids of importance to human metabolism—**deoxyribonucleic acid (DNA)** and **ribonucleic acid (RNA).** DNA is located principally in the nucleus of the cell and serves as the command or control molecule for cell function. DNA contains all the hereditary information representing a cell and, of course, if the cell is a germ cell, all the hereditary information of the whole individual.

RNA is located principally in the cytoplasm, but some is found in the nucleus also. There are two types: messenger RNA (mRNA) and transfer RNA (tRNA). They are distinguished according to their biochemical function. These molecules are involved in the growth and development of the cell through a number of biochemical pathways, notably protein synthesis.

The nucleic acids are very large and extremely complex macromolecules. Fig. 26-5 shows the structural composition of DNA and the manner in which the component molecules are joined. DNA consists of a backbone composed of alternating segments of deoxyribose (a sugar) and phosphate. For each deoxyribose-phosphate conjugate formed, a molecule of water is removed. Attached to each deoxyribose molecule

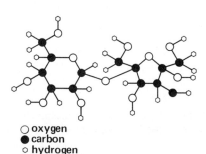

Fig. 26-4. Carbohydrates are structurally different from lipids, even though their compositions are similar. Following is a molecule of sucrose, or ordinary table sugar: ($C_{12}H_{22}O_{11}$).

○ oxygen
● carbon
○ hydrogen

is one of four different nitrogen-containing or nitrogenous organic bases: **adenine, guanine, thymine,** or **cytosine.** Adenine and guanine are **purines;** thymine and cytosine are **pyrimidines.** The base-sugar-phosphate combination is called a **nucleotide,** and the nucleotides are strung together in one long-chain macromolecule. Human DNA exists as two of these long chains attached together in ladder fashion (Fig. 26-6). The side rails of the ladder are the alternating sugar-phosphate molecules, and the rungs of the ladder consist of bases joined together by hy-

drogen bonds. To complete the picture, the ladder is spiraled about an imaginary axis as a spring. This produces a molecule having a **double helix** configuration (Fig. 26-7). The sequence of base bonding is limited to adenines bonded to thymines and cytosines bonded to guanines. **No other base-bonding combinations are possible.**

RNA resembles DNA structurally. The sugar component is ribose rather than deoxyribose, and uracil replaces thymine as a base component.

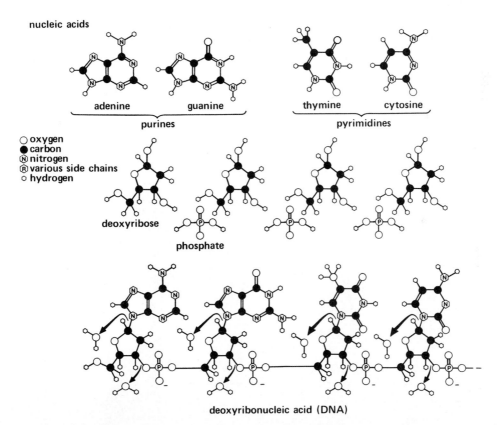

Fig. 26-5. Deoxyribonucleic acid (DNA) is the control center for life. A single molecule consists of a backbone of alternating sugar (deoxyribose) and phosphate molecules. Each sugar molecule has one of the four organic bases attached to it.

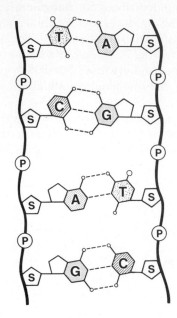

Fig. 26-6. DNA, as found in the cell, consists of two long chains of alternating sugar and phosphate molecules fashioned like the side rails of a ladder with pairs of bases as rungs.

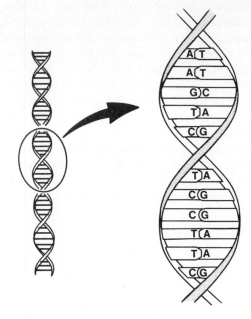

Fig. 26-7. The DNA ladder is twisted about an imaginary axis to form a double helix.

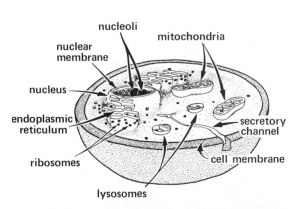

Fig. 26-8. Schematic view of a human cell showing the principal structural components.

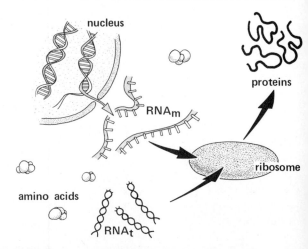

Fig. 26-9. Protein synthesis is a complex process and involves many different molecules and cellular structures.

The human cell

The principal molecular components of the human body are organized intricately into cellular components. These components, or structures, are distributed throughout the cell in assembled fashion much as the parts of an automobile. This assembly ensures proper growth, development, and function of the cell. Fig. 26-8 is a cutaway view of a human cell with its principal parts labeled.

The two major segments of the cell are the **nucleus** and the **cytoplasm.** The principal molecular component of the nucleus is DNA, the genetic material of the cell. The nucleus also contains some RNA, protein, and water. Most of the RNA is contained in a rounded structure, the **nucleolus.** The nucleolus is often attached to the nuclear membrane, a double-walled structure that at some locations is connected to the endoplasmic reticulum. The nature of this connection controls the passage of molecules, particularly RNA, from nucleus to cytoplasm.

The cytoplasm makes up the bulk of the cell and contains all the molecular components in great quantity, except DNA. Found in the cytoplasm are a number of intracellular structures. The endoplasmic reticulum is a channel or series of channels that allows the nucleus to communicate with the cytoplasm. The large bean-shaped structures are **mitochondria.** Macromolecules are digested in the mitochondria to produce energy for the cell. The mitochondria are therefore called the workhorses of the cell. The small dotlike structures are **ribosomes.** Ribosomes are the site of protein synthesis and therefore are essential to the normal cellular function. The small pealike sacs are **lysosomes.** The lysosomes contain enzymes capable of digesting cellular fragments and, in some situations, the cell itself. These are helpful in the control of intracellular contaminants.

All these structures, including the cell itself, are surrounded by membranes. These membranes consist principally of lipid-protein complexes that selectively allow small molecules and water to diffuse from one side to the other. These cellular membranes, of course, also provide structure and form for the cell and its components.

When one irradiates the critical macromolecular cellular components by themselves, a dose of approximately 1 Mrad (10 kGy) is required to produce a measurable change in any physical characteristic of the molecule. When such a molecule, however, is incorporated into the apparatus of a living cell, only a few rad are necessary to produce a measurable biologic response. The dose necessary to produce lethality in some single-cell organisms such as bacteria is measured in kilorad, whereas mammalian cells can be killed with a dose of less than 100 rad (1 Gy).

A number of experiments have been conducted to show that the nucleus is much more sensitive to the effects of radiation than is the cytoplasm. A dose of less than 100 rad (1 Gy) to the nucleus will produce cell death; if only the cytoplasm is irradiated, 1000 rad (10 Gy) or more may be necessary. Such experiments are conducted with either precise microbeams of electrons that can be focused and directed to a precise cell part or through the incorporation of the radioactive isotopes ^{3}H and ^{14}C into cellular molecules that localize exclusively either in the cytoplasm or in the nucleus.

Cell function. Every human cell has a specific function in support of the total body. Some differences are obvious, as with nerve cells, blood cells, and muscle cells. The similarities are also somewhat obvious.

In addition to its specialized function, each cell to some extent performs the function of absorbing through the cell membrane all molecular nutrients and using these nutrients in production of energy and molecular synthesis. If the molecular synthesis is damaged by radiation exposure, the cell may malfunction and die.

Protein synthesis is a good example of a most important and critical cellular function necessary for survival. It is diagrammed in Fig. 26-9. The

DNA, located in the nucleus, contains a molecular code that identifies what proteins that cell will make. This code is determined by the sequence of base pairs adenine-thymine and cytosine-guanine. A series of three base pairs is called a **codon** and identifies one of the twenty-two human amino acids available for protein synthesis. This genetic message is transferred in the nucleus to a molecule of messenger RNA (mRNA). The mRNA leaves the nucleus by way of the endoplasmic reticulum and makes its way to a ribosome, where the genetic message is transferred to yet another RNA molecule called transfer RNA (tRNA). The tRNA searches the cytoplasm for the amino acids for which it is coded. It attaches to the amino acid and carries it to the ribosome, where it is joined with other amino acids in sequence by peptide bonds to form the required protein molecule.

Interference with any phase of this procedure for protein synthesis could result in manifest damage to the cell. Radiation interaction with the molecule having primary control over protein synthesis, DNA, is more effective in producing a response than radiation interaction with other molecules involved in protein synthesis.

Cell proliferation. Although many thousands of rad are necessary to produce physically measurable disruption of macromolecules, single ionizing events at a particularly sensitive site of a critical target molecule are thought to be capable of disrupting cell proliferation. **Cell proliferation** follows growth and development and is the act of a single cell or group of cells reproducing and multiplying in number. This increase in number of cells by reproduction is a result of the process of **cell division,** a mechanism that results in twice the number of cells.

There are two general types of cells in the human body, **somatic cells** and **genetic cells.** The genetic cells are the oogonium of the female and the spermatogonium of the male. All other cells of the body are somatic cells. When somatic cells undergo proliferation, or cell division, they undergo **mitosis.** Genetic cells undergo **meiosis.**

Mitosis. The cell cycle, as visualized by the cell biologist and the geneticist, is diagrammed in Fig. 26-10. Each cycle includes the various states of cell growth, development, and division. The geneticist considers only two phases of the cell cycle: **mitosis (M)** and **interphase.** Mitosis,

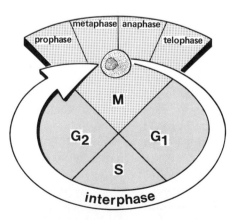

Fig. 26-10. As the cell progresses through one growth cycle, several phases are observed. The cell biologist and the geneticist identify each phase differently.

the division phase, is characterized by four sub-phases: **prophase, metaphase, anaphase,** and **telophase.** The portion of the cell cycle between mitotic events is termed interphase. Interphase is the period of growth of the cell between divisions.

The cell biologist usually identifies four phases of the cell cycle: M, G_1, S, and G_2. These phases of the cell cycle are characterized by the structure of the chromosomes, which contain the genetic material DNA. G_1 is the **gap** in the cell growth between M and S. It is termed the pre-DNA synthesis phase. S is the DNA synthesis phase. During this period, each DNA molecule is replicated into two identical daughter DNA molecules. The chromosome is transformed from a structure with two chromatids attached to a centromere to a structure with four chromatids attached to a centromere (Fig. 26-11). The result is two pairs of homologous chromatids, that is, chromatids having precisely the same DNA content and structure. The G_2 phase is the post-DNA synthesis gap of cell growth.

During interphase, the chromosomes are not visible; however, during mitosis, the DNA slowly takes the form of the chromosome as we know it. Fig. 26-12 shows the process of mitosis schematically. During **prophase,** the nucleus swells and the DNA becomes more prominent and begins to take structural form. At **metaphase** the chromosomes appear and are lined up along the equator of the nucleus. It is during metaphase that mitosis can be stopped and chromosomes studied carefully under the microscope. **Radiation-induced chromosome damage is analyzed during metaphase. Anaphase** is characterized by each chromosome splitting at the centromere so that a centromere and two chromatids are connected by a fiber to the poles of the nucleus. These poles are called **spindles,** and the fibers are **spindle fibers.** The number of chromatids per centromere has been reduced by half, and these newly formed chromosomes migrate slowly toward the nuclear spindle. The final segment of mitosis, **telophase,** is characterized by the disappearance of the structural chromosomes into a mass of DNA and the closing off of the nuclear membrane like a dumbbell into two nuclei. At the same time the cytoplasm is divided into two equal parts, each accompanying one of the new nuclei.

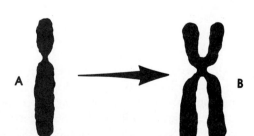

A　　　　　　　　　　　　　　　　B

Fig. 26-11. During the synthesis portion of interphase, the chromosomes replicate from a two-chromatid structure to a four-chromatid structure. **A,** Two-chromatid structure. **B,** Four-chromatid structure.

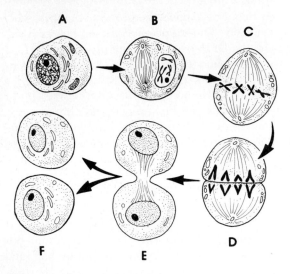

Fig. 26-12. Mitosis is the phase of the cell cycle during which the chromosomes become visible, divide, and migrate to daughter cells. **A**, Interphase. **B**, Prophase. **C**, Metaphase. **D**, Anaphase. **E**, Telophase. **F**, Interphase.

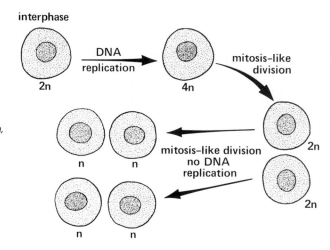

Fig. 26-13. Meiosis is the process of reduction and division, and it occurs only in germ cells. *n*, Number of similar chromosomes.

Cell division is now complete. The two daughter cells appear precisely as the parent and contain exactly the same genetic material.

Meiosis. Changes in genetic material can occur during the division process of genetic cells, called meiosis. The primary genetic cells, the germ cells, begin with the same number of chromosomes as somatic cells (forty-six). But for a germ cell to be capable of marriage with another germ cell, its complement of chromosomes must be reduced in half to twenty-three so that, following conception and the union of two germ cells, the daughter cells will contain forty-six chromosomes. This process of **reduction division** of germ cells is called meiosis (Fig. 26-13).

The primary germ cell begins meiosis with forty-six chromosomes, appearing as a somatic cell having completed G_2 phase. It then progresses through the phases of mitosis into two daughter cells, each containing forty-six chromosomes of two chromatids each. The names of the subphases of meiosis and mitosis are the same. Each of the daughter cells of this first division now progresses through a second division in which all the cellular material is divided, including the chromosomes; however, the second division is not accompanied by an S phase, and therefore there is no replication of DNA and consequently no duplication of the chromosomes. The resulting granddaughter cells contain only twenty-three chromosomes each. Each parent has undergone two division processes, resulting in four daughter cells. During the second division, there is some exchange of chromosomal material among chromatids by a process called **crossing-over,** and this results in changes in genetic constitution and heritable traits.

Tissues and organs

During the development and maturation of a human from the two united germ cells, a number of different types of cells evolve. Collections of cells of similar structure and function form **tissues.** Following is a breakdown of the composition of the body according to its tissue constituents:

Tissue	Abundance
Muscle	43%
Fat	14%
Organs	12.4%
Skeleton	10%
Blood	7.7%
Bone marrow	4.2%
Subcutaneous tissue	5.8%
Skin	2.9%

These tissues in turn are bound together in precise fashion to form **organs.** The tissues and the organs of the body serve as discrete units with specific functional responsibilities. Some tissues and organs will combine into an overall integrated organization known as an **organ system.** The principal organ systems of the body are the nervous system, the digestive system, the endocrine system, and the reproductive system.

The effects of radiation that appear at the whole-body level result from damage to these organ systems, which in turn are a result of radiation injury to the cells of that system.

The cells of a tissue system are identified by their rate of proliferation and their stage of development. Immature cells are called **undifferentiated cells, precursor cells,** or **stem cells.** As a cell matures through growth and proliferation, it can pass through various stages of differentiation into a fully functional and mature cell. The sensitivity of the cell to radiation is determined to some degree by its state of maturity and its functional role. Generally speaking, immature cells are considerably more sensitive to radiation than mature cells. Following is a list of a number of different cell lines in the body according to their degree of radiosensitivity:

Radiosensitivity	Cell type
High	Lymphocytes
	Spermatogonia
	Erythroblasts
	Intestinal crypt cells
Intermediate	Endothelial cells
	Osteoblasts
	Spermatids
	Fibroblasts
Low	Muscle cells
	Nerve cells
	Chondrocytes

The tissues and organs of the body consist of both stem cells and mature cells. There are several types of tissue, and they can be classified according to structural or functional features. These features influence the degree of radiosensitivity of the tissue. **Epithelium** is the covering tissue, and it lines all exposed surfaces of the body, both exterior and interior. Epithelium covers the skin, the blood vessels, the abdominal and chest cavities, and the gastrointestinal tract. **Connective** and **supporting tissues** are high in protein and are composed principally of fibers that usually have a high degree of elasticity. Connective tissue binds tissues and organs together;

bone and cartilage are examples. **Muscle** is a special type of tissue that is capable of contracting. It is found throughout the body and also is high in protein content. **Nervous tissue** is also called **conductive tissue** and consists of specialized cells called **neurons** that have long, thin extensions from the cell to distant parts of the body. Nervous tissue is the avenue through which electrical impulses are transmitted throughout the body for control and response.

When these various types of tissue are combined to form an organ, they are identified according to two parts of the organ. The **parenchymal** part contains tissues that are representative of that particular organ, whereas the **stromal** part is composed of connective tissue and vasculature that provides structure to the organ.

Table 26-1. The relative radiosensitivity of tissues and organs based on clinical radiotherapy

Level of radiosensitivity (rad)*	Tissue or organ	Effects
High: 200 to 1000	Lymphoid tissue	Atrophy
	Bone marrow	Hypoplasia
	Gonads	Atrophy
Intermediate: 1000 to 5000	Skin	Erythema
	Gastrointestinal tract	Ulcer
	Cornea	Cataract
	Growing bone	Growth arrest
	Kidney	Nephrosclerosis
	Liver	Ascites
	Thyroid	Atrophy
Low: >5000	Muscle	Fibrosis
	Brain	Necrosis
	Spinal cord	Transection

*The minimum dose delivered at the rate of approximately 200 rad per day that will produce a response.

When considering the early effects of radiation exposure of high dose levels, it is organ damage that ultimately results in observable effects. The various organs of the body exhibit a wide range of sensitivity to radiation. This radiosensitivity is determined by (1) the function of the organ to the body, (2) the rate at which cells mature and are turned over in the organ, and (3) the inherent radiosensitivity of the cell type.

A precise knowledge of these various organ radiosensitivities is unnecessary; however, knowledge of the general levels of radiosensitivity, as shown in Table 26-1, is helpful in understanding the effects of whole-body radiation exposure and, in particular, the acute radiation syndrome.

LAW OF BERGONIÉ AND TRIBONDEAU

In 1906 two French scientists, Bergonié and Tribondeau, theorized and observed that radiosensitivity was a function of the metabolic state of the tissue being irradiated. This has come to be known as the Law of Bergonié and Tribondeau and has been verified many times. Basically, the law states that the radiosensitivity of living tissue varies as follows:

1. Stem cells are radiosensitive. The more mature a cell is, the more resistant to radiation it is.
2. The younger tissues and organs are, the more radiosensitive they are.
3. When the level of metabolic activity is high, radiosensitivity is also high.
4. As the proliferation rate for cells and the growth rate for tissues increase, the radiosensitivity increases also.

This law is of interest principally as a historical note in the development of radiobiology. However, it has found some application in radiotherapy. In diagnostic radiology it serves to remind us that the fetus is considerably more sensitive to radiation exposure than the child or the mature adult.

PHYSICAL FACTORS AFFECTING RADIOSENSITIVITY

When one irradiates a biologic medium, the response of the medium will be determined principally by the amount of energy deposited per unit mass—the dose in rad (Gy). However, even under controlled experimental conditions, when equal doses are delivered to equal specimens, the response may not be the same because of other modifying factors. There are a number of physical factors that affect the degree of radiation response.

Linear energy transfer

The linear energy transfer (LET) is a measure of the rate at which energy is transferred from ionizing radiation to soft tissue. It is another method of expressing **radiation quality** and determining the value of the **quality factor** used in radiation protection. It has units of keV of energy transferred per micrometer of track length in soft tissue (keV/μm). The ability of ionizing radiation to produce a biologic response increases as the LET of radiation increases. The following list shows the approximate LET of various types of ionizing radiation. The LET of diagnostic x rays is about 3 keV/μm, which is relatively low among all radiations.

Type of radiation	LET (keV/μm)
25 MV x rays	0.2
^{60}Co rays	0.25
1 MeV electrons	0.3
Diagnostic x rays	3.0
10 MeV protons	4.0
Fast neutrons	50.0
5 MeV alpha particles	100.0
Heavy nuclei	1000.0

Relative biologic effectiveness

As the LET of radiation increases, the ability to produce biologic damage also increases. This relative effect is quantitatively described by the relative biologic effectiveness (RBE). The RBE is defined as follows:

(26-1)

$$RBE = \frac{\text{Dose of standard radiation necessary}}{\text{Dose of test radiation necessary}}$$
to produce a given effect over to produce the same effect

The standard radiation, by convention, is orthovoltage x-radiation in the 200 to 250 kVp range. Diagnostic x rays have an RBE of 1. Radiations with lower LET than diagnostic x rays have an RBE less than 1, whereas radiations with higher LET have a higher RBE. Fig. 26-14 shows the relationship between RBE and LET and identifies some of the more common types of radiation. The maximum value of the RBE is approximately 3.

EXAMPLE: When mice are irradiated with 250 kVp x rays, 640 rad (6.4 Gy) are necessary to produce death. If similar mice are irradiated with fast neutrons, only 210 rad (2.1 Gy) are needed. What is the RBE for the fast neutrons?

ANSWER: $RBE = \dfrac{650 \text{ rad}}{210 \text{ rad}}$

$= 3.1$

Fractionation and protraction

If a dose of radiation is delivered over a long period of time rather than quickly, the effect of that dose will be less. Stated differently, if the time of irradiation is lengthened, a higher dose will be required to produce the same effect. This lengthening of time can be accomplished in two ways.

If the dose is delivered continuously but at a lower dose rate, it is said to be **protracted.** Six hundred rad (6 Gy) delivered in 3 minutes (200 rad/min [2 Gy/min]) is lethal for a mouse. However, when 600 rad is delivered at the rate of 1 rad/hr (10 mGy/hr), the mouse will survive. Dose protraction is less effective because of the lower dose rate and the longer irradiation time.

If the 600 rad dose is delivered at the same dose rate, 200 rad/min, but in 12 equal fractions of 50 rad (500 mGy), each separated by 24 hours, the mouse will survive. In this situation the dose

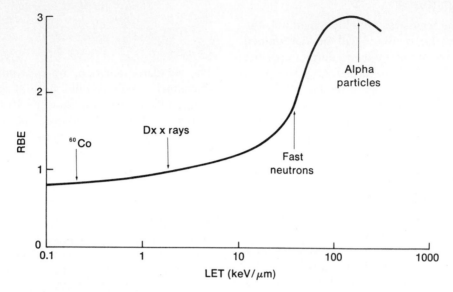

Fig. 26-14. As LET increases, RBE increases also, but a maximum value is reached beyond which the RBE can increase no further.

is said to be **fractionated.** Dose fractionation is less effective because tissue repair and recovery occur between doses. Dose fractionation is employed routinely in radiation therapy.

BIOLOGIC FACTORS AFFECTING RADIOSENSITIVITY

In addition to these physical factors, there are a number of biologic conditions that alter the radiation response of biologic specimens. Some of these factors have to do with the inherent state of the specimen, such as age, sex, and metabolic rate. Other factors are related to artifically introduced modifiers of the biologic system.

Oxygen effect

Biologic tissue is more sensitive to radiation when irradiated in the oxygenated, or aerobic, state than when irradiated under anoxic (without oxygen) or hypoxic (low-oxygen) conditions. This characteristic of biologic tissue is called the oxygen effect and is described numerically by the **oxygen enhancement ratio** (OER). The OER is calculated as follows:

(26-2)

$$OER = \frac{\textit{Dose necessary under anoxic conditions to produce a given effect}}{\textit{Dose necessary under aerobic conditions to produce the same effect}}$$

Generally, the irradiation of biologic tissue is conducted under conditions of full oxygenation. Hyperbaric (high-pressure) oxygen has been used in radiation therapy in an attempt to increase the radiosensitivity of nodular, avascular tumors, which are less radiosensitive than tumors with an adequate blood supply. Diagnostic x rays are administered under conditions of full oxygenation.

EXAMPLE: When experimental mouse mammary carcinomas are clamped and irradiated under hypoxic

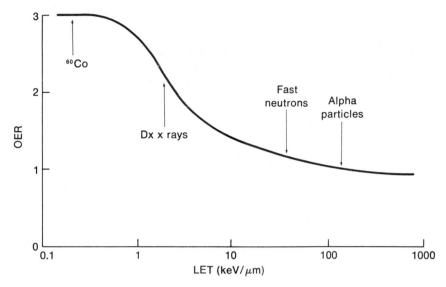

Fig. 26-15. The OER is high for low-LET radiation and decreases in value as the LET increases.

conditions, the tumor control dose is 10,600 rad (106 Gy). When the tumors are not clamped and are irradiated under aerobic conditions, the tumor control dose is 4050 rad (40.5 Gy). What is the OER for this system?

ANSWER:
$$OER = \frac{10,600}{4050}$$
$$= 2.6$$

The OER is LET dependent. As Fig. 26-15 shows, the OER is greatest for low-LET radiation, having a maximum of approximately 3, and decreases to approximately 1 for high-LET radiation.

Age

The age of a biologic structure affects its radiosensitivity. The response of humans is characteristic of this age-related radiosensitivity and is shown in Fig. 26-16. Humans are most sensitive before birth. The sensitivity then decreases until maturity, the time we are most resistant to radiation-induced effects. In old age humans again become somewhat more radiosensitive.

Sex

Many experiments have been conducted to determine which sex is most resistant to the effects of radiation. The results are not all in agreement, nor are they conclusive; however, taken together, the indication is that the female can sustain approximately 5% to 10% more radiation than the male. **Females, therefore, are less radiosensitive than males.**

Recovery

It has been shown without question from experiments in vitro that human cells are capable of recovering from radiation damage. If the radiation dose is not sufficient to kill the cell before its next division (**interphase death**), then given

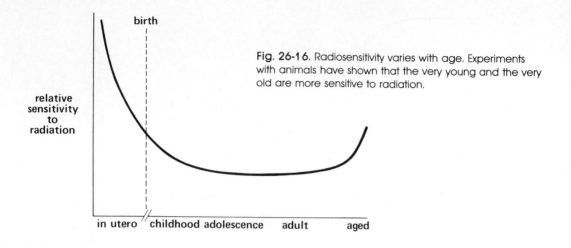

Fig. 26-16. Radiosensitivity varies with age. Experiments with animals have shown that the very young and the very old are more sensitive to radiation.

sufficient time the cell will recover from the **sub-lethal radiation damage** it sustained. This intracellular recovery is due to a **repair** mechanism inherent in the biochemistry of the cell. Some types of cells have greater capacity for repair of this sublethal damage than do others.

At the whole-body level this recovery from radiation damage is assisted through **repopulation** by the surviving cells. If a tissue or organ receives a sufficient radiation dose, it will respond by shrinking in size. This is called **atrophy** and occurs because some cells die, disintegrate, and are carried away as waste products. If a sufficient number of cells sustain only sublethal damage and survive, they may proliferate and repopulate the irradiated tissue or organ. The combined processes of repair and repopulation contribute to **recovery** from radiation damage.

Chemical agents

Some chemicals can modify the response of cells, tissues, and organs to radiation. For the chemical agents to be effective, they generally must be present at the time of irradiation. Post-irradiation application will not usually alter the degree of response.

Radiosensitizers. Agents that enhance the effect of radiation are called **sensitizing agents.** Some examples are halogenated pyrimidines, methotrexate, actinomycin D, hydroxyurea, and vitamin K. The halogenated pyrimidines become incorporated into the DNA of the cell and cause the radiation effects on that molecule to be amplified. All the radiosensitizers have an effectiveness ratio to about 2; that is, if 90% of a cell culture is killed by 200 rad (2 Gy), then in the presence of a sensitizing agent only 100 rad (1 Gy) will be required for the same percent lethality.

Radioprotectors. The radioprotective compounds include molecules containing a sulfhydryl group (sulfur and hydrogen bound together) such as cysteine and cysteamine. Hundreds of others have been tested and found effective to within a ratio of approximately 2. For example, if 500 rad (5 Gy) is a lethal dose to a mouse, then in the presence of a radioprotective agent 1000 rad (10 Gy) would be required to produce lethality. Radioprotective agents have not found human application because, to be effective, they must be administered in a toxic dose level. The protective agent can be worse than the radiation!

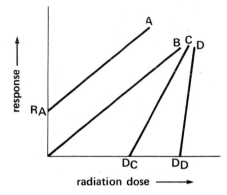

Fig. 26-17. Linear dose-response relationships *A* and *B* are nonthreshold types. *C* and *D* are threshold types.

RADIATION DOSE-RESPONSE RELATIONSHIPS

Radiobiology is a relatively new science. Although some scientists were working with animals to observe the effects of radiation within a few years of the discovery of x rays, these studies were not experimentally sound, nor were their results applied. However, interest in radiobiology increased enormously during the 1940s with the advent of the atomic age.

The object of nearly all radiobiologic research is the establishment of radiation dose-response relationships. A dose-response relationship is a mathematic or graphic relationship between graded levels of radiation dose and the magnitude of the observed response.

Radiation dose-response relationships have two important applications in radiology. First, these experimentally determined relationships are used to design therapeutic treatment routines for patients suffering from malignant disease. Second, radiobiologic studies have been designed to provide information on the effects of low-dose irradiation. These studies and the dose-response relationships obtained are the basis for our radiation control activities and are of particular significance to diagnostic radiology.

Linear dose-response relationships

Every dose-response relationship has two characteristics. It is either linear or nonlinear, and it is either threshold or nonthreshold. These characteristics can be described mathematically or graphically; for the purpose of this discussion the various radiation dose-response relationships will be described graphically.

Fig. 26-17 shows examples of the simplest type. The linear dose-response relationship is so called because the response is directly proportional to the dose. When the radiation dose is doubled, the response to radiation is likewise doubled.

Dose-response relationships *A* and *B* intersect the dose axis at zero or below. These relationships are therefore of the **linear, nonthreshold type.** In a nonthreshold dose-response relationship, any dose, regardless of its size, is expected to produce a response. At zero dose, relationship *A* exhibits a measurable response, R_A. The level R_A is called the **ambient,** or natural, response level and indicates that even without a radiation exposure the response occurs.

Dose-response relationships *C* and *D* are identified as **linear, threshold** because they intercept the dose axis at some value greater than zero. The threshold doses for *C* and *D* are D_C and D_D, respectively. At dose levels below these values, no response would be expected. Relationship *D* has a steeper slope than *C*, and therefore, above the threshold dose, any increment of dose will produce a larger response if it follows relationship *D* rather than *C*.

Nonlinear dose-response relationships

All other dose-response relationships are defined as nonlinear. Fig. 26-18 illustrates some examples of nonlinear dose-response relationships.

Curves *A* and *B* are **nonlinear, nonthreshold.** In relationship *A* a large response will result from very little radiation dose. At high dose levels the radiation is not so efficient, since an incremental dose at high levels results in less relative damage than the same incremental dose at low levels. Relationship *B* is just the opposite. Incremental doses in the low dose range result in very little response. At high doses, however, the same increment of dose will produce a much larger response.

Curve *C* is a **nonlinear, threshold** relationship. At doses below D_C no response will be measured. As the dose is increased above D_C, it becomes increasingly effective per increment of dose until it reaches the dose corresponding to the inflection point of the curve. Above this level, incremental doses become less effective. Relationship *C* is sometimes called an **S-type,** or **sigmoid-type,** dose-response relationship.

We shall refer to these general types of radiation dose-response relationships in discussing the forms of human radiation injury. **Diagnostic radiology is almost exclusively concerned with the late effects of radiation exposure and therefore with linear, nonthreshold dose-response relationships.** However, for completeness, Chapter 28 contains a brief discussion of early radiation damage.

Constructing a dose-response relationship

Determining the dose-response relationship for a whole-body response is tricky. It is very difficult to determine the degree of response, even that of early effects, because the number

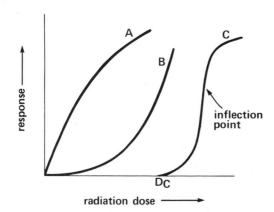

Fig. 26-18. Nonlinear dose-response relationships can assume several shapes.

of experimental animals that can be used is relatively small. It is near impossible to measure low-dose, late effects, and that is the area of greatest interest to radiology.

Therefore we resort to irradiating a limited number of animals to very large doses of radiation in hopes of observing a statistically significant response. Fig. 26-19 shows the results of such an experiment in which four groups of animals were irradiated at a different dose. The observations on each group results in an ordered pair of data—a dose and the associated response.

The error bars in each ordered pair indicate the confidence associated with each data point. The error bars on the dose measurements are very narrow; we can measure dose very accurately. The error bars on the response, however, are very wide because of biologic variability and the limited number of observations at each dose.

Our principal interest in diagnostic radiology is to estimate the response at very low radiation doses. Since this cannot be done directly, we **extrapolate** the dose-response relationship from the high-dose, known region into the low-dose, unknown region. This invariably results in a **linear, nonthreshold** dose-response relationship. Such an extrapolation, however, may not be correct because of the many qualifying conditions on the experiment.

Linear, quadratic dose-response relationship

The Committee on the Biological Effects of Ionizing Radiations (BEIR) of the National Academy of Sciences not long ago completed an exhaustive study of scientific data bearing on the effects of low doses of low-LET radiation. Therefore their findings are directly applicable to diagnostic radiology.

The committee's conclusion was that such effects follow a **linear, quadratic dose-response relationship** such as that shown in Fig. 26-20. The essence of its finding is that the linear, nonthreshold relationship overestimates the risk associated with diagnostic radiation. Although we continue to use the linear, nonthreshold model for establishing radiation protection guidance because that is the conservative approach, it now appears that low doses of low-LET radiation are safer than we previously assumed.

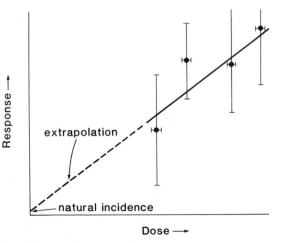

Fig. 26-19. A dose-response relationship is produced by extrapolating high-dose experimental data to low doses.

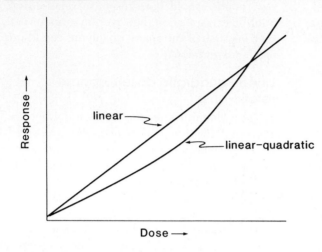

Fig. 26-20. The linear, quadratic dose-response relationship applies to low-dose, low-LET, late radiation effects.

REVIEW QUESTIONS

1. Define or otherwise identify the following:
   a. Robert Hooke
   b. Lipids
   c. Catabolism
   d. Polysaccharides
   e. Mitochondria
   f. Ribosome
   g. Meiosis
   h. Stem cell
   i. Parenchyma
   j. LET
2. Identify three types of proteins and the function of each.
3. Diagram the structural configuration of DNA and include the permitted base pairing.

4. Describe the process of protein synthesis.
5. Identify all the phases of the cell cycle.
6. What are the four statements describing the Law of Bergonié and Tribondeau?
7. Approximately 800 rad (8 Gy) of 220 kVp x rays are necessary to produce death in the armadillo, Cobalt-60 gamma rays have a lower LET than 220 kVp x rays, and therefore 940 rad (9.4 Gy) is required for armadillo lethality. What is the RBE of ^{60}Co compared with 220 kVp?
8. Under fully oxygenated conditions, 90% of human cells in culture will be killed by 150 rad (1.5 Gy) x rays. If the cells are made anoxic, the dose required for 90% lethality is 400 rad (4 Gy). What is the OER?

27

Molecular and cellular radiobiology

IRRADIATION OF MACROMOLECULES
RADIOLYSIS OF WATER
DIRECT AND INDIRECT EFFECT
TARGET THEORY
CELL SURVIVAL KINETICS
LET, RBE, AND OER

Although the initial interaction between radiation and tissue occurs at the atomic level, it is believed that observable human radiation injury results from molecular derangement.

Such molecular derangements or lesions that occur can be conveniently separated into either effects on macromolecules or effects on water. The results of irradiation of macromolecules are quite different from those of irradiation of water. When macromolecules are irradiated **in vitro,** that is, outside the body or outside the cell, a considerable radiation dose is required to produce a measurable effect. **In vivo** irradiation, that is, irradiation of macromolecules in the living cell, demonstrates that molecules are considerably more radiosensitive in their natural state.

IRRADIATION OF MACROMOLECULES

A **solution** is a suspension of particles or molecules in a **fluid** such as water. A mixture of fluids such as water and alcohol is also a solution. When macromolecules are irradiated in solution in vitro, three major effects occur (Fig. 27-1).

Main-chain scission is the breakage of the thread or backbone of the long-chain macromolecule. The result is the reduction of a long single molecule into many smaller molecules, each of which may still be macromolecular in nature. Main-chain scission not only reduces the size of the macromolecule, but also reduces the **viscosity** of the solution. A viscous solution is one that is very thick and slow to flow, such as cold maple syrup. Tap water, on the other hand, has a low viscosity. Measurements of viscosity or sedimentation rates are employed to determine the degree of main-chain scission.

Some macromolecules have small spurlike molecules extending off the main chain. Others produce them as a consequence of irradiation. Following irradiation, these side structures can behave as though they had a sticky substance on

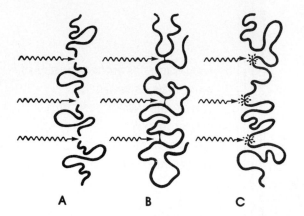

Fig. 27-1. The results of irradiation of macromolecules.
A, Main-chain scission. **B,** Cross-linking. **C,** Point lesions.

the end, and they will attach to a neighboring macromolecule or to another segment of the same molecule. This process is called **cross-linking.** Radiation-induced molecular cross-linking will increase the viscosity of a macromolecular solution. This radiation response has been used to some advantage in the manufacture of stronger fiberboard materials. A high dose of radiation to the cellulose fiber and glue mixture of fiberboard results in considerably more strength and durability.

Finally, radiation interaction with macromolecules can result in disruption of single chemical bonds, producing **molecular lesions** or **point lesions.** Such point lesions are not detectable by current analytic techniques, but they can result in a minor modification of the molecule, which can in turn cause it to malfunction in the cell. **At low radiation doses, point lesions are considered to be the cellular radiation damage resulting in the late radiation effects observed at the whole-body level.**

Laboratory experiments have shown that all these types of radiation effects on macromolecules are reversible through intracellular repair and recovery.

Macromolecular synthesis

Modern molecular biology has developed a generalized scheme for the function of a normal human cell. Molecular nutrients are brought to the cell and diffused through the cell membrane, where they are broken down (**catabolism**) into smaller molecular units with the accompanying release of energy. This energy is expended in several ways, but one of the more important is in the construction, or synthesis, of macromolecules from smaller molecules (**anabolism**). The synthesis of proteins and nucleic acids, both DNA and RNA is critical to the survival of the cell and to its replication.

In Chapter 26 the scheme of protein synthesis and its dependence on nucleic acids was described. Proteins are manufactured by **translation** of the genetic code from tRNA, which in turn was **transferred** from mRNA. The information carried by the mRNA was in turn **transcribed** from the DNA. This chain of events is shown schematically in Fig. 27-2.

Radiation damage to any of these marcomolecules may result in cell death or late effects. Proteins are continuously synthesized throughout the cell cycle and occur in much more abun-

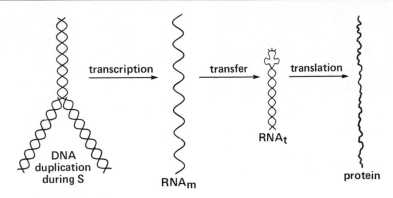

Fig. 27-2. The genetic code of the DNA is transcribed by mRNA and transferred to tRNA, which translates it into a protein at the ribosome.

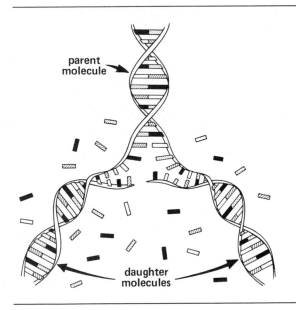

Fig. 27-3. During S phase, the DNA separates like a zipper and two daughter DNA molecules are formed, each alike and each a replicate of the parent molecule.

dance than do the nucleic acids. Furthermore, multiple copies of specific protein molecules are always present in the cell. Consequently, proteins are less radiosensitive than the nucleic acids. Similarly, multiple copies of both types of RNA molecules are present in the cell, though not so many as protein molecules. On the other hand, the DNA molecule, with its unique as-

sembly of bases, is not so abundant. It is therefore **the most radiosensitive of these macromolecules.** RNA radiosensitivity is intermediate between that of DNA and protein.

DNA is synthesized somewhat differently than proteins. During the G_1 portion of interphase, the deoxyribose, phosphate, and base molecules accumulate in the nucleus. These molecules combine to form one large conjugated molecule that, during the S portion of interphase, is attached to an existing single chain of DNA (Fig. 27-3). During G_1, the molecular DNA is in the familiar double helix form. As the cell moves into S phase, the ladder begins to open up in the middle of each rung, much like a zipper. Now the DNA consists of only a single chain, and there is no pairing of bases. However, this state does not exist long because the combined base-sugar-phosphate molecule attaches to the single strand DNA sequence as determined by the permitted base pairing. Consequently, where there was one double helix DNA molecule, there now are two similar molecules, each a duplicate of the original. **In G_2 there is twice as much DNA as in G_1.** The parent DNA is said to be replicated into two duplicate DNA daughter molecules.

Radiation effects on DNA

Deoxyribonucleic acid is the most important molecule in the human body because it contains the genetic information for each cell. Each cell has a nucleus containing DNA complexed with other molecules in the form of chromosomes. The chromosomes therefore control the growth and development of the cell, which in turn determine the characteristics of the individual. This organization is shown in Fig. 27-4.

If radiation damage to the DNA is sufficiently severe, visible chromosome aberrations may be detected. Fig. 27-5 is a representation of a normal chromosome and several distinct types of chromosome aberrations. Radiation-induced **chromosome aberrations,** or **cytogenetic damage,** are discussed more completely in Chapter 28.

The DNA molecule can be damaged without

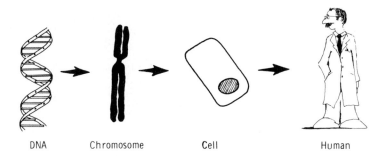

DNA   Chromosome   Cell   Human

Fig. 27-4. DNA is perhaps the most important molecule subject to radiation damage. It forms chromosomes and controls cell and human growth and development.

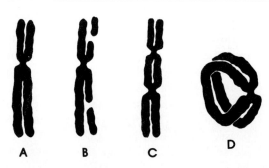

Fig. 27-5. Normal and radiation-damaged human chromosomes. **A,** Normal. **B,** Terminal deletion. **C,** Dicentric formation. **D,** Ring formation.

the production of a visible chromosome aberration. Although such damage is reversible, it can lead to cell death. If enough cells of the same type respond similarly, then a particular tissue or organ can be destroyed. Damage to the DNA can also result in abnormal metabolic activity, such as the uncontrolled rapid proliferation of cells, the principal characteristic of radiation-induced malignant disease. If the damage to the DNA occurs in a germ cell, then it is possible that the manifest response to the radiation exposure will not be observed until the following generation or even later.

The chromosome contains miles of DNA, and therefore, when a visible aberration does appear, it signifies a considerable amount of radiation damage. Unobserved damage to the DNA is also responsible for responses at the cell and whole-body level. The types of damage that can occur in the DNA molecule fall into the categories previously discussed for macromolecules, which follow:

1. Main-chain scission with only one side rail severed
2. Main-chain scission with both side rails severed
3. Main-chain scission and subsequent cross-linking
4. Rung breakage causing a separation of bases
5. A change or loss of a base

Damage types 1 through 4 are diagrammed schematically in Fig. 27-6. Although each of these effects results in a structural change in the DNA molecule, they are all reversible. In some of these types of damage the sequence of bases can be altered, and therefore the triplet code of codons may not remain intact. This represents a genetic mutation at the molecular level.

The fifth type of damage, the change or loss of a base, also destroys the triplet code and may not be reversible. This type of radiation damage is also a type of genetic mutation.

These molecular genetic mutations are called **point mutations** and can be of either minor or major importance to the cell. One critical consequence of such point mutations is the transfer of the incorrect genetic code to one of the two daughter cells. This sequence of events is shown in Fig. 27-7.

In summary, there are three principal observable effects resulting from irradiation of

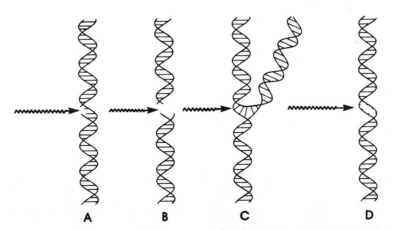

Fig. 27-6. Types of damage that can occur in DNA. A, One side rail severed. B, Both side rails severed. C, Cross-linking. D, Rung breakage.

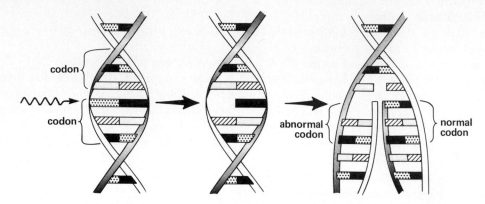

Fig. 27-7. Point mutation results in the change or loss of a base, which creates an abnormal codon and can produce an aberrant gene. This is therefore a genetic mutation that is passed to one of the daughter cells.

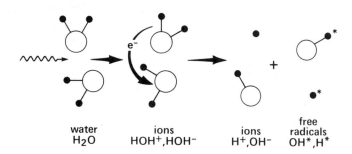

Fig. 27-8. Radiolysis of water results in the formation of ions and free radicals.

DNA: cell death, malignant disease, and genetic damage. The latter two effects **at the molecular level** apparently conform to the **linear, non-threshold** dose-response relationship.

RADIOLYSIS OF WATER

Since the human body is an aqueous solution containing approximately 80% water molecules, irradiation of water represents the principal interaction in the body. When water is irradiated, it dissociates into other molecular products, and this action is termed the **radiolysis of water** (Fig. 27-8).

When an atom of water (H_2O) is irradiated, it is ionized and dissociates into two ions—an ion pair—as shown by the following equation:

(27-1)

$$H_2O + \int \rightarrow HOH^+ + e^-$$

Following this initial ionization, a number of reactions can happen. First, the ion pair may rejoin into a stable water molecule. In this case no damage occurs. Second, if these ions do not rejoin, it is then possible that the negative ion (the electron) would attach to another water molecule by the following reaction and produce yet a third type of ion:

$$(27\text{-}2)$$

$$H_2O + e^- \rightarrow HOH^-$$

The HOH^+ and HOH^- ions are relatively unstable and can dissociate into still smaller molecules as follows:

$$(27\text{-}3)$$

$$HOH^+ \rightarrow H^+ + OH^*$$

$$(27\text{-}4)$$

$$HOH^- \rightarrow OH^- + H^*$$

The final result of the radiolysis of water is therefore the formation of an ion pair, H^+ and OH^-, and two free radicals, H^* and OH^*. The ions can recombine, and therefore no biologic damage would occur. These types of ions are not unusual. Many molecules in aqueous solution exist in a loosely ionized state because of their structure. Salt (NaCl), for instance, easily dissociates into Na^+ and Cl^- ions. Even in the absence of radiation, water can dissociate into H^+ and OH^- ions.

The free radicals are another story. **A free radical is an uncharged molecule containing a single unpaired electron in the valence or outermost shell,** and this causes them to be highly reactive. Free radicals are unstable and therefore exist with a lifetime of less than 1 ms. However, during that time they are capable of diffusion through the cell and of interaction at a distant site. Free radicals contain excess energy that can be transferred to other molecules to disrupt bonds and produce point lesions at some distance from the initial ionizing event.

The H^* and OH^* molecules are not the only free radicals that are produced during the radiolysis of water. The OH^* free radical can join with a similar molecule and form hydrogen peroxide by the following equation:

$$(27\text{-}5)$$

$$OH^* + OH^- \rightarrow H_2O_2$$

Hydrogen peroxide is poisonous to the cell and therefore acts as a toxic agent.

The H^* free radical can interact with molecular oxygen if it is present to form the hydroperoxyl radical:

$$(27\text{-}6)$$

$$H^* + O_2 \rightarrow HO_2^*$$

The hydroperoxyl radical, along with hydrogen peroxide, is considered to be the principal damaging product following the radiolysis of water. Hydrogen peroxide can also be formed by interaction of two hydroperoxyl radicals:

$$(27\text{-}7)$$

$$HO_2^* + HO_2^* \rightarrow H_2O_2 + O_2$$

Some organic molecules, symbolized as RH, can become reactive free radicals as follows:

$$(27\text{-}8)$$

$$RH + \int \rightarrow RH^+ \rightarrow H^+ + R^*$$

When oxygen is present, yet another species of free radical is possible:

$$(27\text{-}9)$$

$$R^* + O_2 \rightarrow RO_2^*$$

DIRECT AND INDIRECT EFFECT

When biologic material is irradiated in vivo, the harmful effects of irradiation occur because of damage to a particular sensitive molecular structure such as DNA. **If the initial ionizing event occurs on that molecule, the effect is said to be direct.** Evidence for the direct effect of radiation comes from in vitro experiments where various molecules can be irradiated in isolation. The effect is produced by ionization of the target molecule.

On the other hand, if the initial ionizing event

occurs on a distant, noncritical molecule that transfers the energy of ionization to the target molecule, the **indirect effect** has occurred. Free radicals, with their excess energy of reaction, are the intermediate molecules. They migrate to the target molecule and transfer their energy, which results in damage to that target molecule.

It is not possible to identify whether the damage to the target molecule resulted from direct or indirect effect. However, since the human body is 80% water, it follows that **the principal action of radiation on humans is indirect.** Most would agree that more than 95% of the effects of radiation in vivo occur via indirect effect. When oxygen is present, as in living tissue, the indirect effects are amplified because of the additional types of free radicals that are formed.

TARGET THEORY

The cell contains many species of molecules, most of which exist in overabundance. Radiation damage to such molecules probably would not result in noticeable injury to the cell because additional similar molecules would be available to continue to support the cell. On the other hand, there are some molecules in the cell that

are considered to be particularly necessary for normal cell function. These molecules are not in abundant supply, and, in fact, there may be only one such molecule. Radiation damage to such a molecule could effect the cell severely, since there would be no similar molecules available as substitutes.

This concept of a sensitive key molecule is the basis for the **target theory.** According to target theory, for a cell to die following radiation exposure, its target molecule must be inactivated (Fig. 27-9). There is considerable experimental evidence in support of the target theory, and it suggests overwhelmingly that the key molecular target is the DNA. Originally, target theory was employed to represent cell lethality. However, it can be employed equally well to describe nonlethal radiation-induced cell abnormalities.

In the nomenclature of the target theory, the target is considered to be an area of the cell occupied by the target molecule or by a sensitive site on the target molecule. This area changes position with time because of intracellular molecular movement. The interaction between radiation and cellular components is random, and therefore, when an interaction does occur with

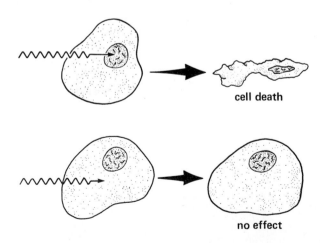

cell death

no effect

Fig. 27-9. According to target theory, cell death will occur only if the target molecule is inactivated.

a target, it occurs randomly. **There is no favoritism of radiation to the target molecule.** Its sensitivity to radiation occurs simply because of its vital function in the cell.

When an interaction does occur between radiation and the target, a **hit** is said to have occurred. Radiation interaction with molecules other than the target molecule does not result in a hit. Some conclude that target theory is applicable only to direct effect. Such is not the case, however, because **hits can occur through both the direct and the indirect effect.** It is not possible to distinguish between a direct and an indirect hit.

When a hit occurs through indirect effect, the size of the target appears considerably larger because of the mobility of the free radicals. This increased target size contributes to the importance of the indirect effect of radiation.

Fig. 27-10 illustrates some of the consequences of using target theory to explain the relationships among LET, the oxygen effect, and direct vs. indirect effect. With low-LET radiation, in the absence of oxygen, the probability of a hit on the target molecule is low because of the relatively large distances between ionizing events. If oxygen is present, reactive free radicals are formed and the volume of effectiveness surrounding each ionization is enlarged. Consequently, the probability of a hit is increased. When high-LET radiation is employed, the distance between ionizations is so close that the probability of a hit by direct effect is high, possibly higher than that for low-LET, indirect effect. When oxygen is added to the system and high-LET radiation employed, the effect of the radiation may not be increased. The added sphere of influence for each ionizing event, although somewhat larger, will not result in additional hits, since the maximum number of hits has already been produced by direct effect with the high-LET radiation.

CELL SURVIVAL KINETICS

Early radiation experiments at the cell level were conducted with simple cells such as bacteria. It was not until the middle 1950s that laboratory techniques were developed to allow the growth and manipulation of human cells in vitro. These techniques required the development of an artifical growth medium that would nourish a human cell. Now cells can be grown in tubes,

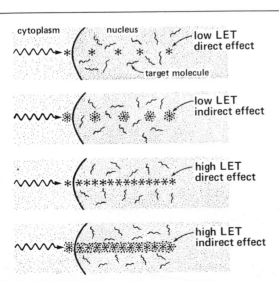

Fig. 27-10. In the presence of oxygen the indirect effect is amplified and the volume of action for low-LET radiation is enlarged. The effective volume of action for high-LET radiation remains unchanged, since maximum injury will have been inflicted by direct effect.

flasks, Petri dishes, or nearly any type of laboratory container.

One technique for measuring the lethal effects of radiation on cells is shown in Fig. 27-11. If normal cells are planted individually in a Petri dish and incubated for 10 to 14 days, they will divide many times and produce a visible **colony** consisting of as many as 1000 cells. This is **cloning.** Following irradiation of such single cells, some will not survive, and therefore fewer colonies will be formed. The higher the radiation dose, the fewer colonies will be formed. This allows us to determine the lethal effects of radiation by observing cell survival.

Employing a mathematic extension of target theory, two models of cell survival result. The models are the radiation dose-response relationships for the cell. The **single target, single hit** model applies to biologic targets such as enzymes, viruses, and simple cells like bacteria. The **multitarget, single hit** model applies to more complicated biologic systems such as human cells. The following discussion concerns the equation of these models. The mathematics of these models is relatively unimportant but is given here for the interested student.

Single target, single hit model

Consider for a moment the situation illustrated in Fig. 27-12. A large concrete runway containing 100 squares is shown, and it is raining. A square is considered wet when one or more raindrops have fallen on it. When the first drop falls in the pavement, 1 of the 100 squares will be wet. When the second drop falls, it is probable that it will fall in a dry square and not

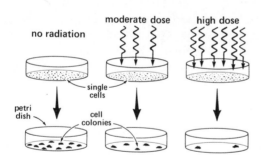

Fig, 27-11. When single cells are planted on a Petri dish, they grow into visible colonies. Fewer colonies will develop if the cells are irradiated.

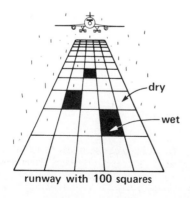

Fig. 27-12. When rain falls on a dry pavement consisting of a large number of squares, the number of squares that remain dry decreases exponentially as the number of raindrops increases.

the one already wet. Consequently, 2 out of 100 squares will be wet. When the third raindrop falls, there will probably be three wet and ninety-seven dry squares. However, as the number of raindrops increases, it will become more probable that a given square will be hit by two or more drops.

Because the raindrops are falling **randomly**, the probability that a square will become wet is governed by a statistical law called the **Poisson distribution**. According to this law, when the number of raindrops is equal to the number of squares (100 in this case), 63% of the squares will be wet and 37% of the squares will be dry. If the raindrops had fallen **uniformly**, all 100 squares would become wet with 100 raindrops. Radiation interacts randomly with matter.

Obviously, many of the sixty-three squares in this example have been hit twice and even more. When the number of raindrops equals twice the number of squares, then 0.37×0.37, or 14, squares will be dry. Following 300 raindrops, only 5 squares will remain dry. A graph of the number of dry squares as a function of the number of raindrops is shown Fig. 27-13. If the number of squares exposed to the rain were large or unknown, the scale on the right, expressed in percent, would be employed.

The wet square analogy can be extended to the irradiation of a large number of biologic specimens—for example, 1000 bacteria. The bacteria presumably contains a single sensitive site, or **target**, that must be inactivated for the cell to die. As the 1000 cells are irradiated with increasing increments of dose, more cells will be killed, as shown in Fig. 27-14. However, just as

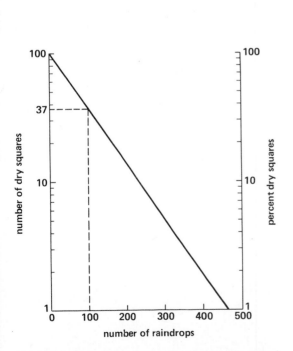

Fig. 27-13. When the number of dry squares is plotted on semilog paper as a function of the number of raindrops, a straight line results because after a few drops some squares will be hit more than once.

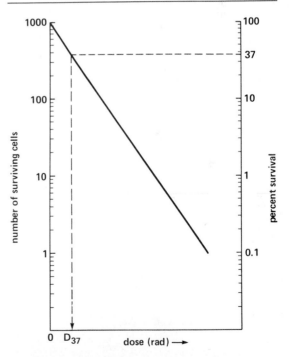

Fig. 27-14. Dose-response relationship following the irradiation of 1000 bacteria with graded doses of radiation is exponential. The D_{37} is that dose that results in 37% survival.

with the wet squares, as the dose increases, some cells will suffer two or more hits. All hits per target in excess of one represent wasted radiation dose, since the bacteria had already been killed by the first hit. Remember, **a hit is not simply an ionizing event, but rather an inactivating ionization in the target molecule.**

When the radiation dose reaches a level sufficient to kill 63% of the cells (37% survival), it is called D_{37}. **D_{37} is that dose which, if fully used so that there were not wasted hits (uniform interaction), would be sufficient to kill 100% of the cells.** Following a dose equal to $2 \times D_{37}$, 14% of the cells would survive, and so on. The D_{37} is a measure of the radiosensitivity of the biologic specimen. A low D_{37} represents a highly radiosensitive specimen, and a high D_{37} represents radioresistance.

The equation that describes the dose-response relationship represented by the graph in Fig. 27-14 is

(27-10)

$$S = N/N_0 = e^{-D/D_{37}}$$

where S is the surviving fraction, N is the number of cells surviving a dose D, N_0 is the initial number of cells, and D_{37} is a constant dose related to the cell radiosensitivity. The equation is the **single target, single hit** model of radiation-induced lethality.

Multitarget, single hit model

Returning to the wet squares analogy, suppose that each pavement square were divided diagonally into two equal parts (Fig. 27-15). By definition, each half must now be hit with a raindrop for the square to be considered wet. The first few raindrops will probably hit only half of any given square, and therefore, following a very light rain, no squares may be wet. Many raindrops must fall before any single square suffers a hit in both halves so that it can be considered wet. This represents a **threshold phenomenon**, since, according to our definition, a number of raindrops can fall and all squares will remain dry.

As the number of raindrops increases, the point will be reached when the first square will have both halves hit and therefore be considered wet. The portion of the curve below this number is represented by region A in Fig. 27-16. When a large number of raindrops has fallen, region C will be reached, where every square will have at least one half wet. When this occurs, each additional raindrop will produce a wet square. In region C the relation between number of raindrops and wet squares is that described by the single target, single hit model. The intermediate region B is the region of accumulation of hits.

Complex biologic specimens such as human cells are thought to have more than a single

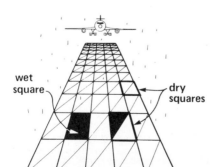

wet square · dry squares

Fig. 27-15. If each pavement square has two equal parts, each will have to be hit for the square to be considered wet.

critical target. Suppose that the human cell has two targets, each of which has to be inactivated for the cell to die. This would be analogous to the square having two halves, each of which had to be hit by rain for it to be considered wet. Fig, 27-17 is a graph of single-cell survival for human cells having two targets.

At very low radiation doses there will be nearly 100% cell survival. As the radiation dose increases, fewer cells will survive because more will have sustained a hit in both target molecules. At some higher radiation dose all cells will have sustained at least one hit in one of its two targets. All cells that survive this dose will have one target hit, and therefore at all higher doses the dose-response relationship would appear as the single target, single hit model.

The model of cell survival just described is the **multitarget, single hit** model. The equation of this model is

(27-11)

$$S = N/N_0 = 1 - (1 - e^{-D/D_0})^n$$

where S is the surviving fraction, N is the number of cells surviving a dose D, N_0 is the initial number of cells, D_0 is the dose necessary to reduce survival by 37% in the straight line portion of the graph, and n is the extrapolation number.

D_0 is called the **mean lethal dose,** and it is a constant related to the radiosensitivity of the cell. It is equal to D_{37} in the linear portion of the curve and therefore represents the dose that would result in one hit per target in the straight line portion of the graph if no radiation were wasted. As with D_{37} of the single target, single

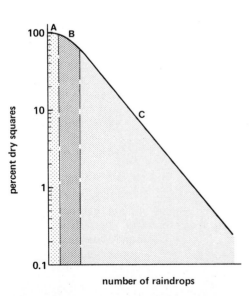

Fig. 27-16. When a square contains two equal parts, both of which have to be hit to be considered wet, three regions of the graphic relationship can be identified.

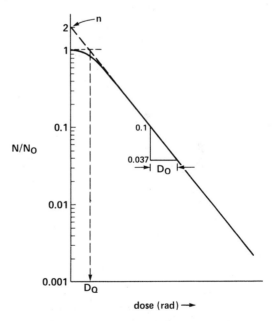

Fig. 27-17. The multitarget, single hit model of cell survival is characteristic of human cells containing two targets.

hit model, a large D_0 indicates a radioresistant cell line, and a small D_0 is characteristic of radiosensitive cells.

The **extrapolation number n** is also called the **target number.** When this type of experiment was first conducted with human cells, the observed extrapolation number was 2. That result agreed with the hypothesis that similar regions on two homologous chromosomes (an identical pair) had to be inactivated to produce cell death.

Table 27-1. The reported mean lethal dose (D_0) and threshold dose (D_Q) for various experimental mammalian cell lines

Cell type	D_0 (rad)	D_Q (rad)
Mouse oocytes	91	62
Mouse skin	135	350
Human bone marrow	137	0
Human fibroblasts	150	160
Mouse spermatogonia	180	270
Chinese hamster ovary	200	210
Human lymphocytes	400	0

Since chromosomes come in pairs, the experimental results confirmed the hypothesis. However, subsequent experiments have resulted in extrapolation numbers ranging from 2 to 12, and therefore the precise meaning of n in unknown.

D_Q is called the **threshold dose.** It is a measure of the width of the shoulder of the multitarget, single hit model and is related to the capacity of the cell to recover from sublethal damage. A large D_Q indicates that the cell can readily recover. Table 27-1 lists reported values for D_0 and D_Q for various experimental cell lines.

Recovery

The shoulder of the graph of the multitarget, single hit model shows that for mammalian cells some damage must be accumulated before the cell dies. This accumulated damage is termed **sublethal damage.** The wider the shoulder, the more sublethal damage that can be sustained and the higher the value of D_Q.

Fig. 27-18 demonstrates the results of a **split-dose technique** designed to describe the capacity of a cell to recover from sublethal damage.

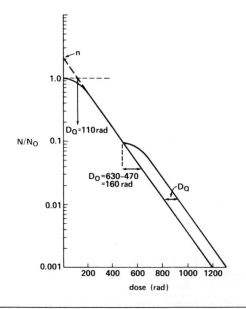

Fig. 27-18. Split dose technique results in a second cell survival curve with the precise characteristics of the first displaced along the dose axis by D_Q.

This illustration shows a rather typical human cell survival curve with D_0 = 160 rad (1.6 Gy), D_Q = 110 rad (1.1 Gy), and n = 2. If one takes those cells that survive any large dose (for example, 470 rad [4.7 Gy]) and reincubates them in a growth medium, they will grow into another large population. This population of cells can then be split into subunits to perform a second cell survival experiment. When the cells that survived the first dose are subsequently subjected to additional incremental doses, a second dose-response curve will be generated that has precisely the same shape as the first. The extrapolation number is the same, the mean lethal dose is the same, and it is separated along the dose axis from the first dose-response curve by D_Q. The time between such split doses must be at least as long as the cell generation time for full recovery to occur.

Such experiments show that cells that survive an initial radiation insult exhibit precisely the same characteristics as nonirradiated cells, and therefore they have fully recovered from the sublethal damage produced by the initial irradiation. Consequently, D_Q is not only a measure of the capacity to accumulate sublethal damage, but it is also a measure of the cells' ability to recover from sublethal damage.

EXAMPLE: From Fig. 27-18 estimate the overall surviving fraction for a cell receiving a split dose of 400 rad followed by 400 rad (4 Gy).

ANSWER: At a dose of 400 rad approximately 0.15 of the cells survive. Therefore, at a split dose of 400 rad and 400 rad, the surviving fraction should equal 0.15 × 0.15 = 0.023. The total dose is 800 rad (8 Gy), and the surviving fraction on the split-dose curve at 800 rad should equal 0.023 and it does. Had the 800 rad been delivered at one time, the surviving fraction would have been 0.012, as shown by the single-dose curve of Fig. 27-18.

Cell cycle effects

When human cells replicate by mitosis, the average time from one mitosis to another is called the **cell cycle time,** or the **generation time.** Most human cells that are in a state of normal proliferation have generation times of 10 to 20 hours. Some specialized cells have generation times extending to hundreds of hours, and some cells, such as neurons (nerve cells), do not normally proliferate. **Longer generation times usually result from a lengthening of the G_1 phase of the cell cycle.**

Techniques are now available for taking a randomly growing population of cells that are uniformly distributed in position throughout the cell cycle and **synchronizing** them. A population

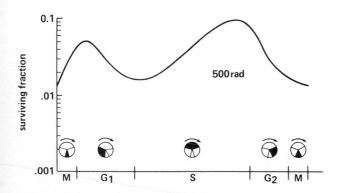

Fig. 27-19. Age-response function for human fibroblasts shows a minimum during the M phase and a maximum during late S phase. Such cells are most radiosensitive during mitosis and most radioresistant during the late S.

of synchronized cells can then be subdivided into smaller populations and irradiated sequentially as they pass through the phases of the cell cycle.

Fig. 27-19 is representative of results that are obtained from human fibroblasts. The fraction of cells surviving a given dose can vary by a factor of ten from the most sensitive to the most resistant phase of the cell cycle. This pattern of change in radiosensitivity as a function of phase in the cell cycle is known as the **age-response function.** It varies from cell type to cell type, but the results illustrated in Fig. 27-19 are characteristic of most human cells. **Cells in mitosis are always most sensitive.** The fraction of surviving cells will be the lowest in this phase. The next most sensitive phase of the cell cycle occurs at the G_1-S transition. **The most resistant portion of the cell cycle occurs in late S phase.**

LET, RBE, AND OER

Mammalian cell survival experiments have been employed extensively to measure the effects of various types of radiation and to determine the magnitude of various dose-modifying factors such as oxygen. Since the mean lethal dose, D_0, is related to radiosensitivity, the ratio of D_0 for one condition of irradiation compared with another will be a measure of magnitude of the dose modifier, whether it is physical or biologic.

If the same cell type is irradiated by two different radiations under identical physical and biologic conditions, results may appear as in Fig. 27-20. At the very high-LET values (as with alpha particles and neutrons), even with mammalian cells, **the cell survival kinetics follow the single target, single hit model.** With low-LET radiation (x rays) the multitarget, single hit mod-

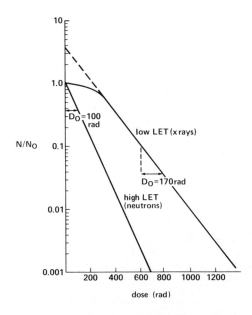

Fig. 27-20. Representative cell survival curves for human fibroblasts following exposure to 200 kVp x rays and 14 MeV neutrons.

el is representative. **The mean lethal dose following low-LET irradiation is always greater than that following high-LET irradiation.** If the low-LET D_0 is representative of x rays, then the ratio of these D_0's will equal the RBE for the high-LET radiation.

(27-12)

$$RBE = \frac{D_0 \ (standard \ radiation)}{D_0 \ (test \ radiation)} \ to \ produce \ the \ same \ effect$$

EXAMPLE: Fig. 27-20 shows the radiation dose-response relationship for human fibroblasts exposed to x rays and to 14 MeV neutrons. The D_0 following x-radiation is 170 rad (1.7 Gy); the D_0 for neutron irradiation is 100 rad. What is the RBE of 14 MeV neutrons relative to x rays?

ANSWER: RBE $= \dfrac{170 \ rad}{100 \ rad}$

$= 1.7$

The most completely studied dose modifier is oxygen. In the presence of oxygen the effect of low-LET radiation is maximum. When hypoxic or anoxic cells are exposed, considerably more dose is required to produce a given effect. When high-LET radiation is employed, there is little difference between the response of oxygenated cells and anoxic cells. Fig. 27-21 shows typical cell survival curves for each of these combinations of LET and oxygen.

Such experiments are designed to measure the magnitude of the oxygen effect. The OER determined from single cell survival experiments is defined as follows:

(27-13)

$$OER = \frac{D_0 \ (anoxic)}{D_0 \ (oxygenated)} \ to \ produce \ the \ same \ effect$$

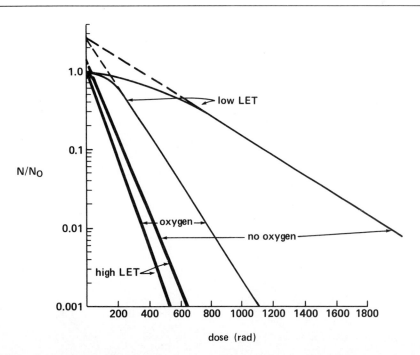

Fig. 27-21. Cell survival curves for human cells irradiated in the presence and absence of oxygen with high- and low-LET radiation.

EXAMPLE: With reference to Fig. 27-21, what is the estimated OER for human cells exposed to low-LET radiation and to high-LET radiation?

ANSWER:

Low LET, now oxygen, D_0 = 340 rad

Low LET, oxygen, D_0 = 140 rad

$$OER = \frac{340 \text{ rad}}{140 \text{ rad}} = 2.4$$

High LET, no oxygen, D_0 = 90 rad

High LET, oxygen, D_0 = 70

$$OER = \frac{90}{70} = 1.3$$

REVIEW QUESTIONS

1. Define or otherwise identify the following:
   a. In vitro
   b. Cytogenetic damage
   c. Point mutation
   d. Free radical
   e. Target theory
   f. D_{37}
   g. Mean lethal dose
   h. Indirect effect
   i. Extrapolation number
   j. D_Q
2. Describe the three types of damage in irradiated macromolecules.
3. Complete the following chemical equations:
   a. H_2O + Radiation
   b. HOH^+ (dissociation)
   c. HOH^- (dissociation)
4. The D_{37} of a cellular species that follows the single target, single hit model is 150 rad (1.5 Gy). What percentage of cells will survive 450 rad (4.5 Gy)?
5. What is the RBE of alpha radiation if the D_0 is 40 rad (400 mGy), compared with 180 rad (1.8 Gy) for x rays?

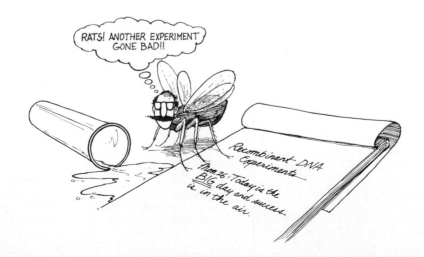

28

Early effects of radiation

To elicit a radiation response at the human level within a few days or even weeks, the dose must be quite substantial. Such a response is called an **early effect** of radiation exposure. A dose of this magnitude is not encountered in diagnostic radiology today. However, many years ago some of these early effects were the principal hazards to radiologists, technologists, and patients involved in diagnostic x-ray examinations.

These early effects have been studied rather completely with animals in the laboratory, and there is even a modest quantity of data available from observations on humans. Only the more important will be considered here, and these are identified in Table 28-1, along with the minimum radiation dose necessary to produce each.

ACUTE RADIATION LETHALITY

Death is of course the most devastating human response to radiation exposure. No cases of death following diagnostic x-ray exposure have been recorded, although some early x-ray pioneers died from the late effects of x-ray exposure. In each of these cases, however, the total radiation dose was extremely high by today's standards.

Table 28-1. The principal early effects of radiation exposure on humans and the approximate minimum radiation dose necessary to produce them

Effect	Anatomic site	Minimum dose (rad)
Death	Whole body	100
Hematologic depression	Whole body	25
Skin erythema	Small field	300
Epilation	Small field	300
Chromosome aberration	Whole body	5
Gonadal dysfunction	Local tissue	10

Acute radiation-induced human lethality is only of academic interest in diagnostic radiology. Diagnostic x-ray beams are neither sufficiently intense nor sufficiently large to cause death. Diagnostic x-ray beams always result in partial-body exposure, which is much less effective than whole-body exposure.

Some accidental exposures of persons in the nuclear weapons and nuclear energy fields have resulted in immediate death, but the number of such accidents has been small considering the length of the atomic age. The unfortunate incident at Chernobyl in April 1986 is the one notable exception. Thirty people died of the acute radiation syndrome, and a number of late effects are expected. No one died or was even seriously irradiated in the March 1979 meltdown at the nuclear power reactor of Three Mile Island. Employment in the nuclear industry is still considered one of the safest occupations.

The sequence of events following high-level radiation exposure leading to death within days or weeks is called the **acute radiation syndrome.** There are, in fact, three separate syndromes that are dose related and that follow a rather distinct course of events. These syndromes are called **hematologic death, gastrointestinal (GI) death,** and **central nervous system (CNS) death.** The clinical signs and symptoms of each are outlined in Table 28-2. Table 28-2 also shows that CNS death requires radiation doses in excess of 5000 rad (50 Gy) and results in death within hours.

GI death and hematologic death follow lower exposures and require a long time for death to occur.

In addition to the three lethal syndromes, there are two other stages to acute radiation lethality. The **prodromal syndrome** consists of acute clinical symptoms that occur within hours of the exposure and continue for up to a day or two. Following the prodromal syndrome, there may be a **latent period,** during which time the subject will be free of visible effect.

The clinical signs and symptoms of the **manifest illness** stage of acute radiation lethality can be classified into three principal groups: hematologic, gastrointestinal, and neuromuscular. The hematologic signs relate to changes in the cells of the peripheral blood. Red cells (erythrocytes), white cells (leukocytes), and platelets (thrombocytes) are reduced in number in the blood following exposure. The gastrointestinal symptoms are nausea, vomiting and diarrhea, anorexia, intestinal cramps, dehydration, and weight loss. Neuromuscular symptoms are listlessness, apathy, sweating, fever, headache, and hypertension.

Prodromal syndrome

At radiation doses above approximately 100 rad delivered to the total body, the signs and symptoms of radiation sickness may appear within a matter of minutes to hours following exposure. The symptoms of this early radiation

---

Table 28-2. Summary of acute radiation lethality

Stage	Dose (rad)	Mean survival time (days)	Clinical signs and symptoms
Prodromal	>100	—	Nausea, vomiting, diarrhea
Latent	100-10,000	—	None
Hematologic	200-1000	10-60	Nausea, vomiting, diarrhea, anemia, leukopenia, hemorrhage, fever, infection
Gastrointestinal	1000-5000	4-10	Same as hematologic, electrolyte imbalance, lethargy, fatigue, shock
Central nervous system	>5000	0-3	Same as GI, ataxia, edema, vasculitis, meningitis

sickness most often take the form of nausea, vomiting, diarrhea, and a reduction in the white cells of the peripheral blood (leukopenia). **This immediate radiation sickness is the prodromal syndrome.**

The prodromal syndrome may last from hours to a couple of days. The severity of the symptoms is dose related, and at doses in excess of 1000 rad (10 Gy) the symptoms can be rather violent. At still higher doses the duration of the prodromal syndrome becomes shorter, until it is difficult to separate the prodromal syndrome from the stage of manifest illness.

Latent period

Following the period of initial radiation sickness, there is a period of apparent well-being. **This is the latent period, during which time there is no sign of radiation sickness.** The latent period will extend from hours or less (at doses in excess of 5000 rad) to weeks (at doses from 100 to 500 rad). The latent period is sometimes mistakenly thought to indicate the early recovery from a moderate radiation dose. It may be quite different, however, giving no indication of the extensive radiation response yet to follow.

Hematologic syndrome

Radiation doses in the range of approximately 200 to 1000 rad produce the **hematologic syndrome.** The subject will initially experience mild symptoms of the prodromal syndrome, which will appear in a matter of a few hours and may persist for several days. The latent period that follows can extend as long as 4 weeks and is characterized by a general feeling of well-being. There are no obvious signs of illness, although the number of cells in the peripheral blood will be declining during this time. The period of **manifest illness** is characterized by possible vomiting, mild diarrhea, malaise, lethargy, and fever. The signs that characterize the hematologic syndrome are the reduction in numbers of white cells, red cells, and platelets in the circulating blood. Each of these types of cells fol-

lows rather characteristic patterns of cell depletion. If the dose is not lethal, recovery begins in 2 to 4 weeks, but it may take as long as 6 months for full recovery.

If the radiation injury is sufficiently severe, the reduction in blood cells will continue unchecked until the body's defense against infection is nil. Just before death, hemorrhage and dehydration may be pronounced. Death occurs because of generalized infection, electrolyte imbalance, and dehydration.

The dose necessary to produce a given syndrome and the mean survival time are the principal quantitative measures of human radiation lethality, as indicated in Table 28-2. Although ranges of effective dose and resulting mean survival times are given, it should be clear that there is rarely a precise difference in the dose- and time-related sequence of events associated with each syndrome. At very high radiation doses the latent period will disappear altogether. At very low radiation doses there may be no prodromal syndrome and consequently no associated latent period.

Gastrointestinal (GI) syndrome

Following radiation doses extending from approximately 1000 to 5000 rad (10 to 50 Gy), the **gastrointestinal (GI) syndrome** will occur. The prodromal symptoms of vomiting and diarrhea occur within hours of exposure and persist for hours to as long as a day. Thereafter follows a latent period of 3 to 5 days, during which time no symptoms are present. The manifest illness stage begins with a second wave of nausea and vomiting, followed by diarrhea. The individual will experience a loss of appetite (anorexia) and may become lethargic. The diarrhea will persist and increase in severity, leading to loose and then watery and bloody stools. Supportive therapy is unable to prevent the rapid progression of symptoms that ultimately leads to death within 4 to 10 days of exposure.

Death occurs principally because of severe damage to the cells lining the intestines. These cells are normally in a rapid state of proliferation and are continuously being replaced by new cells. The turnover time for this cell renewal system in a normal individual is 3 to 5 days. Radiation exposure kills the most sensitive cells—the stem cells—and this controls the length of time until death. When the intestinal lining is completely denuded of functional cells, there is uncontrolled passage of fluids across the intestinal membrane, a severe destruction of electrolyte balance, and conditions promoting infection.

At doses consistent with the GI syndrome, damage to the hematologic system will also occur. The cell renewal system of the blood takes a longer time for development into mature cells from the stem cell population, and therefore sufficient time is not provided for maximum hematologic effects to occur. There will be measurable and even severe hematologic changes accompanying gastrointestinal death.

Central nervous system (CNS) syndrome

Following a radiation dose in excess of approximately 5000 rad (50 Gy), a series of signs and symptoms occur that lead to death within a matter of hours to 3 days. First, there is an onset of severe nausea and vomiting, usually within a few minutes of exposure. During this time, the individual may become extremely nervous and confused, complain of a burning sensation in the skin, lose vision, and even lose consciousness within the first hour. This may be followed by a latent period lasting up to 6 to 12 hours, during which time the earlier symptoms subside or disappear. Following the latent period is the period of manifest illness, during which time the symptoms of the prodromal stage return but more severely. The person becomes disoriented, loses muscle coordination, has difficulty breathing, may go into convulsive seizures, experiences loss of equilibrium, ataxia, and lethargy, lapses into a coma, and dies.

Regardless of the medical attention given the subject, the symptoms of manifest illness appear rather suddenly and always with extreme severity. At radiation doses sufficiently high to produce central nervous system effects, the outcome has always been death within a few days of exposure.

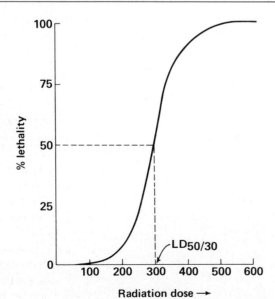

Fig. 28-1. Radiation-induced death in humans follows a nonlinear, threshold dose-response relationship. The $LD_{50/30}$ can be determined from a graph of radiation dose vs. percent lethality, as shown.

The cause of death in CNS syndrome is apparently the elevated fluid content of the brain, resulting in increased intracranial pressure, inflammatory changes in the blood vessels of the brain (vasculitis), and inflammation of the meninges (meningitis). At doses sufficient to produce CNS damage, damage to all other organs of the body would be equally as severe. The classical radiation-induced changes in the gastrointestinal tract and the hematologic system cannot occur because sufficient time between exposure and death is not available for their appearance.

LD$_{50/30}$

If one irradiates experimental groups of animals with varying doses of radiation, for example, 100 to 1000 rad (1 to 10 Gy), a plot of the percentage of animals that die as a function of the radiation dose would appear as in Fig. 28-1. This figure illustrates the radiation dose-response relationship for acute human lethality. Note that it is a threshold relationship and nonlinear. At the lower dose of approximately 100 rad (1 Gy) no one is expected to die, whereas above approximately 600 rad (6 Gy) all those so irradiated would die unless vigorous medical support were available. Above 1000 rad (10 Gy) even vigorous medical support will not prevent death.

If death is to occur, it will usually happen within 30 days of exposure. Acute radiation lethality is measured quantitatively by the LD$_{50/30}$. **The LD$_{50/30}$ is the dose of radiation to the whole body that will result in death within 30 days to 50% of the subjects so irradiated.** The LD$_{50/30}$ for humans is estimated to be approximately 300 rad (3 Gy). With clinical support humans can tolerate much higher doses, the maximum reported being 850 rad (8.5 Gy). Table 28-3 lists values of LD$_{50/30}$ for various experimental species and humans.

Sometimes additional measures of acute lethality are identified. The LD$_{10/30}$ or LD$_{90/30}$ would indicate the dose resulting in 10% lethality or 90% lethality within 30 days, respectively. The LD$_{50/60}$ is the lethal dose to 50% when the observed survival time is extended for 60 days. Normally, this is not much different from the LD$_{50/30}$.

EXAMPLE: From Fig. 28-1 estimate the radiation dose that will produce 25% lethality in humans within 30 days.

ANSWER: First draw a horizontal line from the 25% level on the y axis until it intersects the S curve. Now drop a vertical line from this point to the x axis. This intersection with the x axis occurs at the LD$_{25/30}$, which is approximately 250 rad (2.5 Gy).

Mean survival time

As the whole-body radiation dose increases, the average time between exposure and death decreases. This time is known as the **mean survival time.** A plot of radiation dose vs. mean survival time is shown in Fig. 28-2. There are three distinct regions to this plot, and they are associated with the three radiation syndromes.

As the radiation dose increases from 200 to 1000 rad (2 to 10 Gy), the mean survival time decreases from approximately 60 to 4 days, and this region is consistent with death resulting from the hematologic syndrome. Mean survival time is dose dependent with the hematologic

---

Table 28-3. LD$_{50/30}$ for various species following whole-body x-radiation

Species	LD$_{50/30}$ (rad)
Pig	250
Dog	275
Human	300
Guinea pig	425
Monkey	475
Opossum	510
Mouse	620
Goldfish	700
Hamster	700
Rat	710
Rabbit	725
Gerbil	1050
Turtle	1500
Armadillo	2000
Newt	3000

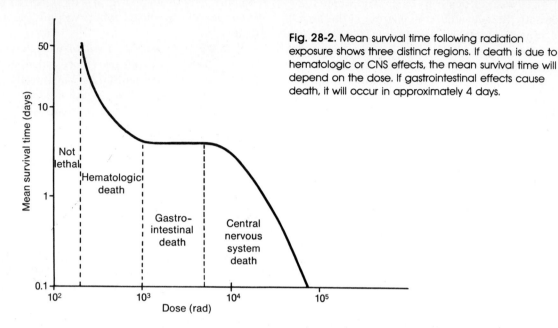

Fig. 28-2. Mean survival time following radiation exposure shows three distinct regions. If death is due to hematologic or CNS effects, the mean survival time will depend on the dose. If gastrointestinal effects cause death, it will occur in approximately 4 days.

syndrome. In the dose range associated with the GI syndrome, however, the mean survival time remains relatively constant at 4 days. With larger doses, those associated with the CNS syndrome, the mean survival time is again dose dependent, varying from approximately 3 days to a matter of hours.

LOCAL TISSUE DAMAGE

When only part of the body is irradiated, compared with whole-body irradiation, a higher dose is required to produce a response. Every organ and tissue of the body can be affected by partial-body irradiation. The effect is cell death, resulting in a shrinkage, or reduction in size (**atrophy**), of the tissue or organ. This can lead to a total nonfunction of that tissue or organ, or it can be followed by recovery.

There are many examples of local tissue damage immediately following radiation exposure. In fact, if the dose is high enough, any local tissue will respond. The manner in which local tissues respond depends on their intrinsic ra-

diosensitivity and the kinetics of cell proliferation and maturation. Examples of local tissues that can be affected immediately are gonads, bone marrow, and skin.

Skin

The tissue with which we have most experience at the human level is the skin. Normal skin consists of three layers: an outer layer (the epidermis), an intermediate layer of connective tissue (the dermis), and a subcutaneous layer of fat and connective tissue. There are additional accessory structures in the skin, such as hair follicles, sweat glands, and sensory receptors. All the cell layers and the accessory structures participate in the response to radiation exposure.

The skin, like the lining of the intestine, represents a continuing cell renewal system, only at a much slower rate than that experienced by intestinal cells. Almost 50% of the cells lining the intestine are replaced every day, whereas the skin cells are replaced at the rate of only 2% per day. The outer skin layer, the epidermis,

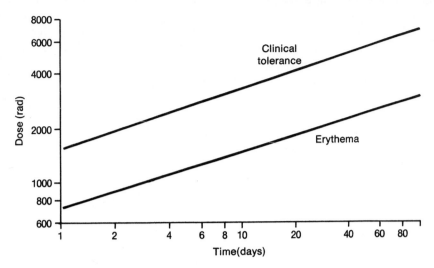

Fig. 28-3. These isoeffect curves show the relationship between the number of daily fractions and the total radiation dose that will produce erythema or moist desquamation. As the fractionation of the dose increases, so will the total dose required.

consists of several layers of cells, the lowest layer being the **basal cells. The basal cells are the stem cells** that mature as they slowly migrate to the surface of epidermis. Once these cells arrive on the surface as mature cells, they are slowly lost and have to be replaced by new cells from the basal layer. It is damage to these basal cells that results in the earliest manifestation of radiation injury to the skin.

Before the advent of cobalt teletherapy, the limitations of radiation therapy with **orthovoltage x rays** (200 to 300 kVp x rays) were determined by the tolerance of the patient's skin. The object of x-ray therapy is to deposit x-ray energy in the tumor while sparing the surrounding normal tissue. Since the x rays must pass through the skin to reach the tumor, the skin was often necessarily subjected to higher radiation doses than the tumor. The resultant skin damage was **erythema** (a sunburnlike reddening of the skin), followed by **desquamation** (ulceration and denudation of the skin), and often required that the therapy be interrupted.

Following a single dose of 300 to 1000 rad (3 to 10 Gy), an initial mild erythema may occur within the first or second day. This first wave of erythema will then subside, only to be followed by a second wave that reaches maximum intensity in about 2 weeks. At higher doses, this second wave of erythema will be followed by a moist desquamation, which in turn may lead to a dry desquamation. Moist desquamation is known as **clinical tolerance** for radiation therapy.

In the clinical situation, radiation exposure of the skin is delivered in a fractionated scheme, usually approximately 200 rad per day (2 Gy per day), 5 days a week. To assist the radiotherapist in planning patient treatments, isoeffect curves have been generated that accurately project the dose necessary to produce a skin erythema or clinical tolerance following a prescribed treatment routine. Sample isoeffect curves are shown in Fig. 28-3.

Erythema was perhaps the first observed biologic response to radiation exposure. Many of the early x-ray pioneers, including Roentgen, suffered x-ray–induced skin burns. One of the hazards to the patient during the early years of radiology was x-ray–induced erythema. During those years, x-ray tube potentials were so low that it was usually necessary to position the tube very close to the patient's skin, and not uncommonly 10- to 15-minute exposures were required to obtain a suitable radiograph. Often the patient would return several days later suffering from an x-ray burn.

These skin effects follow a nonlinear, threshold dose-response relationship similar to that described for radiation-induced lethality. Small doses of x-radiation do not cause erythema. Extremely high doses of radiation cause erythema in all persons so irradiated. Whether intermediate radiation doses produce erythema depends on the individual's radiosensitivity, the dose rate, and the size of the skin field irradiated. Analysis of persons irradiated therapeutically with superficial x rays has shown that the **skin erythema dose** required to affect 50% of persons so irradiated (**SED$_{50}$**) is about 600 rad (6 Gy).

Before the definition of the roentgen and the development of accurate radiation measuring apparatus, the skin was observed and its response to radiation used in formulating radiation protection practices. The unit used was the SED$_{50}$, and permissible radiation exposures were specified in fractions of SED$_{50}$.

Another response of the skin to radiation exposure is **epilation,** or loss of hair. For many years soft x rays (10 to 20 kVp), called **grenz rays,** were used as the treatment of choice for skin diseases such as ringworm. Ringworm of the scalp, not uncommon in children, was successfully treated by grenz radiation, but unfortunately the patient's hair would fall out for weeks or even months. In some instances, where an unnecessarily high dose of grenz rays was employed, the epilation was permanent.

Gonads

The human gonads are critically important target organs for irradiation. As an example of local tissue effects, they are particularly sensitive to radiation. Responses to doses as low as 10 rad have been observed. Since these organs produce the germ cells that control fertility and heredity, their response to radiation has been studied extensively.

Much of what is known in the area of both type of radiation response and dose-response relationships has been derived from numerous animal experiments. However, some significant data are also available from human populations. Radiotherapy patients, radiation accident victims, and volunteer convicts have all provided data at the human level to allow a rather complete description of the response of the gonads to radiation.

The cells of the testes, the male gonads, and the ovaries, the female gonads, respond differently to radiation because of differences in progression of the germ cells from the stem cell phase to the mature cell. Fig. 28-4 describes this progression, indicating the most radiosensitive phase of cell maturation.

Germ cells are produced by both ovaries and testes, but they develop from the stem cell phase to the mature cell phase at different rates and at different times. The stem cells of the ovaries are the **oogonia,** and they multiply in number only during fetal life. The oogonia reach a maximum number of about 7 million during midpregnancy and then begin to decline because of spontaneous degeneration. During late fetal life many **primordial follicles** grow to encapsulate the oogonia, which become **oocytes.** These follicle-containing oocytes remain in a suspended state of growth until puberty. In prepuberty the number of oocytes has been reduced to only several hundred thousand. Commencing at puberty, the follicles rupture with regularity, ejecting a mature germ cell, the **ovum.** There will be only 400 or 500 such ova available for fertilization (number of years of menstruation times thirteen per year).

The germ cells of the testes are continually being produced from stem cells progressively through a number of stages to maturity, and,

male:

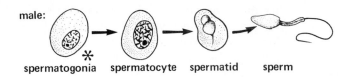

spermatogonia   spermatocyte   spermatid   sperm

female:

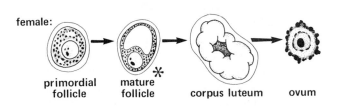

primordial   mature   corpus luteum   ovum
follicle   follicle

*most radiosensitive

Fig. 28-4. Progression of germ cells from the stem cell phase to the mature cell.

like the ovaries, the testes provide a sustaining cell renewal system. The male stem cell is the **spermatogonia,** which matures into the **spermatocyte.** The spermatocyte in turn multiplies and develops into a spermatid, which finally differentiates into the functionally mature germ cell, the **spermatozoa,** or **sperm.** This maturation process from stem cell to spermatozoa requires 3 to 5 weeks.

Ovaries. Irradiation of the ovaries early in life will cause a reduction in their size (atrophy) by germ cell death. After puberty such irradiation will, in addition, cause a suppression and delay of menstruation. The most radiosensitive cell in the scheme of female **gametogenesis** (development of the gametes, or germ cells) is the **oocyte in the mature follicle.** Radiation effects on the ovaries are somewhat age dependent. At fetal life and early childhood the ovaries are especially radiosensitive. They decline in sensitivity, reaching a minimum in the 20- to 30-year age range and then increase continually with age. Doses as low as 10 rad (100 mGy) in the mature female may result in the delay or suppression of menstruation. A dose of approximately 200 rad (2 Gy) will produce a pronounced temporary sterility; approximately 500 rad (5 Gy) to the ovaries is necessary to produce permanent sterility.

In addition to the destruction of fertility, irradiation of the ovaries of experimental animals has been shown to produce genetic mutations. Even moderate doses such as 25 to 50 rad (250 to 500 mGy) have been associated with measurable increases in genetic mutations. There is also some evidence to indicate that oocytes surviving such a modest dose are capable of repairing some genetic damage as they mature into ova. On the basis of those data, some radiation scientists advise women to abstain from procreation for a period of several months following ovarian doses in excess of 10 rad (100 mGy). The object is to minimize the possibility of genetic mutations in offspring. This is by no means a consensus view.

Testes. The testes, like the ovaries, atrophy after high doses of radiation. Many data on testicular damage have been gathered from observations of volunteer convicts and radiotherapy patients treated for testicular carcinoma in one testis while the other was shielded. Many investigators have recorded normal births to such patients whose remaining functioning testis received a radiation dose between 50 and 300 rad (0.5 and 3 Gy). Nevertheless, procreation at any time following such testicular irradiation is ill advised.

The spermatogonial stem cells are the most sensitive phase in the gametogenesis of the spermatozoa. Following irradiation of the testes, the maturing cells, spermatocytes and spermatids, are relatively radioresistant and continue to mature. Consequently, there is no significant reduction in spermatozoa until several weeks after exposure, and therefore fertility continues during this time. At this time the irradiated spermatogonia would have developed into mature spermatozoa had they survived.

Radiation doses as low as 10 rad (100 mGy) can result in a reduction in the number of spermatozoa. With increasing dose the depletion of spermatozoa becomes greater and extends over a longer period of time. Two hundred rad (2 Gy) will produce temporary sterility, which will commence approximately 2 months after irradiation and persist for up to 12 months. Five hundred rad (5 Gy) to the testes will produce permanent sterility. Even following doses sufficient to produce permanent sterility, the male will normally retain his potency and ability to engage in sexual intercourse.

Since male gametogenesis is a self-renewing system, there is some evidence to suggest that genetic mutations induced in surviving postspermatogonial cells represent the most hazardous mutations. Consequently, following testicular irradiation to doses above approximately 10 rad (100 mGy), the male should refrain from procreation for 2 to 4 months until all cells in the spermatogonial and postspermatogonial stages at the time of irradiation have matured and disappeared. This will reduce but probably not eliminate any increase in genetic mutations because of the persistence of the stem cell. Evidence from animal experiments suggests that there is some repair of genetic mutations even when the stem cell is irradiated.

HEMATOLOGIC EFFECTS

If you were a radiologic technologist in practice during the early years of this century (for example, the 1920s and the 1930s), it would not have been unusual for you to visit the hematology lab once a week for a routine blood examination. Before the introduction of personnel radiation monitors, the only monitoring performed on x-ray and radium workers was a periodic blood examination. The examination included total cell counts and a white cell (leukocyte) differential count. Most institutions had a radiation safety regulation such that, if the leukocytes were depressed by greater than 25% of normal level, the employee was either given time off or assigned to nonradiation activities until the count returned to normal. What was not entirely understood at this time was that the minimum whole-body dose necessary to produce a measurable hematologic depression was approximately 25 rad (250 mGy). These workers were being heavily irradiated by today's standards. **Under no circumstances is a periodic blood examination recommended as a feature of any current radiation protection program.**

Hemopoietic system

The hemopoietic system consists of bone marrow, circulating blood, and lymphoid tissue. Lymphoid tissues are the lymph nodes, spleen, and thymus. The principal effect of radiation on this system is to depress the number of blood cells in the peripheral circulation. The time- and dose-related effects on the various types of circulating blood cells are determined by the normal growth and maturation of these cells.

As shown in Fig. 28-5, all cells of the hemopoietic system apparently develop from a single type of stem cell. This stem cell is called a **pluripotential stem cell** because it has the ability to develop into several different types of mature cells. Although the spleen and thymus manufacture one type of leukocyte (the lymphocyte), most circulating blood cells, including lymphocytes, are manufactured in the bone marrow. In a child the bone marrow is rather uniformly distributed throughout the skeleton. In an adult the active bone marrow responsible for producing circulating cells is restricted to flat bones, such as the ribs, sternum, and skull, and the ends of long bones.

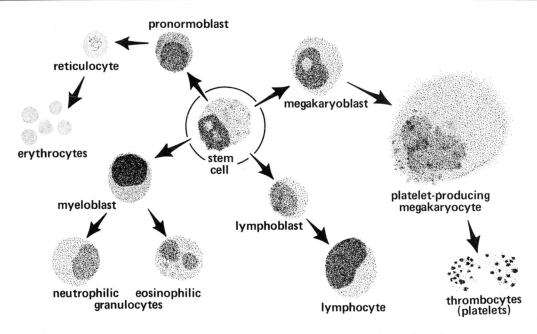

Fig. 28-5. Four principal types of blood cells—lymphocytes, granulocytes, erythrocytes, and thrombocytes—develop and mature from a single pluripotential stem cell.

From the single pluripotential stem cell a number of cell types are produced, but principally these are the **lymphocytes** (those involved in the immune response), the **granulocytes** (scavenger-type cells used to fight bacteria), **thrombocytes** (also called platelets and involved in the clotting of blood to prevent hemorrhage), and **erythrocytes** (red blood cells that are the transportation agents for oxygen). These cell lines develop at different rates in the bone marrow and are released to the peripheral blood as mature cells. While in the bone marrow, the cells proliferate in number, differentiate in function, and mature. The developing granulocytes and erythrocytes spend about 8 to 10 days in the bone marrow. Thrombocytes have a lifetime of about 5 days in the bone marrow. Lymphocytes are produced over varying times and have varying lifetimes in the peripheral blood. Some are thought to have lives measured in terms of hours

and others in terms of years. In the peripheral blood the granulocytes have a lifetime of only a couple of days. Thrombocytes have a lifetime of approximately 1 week, and erythrocytes a lifespan of nearly 4 months.

The hemopoietic system, therefore, is another example of a cell renewal system. The effect of radiation on this system is determined by the normal cell growth and development.

Hemopoietic cell survival

The principal response of the hemopoietic system to radiation exposure is a decrease in the number of all types of blood cells in the circulating peripheral blood. Lethal injury to the precursor cells causes the depletion of these mature circulating cells.

Fig. 28-6 shows the radiation response of the four principal circulating cells. Examples are given for low, moderate, and high radiation

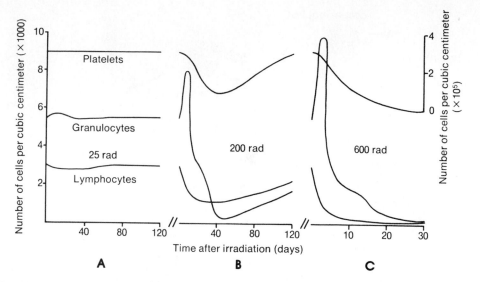

Fig. 28-6. These graphs show the response of the major circulating blood cells to radiation following different approximate doses. **A,** Twenty-five rad. **B,** Two hundred rad. **C,** Six hundred rad.

doses, and it is seen that the degree of cell depletion increases with increasing dose. These figures are the results of observations on experimental animals, radiotherapy patients, and the few radiation accident victims.

Following exposure, the first cells to become affected are the lymphocytes. These cells are reduced in number (lymphopenia) within minutes or hours following exposure, and they are very slow to recover. **The lymphocytes and the spermatogonia are considered the most radiosensitive cells in the body.** Because their response is so immediate, the radiation effect is apparently a direct one on the lymphocytes themselves, rather than on the precursor cells.

Granulocytes experience a rapid rise in number (granulocytosis), followed first by a rapid decrease and then a slower decrease in number (granulocytopenia). If the radiation dose is moderate, then approximately 15 to 20 days after irradiation an abortive rise in granulocyte count

may occur. Minimum granulocyte levels are reached approximately 30 days after irradiation. If recovery is to occur, return to normal will take approximately 2 months.

The depletion of platelets (thrombocytopenia) following irradiation develops more slowly, again because of the time required for the more sensitive precursor cells to reach maturity. Thrombocytes reach a minimum in about 30 days and exhibit recovery in about 2 months, similar to the response kinetics of granulocytes.

The erythrocytes are less sensitive than the other blood cells. This occurs apparently because of the very long lifetime they experience in the peripheral blood. Injury of these cells is not apparent for a matter of weeks. Total recovery may take 6 months to a year.

CYTOGENETIC EFFECTS

Cytogenetics is the study of the genetic aspects of cells, in particular, cell chromosomes.

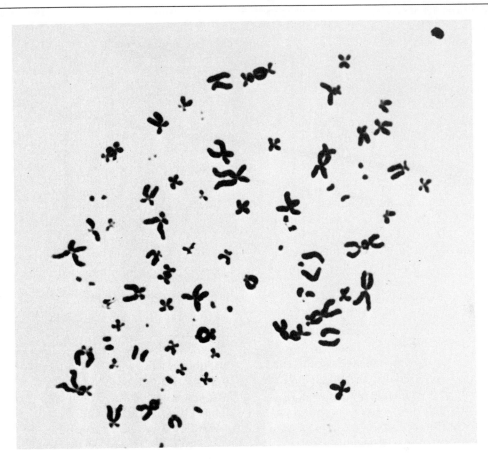

Fig. 28-7. Chromosome damage in an irradiated human cancer cell.

When a cell is irradiated, damage to its chromosomes can occur and this damage takes several characteristic forms.

A technique developed in the early 1950s contributed enormously to human genetic analysis and radiation genetics. The technique calls for a culture of human cells to be prepared and treated so that the chromosomes of each cell can be easily observed and studied. This has resulted in many observations on human radiation-induced chromosome damage. Fig. 28-7 is a photomicrograph of the chromosomes of a human cancer cell following radiation therapy. The many chromosome aberrations seen represent a high degree of damage. Radiation cytogenetic studies have shown that nearly every type of chromosome aberration can be radiation induced and that some may be specific to radiation. The rate of induction of chromosome aberrations is related in a complex way to the radiation dose, but in every case it is apparently of the **nonthreshold form.**

Attempts to measure chromosome aberrations in patients following diagnostic radiographic examination have been largely unsuccessful. Some studies involving higher-dose fluoroscopic special procedures have shown the presence of radiation-induced chromosome aberrations soon after the examination.

High doses of radiation, without question, cause chromosome aberrations. Low doses, no doubt, do also. But it is difficult technically to observe aberrations at doses less than approximately 5 rad (50 mGy). An even more difficult task is the identification of the link between radiation-induced chromosome aberrations and latent illness or disease.

When the body is irradiated, all cells can suffer cytogenetic damage. Such damage is classified here as an early response to radiation because, if the cell survives, the damage will be manifested during the next mitosis following the radiation exposure. Human peripheral lymphocytes are most often used for cytogenetic analysis, and these lymphocytes do not move into mitosis until stimulated in vitro by an appropriate laboratory technique. Cytogenetic damage to the stem cells will be sustained immediately but may not be manifested for the considerable time required for that stem cell to reach maturity as a circulating lymphocyte. Consequently, although chromosome damage is produced at the time of irradiation, it can be months and even years before the damage is measured. For this reason some workers who were irradiated in industrial accidents 20 years ago continue to show chromosome abnormalities in their circulating lymphocytes.

The normal karyotype

The human chromosome consists of considerable strings of DNA conjugated with a protein and folded back on itself many times. A normal chromosome was shown in Fig. 26-11 as it would appear in the G_1 phase of the cell cycle, when only two chromatids are present, and in the G_2 phase of the cell cycle following DNA replication. The chromosome structure represented for the G_2 phase is that which is visualized in the metaphase portion of mitosis.

For certain types of cytogenetic analyses of the chromosomes, photographs are taken and enlarged so that each individual chromosome can be cut out and paired with its sister into a chromosome map, which is called a **karyotype.** Fig. 28-8 is an example of a normal karyotype for a human somatic cells. There are twenty-two pairs of **autosomes** and one pair of **sex chromosomes,** the X chromosome from the female and the Y chromosome from the male.

Structural radiation damage to individual chromosomes can be visualized without constructing a karyotype. These are the single- and double-hit chromosome aberrations. Reciprocal translocations generally require a karyotype for detection. Point genetic mutations are undetectable even with karyotype construction.

Single-hit chromosome aberrations

When radiation interacts with chromosomes, the interaction can be through direct or indirect effect. In either mode these interactions result in a **hit.** The hit, however, is somewhat different from the hit described previously in radiation interaction with DNA. The DNA hit resulted in an invisible disruption of the molecular structure of the DNA. A chromosome hit, on the other hand, produces a visible derangement of the chromosome. This indicates that such a hit has disrupted many molecular bonds and severed many chains of DNA. A chromosome hit represents severe damage to the DNA.

Single-hit effects produced by radiation during the G_1 phase of the cell cycle are shown in Fig. 28-9. The breakage of a chromatid is called **chromatid deletion.** During S phase, both the remaining chromosome and the deletion are replicated. The chromosome aberration visualized at metaphase consists of a normal-looking chromosome with material missing from the ends of two sister chromatids and two acentric fragments (without a centromere). These fragments are called **isochromatids.**

Chromosome aberrations could also be pro-

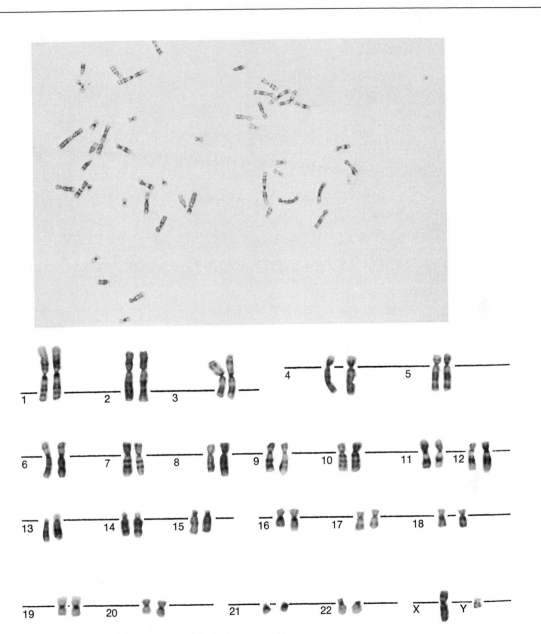

Fig. 28-8. Enlarged photomicrograph of the human cell nucleus at metaphase showing each chromosome distinctly. The karyotype is made from the photograph by cutting and pasting. (Courtesy V. Riccardi, Baylor College of Medicine, Houston, Tex.)

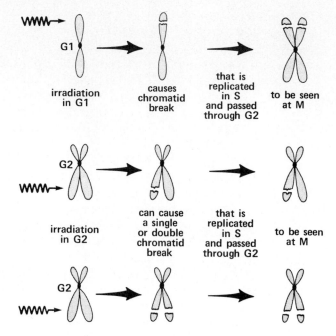

Fig. 28-9. Single-hit chromosome aberrations following irradiation in G_1 and G_2. The aberrations are visualized and recorded at M.

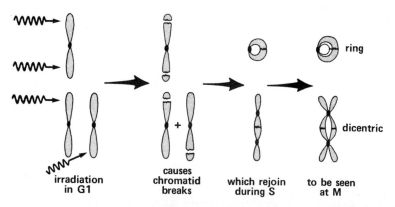

Fig. 28-10. Multihit chromosome aberrations following irradiation in G_1 phase result in ring and dicentic chromosomes in addition to chromatid fragments. Similar aberrations can be produced by irradiation during G_2, but they are rarer.

duced by single-hit events during the G_2 phase of the cell cycle (Fig. 28-9). The probability of ionizing radiation passing through sister chromatids to produce isochromatids is low. Usually the radiation will produce a chromatid deletion in only one arm of the chromosome. The result is a chromosome with an arm obviously missing genetic material and a chromatid fragment.

Multihit chromosome aberrations

It is possible that a single chromosome will sustain more than one hit. Multihit aberrations are not uncommon (Fig. 28-10). In the G_1 phase of the cell cycle, ring chromosomes are produced if the two hits occur on the same chromosome. Dicentrics are produced when adjacent chromosomes each suffer one hit and recombine as shown. The mechanism for the joining of chromatids depends on the quality of **stickiness** that appears at the site of the severed chromosome.

In the G_2 phase of the cell cycle, similar aberrations can be produced; however, such aberrations again require that (1) either the same chromosome be hit two or more times or (2) adjacent chromosomes be hit and joined together. These are rare.

Reciprocal translocations. The multihit chromosome aberrations previously described represent rather severe damage to the cell. At mitosis the acentric fragments will either be lost or be attracted to only one of the daughter cells, since they are unattached to a spindle fiber. Consequently, one or both of the daughter cells will be missing considerable genetic material.

Reciprocal translocations are multihit chromosome aberrations that require karyotypic analysis for their detection. The process of reciprocal translocation is diagramed in Fig. 28-11. Radiation-induced reciprocal translocations result in no loss of genetic material, simply a rearrangement of the genes. Consequently, all or nearly all genetic codes are available; they simply may be organized in an incorrect sequence.

Kinetics of chromosome aberration

At very low doses of radiation, only single-hit types of aberrations are observed. When the radiation dose exceeds perhaps 100 rad (1 Gy), the frequency of multihit aberrations increases more rapidly. Fig. 28-12 shows the general dose-response relationship for production of single- and multihit aberrations. Single-hit aberrations are produced with a **linear, nonthreshold** dose-response relationship. Multihit aberrations are produced following a **nonlinear, nonthreshold** relationship. These relationships have been determined experimentally by a number of investigators. The approximate equations for each of these relationships are

(28-1)

$$\textit{Single hit: } Y = a + bD$$

(28-2)

$$\textit{Multihit: } Y = a + bD + cD^2$$

where Y is the number of single- or multihit chromosome aberrations, a is the naturally occurring frequency of chromosome aberrations,

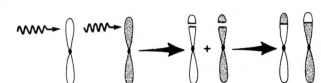

Fig. 28-11. Radiation-induced reciprocal translocations are multihit chromosome aberrations that require karyotypic analysis for detection.

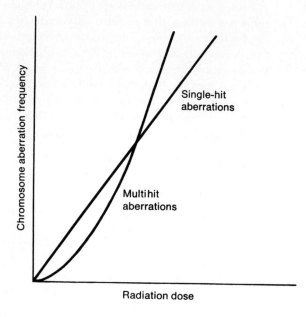

Fig. 28-12. Dose-response relationship for single-hit aberrations is linear, nonthreshold, whereas that for multihit aberrations is nonlinear, nonthreshold.

and b and c are coefficients of damage for single- and multihit aberrations, respectively. The variable, radiation dose, is represented by D.

Some laboratories are currently attempting to exploit cytogenetic analysis as a biologic radiation dosimeter. **The multihit aberrations are considered to be the most significant in terms of latent human damage.** If the radiation dose is unknown yet not life threatening, the approximate chromosome aberration frequency will be two single-hit aberrations per rad per 1000 cells and one multihit aberration per 10 rad per 1000 cells. This approximation holds through a total dose of perhaps 200 rad.

REVIEW QUESTIONS

1. Define or otherwise identify the following:
   a. Gastrointestinal death
   b. Latent period
   c. $LD_{50/30}$
   d. Erythema
   e. Clinical tolerance
   f. Primordial follicle
   g. Erythrocyte
   h. Karyotype
   i. Epilation
   j. Multihit aberration
2. Describe the changes in mean survival time with increasing dose.
3. What are the approximate values for $LD_{50/30}$ and SED_{50} in humans?
4. Describe the stages of gametogenesis in the male and the female and identify the most sensitive phases.
5. What are the four principal blood cell lines and the function of each?
6. Diagram the mechanism for the production of a reciprocal translocation.

29

Late effects of radiation

Unlike the early effects of radiation exposure that are produced by relatively high radiation doses, the delayed, or so-called late, effects can follow low doses delivered over a long time period. That is not to say that the late effects cannot be produced by high-dose, short-term exposure, since they can; but in diagnostic radiology, when one considers the exposure of both patient and personnel, the late effects are of particular importance. The radiation exposures that we experience in diagnostic radiology are low, and they are chronic in nature because they are delivered intermittently over long periods of time.

The principal late effects are radiation-induced malignancies and genetic effects. Life span shortening and effects on local tissues have also been reported as late effects. Our radiation protection guides are based on the suspected or observed late effects of radiation and on an **assumed linear, nonthreshold dose-response relationship.**

Studies of the responses of large numbers of persons to a stress require considerable statistical manipulation of data. Such studies are called **epidemiologic studies,** and they are required when the percentage of persons responding is small. Epidemiologic studies of persons exposed to radiation are difficult because (1) the dose is usually not known but presumed to be

Table 29-1. Minimum population sample required to show that the given radiation dose significantly elevated the incidence of leukemia

Dose (rad)	Required sample size (number of persons)
5	6,000,000
10	1,600,000
15	750,000
20	500,000
50	100,000

low and (2) the frequency of response is very low. Consequently, the results of radiation epidemiologic studies do not carry the statistical surety that observations of early radiation effects do.

Table 29-1 illustrates the difficulty of the problem. It shows the minimum number of persons that must be observed as a function of radiation dose to definitely link an increase in the incidence of leukemia with the radiation dose in question.

LOCAL TISSUE EFFECTS
Skin

In addition to the acute effects of erythema and desquamation and late developing carcinoma, chronic irradiation of the skin can result in severe nonmalignant changes. Early radiologists who performed fluoroscopic examinations without protective gloves developed a very calloused, discolored, and weathered appearance to the skin of their hands and forearms. In addition, the skin would be very tight and brittle and sometimes severely crack or flake. The dose necessary to produce such an effect would of course be very high. No such effects occur in the current practice of radiology.

Chromosomes

Irradiation of blood-forming organs can produce a hematologic depression as an early response or leukemia as a late response. Chromosome damage in the circulating lymphocytes can be produced as both an early and a late response. The types and frequency of chromosome aberrations have previously been described. It is important to point out here, however, that even a low dose of radiation can produce chromosome aberrations that may not be apparent until many years after the radiation exposure. For example, individuals irradiated accidentally with rather high radiation doses continue to show chromosome abnormalities in their peripheral lymphocytes as long as 20 years afterward. This presumably occurs because of

radiation damage to the lymphocytic stem cells. These cells may not be stimulated into replication and maturation for many years.

Cataracts

In 1932 E.O. Lawrence of the University of California developed the first **cyclotron,** a machine capable of accelerating charged particles to very high energies. These charged particles are used as bullets and are shot at the nuclei of target atoms in the study of nuclear structure. By 1940 every university physics department of any worth had built its own cyclotron and was engaged in what has come to be called high-energy physics.

A modern cyclotron is shown in Fig. 29-1. Early machines might be located in one room and a beam of high-energy particles would be extracted through a tube and steered and focused by electromagnets onto the target material in the adjacent room. At that time sophisticated electronic equipment was not available for controlling this high-energy beam. The cyclotron physicists used a tool of the radiologists, the fluorescent screen, to aid in steering the high-energy beam. Unfortunately, in so doing, the physicists would receive high radiation exposures to the lens of the eye because the beam-steering maneuver required that they look into the beam nearly directly.

In 1949 the first paper reporting cataracts in cyclotron physicists was presented. By 1960 several hundred such cases of radiation-induced cataracts had been reported. This was particularly tragic, since there were few high-energy physicists.

On the basis of these observations and animal experimentation, several conclusions can be drawn regarding radiation-induced cataracts. The radiosensitivity of the lenses of the eyes is age dependent. The older the individual, the greater the radiation effect and the shorter the latent period. Latent periods varying from 5 to 30 years have been observed in humans, and the average latent period is approximately 15 years.

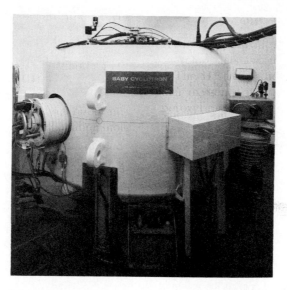

Fig. 29-1. Modern cyclotron used to produce radionuclides for nuclear medicine applications. (Courtesy Japan Steel Works America, Inc.)

High-LET radiation, such as neutrons, has a high RBE for the production of cataracts.

The dose-response relationship for radiation-induced cataracts is apparently threshold, non-linear. If the local tissue dose is high enough, in excess of approximately 1000 rad (10 Gy), nearly 100% of those who are irradiated will develop cataracts. The precise level of the threshold dose is difficult to assess. Most investigators would suggest that the threshold following an acute x-ray exposure is approximately 200 rad (2 Gy). The threshold following fractionated exposure, such as that in radiology, is probably in excess of 1000 rad (10 Gy).

Occupational exposures to the lens of the eye are too low to require protective lens shields for technologists or radiologists. It is nearly impossible for a medical radiation worker to reach the threshold dose.

The radiation level to patients undergoing head and neck examination by either conventional or computed tomographic techniques can be rather significant. In multidirectional conventional tomography the dose to the lens of the eyes can easily be 1 rad per view. Many such examinations require twenty views or more. In computed tomography the lens dose can likewise be 1 rad per slice. However, in this situation usually no more than one or two slices intersect the lens. In either case **protective lens shields should be employed when the use of such devices does not interfere with obtaining the required diagnostic information.**

LIFE SPAN SHORTENING

There have been several dozen experiments conducted with animals following both acute and chronic irradiation that show that such animals die young. Fig. 29-2 is redrawn from several such representative experiments and shows that the relationship between life span shortening and dose is apparently linear, nonthreshold. When all the animal data are considered collectively and a meaningful extrapolation to humans

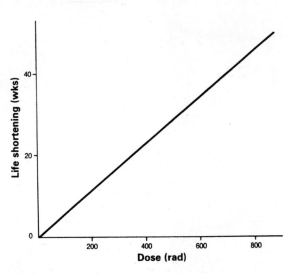

Fig. 29-2. In chronically irradiated animals the extent of life shortening appears linear, nonthreshold. This graph shows the representative results of several such experiments with mice.

Table 29-2. Risk of life span shortening as a consequence of occupation, disease, or various other conditions

Risky condition	Expected days of life lost
Being male rather than female	2800
Heart disease	2100
Being unmarried	2000
One pack of cigarettes a day	1600
Working as a coal miner	1100
Cancer	980
30 pounds overweight	900
Stroke	520
All accidents	435
Service in Vietnam	400
Motor vehicle accidents	200
Average occupational accidents	74
Speed limit increase from 55 to 65 mph	40
Radiation worker	12
Airplane crashes	1

is attempted, it is concluded that, **at worst, humans can expect a reduced life span of 10 days for every rad.**

Review the data presented in Table 29-2, which was compiled by Bernard L. Cohen of the University of Pittsburgh and extrapolated from various statistical sources of mortality. The expected loss of life in days is given as a function of occupation, disease, or other condition. As one can see, the most grievous risk is being male rather than female. Whereas the average life shortening caused by occupational accidents is 74 days, that for radiation workers is only 12 days. **Radiologic technology is a safe occupation.**

This radiation-induced life span shortening is nonspecific, that is, there are no characteristic disease entities associated with it, and it does not include late malignant effects. It is simply accelerated premature aging and death.

Observations on human populations have not been totally convincing. No life span shortening has been observed in the atomic bomb survivors, and some received rather substantial radiation doses. Life span shortening in watch-dial painters, x-ray patients, and other human radiation populations does not exist.

One population that has been rather extensively studied by a number of investigators is the American radiologists. Such a study has many shortcomings, not the least of which is the fact that it is retrospective in nature. Fig. 29-3 shows the results obtained when the age at death for radiologists was compared with the age at death for the general population. Radiologists dying in the early 1930s were approximately 5 years younger than the average age at death of the general population. However, as shown in Fig. 29-3, this difference in age at death had shrunk to zero by 1965.

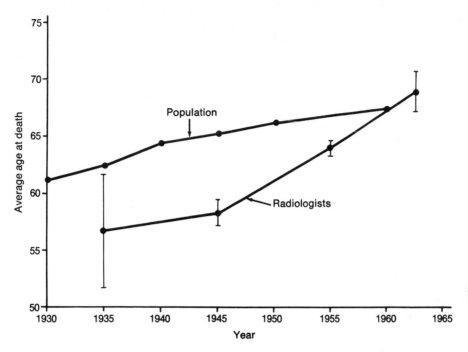

Fig. 29-3. Radiation-induced life span shortening is shown for American radiologists. The age at death in the radiologists has been less than that of the general population, but this difference has disappeared.

A more recent study used two other physician groups as controls rather than the general population. Table 29-3 summarizes the results of this investigation. The three physician groups observed in this study were members of the radiological society of North America (RSNA) as the high-risk group, members of the American College of Physicians (ACP) as the intermediate-risk group, and members of the American Academy of Ophthalmology and Otolaryngology (AAOO) as the low-risk group. A comparison of the median age at death and age-adjusted death rates for these three physician specialties demonstrates a significant difference in age at death during the early years of radiology. This difference has disappeared in the contemporary practice of radiology, presumably because of better

Table 29-3. Death statistics for three groups of physicians

	Median age at death	Age-adjusted deaths per 1000
1935 to 1944		
RSNA	71.4	18.4
ACP	73.4	15.4
AAOO	76.2	13.0
1945 to 1954		
RSNA	72.0	16.4
ACP	74.8	13.7
AAOO	76.0	11.9
1955 to 1958		
RSNA	73.5	13.6
ACP	76.0	11.4
AAOO	76.4	10.6

attention to radiation protection through proper procedures and equipment design.

When these differences in mortality were first described, British investigators began looking for similar effects in British radiologists. To date none has been found, which raises some questions about the validity and significance of the findings in American radiologists.

One investigator has evaluated the death records of radiologic technologists who operated field x-ray machines during World War II. These machines were poorly designed and inadequately shielded so that the technologists received higher than normal exposures. Seven thousand such technologists have been studied, and no radiation effects have been observed.

RISK ESTIMATES

The early effects of high-dose radiation exposure are usually easy to observe and measure. The late effects are also easy to observe, but it is difficult if not impossible to associate a particular late response with a previous radiation exposure history. Consequently, precise dose-response relationships are often not possible, and we therefore resort to **risk estimates.** There are three types of risk estimates, and they each represent different statements of risk and have different dimensions.

Relative risk

If one observes a large population for late radiation effects without having any precise knowledge of the radiation dose to which they are exposed, then the concept of **relative risk** is employed. The relative risk is computed by comparing the number of persons in the exposed population showing a given late effect with the number who developed the same late effect in an unexposed population. For instance, a relative risk of 1 would indicate no risk at all. A relative risk of 1.5 indicates that the frequency of the late response under observation is 50% higher in the irradiated group compared with the nonirradiated population.

Relative risk factors for radiation-induced late effects in humans range from 1 to 10 and sometimes even higher. For the late effects of particular importance observed in human populations, most are reported in the range from 1 to 2. Occasionally, an investigation will result in a relative risk of less than 1. This would indicate that the exposed population receives some protective benefit, but of course this is not likely. The consistent interpretation of such studies is that the results are not statistically significant either because of the small number of observations or because of inadequate identification of irradiated and control populations.

EXAMPLE: In a study of radiation-induced leukemia following diagnostic levels of radiation, 227 cases were observed in 100,000 persons so irradiated. The normal incidence of leukemia in the United States is 150 cases per 100,000. If this normal incidence was assumed to occur in a completely nonirradiated population, what would be the relative risk of radiation-induced leukemia?

ANSWER: $\dfrac{\dfrac{227}{100,000}}{\dfrac{150}{100,000}} = \dfrac{0.00227}{0.00150} = 1.51$

Absolute risk

If some information is available regarding the radiation dose and if at least two different dose levels are involved, then it may be possible to determine an absolute risk factor. Unlike the relative risk, which is a dimensionless ratio, the absolute risk has units of **number of cases/10^6 persons/rad/year.** Absolute risk values range from approximately one to ten cases/10^6 persons/ rad/yr. To determine the absolute risk factor, one must assume a linear dose-response relationship. If the dose-response relationship is assumed nonthreshold, then only one dose level is required. The value of the absolute risk factor is equal to the slope of the dose-response relationship (Fig. 29-4). The error bars on each data point indicate the precision of the observation of response.

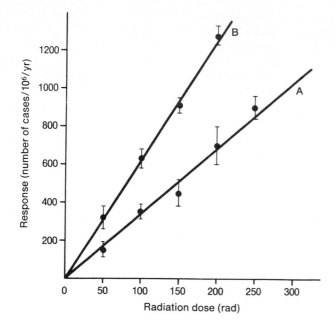

Fig. 29-4. Slope of the linear, nonthreshold dose-response relationship is equal to the absolute risk. *A* and *B* show absolute risks of 3.4 and 6.2 cases/10^6 persons/rad/yr, respectively.

EXAMPLE: The absolute risk for radiation-induced breast cancer is considered to be six cases/10^6 persons/rad/yr for a 20-year at-risk period. If 100,000 women receive 1 rad during mammography, what total number of cancers would be expected to be induced?

ANSWER: (Six cases/10^6 persons/rad/yr) (10^5 persons) (1 rad) (20 yr) = twelve cases

Excess risk

Often when an investigation of human radiation response indicates the induction of some late effect, the magnitude of the effect will be expressed by the **excess cases induced.** Leukemia, for instance, is known to occur spontaneously in nonirradiated populations. If the leukemia incidence in an irradiated population exceeds that which is expected, then the difference between the observed number of cases and the expected number would be excess cases. The excess cases in this instance are assumed to be radiation induced. To determine the number of excess cases, one must be able to measure the observed number of cases in the irradiated population and compare them with the number that would have been expected on the basis of known population levels.

EXAMPLE: Twenty-three cases of skin cancer were observed in a population of 1000 radiologists. The incidence in the general population is 0.5/100,000. How many excess skin cancers were produced in the population of radiologists?

ANSWER:

$$\text{Excess cases} = \text{Observed} - \text{Expected}$$
$$= 23 - 0.005$$
$$\approx 23$$

Since none would be expected, all twenty-three cases represent risk.

RADIATION-INDUCED MALIGNANCY

All the late effects, including radiation-induced malignancy, have been observed in experimental animals, and from these animal experiments dose-response relationships have been developed. At the human level these late effects have been observed, but often there are insufficient data to precisely identify the dose-response relationship. Consequently, some of the conclusions drawn regarding human responses are based in part on animal data.

Leukemia

When one considers radiation-induced leukemia in laboratory animals, there is no question that this response is real and that the incidence increases with increasing radiation dose. The form of the dose-response relationship is apparently linear and nonthreshold. A number of human population groups have exhibited an elevated incidence of leukemia following radiation exposure: A-bomb survivors, radiotherapy patients, American radiologists, and children irradiated in utero, to name a few.

A-bomb survivors. Probably the greatest wealth of information that we have on radiation-induced leukemia in humans results from observations of the survivors of the atomic bombings of Hiroshima and Nagasaki. At the time of the bomb (**ATB**), approximately 300,000 persons were living in those two cities. Nearly 100,000 were killed from the blast and early effects of radiation. Another 100,000 persons received significant doses of radiation and survived. The remainder were unaffected since their radiation exposure was very low.

Following World War II, scientists of the Atomic Bomb Casualty Commission (**ABCC**), now known as the Radiation Effects Research Foundation (**RERF**), attempted to determine the radiation dose received by each of the A-bomb survivors in both cities. They first estab-

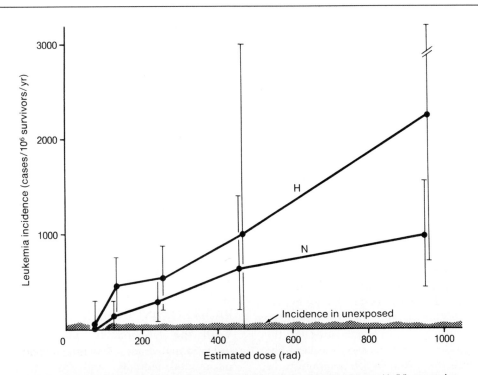

Fig. 29-5. Data from the atomic bomb survivors of Hiroshima *(H)* and Nagasaki *(N)* suggest a linear, nonthreshold dose-response relationship.

lished the position of each individual ATB and estimated the dose to that survivor by considering not only distance from the hypocenter (the point at ground level where the bomb exploded) but also terrain, type of bomb, type of construction if the survivor were inside, and other factors

Table 29-4. Summary of the incidence of leukemia in A-bomb survivors

	Hiroshima	Nagasaki	Total
Total number of survivors in study	74,356	25,037	99,393
Observed cases of leukemia	102	42	144
Expected cases of leukemia	39	13	52

that might influence dose. To assist in these dose estimations, simulated explosions were carried out on the Nevada desert where various Japanese structures had been erected.

A summary of the data obtained by these investigations is given in Table 29-4. The results of the data analysis are shown in Fig. 29-5. The spontaneous incidence of leukemia in the Japanese ATB was approximately twenty-five cases/ 10^6 persons/yr. Following high doses, the leukemia incidence is as much as 100 times that in the nonirradiated population. Even though there are large error bars at each dose increment, it is clear that the response appears linear, nonthreshold. However, if one expands the data in the low-dose region (for example, below 200 rad), one could conclude that a threshold exists and is in the neighborhood of 50 rad. Never-

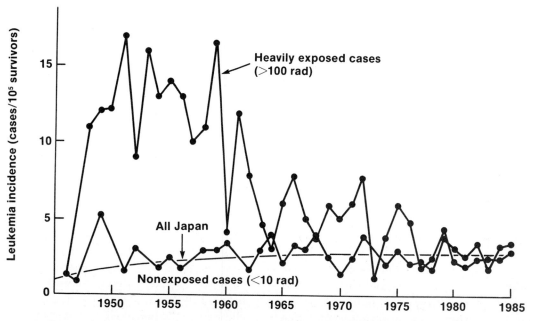

Fig. 29-6. Incidence of leukemia in the A-bomb survivors increased rapidly for the first few years and has slowly declined since.

theless, neither this information nor other available information is interpreted to support a threshold response. **Radiation-induced leukemia is considered linear, nonthreshold.**

Fig. 29-6 demonstrated the temporal distribution of the onset of leukemia in the A-bomb survivors since August 1945. The data are presented as cases per 100,000 and include for comparison the leukemia rate in the population at large and in the nonexposed populations of the bombed cities. There was a rather rapid rise in leukemia incidence that reached a plateau after about 5 years. The incidence has been declining slowly since that time. Based on this analysis, **radiation-induced leukemia is considered to have a latent period of 4 to 7 years and an at-risk period of approximately 20 years.** The at-risk period is that time following irradiation during which one might expect the radiation effect to occur.

The data from the A-bomb survivors show without a doubt that the radiation exposure to those survivors caused the later development of leukemia. However, it is interesting to reflect on some additional aspects of these events. The first bomb was dropped on Hiroshima; it was fueled with uranium, so the radiation dose was about equally distributed between gamma rays and neutrons. The Nagasaki bomb was a plutonium bomb. Ninety percent of its radiation was caused by gamma rays and only 10% by neutrons. Neutron radiation has a higher RBE than gamma rays, and this difference contributes to the difficulties in assessing the dose for each survivor.

Of the 300,000 total resident population, 335 persons are estimated to have survived doses in excess of 600 rad. Through 1975 there had been only 144 cases of leukemia in the total exposed population. Acute Leukemia and chronic myelocytic leukemia were observed most often in the A-bomb survivors. Chronic lymphocytic leukemia is rare and therefore not considered to be a form of radiation-induced leukemia.

Taken to the final analysis, the data from the A-bomb survivors pointed to an absolute risk factor of 1.5 cases/10^6 persons/rad/yr. The overall relative risk based on the total number of observed leukemia deaths (144) vs. the number of expected leukemia deaths (52) is approximately 2.8:1.

Radiologists. By the second decade of radiology, reports of pernicious anemia and leukemia in radiologists were not uncommon. In the early 1940s several investigators had reviewed the incidence of leukemia in American radiologists and found it alarmingly high. These early radiologists functioned without the benefit of modern radiation protection devices and procedures, and many served as both radiotherapists and diagnostic radiologists. In radiotherapy activities they received substantial radiation exposures from radium applications. It has been estimated that some of these early radiologists received doses exceeding 100 rad/yr (1 Gy/yr).

A report of the death records of medical specialists dying between 1929 and 1943 showed that 8 out of 175 deaths in radiologists were caused by leukemia. In nonradiologist physicians there were 221 leukemia deaths in a total of 55,160 total deaths. These data indicate a relative risk of 10.3:1. In a more recent study covering the years 1948 to 1963 and based on a total of 12 leukemia cases in 425 radiology-related deaths, a relative risk of 4:1 was obtained. Currently, American radiologists do not exhibit an elevated incidence of leukemia when compared with other physician specialists.

It must be pointed out that a rather exhaustive study of mortality in radiologists in Great Britain covering the period from the turn of the century to 1960 did not show such an elevated risk of leukemia. The reasons for such a different experience between American and British radiologists is unknown. Some suggest that it is because the radiation therapy activities in Great Britain have always been attended by radiologic physicists, who presumably were more radiation safety conscious.

Studies of radiation-induced leukemia in American radiologic technologists have been conducted, and they consistently show no evidence of such an effect.

Ankylosing spondylitis patients. In the 1940s and 1950s, in Great Britain particularly, it was common practice to treat ankylosing spondylitis patients with radiation. Ankylosing spondylitis is an arthritic-like condition along the vertebral column that causes one to hunch over. Such patients cannot walk upright or move except with great difficulty. For relief they would be given rather high doses of radiation to the spinal column, and the treatment was quite successful.

Patients who previously had to walk hunched over could now stand erect. It was a permanent cure and remained the treatment of choice for approximately 20 years, until it was discovered that some who had been cured by radiation were dying from leukemia. The graphic results on the observations of these patients are shown in Fig. 29-7. During the period from 1935 to 1955, 14,554 male patients were treated at eighty-one different radiation therapy centers in Great Britain. Review of the treatment records showed the dose to the bone marrow of the spinal column to range from 100 to 4000 rad (1 to 40 Gy). Fifty-two cases of leukemia occurred in this population.

The rate of leukemia in patients receiving more than 2000 rad was 17 cases/10,000 persons; in Great Britain the normal incidence of leukemia was 0.5 cases/10,000. The relative risk, therefore, is approximately 34:1. When one considers all 52 cases and compares the incidence of leukemia with that of the general population, the relative risk is 9.5:1.

The absolute risk can be obtained from these data by determining the slope of the best fit line through the data points, as shown in Fig. 29-7. Such an analysis results in approximately 0.8 cases/10^6 persons/rad/yr. If 95% confidence limits are placed on the data, one could not rule out the possibility of a threshold dose at approximately 300 rad.

Leukemia in other populations. There have been a number of studies designed to link leukemia incidence with environmental factors. Background radiation levels increase in general with altitude and with latitude, but the range of levels observed is not sufficient to demonstrate a relationship with leukemia.

Other population groups that have provided

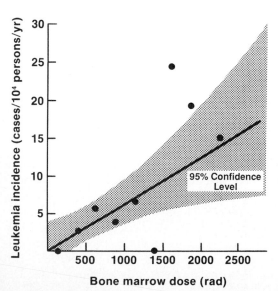

Fig. 29-7. Results of observations of leukemia in ankylosing spondylitis patients treated with x-ray therapy suggest a linear, nonthreshold dose-response relationship. The line is the best fit to the observed data, and it has a slope of approximately 0.8 cases/10^6 persons/rad/yr.

evidence, both positive and negative, regarding the leukemia-inducing action of radiation are radium watch-dial painters, children receiving superficial x-ray treatment, and some additional adult radiotherapy groups.

Cancer

What has been discussed regarding radiation-induced leukemia can be reported also for radiation-induced cancer. We do not have quite as much human data concerning cancer as for leukemia; nevertheless, it can be said without question that radiation can cause cancer. Nearly all types of human cancer have been implicated as capable of being radiation induced. The relative risk factors and absolute risks are shown to be similar to those reported for leukemia. Many types of cancer have been implicated as radiation induced, and a discussion of the more important ones is in order.

It is difficult to ascribe any case of cancer to a previous radiation exposure, regardless of its magnitude, because cancer is so common. Approximately 20% of all deaths are caused by cancer; therefore any radiation-induced cancers are obscured. Leukemia, on the other hand, is a rare disease that makes analysis of radiation-induced leukemia easier.

Thyroid cancer. Neoplasms of the thyroid gland have developed in three groups of patients whose thyroid glands were irradiated in childhood. The first two groups, called the Ann Arbor series and the Rochester series, consist of individuals who, in the 1940s and early 1950s, were treated shortly after birth for thymus gland enlargement. The thymus is a gland just below the thyroid gland that can enlarge shortly after birth in response to infection. At these facilities, radiotherapy was often the treatment of choice. Following a dose of up to 500 rad (5 Gy), the thymus gland would shrink so that all enlargement disappeared. No further problems were evident until up to 20 years later, when some of these patients began to develop thyroid nodules

and some cases of thyroid cancer. In the Ann Arbor series several thousand children were involved. The dose to the thyroid gland was estimated to be 20 to 30 rad (200 to 300 mGy) and received mainly from scatter radiation from the adjacent useful beam to the thymus gland. Reasonable beam collimation was practiced. In the Rochester series there was a smaller number of cases, but the practice was to irradiate a rather large area so that the thymus gland and thyroid gland were equally irradiated. The estimated thyroid dose was approximately 300 rad (3 Gy).

The final group included twenty-one children who were natives of the Rongelap Atoll in 1954; they were subjected to high levels of fallout during an atomic bomb test. The winds shifted during the test, carrying the fallout over the adjacent inhabited island rather than one that had been evacuated. These children received radiation doses to the thyroid gland from both external exposure and internal ingestion of about 1200 rad (12 Gy).

If one computes the incidence of thyroid nodularity, considered preneoplastic, in these three groups and plots this incidence as a function of estimated dose, the result will be that shown in Fig. 29-8. Admittedly, the error bars on both the dose data and the incidence levels are large. Still, the implication of a linear, nonthreshold dose-response relationship is clear.

In a similar population of children irradiated for thymic enlargement, 24 thyroid carcinomas were reported in nearly 3000 irradiated patients; none was reported in 5000 nonirradiated siblings. The absolute risk factor was reported as 2.5 cases/10^6 persons/rad/yr.

Bone cancer. There are two population groups that have contributed an enormous amount of data showing that radiation causes bone cancer. The first group consists of the radium watch-dial painters. In the 1920s and 1930s there were various small laboratories whose employees, mostly female, worked at benches with luminous paints containing radium sulfate. The

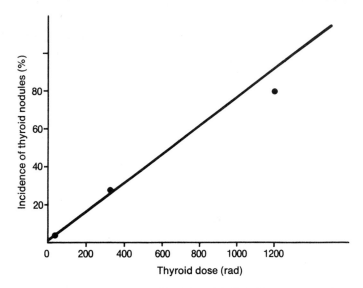

Fig. 29-8. Radiation-induced preneoplastic thyroid nodularity in three groups of persons whose thyroid glands were irradiated in childhood.

job involved painting watch dials with paint laden with radium salt. To prepare a fine point on the paintbrushes, the employees would touch the tip of the brush to the tongue. In this manner substantial quantities of radium were ingested.

Radium salts were used because the emitted radiation, principally alpha and beta particles, would continuously excite the luminous compounds so they would glow in the dark. Current technology uses harmlessly low levels of tritium (^{3}H) and promethium (^{147}Pm) for this purpose.

When ingested, the radium would behave metabolically like calcium and deposit in bone structures. Because of radium's long half-life (1620 years) and alpha emission, the employees received radiation doses up to 50,000 rad (500 Gy) to bone. Seventy-two bone cancers in some 800 persons have been observed during a follow-up period in excess of 50 years. Analysis of these data has resulted in an overall relative risk of 122:1. The absolute risk is equal to 0.11 cases/ 10^6 persons/rad/yr.

Another population to develop excess bone cancer is patients treated with radium salts for a variety of diseases from arthritis to tuberculosis. Such treatments were common practice in many parts of the world until about 1950.

Skin cancer. Skin cancer usually begins with the development of a radiodermatitis. Significant data have been developed from several reports of skin cancer induced in radiotherapy patients treated with orthovoltage (200 to 300 kVp) or superficial x rays (50 to 150 kVp). From these data we conclude that the latent period is approximately 5 to 10 years. **Radiation-induced skin cancer follows a threshold dose-response relationship,** but we do not have enough data with which to develop absolute risk values. When the dose delivered to the skin was in the range of 500 to 2000 rad (5 to 20 Gy), the relative risk of developing skin cancer was 4:1. If the dose were 4000 to 6000 rad (40 to 60 Gy) or 6000 to 10,000 rad (60 to 100 Gy), the relative risks were 14:1 and 27:1, respectively.

Breast cancer. In Chapter 19 some of the radiographic techniques employed in mammography were discussed. The radiation dose to mammography patients is considered in a later chapter. At this time a discussion of the risk of radiation-induced breast cancer will be considered.

There is a continuing controversy regarding the risk of radiation-induced breast cancer, and the implications of this controversy carry to breast cancer detection by x-ray mammography. The concern of such risk first surfaced in the middle 1960s following the published reports of breast cancer developing in tuberculosis patients. Tuberculosis was for many years treated by isolation in a sanitorium. During the patient's stay, one mode of therapy was to induce an artificial pneumothorax in the affected lung, and this was done under fluoroscopy. Many patients received multiple treatments and up to several hundred fluoroscopic examinations. Precise dose determinations are not possible, but levels of several hundred rad would have been common. In some of these patient populations the relative risks for radiation-induced breast cancer were shown to be as high as 10:1.

One such population exhibited no excess risk. This finding, however, was explained as a consequence of the fluoroscopic technique. In the positive studies previously mentioned the patient faced away from the radiologist, toward the fluoroscopic x-ray tube, during exposure. In the study that reported negative findings, the patients were fluoroscoped facing the radiologist so that the radiation beam entered posteriorly. The breast tissue was exposed only to the low-intensity beam exiting the patient.

Additional studies have produced results suggesting radiation-induced breast cancer in patients treated with x rays for acute postpartum mastitis. The dose to these patients ranged from 75 to 1000 rad (0.75 to 10 Gy). The relative risk factor in this population was approximately 2.5:1.

Radiation-induced breast cancer has also been observed in the atomic bomb survivors. Through 1980, observations on nearly 12,000 women who received radiation doses to the breasts of 10 rad or more exhibited a relative risk of 4:1.

In some of these studies only one breast was irradiated. In nearly every such case breast cancer developed only in the irradiated breast. These patients have now been followed for up to 25 years. On the basis of all available data regarding radiation-induced breast cancer, the best estimate for absolute risk is six cases/10^6 persons/rad/yr.

Lung cancer. Early in this century it was observed that approximately 50% of the workers in the Bohemian pitchblende mines died of lung cancer. Lung cancer incidence in the general population was negligible by comparison. The dusty mine environment was considered to be the cause of this lung cancer. Now it is known that radiation exposure from radon in the mines contributed to the incidence of lung cancer in these miners.

Recently, observations on the American uranium miners active in the Colorado plateau in the 1950s and 1960s have also pointed out elevated levels of lung cancer. The peak of this activity occurred in about 1961 when there were approximately 4000 miners active in nearly 500 underground mines and 150 open pit mines. Most of the mines were worked by less than ten men; therefore, for such a small operation, one could expect a lack of proper ventilation.

The radiation exposure of these miners occurred because of the high concentration of uranium ore. Uranium, which is radioactive with a very long half-life of 10^9 years, decays through a series of radioactive nuclides by successive alpha and beta emissions, each accompanied by gamma radiation. One of the decay products of uranium is radon (^{222}Rn). This radionuclide is a gas that emanates through the rock to produce a high concentration in the air. When breathed, the radon can be deposited in the lung spaces where it undergoes additional successive series decay to a stable isotope of lead. During these subsequent decay actions, several alpha particles are released, and these result in a rather high local dose. Also, alpha particles are high-LET radiation and therefore have a high RBE.

To date more than 4000 uranium miners have been observed, and they have received estimated doses to lung tissue as high as 3000 rad, and on this basis the relative risk was approximately 8:1. Interestingly, smoking uranium miners have a relative risk of approximately 20:1.

The available data indicate a dose-response relationship that is linear, nonthreshold with an absolute risk of 1.3 cases/10^6 persons/rad/yr.

Liver cancer. Thorium dioxide (ThO_2) in a colloidal suspension known as **Thorotrast** was widely used in diagnostic radiology between 1925 and 1945 as a contrast agent for angiography. Thorotrast was about 25% by weight ThO_2, and it contained the several radioactive isotopes of thorium and its decay products. Radiation that was emitted produced a dose in the ratio of about 100:10:1 of alpha, beta, and gamma radiation, respectively. The use of Thorotrast has been shown to be responsible for several types of carcinoma following a latent period of about 15 to 20 years. Following extravascular injection, it is carcinogenic at the site of the injection. Following intravascular injection, thorium dioxide particles are deposited in phagocytic cells of the reticuloendothelial system and are concentrated in the liver and spleen. Its long half-life and high alpha radiation dose has resulted in many cases of cancer in these organs.

TOTAL RISK OF MALIGNANCY

From the basis of many of these observations on human population groups following exposure to low-level radiation, and considering all the risk estimates taken collectively for leukemia and cancer, a number of simplified conclusions can be made. The overall absolute risk for in-

duction of malignancy probably lies in the range of two to six cases/10^6 persons/rad/yr with the at-risk period extending for 20 to 25 years following exposure. This is approximately 50 to 150 deaths from radiation-induced malignancy following an exposure of 1 rad to 1,000,000 persons when all such cases occurring within 25 years of exposure are counted.

To make these values somewhat more meaningful, we can consider the celebrated Three Mile Island incident. There are approximately 2,000,000 people residing within a 80 km (50-mile) radius of Three Mile Island. On the basis of our total population statistics, one would expect to observe approximately 330,000 cancer deaths in these persons. During the total period of the radiation incident, the average dose to persons living within a 160 km (100 mile) radius was 8 mrad; to those within the 80 km (50 mile) radius it was 1.5 mrad. Applying the upper limit estimate just cited, one would predict that the Three Mile Island incident will result in no more than one additional malignant death as a result of this population radiation exposure.

The Committee on the Biologic Effects of Ionizing Radiation (BEIR), an arm of the National Academy of Sciences, has reviewed the late effects of low-dose, low-LET radiation. Their results are shown in Table 29-5, and they are accepted by most.

The BEIR Committee examined two situations. First, they estimated the excess cases of malignant disease following a one-time acciden-

Table 29-5. BEIR Committee estimated excess mortality from malignant disease in 1 million persons

	Absolute risk	Relative risk
Normal expectation	163,800	163,800
Excess cases		
Single exposure to 10 rad	766	2255
1 rad/yr for life	4751	11,970

tal exposure to 10 rad; such a situation is highly unlikely in radiology. Second, they considered the response to a dose of 1 rad/yr for life; this situation is possible in diagnostic radiology but is certainly rare. The dose-response relationship most likely to be true is the linear, quadratic model. These analyses showed an additional 766 to 2255 cases of malignant disease in a population of 1 million following 10 rad and an additional 4751 to 11,970 cases following 1 rad/yr. These cases are in addition to the normal incidence of cancer, which is 163,800 cases per 1 million persons. The BEIR Committee has further stated that **less than 1 rad/yr may not be harmful.**

RADIATION AND PREGNANCY

Since the first medical applications of x-radiation, there has been concern and apprehension regarding the effects of radiation before, during, and after pregnancy. Before pregnancy, the concern is interrupted fertility. During pregnancy, concern is directed to the possible congenital effects in newborns. The postpregnancy concerns are related to the suspected genetic effects. All these effects have been demonstrated in animals, and some have been observed in humans.

Effects on fertility

The early effect of high-level radiation on the interruption of fertility in both males and females has been discussed, and there is ample evidence to show that such an effect does exist and is dose related. However, the effects of low-dose, long-term irradiation on fertility are less well defined.

Animal data in this area are lacking. Those that are available indicate that, even when radiation is delivered at the rate of 100 rad per year, there is no noticeable depression in fertility.

There have been two national surveys of American radiologists, one reported in 1927 and the other in 1955. In each case a finding of depressed fertility and increased congenital abnormalities in the offspring of radiologists was reported. Both these studies have been questioned because of the experimental methods involved. The conclusions reported are not generally accepted.

Irradiation in utero

Irradiation in utero concerns two types of exposures: that of the radiation worker and that of the patient. The recommended techniques and radiation control procedures associated with these exposed persons are considered fully in Chapter 32. At this time the biologic effects of such irradiation will be considered.

There are substantial animal data to describe rather completely the effects of relatively high doses of radiation delivered during various periods of gestation. Because the embryo is a rapidly developing cell system, it is particularly sensitive to radiation. With age the embryo (and then the fetus) becomes less sensitive to the effects of radiation, and this pattern continues into adulthood. After maturity, however, mammalian radiosensitivity increases with age. Fig. 29-9 is a summary of the observed $LD_{50/30}$ in mice exposed at various times, showing this age-related radiosensitivity.

All observations point to the first trimester during pregnancy as the most sensitive period. Such findings are of particular concern because an x-ray exposure often occurs when pregnancy is unknown.

The effects of radiation in utero are time related and dose related. They include prenatal death, neonatal death, congenital abnormalities, malignancy induction, general impairment of growth, genetic effects, and mental retardation. Fig. 29-10 is redrawn from studies designed to observe the effects of a 200 rad (2 Gy) dose delivered at various stages in utero in mice. The scale along the x axis indicates the approximate comparable time in humans.

Within **2 weeks** of fertilization, the most pronounced effect of a high radiation dose is prenatal death, which is manifested as a sponta-

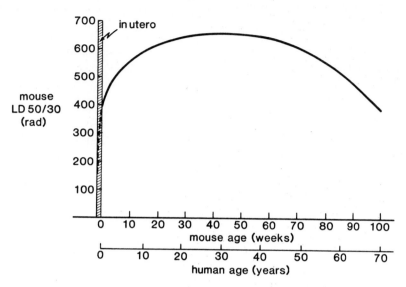

Fig. 29-9. LD$_{50/30}$ of mice in relation to age at time of irradiation.

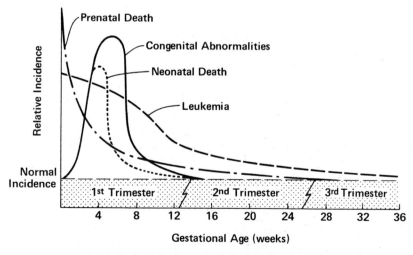

Fig. 29-10. Following 200 rad delivered at various times in utero, a number of effects can be observed. The incidence of these effects in nonirradiated persons is shown by the horizontal dashed line.

neous abortion. Observations in radiotherapy patients have confirmed this effect but only after rather high doses.

On the basis of animal experimentation, it would appear that this response is very rare. Our best estimate is that a 10 rad (0.1 Gy) dose during the first 2 weeks will induce perhaps 0.1% spontaneous abortions. This is in addition to the 25% to 50% normal incidence of spontaneous abortions. Fortunately, this response is of the all-or-none variety. Either there is a radiation-induced abortion or the pregnancy will carry to term with no ill effect. The first 2 weeks of pregnancy may indeed be the safest.

During the period of **major organogenesis,** from the second through the eighth week, two effects are likely to occur. Early in this period, skeletal abnormalities can be induced. As major organogenesis continues, congenital abnormalities of other organs can be observed if the pregnancy is carried to term. If the radiation-induced congenital abnormalities are severe enough, the result will be neonatal death. Following a dose of 200 rad (2 Gy) to the mouse, nearly 100% of the fetuses suffered significant abnormalities. In 80% it was sufficient to cause neonatal death. Such effects are rare following diagnostic levels of exposure and are essentially undetectable after radiation doses less than 10 rad (0.1 Gy). A dose of 10 rad (0.1 Gy) during this time is expected to increase the incidence of congenital abnormalities by 1% above the natural incidence. To complicate matters, there is a 4% to 10% incidence of naturally occurring congenital abnormalities in the unexposed population.

Irradiation in utero at the human level has been associated with childhood malignancy by a number of investigators. Perhaps the most complete study of this effect was conducted by Alice Stewart and her co-workers in a project known as the Oxford Survey, a study of childhood malignancies, in England, Scotland, and Wales. Nearly every case of such childhood ma-

Table 29-6. Relative risk of childhood leukemia following irradiation in utero by trimester

Time of x-ray examination	Relative risk
First trimester	8.3
Second trimester	1.5
Third trimester	1.4
TOTAL	1.5

lignancy in these countries since 1946 has been investigated. Each case was first identified and then investigated by way of interview with the mother, review of the hospital charts, and review of the physician records. Each "case" of childhood malignancy was matched with a "control" for age, sex, place of birth, socioeconomic status, and other demographic factors. The control was a child who matched with the "case" in all respects except for the development of a malignancy. The Oxford Survey is being continued at this time and has now considered in excess of 8000 cases and a like number of matched controls.

Although the Oxford Survey has reviewed all malignancies, it is the findings of radiation-induced leukemia that have been of particular importance. Table 29-6 shows the results of this survey in terms of relative risk. A relative risk of the development of childhood leukemia following irradiation in utero of 1.5 is significant. This indicates an increase of 50% over the presumed nonirradiated rate. However, the number of cases involved is small. The incidence of childhood leukemia in the population at large is approximately 9 cases per 100,000 live births. According to the Oxford Survey, if all 100,000 had been irradiated in utero, perhaps 14 cases of leukemia would have resulted. Although these findings have been substantiated in several American populations, there is no consensus among radiation scientists that this effect follow-

Table 29-7. Summary of effects following 10 rad in utero

Time of exposure	Type of response	Natural occurrence	Radiation response
0-2 weeks	Spontaneous abortion	25%-50%	0.1%
2-8 weeks	Congenital abnormalities	4%-10%	1%
0-9 months	Malignant disease	16/100,000	24/100,000
0-9 months	Impaired growth and development	1%	nil
0-9 months	Genetic mutations	10%	nil

ing such low doses is indeed real.

There are other effects following irradiation in utero that have been studied rather fully in animals and have been observed in some human populations. Radiation exposure in utero does retard the growth and development of the newborn. Not only are the physical growth and development affected but the mental growth as well. Irradiation in utero, principally during the period of major organogenesis, has been associated with microcephaly (small head) and mental retardation. The human data bearing on these effects are obtained from patients irradiated medically, the atomic bomb survivors, and the residents of the Marshall Islands who were exposed to radioactive fallout in 1954 during weapons testing. For instance, the heavily irradiated children at Hiroshima are, on the average, 2.25 cm (0.9 in) shorter, 3 kg (6.6 lb) lighter, and 1.1 cm (0.4 in) smaller in head circumference than members of the nonirradiated control groups. These effects, as well as mental retardation, have been observed principally in those receiving doses in excess of 100 rad (1 Gy) in utero. The lack of appropriate and sensitive tests of mental function make it impossible to draw similar conclusions at doses below 100 rad (1 Gy).

A summary of the effects of irradiation in utero is shown in Table 29-7. There are three responses of concern in radiology—spontaneous abortion, congenital abnormalities, and childhood malignancy. Spontaneous abortion causes

the least concern of the three, since it is an all-or-none effect. Congenital abnormalities and childhood malignancy are of real concern, but it should be recognized that the probability of such a response following a fetal dose of 10 rad (0.1 Gy) is nil. Furthermore, 10 rad to the fetus is very rarely ever experienced in radiology.

The form of the dose-response relationship for each of these effects is unknown. However, they do appear to be linear and nonthreshold when based on doses greater than 100 rad (1 Gy). When large experimental animal populations were acutely exposed, the minimum reported dose for observing such effects as statistically significant was approximately 10 rad (0.1 Gy). There is no evidence at either the human or the animal level to indicate that the levels of radiation exposure currently experienced occupationally and medically are responsible for any such effects on growth and development.

Although our efforts for protecting the unborn from the harmful effects of radiation are principally directed at diagnostic x-ray exposures, we must also be aware of similar hazards from radioisotope examinations. For example, radioiodine is known to concentrate principally in the thyroid gland. Following an administration of radioactive iodine, the dose to thyroid tissue will be several orders of magnitude higher than the whole-body dose because of this organ concentration effect. The thyroid gland begins to function at approximately 10 weeks of gestation, and, since radioiodine readily crosses the placental barrier from the mother's blood to the fetal circulation, radioiodine should be administered during pregnancy only in trace doses and before the 10-week gestation period. At any time thereafter the hazard of such an administration increases. This is quite the opposite from what we observe with external x-ray exposure.

Genetic effects

Unfortunately, our weakest area of knowledge in radiation biology is the area of radiation genetics. Essentially all the data indicating that radiation causes genetic effects have come from rather large-scale experiments with either flies or mice. **We do not have any substantive data on humans.** Observations of the atomic bomb survivors have shown no radiation-induced genetic effects, and we are now into the third generation. Other human populations have likewise provided only negative observations. Consequently, in the absence of accurate human data we have no choice but to rely on information

from experimental laboratory irradiations.

In 1927 the Nobel prize–winning geneticist H.J. Muller from the University of Texas reported the results of his irradiation of *Drosophila*, the fruit fly. He irradiated mature flies before procreation and then measured the frequency of lethal mutations in the offspring. The radiation doses employed were thousands of rad, but, as the data of Fig. 29-11 show, the dose-response relationship for radiation-induced genetic damage is unmistakably linear, nonthreshold. From Muller's studies other conclusions were drawn. Radiation does not alter the quality of mutations but rather increases the frequency of those mutations that are observed spontaneously. Muller's data showed no dose rate or dose fractionation effects. Hence he concluded that such mutations were single-hit phenomena.

It was principally on the basis of Muller's work that the National Council on Radiation Protection in 1932 lowered the maximum permissible dose and acknowledged officially for the first

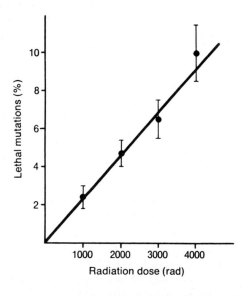

Fig. 29-11. Irradiation of flies by H.J. Muller shows the genetic effects to be linear, nonthreshold. Note that the doses were exceedingly high.

time the existence of nonthreshold radiation effects. Since that time, all radiation protection guides have assumed a linear, nonthreshold dose-response relationship and have been based on the suspected genetic, as well as somatic, effects of radiation.

The only other experimental work of any significance is that of Russell. Beginning in 1946, he commenced to irradiate a rather large mouse colony with radiation dose rates that varied from 0.001 to 90 rad per minute and total doses up to 1000 rad (10 Gy). These studies are continuing, and observations have now been made on over 7 million mice. The experiment requires the observation of seven specific genes that control readily recognizable characteristics such as ear shape, coat color, and eye color.

Russell's data show that a dose rate effect does exist, which would indicate that the mammal has some capacity to repair genetic damage. Significant differences between irradiation of males and of females were observed. He has confirmed the linear, non-threshold form of the dose-response relationship and has not detected any types of mutations that did not occur naturally.

The average mutation rate per unit dose in the mouse is approximately fifteen times that observed in the fruit fly. Whether an increased sensitivity exists in humans relative to the mouse is unknown.

From these experimental studies has developed the concept of doubling dose. **The doubling dose is that dose of radiation that will produce twice the frequency of genetic mutations as would have been observed without the radiation.** The doubling dose in humans is estimated to lie in the range between 50 and 250 rad (0.5 and 2.5 Gy).

Some additional conclusions drawn from these experimental studies follow:

1. Radiation-induced mutations are usually harmful.
2. Any dose of radiation, however small,

to germ cell results in some genetic risk.
3. The frequency of radiation-induced mutations is directly proportional to dose so that a linear extrapolation of data obtained at high doses provides a valid estimate for low-dose effects.
4. The effect is dependent on the rate at which the radiation is delivered (protraction) and on the time between exposures (fractionation).
5. For most of prereproductive life the female is less sensitive to the genetic effects of radiation than the male.
6. Most radiation-induced mutations are recessive. These require that the mutant genes be present in both the male and the female to produce the trait. Consequently, such mutations may not be expressed for many generations.
7. The frequency of radiation-induced genetic mutations is extremely low. It is approximately 10^{-7} mutation/rad/gene.

So what is the significance of all this in our daily practice to either patients or radiation employees? First, it can be said with certainty that radiation-induced genetic mutations following the levels of exposure experienced in diagnostic medicine are extremely low and the probability of such an effect is extremely rare. Under nearly all such exposures no action is required; however, should a high radiation dose be experienced preconceptionally (for example, an excess of 10 rad), some protective action may be required. The prefertilized egg, in its various stages, exhibits a constant sensitivity to radiation; however, it also demonstrates some capacity for repair of genetic damage. If repair occurs, it is rapid, and therefore a delay in procreation of only a few days is called for. In the male, on the other hand, it might be prudent to refrain from procreation for a period of 60 days to allow cells that were in a resistant stage of development at the time of exposure to mature to functioning spermatids.

REVIEW QUESTIONS

1. Define or otherwise identify the following:
   a. Epidemiology
   b. In utero
   c. ABCC-RERF
   d. Thorotrast
   e. Major organogenesis
   f. The Oxford Survey
   g. H.J. Muller
   h. Doubling dose
   i. Radon (^{222}Rn)
   j. Radium watch-dial painters
2. Discuss the three principal methods of identifying risk and the limitations of each.
3. In a population of 30,367 irradiated persons, 13 cases of leukemia developed; in a control population of 86,672 persons, 31 cases of leukemia developed. What was the relative risk?
4. What is the absolute risk if 3 cases of leukemia develop per year in 100,000 persons following an average dose of 2 rad?
5. Discuss the experience of radiation-induced leukemia in ankylosing spondylitis patients.
6. Discuss the shape of the radiation dose-response relationship as it represents the following:
   a. Leukemia
   b. Cancer
   c. Cataracts
   d. Life span shortening
   e. Genetic mutations

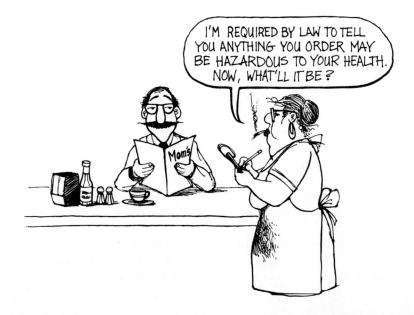

30

Health physics

CARDINAL PRINCIPLES OF
RADIATION PROTECTION
MAXIMUM PERMISSIBLE DOSE
X RAYS AND PREGNANCY

Immediately following their discovery, x rays were applied to the healing arts. It was recognized within months that they could cause harmful effects. Since that time, a great deal of effort has been devoted to developing equipment, techniques, and procedures to control radiation levels and reduce unnecessary radiation exposure.

Health physics is concerned with providing radiation protection for persons employed in radiation industries and for the population at large. The term "health physicist" was coined during the early days of the Manhattan Project (the secret wartime effort to develop the atomic bomb) to describe the group of physicists and physicians who were given the responsibility of ensuring the radiation safety of persons involved in the production of material for use in atomic bombs. The health physicist thus is a radiation scientist, engineer, or physician concerned with the research, teaching, or operational aspects of radiation safety.

CARDINAL PRINCIPLES OF RADIATION PROTECTION

All health physics activity in radiology is designed to minimize radiation exposure of patients and personnel. Three cardinal principles of radiation protection developed for nuclear activities find equally useful application in diagnostic radiology: **time, distance,** and **shielding.** By observing the following principles, one can minimize radiation exposure:

1. Keep the time of exposure to radiation short.
2. Maintain a large distance between the source of radiation and the exposed person.
3. Insert shielding material between the source and the exposed person.

Minimize time

The dose to an individual is directly related to the duration of exposure. If the time during which one is exposed to radiation is doubled, the exposure will be doubled. The equation for this relationship is

(30-1)

$$Exposure = Exposure\ rate \times Time$$

EXAMPLE: A radiation source has an exposure rate of 225 mR/hr (0.58 μC/kg – hr) at a position occupied by a radiation worker. If the worker remains at that position for 36 minutes, what will be the total occupational exposure?

ANSWER:

$$Occupational\ exposure = (225 mR/hr)\left(\frac{36\ min}{60\ min/hr}\right)$$

$$= 135\ mR$$

During radiography, the time of exposure is kept to a minimum to reduce motion unsharpness. During fluoroscopy, the time of exposure should also be kept to a minimum to reduce patient and personnel exposure. This is an area of radiation protection not directly controlled by the radiologic technologist. Radiologists are trained to depress the fluoroscopic foot switch in an alternating fashion, sequencing **on-off** rather than continuous **on** during the course of the examination. A repeated up-and-down motion on the fluoroscopic foot switch permits a high-quality examination to be made with a considerably reduced exposure to the patient.

The **5-minute reset timer** on all fluoroscopes reminds the radiologist that a considerable fluoroscopic time has elapsed. The timer records the amount of x-ray beam on-time. Most fluoroscopic examinations take less than 5 minutes. Only during difficult special procedures should it be necessary to exceed 5 minutes of exposure time.

EXAMPLE: A fluoroscope emits 1.2 R/min (31 mC/kg-min) at the tabletop for every milliampere of operation (1.2 R/mA-min). What is the patient exposure in a barium enema examination that is conducted at 1.8 mA and requires 2.5 minutes of fluoroscopic time?

ANSWER:

$$Patient\ exposure = \left(\frac{1.2R}{mA - min}\right)(1.8\ mA)\ (2.5\ min)$$

$$= 5.4\ R$$

Maximize distance

As the distance between the source of radiation and a person increases, the radiation exposure decreases rapidly. The decrease in exposure can be calculated using the inverse square law (equation 4-3) if the source of radiation can be considered a point source. Most radiation sources are point sources; the x-ray tube target for example, is a point source of radiation. However, the scattered radiation generated within a patient appears to come not from a point but rather from an extended area. As a rule of thumb, even an extended source can be considered a point source **if the distance from the source exceeds seven times the source diameter.**

EXAMPLE: An x-ray tube has an output intensity of 2.6 mR/mAs (0.7 μC/kg – mAs) when operated at 70 kVp at 100 cm SID. What would be the radiation exposure 350 cm from the target?

ANSWER: $\dfrac{I_1}{I_2} = \dfrac{d_2^2}{d_1^2}$

$$I_1 = I_2\left(\frac{d_2}{d_1}\right)^2$$

$$= (2.6\ mR/mAs)\left(\frac{100}{350}\right)^2$$

$$= (2.6\ mR/mAs)\ (0.082)$$

$$= 0.21\ mR/mAs$$

In radiography, the distance from radiation source to patient is generally fixed by the type of examination, and the technologist is positioned behind a protective barrier.

During fluoroscopy, the radiologic technologist can exercise good radiation protection procedures. Fig. 30-1 shows the approximate radiation exposure levels waist high during a fluoroscopic examination. The lines on the plot plan are called **isoexposure lines** and represent positions of equal exposure in the examining

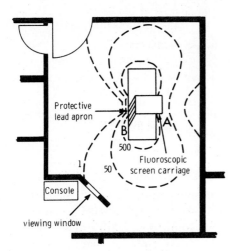

Fig. 30-1. Typical isoexposure contours during fluoroscopic examination. *A* represents the location of the technologist providing backloaded spot films. *B* represents the probable position of the radiologist.

Table 30-1. Approximate half-value and tenth-value layers of lead and concrete at various tube potentials

Tube potential	HVL Lead (mm)	HVL Concrete (in)	TVL Lead (mm)	TVL Concrete (in)
40 kVp	0.03	0.13	0.06	0.40
60 kVp	0.11	0.25	0.34	0.87
80 kVp	0.19	0.42	0.64	1.4
100 kVp	0.24	0.60	0.80	2.0
120 kVp	0.27	0.76	0.90	2.5
140 kVp	0.28	0.86	0.95	2.8
250 kVp	0.9	1.1	3.0	3.7
^{60}Co	12.0	2.5	40.0	8.1
4 MV	16.5	3.6	54.8	12.0

room. Point *A* indicates the normal position for a technologist during a fluoroscopic examination with equipment using a cassette spot film loaded from the back. The exposure rate at this position is approximately 300 mR/hr (77 μC/kg-hr). During portions of the examination, it might not be necessary for the technologist to remain in that position. Two steps back the exposure rate is only 20 mR/hr (5 μC/kg-hr). This reduction in exposure does not follow the inverse square law since during fluoroscopy the patient serves as an extended source of radiation because of scattered x rays generated within the body. Therefore, during fluoroscopy, **the technologist should remain as far from the examining table as practical.**

EXAMPLE: Using the exposure levels shown in Fig. 30-1, determine the approximate occupational exposure of a radiologic technologist at position A and at a position A', two steps farther back, during a fluoroscopic examination requiring 4 minutes, 15 seconds.

ANSWER: Occupational exposure equals

Position *A:* (300 mR/hr) (4.25 min) (1 hr/60 min)
= 21.25 mR

Position *A':* (20 mR/hr) (4.25 min) (1 hr/60 min)
= 1.4 mR

Maximize shielding

Placing shielding material between the radiation source and persons exposed reduces the level of exposure. Shielding used in diagnostic radiology usually consists of lead, although sometimes concrete is used. The amount a protective barrier reduces radiation intensity can be estimated if the half-value layer (HVL) or the tenth-value layer (TVL) of the barrier material is known. The HVL was defined and discussed in Chapter 10. The TVL is similarly defined. **One TVL is the thickness of material that will reduce the radiation intensity to one-tenth its original value.** One TVL is equal to 3.3 HVLs. Table 30-1 shows approximate half-value and tenth-value layers for lead and concrete for diagnostic x-ray facilities operated between 40 and 140 kVp. For comparison, the HVL and TVL for several therapeutic sources of radiation are also shown.

EXAMPLE: When operated at 70 kVp, an x-ray machine has a radiation intensity of 3.6 mR/mAs (9 μC/kg-mAs) at a distance of 100 cm. How much shielding material, concrete and lead, would be required to reduce the intensity to less than 0.25 mR/mAs?

ANSWER: The amount of shielding material in the first or second column of the date below will reduce the beam intensity to the value in the third column.

Pb (mm)	Concrete (in)	Beam Intensity (mR/mAs)
0	0	3.60
0.15	0.33	1.80
0.30	0.67	0.90
0.45	1.00	0.45
0.60	1.33	0.23

EXAMPLE: An x-ray machine used strictly for chest radiography that never exceeds 125 kVp is pointed to a wall containing 1.6 mm Pb shielding. How much additional shielding will be required if the work load for this unit doubles and the exposure rate on the other side of the wall is to remain constant?

ANSWER: One HVL, or 0.27 mm Pb, will be necessary.

Time, distance, and shielding

Usually, applications of the cardinal principles of radiation protection involve a consideration of all three. The typical problem involves a known radiation level at a given distance from the source. One can calculate the level of exposure at any other distance, behind any shielding, for any length of time. The order in which these calculations are made makes no difference.

EXAMPLE: A radiographic installation is designed exclusively for chest radiography at 120 kVp. The output intensity is 4.6 mR/mAs (1.2 μC/kg-mAs) at 100 cm SID. The distance to a secretary's desk on the other side of the wall to which the x-ray beam is directed is 200 cm. The wall contains 0.96 mm Pb, and 300 mAs is anticipated daily. If the secretary is to be restricted to 2 mR exposure per day, how long each day may she remain at her desk?

ANSWER:
Daily x-ray output at 100 cm =
$$(4.6 \text{ mR/mAs}) (300 \text{ mAs}) = 1380 \text{ mR}$$

Daily output at 200 cm =
$$(1380) (100/200)^2 = 345 \text{ mR}$$

Daily output behind 0.96 mm Pb, or 4 HVLs =
$$22 \text{ mR}$$

$$\text{Time allowed} = \frac{2 \text{ mR}}{22 \text{ mR/day}} = 0.09 \text{ day} =$$

$$2.16 \text{ hr} = 130 \text{ min}$$

MAXIMUM PERMISSIBLE DOSE

A continuing effort of health physicists has been the description and identification of a **maximum permissible dose (MPD)**. The MPD is the maximum dose of radiation that in light of present knowledge would not be expected to produce significant radiation effects. At radiation doses below the MPD, neither somatic nor genetic responses should occur. At doses at the level of the MPD, the risk is not zero, but it is small—lower than the risks associated with other occupations and reasonable in light of the benefits derived.

Consequently, particular care is taken to make certain that no **radiation worker** receives a radiation dose in excess of the MPD. The MPD is specified only for occupational exposure. It should not be confused with medical x-ray exposure received as a patient.

In the early years of radiology, the MPD was termed the "tolerance dose" because it was considered the dose of radiation below which no effect could be observed. Above the tolerance dose, a response would be expected. In 1902 the first maximum permissible dose, 50,000 mrem/wk (500 mSv/wk), was recommended. The current MPD is 100 mrem/wk (1 mSv/wk). Through the years there has been a downward revision of the MPD, and this downward trend will no doubt continue. The history of these continuing recommendations is shown in Table 30-2.

In the early years of radiology, the MPD consisted of a single value considered the safe work-

Table 30-2. Historical review of the maximum permissible dose for occupational exposure

Year	Recommendation	Approximate daily dose (mrem)	Recommender
1902	Dose limited by fogging of a photographic plate following 7-minute contact exposure	10,000	Rollins
1915	Lead shielding of tube needed (no numeric exposure levels given)		British Roentgen Society
1921	General methods to reduce exposure		British X-ray and Radium Protection Committee
1925	"It is entirely safe if an operator does not receive every thirty days a dose exceeding $1/_{100}$ of an erythema dose."	200	Mutscheller
1925	10% of an SED* per year	200	Sievert
1926	One SED per 90,000 working hours	40	Dutch Board of Health
1928	0.00028 of an SED per day	175	Barclay and Cox
1928	0.001 of an SED per month 5 R per day permissible for the hands	150	Kaye
1931	Limit exposure to 0.2 R per day	200	Advisory Committee on X-ray and Radium Protection of the United States
1932	0.001 of an SED per month	30	Failla
1934	5 R per day permissible for the hands		Advisory Committee on X-ray and Radium Protection of the United States
1936	0.1 R per day	100	Advisory Committee on X-ray and Radium Protection of the United States
1941	0.02 R per day	20	Taylor
1943	200 mR per day is acceptable	200	Patterson
1959	0.1 R per week	20	National Council on Radiation Protection and Measurements

*SED, Skin erythema dose.

ing level for whole-body exposure. It was based primarily on the known acute response to radiation exposure and presumed that a **threshold dose** existed. Today the MPD is specified not only for whole-body exposure but also for partial-body exposure, organ exposure, and exposure of the general population (again, excluding medical exposure as a patient). These MPD values are known as **dose-limiting recommendations** and are summarized in Table 30-3.

Current dose-limiting recommendations were developed with consideration for both the genetic and somatic responses to radiation exposure. Based on a **linear, nonthreshold dose-response relationship,** they are considered the level of exposure acceptable as an occupational hazard. In practice, at least in diagnostic radiology, it is seldom necessary to exceed even one-fourth the appropriate MPD. Since the basis for the MPD assumes a linear, nonthreshold dose-response relationship, **all unnecessary** radiation exposure should be avoided.

Table 30-3. Maximum permissible dose

Group	MPD
Radiation workers	
Combined whole-body occupational exposure	
Prospective annual limit	5 rem in any given year
Retrospective annual limit	10 to 15 rem in any given year
Long-term accumulation to age N years	$5(N - 18)$ rem
Skin	15 rem in any given year
Hands	75 rem in any given year (25 rem per quarter)
Forearms	30 rem in any given year (10 rem per quarter)
Other organs, tissues, and organ systems	15 rem in any given year (5 rem per quarter)
Pregnant women (with respect to fetus)	0.5 rem in gestation period
Public or occasionally exposed individuals	0.5 rem in any given year
Students	0.1 rem in any given year
General population	
Genetic	0.17 rem average per year
Somatic	0.17 rem average per year

Whole-body occupational exposure

The cumulative MPD for occupationally exposed persons is determined by

(30-2)

$$MPD = 5(N - 18) \ rem$$

where N is age in years.

This results in an annual MPD of 5 rem, or 5000 mrem (50 mSv). One consequence of this specification for MPD is that persons less than 18 years of age should not be employed in radiation occupations. Older workers who have not been exposed previously to radiation may be allowed to receive radiation exposure at a rate exceeding the 5000 mrem/yr (50 mSv/yr) limit so long as the cumulative limit of equation 30-2 is not exceeded. Some recommendations will allow annual exposures of up to 12 rem (0.12 Sv) so long as the cumulative MPD is not exceeded. In practice, this administrative procedure never is justified in diagnostic radiology and only seldom is justified in other radiation industries.

EXAMPLE: A 23-year-old worker who has never before been occupationally exposed to ionizing radiation is employed in a radiology department. What are his cumulative MPD and annual MPD levels?

ANSWER:

$$
\begin{aligned}
Cumulative \ MPD &= 5(23 - 18) \\
&= 5 \times 5 \\
&= 25 \ rem \\
Annual \ MPD &= 5 \ rem, \ unless \ allowance \ is \ made \\
&\quad to \ exceed \ this
\end{aligned}
$$

There are several special situations associated with the whole-body occupational MPD. Students under the age of 18 may not receive more than 100 mrem/yr (1 mSv/yr) during the course of their educational activities. This is included in and not in addition to the 500 mrem (5 mSv) permitted each year as a nonoccupational exposure. Consequently, student radiologic technologists under the age of 18 may be engaged in departments of radiology, but their personnel exposure must be monitored and should remain below 100 mrem/yr. Because of this, it is general practice not to accept underage persons into schools of radiologic technology unless their eighteenth birthday is only a few months away.

Female radiologic technologists who become pregnant are subject to a different MPD. During her pregnancy, an employee's exposure should not exceed 500 mrem (5 mSv) because the MPD for the fetus is 500 mrem. In most radiology departments this does not present a problem. **Pregnancy should never be considered sufficient reason for terminating employment, either voluntarily or involuntarily.**

Whole-body nonoccupational exposure

The MPD established for nonoccupationally exposed persons is one tenth of that for the radiation worker. Individuals in the general population are limited to 500 mrem/yr (5 mSv/yr). Radiation exposure of the general population or individuals in the population is rarely measured, and therefore the application of this MPD is limited. In radiology the population MPD of 500 mrem/yr is used in designing radiation barriers for diagnostic rooms. In general, if a barrier separates an x-ray examining room from an area occupied by radiation workers, then the shielding is designed so that the annual exposure in the adjacent area cannot exceed 5000 mR (1.3 mC/kg). If the adjacent area is occupied by others, then the shielding must be sufficient to maintain an annual exposure level less than 500 mR (0.13 mC/kg).

The MPD currently established for the population as a whole is one-third that established for any individual in the population. The population MPD is therefore 170 mrem/yr (1.7 mSv/yr). This dose-limiting recommendation is used in designing large radiation facilities such as nuclear reactors or nuclear fuel processing plants.

Partial-body occupational exposure

The whole-body MPD of 5000 mrem/yr (50 mSv/yr) applies also to the following parts of the body: head, neck, trunk, lens of the eye, blood-forming organs, and gonads. In other words, in addition to a limitation of 5000 mrem/yr for the whole body, the dose to any of these parts of the body may not exceed the same limit. This interpretation is accepted because irradiation of any of these parts carries a presumed risk of late effects equal to the risk associated with whole-body irradiation.

Skin. Some organs of the body have a higher MPD than the whole-body MPD. The MPD for the skin is 15,000 mrem/yr (150 mSv/yr). This limit is not normally of concern in diagnostic radiology, since it applies to nonpenetrating radiation such as alpha and beta radiation and very soft x rays. Radiologic technologists exclusively engaged in soft tissue radiography are highly unlikely to sustain radiation exposures to the skin in excess of 15,000 mrem/yr (150 mSv/yr). Were this to occur, the MPD would have been violated.

Extremities. Radiologic technologists often have their hands near the primary radiation beam, and therefore extremity exposure is of considerable concern. The MPD for the forearms is 30,000 mrem/yr (300 mSv/yr), and the MPD for the hands is 75,000 mrem/yr (750 mSv/yr). These radiation levels are quite high and under normal circumstances should not even be approached. For certain occupational groups, such as special procedures radiologic technologists and nuclear medicine technologists, extremity personnel monitors should be provided. Such devices are worn on the wrist or the finger.

X RAYS AND PREGNANCY

There are two situations in diagnostic radiology that require particular care and action. Both are associated with pregnancy. Their importance is obvious from both a physical and an emotional standpoint.

Radiobiologic considerations

The severity of the potential response to radiation exposure in utero is both time related and intensity related. This was discussed briefly in Chapter 29. Unquestionably the most sensitive period to radiation exposure in our lives occurs before birth. Furthermore, we are more sensitive early in pregnancy than late in pregnancy. As a general rule, the higher the radiation dose, the more severe will be the radiation response.

Time dependence. There is a grave misconception that the most critical time for irradiation is during the first two weeks when it is most unlikely that the expectant mother knows of her condition. In fact, this is probably the safest time for such irradiation. The biologic response to irradiation during the first two weeks of pregnancy is **resorption of the embryo**—a spontaneous abortion. No other type of response is likely. One should not be concerned with the possibility of the induction of congenital abnormalities during the first two weeks of pregnancy, because such a response has not been demonstrated in experimental animals or humans following any radiation dose.

The time from approximately the second week to the eighth week of pregnancy is called the period of **major organogenesis.** During this time the major organ systems of the body are developing. If the radiation dose is sufficient, congenital abnormalities will result. Early in this interval, the most likely congenital abnormalities are associated with skeletal deformities. Later in this period, neurologic deficiencies are more likely to occur.

During the second and third trimesters of pregnancy, the responses previously noted are unlikely. Results of numerous investigations strongly suggest that if a response occurs following irradiation during the latter two trimesters, the only one possible would be the appearance during childhood of malignant disease: leukemia or cancer. Malignant disease induction in childhood is also a possible response during the first trimester.

These responses to irradiation during pregnancy require a very high radiation dose before there is a significant risk of occurrence. No such responses would occur at less than 25 rad (250 mGy). Such dose levels are possible with patients who receive multiple x-ray examinations of the abdomen or pelvis. They are essentially impossible with radiologic technologists. There are no other significant responses following irradiation in utero.

Dose dependence. As one might imagine, virtually no information is available at the human level to construct dose-response relationships for irradiation in utero. There is, however, a large body of data from animal irradiation, particularly rats and mice, from which we can estimate such relationships. The statements that follow, although attributed to human exposure, represent estimates based on extrapolation from animal studies.

Following an in utero radiation dose of 200 rad (2 Gy), it is nearly certain that each of the effects noted previously will occur. However, the likelihood that an exposure of this magnitude would be experienced in diagnostic medicine is nil.

Spontaneous abortion following irradiation during the first two weeks of pregnancy is not likely to occur at radiation doses less than 25 rad (250 mGy). The precise nature of the dose-response relationship is unknown, but a reasonable estimate of risk suggests that 0.1% of all conceptions would be resorbed following a dose of 10 rad (100 mGy). The response at lower doses would be proportionately lower. Keep in mind, however, that the incidence of spontaneous abortion in the absence of radiation exposure is estimated to be in the 25% to 50% range.

When assessing the risk of inducing congenital abnormalities, one should be aware that in the absence of radiation exposure, approximately 5% of all live births exhibit a manifest congenital abnormality. A 1% increase in congenital abnormalities is estimated to follow a 10 rad (100 mGy) fetal dose and a proportionately lower increase at lower doses.

The induction of a childhood malignancy following irradiation in utero is difficult to assess.

Risk estimates are even lower than those reported for spontaneous abortion and congenital abnormalities. Our best approach to assessing risk of childhood malignancy is to employ a relative risk estimate.

During the first trimester, the relative risk of childhood malignancy is in the range of 5 to 10, it drops to about 1.3 during the third trimester. The overall risk is accepted to be 1.5, a 50% increase over the naturally occurring incidence.

The pregnant technologist

When a technologist becomes pregnant, she should notify her supervisor. The supervisor should then review her previous radiation exposure history, since this will aid in deciding what protective actions are necessary. The maximum permissible dose for the fetus is 500 mrem (5 mSv) for the period of pregnancy, a dose level that most technologists will not reach. Although some technologists may exceed 1000 mrem/yr (10 mSv/yr), most receive less than 100 mrem/yr (5 mSv/yr), as indicated with the personnel monitoring device positioned at the collar above the protective apron. The exposure at the waist under the protective apron will not normally exceed 10% of these values, and therefore, under normal conditions, specific protective action may not be necessary.

However, to be prudent, there are several ways to protect the fetus with minimum interference to clinical activity. In a large hospital where many technologists are to be assigned, **a pregnant technologist should be removed from fluoroscopy, special procedures, and portable work,** activities that have been shown to result in the bulk of the exposure that a technologist receives.

In a small community hospital or in a private office, situations in which it may not be possible to reassign the technologist, efforts should be made to provide adequate protective apparel. Most lead aprons are 0.5 mm lead equivalent. These provide approximately 88% attenuation

at 75 kVp, which is sufficient. One millimeter lead equivalent protective aprons are available, but such thickness is not necessary, particularly in view of the additional weight. Back problems during pregnancy constitute a greater hazard than radiation exposure. The length of the apron need not extend to the knees or below. If necessary, a special effort should be made to provide an apron of proper size because of its weight.

After these protective measures have been instituted, it is reasonable **to provide the pregnant technologist with a second personnel monitoring device** to be positioned under the protective apron at waist level. The exposure reported on the second monitor should be maintained on a separate record and identified as exposure to the fetus.

The use of such an additional monitor shows consistently that exposures to the fetus are insignificant. Suppose, for instance, that a pregnant technologist wearing a single radiation monitor at collar level receives 1000 mrem (10 mSu) during the 9-month period. The dose at waist level under a protective apron would be approximately 5% of the collar dose, or 50 mrem (500 μSu). Because of attenuation by the maternal tissues overlying the fetus, the dose to the fetus would be approximately 30% of the abdominal skin dose, or 15 mrem (150 μSu). Consequently, when adequate protective measures are taken, it is nearly impossible for a technologist to even approach the fetal MPD.

When pregnancy is reported, regardless of the nature of the x-ray facilities or the technologist's work experience, the supervisor should review acceptable practices of radiation protection. This review should emphasize the cardinal principles of radiation protection: minimize time, maximize distance, and use available shielding.

Management principles

It should be clear that the probability of an untoward effect following any radiation exposure received in medicine is nil. A biologic response is very rarely expected and has not been ob-

Table 30-4. Pregnancy in diagnostic radiology

Human responses to low-level x-ray exposure

Life span shortening	10 days/rad
Cataracts	None below 200 rad
Leukemia	0.2-55 cases/10^6/rad
Cancer	67-169 cases/10^6/rad
Genetic effects	Doubling dose = 50 rad
Death from all causes	1:10,000/rad

Effects of irradiation in utero

0-14 days	Spontaneous abortion: 25%-50% natural incidence; 0.1% increase/10 rad
2-8 weeks	Congenital abnormalities: 5%-10% natural incidence; 1% increase/10 rad
	Cell depletion: no effect at less than 50 rad
2nd-3rd trimester	Latent malignancy: 4:10,000 natural incidence; 6:10,000/rad
0-9 months	Genetic effects: 10% natural incidence; 5×10^{-7} mutations/rad

Protective measures for the technologist

No fluoroscopy
No special procedures
No portable radiography
Two personal radiation monitors
Maximum permissible dose: 500 mrem/9 months

---

served in radiologic personnel for the past 50 years or so. Unfortunately, because of lack of knowledge and improper counseling, apprehension and despair occur much too frequently among radiologic personnel. Consequently, it is essential for the director of radiology to incorporate three steps into the radiation protection program: (1) new employee indoctrination, (2) periodic in-service training, and (3) counseling during pregnancy.

New employee indoctrination. The initial step for any administrative protocol dealing with pregnant employees involves orientation and indoctrination. During these orientation discussions, which would normally occur during the first week of employment, all female employees should be instructed as to their responsibility regarding pregnancy and radiation. Each technologist should be provided with a copy of the facility radiation protection manual and other appropriate material. This material might include a one-page summary of doses, responses, and proper radiation control working habits, such as shown in Table 30-4.

The new employee should then be required to read and sign a form, such as that shown in the box on p. 545, indicating that she has been instructed in this area of radiation protection. An important point to be made by signing this document is that she has been instructed that it is her responsibility to notify her supervisor when she is pregnant or suspects she is pregnant.

In-service training. Every well-run radiology service maintains a regular schedule of in-

---

New employee notification

This is to certify that _____ , a new employee of this radiologic facility, has received instructions regarding mutual responsibilities should she become pregnant during this employment.

In addition to personal counseling by _____ , she has been given to read several documents dealing with pregnancy in diagnostic radiology. Furthermore, the additional reading material that follows is available in the departmental office:

1. Instruction concerning prenatal radiation exposure, NRC Regulatory Guide 8:13, Washington, D.C., 1980, U.S. Nuclear Regulatory Commission.
2. Review of NCRP radiation dose limit for embryo and fetus in occupationally-exposed women, NCRP Report No. 53, Washington, D.C., 1977, National Council on Radiation Protection and Measures.
3. Medical radiation exposure of pregnant and potentially pregnant women, NCRP Report No. 54, Washington, D.C., 1977, National Council on Radiation Protection and Measures.
4. The effects on populations of exposure to low levels of ionizing radiation, Washington, D.C., 1980, National Academy of Sciences.

I understand that should I become pregnant, it is my responsibility to inform my supervisor of my condition immediately so that additional protective measures can be taken.

_____   _____
Supervisor   Employee

_____
Date

---

service training. Usually these are conducted at monthly intervals but sometimes more often. At least twice each year such training should be devoted to radiation protection, and a portion of these sessions should be directed at the potentially pregnant employee.

The material to be covered in such sessions is outlined in Table 30-4. Although it is good to review doses and responses, it is probably more appropriate to emphasize radiation control procedures. These, of course, affect the radiation safety of all technologists, not just the pregnant technologist.

A review of personnel monitoring records is particularly important. All too often technologists are unaware of their radiation exposure because of their inability to interpret the radiation monitoring report. A helpful procedure is to post the most recent radiation monitoring report for all to see. The year-end report should be initialed by each technologist, and the director of radiology should be sure that all technologists understand the nature and magnitude of their annual exposure.

Through such training, radiologic personnel will realize that the extent of their occupational exposure is minimal, usually much less than 10% of the MPD. It should be emphasized that (1) the MPD is 5000 mrad/yr (50 mSv/yr), (2) environmental background radiation is approximately 100 mrad/yr (1 mSv/yr), and (3) occupational exposures are closer to the latter than the former.

Counseling during pregnancy. The next point for action on the part of the director of

---

Acknowledgment of radiation risk during pregnancy

I, _____ , do acknowledge that I have received counseling from _____ regarding my employment responsibilities during my pregnancy.

It is clear to me that there is a vanishly small probability that my employment will in any way adversely affect my pregnancy. The reading material listed below has been made available to me to demonstrate that the additional risk during my pregnancy is much less than that for most occupational groups. I further understand that, although I may be assigned to low-exposure duties and provided with a second radiation monitor, these are simply added precautions and do not in any way convey that any assignment in this department is especially hazardous during pregnancy.

1. Instruction concerning prenatal radiation exposure, NRC Regulatory Guide 8:13, Washington, D.C., 1980, U.S. Nuclear Regulatory Commission.
2. Review of NCRP radiation dose limit for embryo and fetus in occupationally-exposed women, NCRP Report No. 53, Washington, D.C., 1977, National Council on Radiation Protection and Measures.
3. Medical radiation exposure of pregnant and potentially pregnant women, NCRP Report No. 54, Washington, D.C., 1977, National Council on Radiation Protection and Measures.
4. The effects on populations of exposure to low levels of ionizing radiation, Washington, D.C., 1980, National Academy of Sciences.

_____   _____
Supervisor   Employee

_____
Date

---

radiology occurs when the technologist discloses her state of pregnancy. First, the administrator should counsel the employee, including a review of her radiation exposure history and any future restrictions to her schedule that are appropriate. **Under no circumstances should termination or involuntary leave-of-absence occur.** In all likelihood, a review of the employee's previous radiation exposure history will show an exceedingly low exposure profile. Those who wear the radiation monitor positioned at the collar, as recommended, and who are heavily involved in fluoroscopy and special procedures, may receive an exposure greater than 1000 mrem/yr (10 mSv/yr). Such employees, however, are protected by lead-lined aprons so that exposure to the trunk of the body would not normally exceed 100 mrem/yr (1 mSv/yr). However, 95% of all such employees will exhibit a reported exposure less than 500 mrem/yr (5 mSv/yr).

This review of personnel radiation exposure is the appropriate time to emphasize that the MPD during pregnancy is 500 mrem (5 mSv). Furthermore, it should be shown that this MPD level refers to the fetus and not to the worker herself. This level of 500 mrem (5 mSv) to the fetus during gestation is considered an absolutely safe radiation exposure level.

In view of this discussion, the director of radiology should point out to the technologist that an alteration in her work schedule is not essential; however, for her peace of mind she may be rotated out of fluoroscopy and portable radiography if it is within the resources of the department. Under no circumstances should she be allowed to hold patients during x-ray procedures.

It is also appropriate, although not necessary, to provide the pregnant technologist with an additional monitor. This requires precise instructions that the monitor be worn at waist level under protective apparel, that the monitor be cycled in a timely fashion, and that it not be mixed up with the collar monitor. This monitor should be labeled "baby badge," or "fetal dose," or something similar. Additional or thicker lead aprons are unnecessary.

For technologists involved in radiation oncology, nuclear medicine, or ultrasound, a similar consultation and level of restriction is appropriate. In radiation oncology the pregnant technologist may continue her normal work load but should not be allowed to participate in brachytherapy applications.

In nuclear medicine the pregnant technologist should handle only small quantities of radioactive material. She should not be permitted to elute radioisotope generators or inject millicurie quantities of radioactive material.

Ultrasound technologists are not normally classified as radiation workers. However, a sizable portion of ultrasound patients have previously been nuclear medicine patients and therefore become a source of exposure to the ultrasonographer. Proper patient scheduling can remove this potential hazard. It may be advisable during the pregnancy to provide the ultrasonographer with a radiation monitor.

Finally, the pregnant technologist should be required to read and sign a form, such as that shown in the boxed material on p. 546, attesting to the fact that she has been given proper attention and that she understands that the level of risk associated with her employment is much less than that experienced by nearly all occupational groups.

The pregnant patient

Safeguards against accidental irradiation early in pregnancy are administrative problems. This situation is particularly critical during the first two months of pregnancy, when such a condition may not be suspected and when the fetus is particularly sensitive to radiation exposure. After a couple of months the risk of irradiating an unknown pregnancy becomes small because the patient is generally aware of her condition. If the state of pregnancy is known, then under many circumstances the radiologic examination should not be conducted.

A number of techniques can be employed to reasonably ensure that irradiation of an unknown pregnancy does not occur. The following is a statement from the International Commission on Radiation Protection (ICRP)*:

The ICRP has for a number of years called attention to the embryonic and fetal sensitivity to ionizing radiation. The possibility of pregnancy must be taken into account by the attending physician when he is deciding on examinations that involve the lower abdomen and pelvis of women of reproductive capacity. The commission has pointed out that the ten-day interval following the onset of menstruation is the time when it is most improbable that such women could be pregnant. **Therefore, it is recommended that all lower-abdomen and pelvic radiological examinations of women of reproductive capacity which are not of importance in connection with the immediate illness of the patient be limited to this period,** when pregnancy is improbable. The examinations that will be appropriate to delay until the onset of the next menstruation are the few that could without detriment be postponed until the conclusion of a pregnancy or at least until its later half.

This recommendation is called the **10-day rule.** Of course, the x-ray examination should be conducted if the health of the mother or the fetus would be compromised by failure to perform it when requested. However, every care should be taken, when appropriate, to shield the fetus from the primary beam and from scatter radiation. Following is a list of some x-ray examinations that should be scheduled according to the 10-day rule.

---

*International Commission on Radiation Protection: Protection of the patient in x-ray diagnosis, publication no. 16, Oxford, England, 1970, Pergamon Press.

X-ray consent for women of childbearing age*

X-ray examinations of abdomen and pelvis exposing the uterus to radiation are:

Abdomen (KUB)	Colon (barium enema)	Pyelograms (IVP and retrograde)
Stomach (UGI)	Gallbladder	Cystograms
Small intestine (s1)	Hips, sacrum, coccyx	Lumbar spine and pelvis

All nuclear medicine studies

The 10 days following onset of menstrual period are generally considered safe for x-ray examinations.

Onset of last menstrual period, Date: _____   Date today: _____

I am pregnant	Yes _____	No _____	Don't know _____
I have had a hysterectomy	Yes _____	No _____	Don't know _____
I use an IUD	Yes _____	No _____	Don't know _____

I recognize that if I am pregnant and have radiation to the abdomen, there is a possibility of injury to the fetus. However, I understand that the likelihood of such injury is slight and that my physician feels that the information to be gained from this examination is important to my health. I therefore wish to have this x-ray examination performed now.

_____
Name of examination

_____   _____
Witness   Signature of patient

*A simple yet effective patient questionnaire for implementing the 10-day rule. (Courtesy Vincent P. Collins, M.D., Houston, Tex.)

Radiologic examinations that should be postponed if pregnancy is known

Lumbar spine	Urethrocystography
Pelvis and abdomen	Pelvimetry
Hip and femur	Hysterosalpingography
Urography	Barium enema
Pyelography	

When the 10-day rule cannot be accommodated and the examination is conducted, it should be done with precisely collimated beams and carefully positioned protective shields.

Some radiation scientists do not agree with implementation of the 10-day rule, since they would contend that x-ray examinations would not be ordered if not essential. Still most would agree that this is the safest approach to patient management. The administrative protocols that can be employed to effect the 10-day rule vary from simple to complex, with the degree of success proportionally observed.

Elective booking. The most direct way to ensure against the irradiation of an unsuspected pregnancy is to institute the 10-day rule positively. This **elective booking** requires that the clinician or radiologist determine the time of the patient's previous menstrual cycle. All examinations of the lower abdomen and pelvis that do not fall within the 10-day period following onset of the previous menstruation must then be postponed unless absolutely essential. X-ray examinations in which the fetus is not in or near the primary beam may be allowed outside this 10-day period, but they should be accompanied by pelvic shielding.

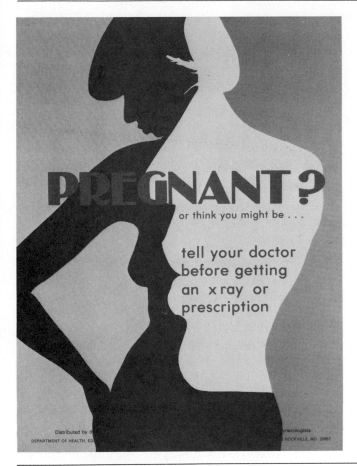

PREGNANT?

or think you might be . . .

tell your doctor
before getting
an x ray or
prescription

Distributed by th... ...ynecologists
DEPARTMENT OF HEALTH, ED... ...ROCKVILLE, MD. 20857

Fig. 30-2 Wall posters and cardboard table centers with warnings concerning possible pregnancy are available from the National Center for Devices and Radiological Health. (Courtesy National Center for Devices and Radiological Health.)

The 10-day rule has been successfully demonstrated in small hospitals and clinics where the relationship between the radiologist and the referring physician is close. In large general hospitals and teaching hospitals, such procedures are a little more difficult because of the loss of close contact among the staff and the frequent rotation of interns and residents. Ideally, the referring physician should be responsible for determining the menstrual cycle and for withholding the examination request if the time is not right. This requires a radiologist-sponsored educational program that can be easily conducted at regularly scheduled medical staff meetings.

Patient questionnaire. An alternative procedure is to have the patient herself indicate her menstrual cycle. In many radiology departments the patient must complete an information form before examination. These forms often include questions such as "Are you or could you be pregnant?" and "What was the date of your last menstrual period?" An example of such a form is shown in the boxed material.

Posting. If neither elective booking nor the request form seems appropriate to any radiology service, a moderately successful method of implementing the 10-day rule is to post signs of caution in the radiology waiting room. Such

Table 30-5. Representative entrance exposures and fetal doses for frequently performed radiographic examinations with a 200-speed image receptor

Examination	Entrance exposure (mR)	Fetal dose (mrad)
Skull (lateral)	70	0
Cervical spine (AP)	110	0
Shoulder	90	0
Chest (PA)	10	0
Thoracic spine (AP)	180	1
Cholecystogram (PA)	150	1
Lumbosacral spine (AP)*	250	80
Abdomen or KUB (AP)*	220	70
Intravenous pyelogram (IVP)*	210	60
Hip*	220	50
Wrist or foot	5	0

*Gonadal shields should be used if possible.

signs could read "Are you pregnant or could you be? If so, inform the radiologic technologist," or "Warning—special precautions are necessary if you are pregnant," or "Caution—if there is any possibility that you are pregnant, it is very important that you inform the radiologic technologist before you have an x-ray examination." Fig. 30-2 is a helpful poster available from the National Center for Devices and Radiological Health.

What if?

It has been estimated that fewer than 1% of all females referred for x-ray examination are subject to the 10-day rule; therefore, a considerably lower percentage will be refused examination. However, if a pregnant patient escapes detection and is irradiated, what is the subsequent responsibility of the radiology service to the patient, and what should be done?

The first step is to estimate the fetal dose. The radiologic physicist should be consulted immediately and requested to estimate the fetal dose. If a preliminary review of the examination techniques employed (for example, type of examination, kVp, and mAs) determines that the dose may have exceeded 1 rad (10 mGy), a more com-

plete dosimetric evaluation should be conducted. Table 30-5 presents representative radiation levels for many examinations. With a knowledge of the types of examinations performed and the techniques and apparatus employed, the physicist can accurately measure the fetal dose. There are phantoms and dosimetry materials available to ensure that this determination can be made with confidence.

Once the fetal dose is known, the referring physician and radiologist should determine the stage of gestation at which the x-ray exposure occurred. With this information there are only two alternatives: allow the patient to continue to term or terminate the pregnancy.

There are few authoritative recommendations regarding whether abortion is indicated. Since the natural incidence of congenital anomalies is approximately 5%, such effects are undetectable at low x-ray doses. Manifest damage to the newborn is unlikely at fetal doses below 25 rad (250 mGy), although some suggest that lower doses may cause mental developmental abnormalities. In view of the available evidence, a reasonable approach is to apply a 10 to 25 rad rule. Below 10 rad (100 mGy) a therapeutic abortion is not indicated unless there are additional mitigating circumstances. Above 25 rad (250 mGy) the risk of latent injury may justify a therapeutic abortion. Between 10 and 25 rad one must carefully consider the precise time of irradiation, the emotional state of the patient, the effect an additional child would have on the family, and other social and economic factors.

Fortunately, experience with such situations has shown that fetal doses have been consistently low. The fetal dose is usually in the 1 to 5 rad (10 to 50 mGy) range following a series of conventional x-ray examinations.

REVIEW QUESTIONS

1. Define or otherwise identify the following:
   a. Health physics
   b. TVL
   c. Cumulative total exposure
   d. Fetal radiation risk
   e. MPD
   f. 10-day rule
   g. Fetal MPD
   h. Extremity monitor
   i. Major organogenesis
   J. Elective booking
2. The output intensity of a radiographic unit is 4.2 mR/mAs. What is the total output following a 200 ms exposure at 300 mA)(1.1 μC/kg-mAs)?

3. What is the approximate patient skin dose following a 3.2-minute fluoroscopic examination of 1.5 mA?
4. Calibration of a radiographic unit shows the patient skin dose to be 5.4 mrad/mAs (54 μGy/mAs) at 70 kVp. What will be the approximate skin dose following a technique of 84 kVp, 120 mAs?
5. What steps should be taken in the event that a fetus was accidentally irradiated?
6. List five procedures that should be scheduled according to the 10-day rule.
7. What are the three cardinal principles of radiation protection, and how can they best be applied in diagnostic radiology?
8. At 60 cm from the side of a fluoroscopic table (assume 90 cm from a point source) the exposure rate is 50 mR/hr (135 mC/kg-hr). What is the exposure rate at 180 cm from the source?
9. In question B, if a technologist remained 30 cm from the table (60 cm from the source) for a total of 150 minutes of beam-on time during a week, what would be the expected personnel exposure?
10. What exposure will a technologist receive when exposed for 10 minutes at 4 m to a source with intensity of 100 mR/hr at 1 m while wearing a protective apron equivalent to 2 HVLs?

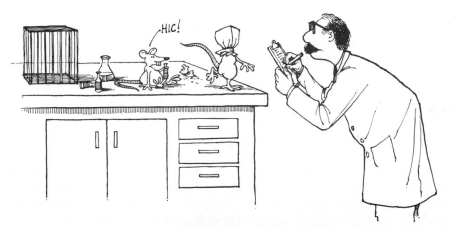

AND THEN, WITH GOVERNMENTAL FUNDS DWINDLING, THE BREAKTHROUGH CAME — A CURE FOR HICCUPS IN LABORATORY ANIMALS.

31

Designing for radiation protection

DESIGN OF X-RAY APPARATUS
DESIGN OF PROTECTIVE BARRIERS
RADIATION DETECTION AND MEASUREMENT

DESIGN OF X-RAY APPARATUS

A number of features of modern x-ray equipment designed to improve radiographic quality have been previously discussed. Many of these features and a number of additional ones are also designed to reduce patient dose during x-ray examination. For instance, proper beam collimation is very effective in reducing patient dose, and it is also a primary contributor to improved image quality. Filtration, on the other hand, is added to the x-ray beam only to reduce the patient dose.

More than 100 individual radiation protection devices and accessories are associated with modern x-ray equipment. Some are characteristic of either radiographic or fluoroscopic assemblies, and some are required for all diagnostic x-ray equipment. A few of those appropriate for all diagnostic x-ray equipment follow.

Diagnostic-type protective tube housing. Every x-ray tube must be contained within a protective housing that reduces the **leakage radiation** to less than 100 mR/hr (26 μC/kg-hr) at a distance of 1 m from the housing.

Control panel. The control panel must indicate the conditions of exposure and positively indicate when the x-ray tube is energized. These requirements are usually satisfied with kVp and mA meters. Sometimes visible or audible signals will indicate when the beam is on.

Radiographic equipment

Some of the more important aspects of radiation protection when using radiographic equipment are discussed next.

Source–to–image receptor distance (SID) indicator. An SID indicator must be provided. It can be as simple as a tape measure attached to the tube housing or as advanced as laser lights, but it must be accurate to within 2% of the indicated SID.

Collimation. Light-localized variable-aperture rectangular collimators should be provided. The x-ray beam and light beam must coincide to within 2% of the SID. Cones and diaphragms may replace the collimator for special examination. The attenuation of the useful beam by the collimator leaves must be equivalent to that by the protective housing.

EXAMPLE: Most radiographs are taken at an SID of 100 cm. How much difference is allowed between the projection of the light field and the x-ray beam at the image receptor?

ANSWER: 2% of 100 cm = 2 cm

Positive beam limitation (PBL). Automatic light-localized variable-aperture collimators are now required on all but special equipment in the United States. These PBL devices must be adjusted so that with any film size in use and at all standard SIDs the collimator leaves are automatically adjusted to provide an x-ray beam equal to the image receptor. The PBL must be accurate to 2% of the SID.

Beam alignment. In addition to proper collimation, each radiographic tube head should be provided with a mechanism to ensure proper alignment of the x-ray beam and the film. It does no good to align the light beam and the x-ray beam but have the film partly out of the beam.

Filtration. All general-purpose diagnostic x-ray beams must have a total filtration (inherent plus added) of at least 2.5 mm Al when operated above 70 kVp. Radiographic tubes operated between 50 and 70 kVp must have at least 1.5 mm Al. Below 50 kVp, a minimum of 0.5 mm Al total filtration is required. X-ray tubes with a molybdenum target for mammography will usually have 30 μm Mo filtration and that is adequate below 50 kVp.

Reproducibility. For any given radiographic technique the output radiation intensity should be constant from one exposure to another. This is checked by making 10 repeated exposures at the same technique and observing that the average variation in radiation intensity does not exceed 5%.

Linearity. When adjacent mA stations are employed, for example, 100 and 200 mA, and exposure time is adjusted for constant mAs, the output radiation intensity must remain constant. The radiation intensity is measured in units of milliroentgens per milliampere-seconds (mR/mAs), and the maximum acceptable variation in this linearity is 10%.

Personnel shield. It must not be possible to expose a radiograph while the technologist stands outside a fixed protective barrier, usually the console booth. The exposure control should be fixed to the operating console and not a long cord.

Portable x-ray unit. A protective lead apron should be assigned to each portable x-ray unit. The exposure switch of such a unit must allow the operator to remain at least 180 cm from the x-ray tube during exposure.

Fluoroscopic equipment

The features of fluoroscopic equipment discussed below are designed primarily to reduce patient and personnel exposure.

Source-to-tabletop distance. The source-to-tabletop distance must be not less than 38 cm on stationary fluoroscopes and not less than 30 cm on mobile fluoroscopes. Increasing the distance between the fluoroscopic tube and the patient results in reduced patient dose because of the corresponding decrease in the difference between the entrance and exit dose to the patient. This is illustrated in Fig. 31-1.

Primary protective barrier. The image-intensifier assembly serves as a primary protective barrier and must be 2 mm Pb equivalent for

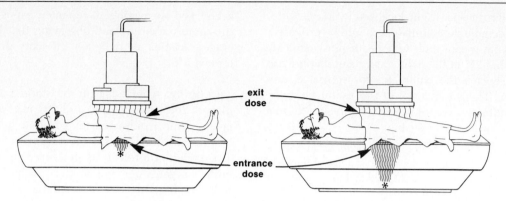

Fig. 31-1. Patient dose is higher and magnification greater when the fluoroscopic tube is close to the tabletop.

equipment capable of operating above 125 kVp. It must be coupled with the x-ray tube and interlocked so that the fluoroscopic tube cannot be energized when in the parked position.

Filtration. The total filtration of the fluoroscope must be at least 2.5 mm Al equivalent. The tabletop, patient cradle, or other material positioned between the tube and the tabletop should be included as part of the total filtration. When the filtration is unknown, the half-value layer should be measured. If the half-value layer is not less than 2.4 mm Al when operated at 80 kVp, adequate filtration may be assumed.

Collimation. The fluoroscopic beam collimators must be adjusted so that an unexposed border is visible on the monitor when the input phosphor of the image intensifier is positioned 35 cm above the tabletop and the collimators are fully open. For automatic collimating devices, such an unexposed border should be visible at all heights above the tabletop.

Exposure switch. The fluoroscopic exposure switch should be the dead-man type; that is, if the operator should drop dead, the exposure would be terminated—unless, of course, he or she falls on the switch. The conventional foot pedal satisfies this condition.

Bucky slot cover. During fluoroscopy, the Bucky tray is moved to the end of the examining table, leaving an opening in the side of the table approximately 5 cm wide at gonadal level. This opening should be automatically covered with at least 0.25 mm Pb equivalent.

Protective curtain. A protective curtain or panel of at least 0.15 mm Pb equivalent should be positioned between the fluoroscopist and the patient. Fig. 31-2 shows the typical vertical iso-exposure distribution for a fluoroscope. Without the curtain and Bucky slot cover, the exposure of radiology personnel is many times higher.

Cumulative timer. A cumulative timer that produces an audible signal or temporarily interrupts the x-ray beam when the fluoroscopic time has exceeded 5 minutes must be provided. This device is designed to make sure the radiologist is aware of the relative beam-on time during each procedure.

X-ray intensity. The intensity of the x-ray beam at the tabletop of a fluoroscope should not exceed 2.1 R/min (0.54 mC/kg-min) for each

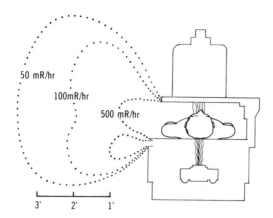

Fig. 31-2. Isoexposure profile for typical fluoroscope demonstrating need for protective curtains and Bucky slot covers.

50 mR/hr

100mR/hr

500 mR/hr

3'   2'   1'

mA of operation at 80 kVp. Under no conditions should the intensity exceed 10 R/min (2.6 mC/kg-min) during fluoroscopy. Tabletop intensities may exceed this level during cineradiography.

DESIGN OF PROTECTIVE BARRIERS

When one is designing radiology departments or individual x-ray examination rooms, it is not sufficient to consider only the general architectural characteristics described in Chapter 25. Great attention must be given to the location of x-ray machines within the examination room and to the use of adjoining rooms. It is nearly always necessary to insert protective barriers, usually sheets of lead, in the walls of x-ray examining rooms. If the radiology facility is located on an upper floor, then it may be necessary to shield the floor as well. For these reasons it can be desirable to locate the radiology facility on the ground or basement level, with the examining rooms positioned along outside walls.

A great number of factors should be considered in designing a protective barrier. This discussion will touch on only the fundamentals and some basic definitions. Any time new x-ray facilities are being designed or old ones renovated, a certified physicist must be consulted for assistance in designing proper radiation shielding.

Types of radiation

For the purpose of designing protective barriers, three types of radiation are considered. These are shown diagramatically in Fig. 31-3. Primary radiation is the most intense and therefore the most hazardous and the most difficult to protect against. **Primary radiation is the useful beam.** When a chest board is positioned on a given wall, it can be assumed that it will intercept the useful beam frequently. Therefore, it is sometimes necessary to provide shielding directly behind the chest board in addition to that specified for the rest of the wall. Any wall to which the useful beam can be directed is designated a **primary protective barrier.**

Lead bonded to sheet rock or wood paneling is most often employed as a primary protective barrier. Such lead shielding is available in various thicknesses, and it is specified for architects and contractors in units of pounds per square foot (lb/ft²). Rarely is it necessary to use in excess of 4 lb/ft² in a diagnostic room. Concrete, concrete block, or brick may be used instead of lead. As a rule of thumb, 4 inches of masonry is equivalent to 1/16 inch of lead. Table 31-1 shows available lead thicknesses and equivalent thicknesses of concrete. The thinnest available shielding is 1 lb/ft², but because of some difficulties in fabrication, 2 lb/ft² lead is often no more costly.

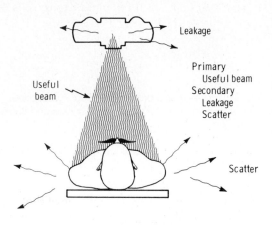

Fig. 31-3. Three types of radiation—the useful beam, leakage radiation, and scatter radiation—must be considered in designing the protective barriers of an x-ray room.

Table 31-1. Lead and concrete equivalents for primary protective barriers

	Lead		Concrete	
(mm)	(in)	(lb/ft²)	(cm)	(in)
0.4	1/64	1	2.4	1⅜
0.8	1/32	2	4.8	1⅞
1.2	3/64	3	7.2	2⅞
1.6	1/16	4	9.6	3¾

Table 31-2. Equivalent material thicknesses for secondary barriers

Computed lead requirement (mm)	Substitutes		
	Gypsum board (in × ⅝ in)	Glass (in)	Lead acrylic (mm)
0.1	2	½	2
0.2	4	1	5
0.3	6	1½	7
0.4	8	2	9

There are two types of **secondary radiation: scatter radiation** and **leakage radiation.** Scatter radiation results when the useful beam intercepts any object so that some x rays are scattered. For the purpose of protective shielding calculations, the scattering object can be considered as a new source of radiation. During both radiography and fluoroscopy, the patient is the single most important scattering object. As a general rule of thumb, **the intensity of scatter radiation 1 m from the patient is 0.1% of the intensity of the useful beam at the patient.**

EXAMPLE: The output intensity of a radiographic unit at patient position is 410 mR (0.1 mC/kg) for a kidney, ureter, and bladder (KUB) examination. What will be the approximate radiation exposure 1 m from the patient? 3 m from the patient?

ANSWER:

At 1 m: 410 mR × 0.1% = 410 mR × 0.001
$$= 0.41 \text{ mR}$$

At 3 m:
$$= 0.41 \text{ mR } (⅓)^2$$
$$= 0.41 \text{ mR } (⅑)$$
$$= 0.036 \text{ mR}$$
$$= 36 \text{ μR}$$

Leakage radiation is radiation emitted from the x-ray tube housing assembly in all directions other than that of the useful beam. If the tube housing is properly designed, the leakage radiation will never exceed the regulatory limit of 100 mR/hr (26 μC/kg-hr) at 1 m. Although in practice leakage radiation levels are much less than this limit, 100 mR/hr at 1 m is used for barrier calculations.

Barriers designed to shield areas from secondary radiation are called **secondary radiation barriers.** Secondary radiation barriers are always less thick than primary protective barriers.

Lead is rarely required for secondary barriers because the computation usually results in less than 0.4 mm Pb. In such cases, conventional gypsum board, glass, or lead acrylic is adequate. Many walls that are secondary barriers can be adequately protected with four thicknesses of ⅝-inch gypsum board. Most control booth barriers are secondary protective barriers—the useful beam is never directed at the control booth. Four thicknesses of gypsum board and ½-inch plate glass may be all that is necessary. Sometimes glass walls ½- to 1-inch thick can be used for control booth barriers. Table 31-2 contains equivalent thicknesses for secondary barrier material.

EXAMPLE: What percentage of the maximum permissible dose (100 mR/wk) will be incident on a control booth barrier located 3 m from the x-ray tube and patient? Assume the x-ray output is 3 mR/mAs and that the weekly beam-on time is 5 minutes, at an average 100 mA, a generous assumption.

ANSWER: From scatter radiation the barrier will receive:

$$\text{Total primary beam} = 3 \text{ mR/mAs} \times 100 \text{ mA} \times 5\text{m} \times 60 \text{ s/m}$$
$$= 90{,}000 \text{ mR}$$
$$\text{Scatter radiation} = 90{,}000 \text{ mR} \times \frac{1}{1000} \times (\frac{1}{3})^2$$
$$= 10 \text{ mR}$$

From leakage radiation, the barrier will receive:

$$\text{Leakage radiation at 1 m} = 100 \text{ mR/hr} \times \frac{5}{60} \text{ hr}$$
$$= 8.3 \text{ mR}$$
$$\text{Leakage radiation} = 8.3 \text{ mR} (\frac{1}{3})^2$$
$$= 0.9 \text{ mr}$$
$$\text{Total secondary radiation} = 10 \text{ mR} \times 0.9 \text{ mR}$$
$$= 10.9 \text{ mR or 11\% of the MPD}$$

This analysis is representative of the clinical environment. The estimated exposure is to the control booth barrier, not to the technologist. The composition of the barrier and the additional distance will reduce technologist exposure even more. This is the reason that personnel radiation exposure during radiography is very low. We get most of our exposure during fluoroscopy.

Factors affecting barrier thickness

Many factors must be taken into consideration when calculating the required protective barrier thickness. A thorough discussion of these factors is beyond the scope of this book; however, a definition of each will be useful for understanding the problems involved.

The thickness of a barrier naturally depends on the **distance** between the source of radiation and the barrier. The distance is that to the adjacent occupied area, not to the inside of the wall of the x-ray room. A wall along which an x-ray machine is positioned will probably require more shielding than the other walls of the room. In such a case, the leakage radiation may be more hazardous than the scatter radiation or even the useful beam. It is usually desirable to position the x-ray machine in the middle of the room because then no single wall is subjected to especially intense radiation exposure.

The use of the area being protected is of principal importance. If the area were a rarely occupied closet or storeroom, the required shielding would be less than if it were an office or laboratory occupied 40 hours per week. This reflects the **occupancy factor (T).** Table 31-3 reports the occupancy levels of various areas as suggested by the National Council on Radiation Protection and Measurements (NCRP). An area occupied primarily by radiation workers is called a **controlled area.** The design limits for a controlled area require that the barrier shielding confine the exposure rate in the area to less than 100 mR/wk (26 μC/kg-wk). An **uncontrolled area** can be occupied by anyone, and therefore

Table 31-3. Levels of occupancy of areas that may be adjacent to x-ray rooms, as suggested by the NCRP

Occupancy	Area
Full	Work areas (for example, offices, laboratories, shops, wards, nurses' stations), living quarters, children's play areas, occupied space in nearby buildings
Partial	Corridors, restrooms, elevators using operators, unattended parking lots
Occasional	Waiting rooms, stairways, unattended elevators, janitors' closets, outside areas

the maximum exposure rate allowed in such an area is 10 mR/wk (2.6 μC/kg-wk). Consequently, a wall protecting an uncontrolled area must have approximately a tenth-value layer more lead than one protecting a controlled area.

The shielding required for an x-ray examining room is dependent on the level of radiation activity in that room. The greater the number of examinations performed each week, the thicker the shielding required. This characteristic is called **workload (W)** and has units of milliampere-minutes per week (mA-min/wk). A busy general-purpose x-ray room may have a workload as high as 500 mA-min/wk. Rooms that handle no more than five patients per day have workloads of less than 100 mA-min/wk.

EXAMPLE: The plans for a small community hospital call for two x-ray rooms. The estimated patient load for each room is fifteen patients per day, and each patient will average three films taken at 80 kVp, 70 mAs. What is the projected workload of each room?

ANSWER:

$$15 \text{ pts/day} \times 5 \text{ days/wk} = 75 \text{ pts/wk}$$
$$75 \text{ pts/wk} \times 3 \text{ films/pt} = 225 \text{ films/wk}$$
$$225 \text{ films/wk} \times 70 \text{ mAs/film} = 15750 \text{ mAs/wk}$$
$$15,750 \text{ mAs/wk} \times \frac{1 \text{ min}}{60 \text{ sec}} = 262.5 \text{ mA-min/wk}$$

For combination radiographic-fluoroscopic x-ray rooms, usually only the radiographic workload need be considered for barrier calculations. When the fluoroscopic x-ray tube is energized, a primary barrier in the form of the fluoroscopic screen always intercepts the useful x-ray beam. Consequently, the room shielding requirements are always much less for fluoroscopic beams than for radiographic beams.

The percentage of time during which the x-ray beam is on and directed toward a particular wall is called the **use factor (U)** for that wall. The NCRP recommends that walls be assigned a use factor of ¼ and the floor a use factor of 1. If an x-ray room has a special design, other use factors may be assigned. A room designed strictly for chest radiography has one wall with a use factor of 1. All others have a use factor of 0 for primary radiation and thus would be considered secondary radiation barriers. The ceiling is nearly always considered a secondary protective barrier. **The use factor for secondary barriers is always 1,** since leakage and scatter radiation are present 100% of the time that the tube is energized.

The final consideration in the design of an x-ray protective barrier is the penetrability of the x-ray beam. For protection calculations, **kVp is used as the measure of penetrability.** Most modern x-ray machines are designed to operate at up to 150 kVp. However, most examinations are conducted at less than 100 kVp. One usually assumes constant operation at penetrability greater than that actually used. An operating potential of 100 kVp is usually assumed. Therefore, it is more likely that the protective barrier will be too thick than too thin.

Measurements of radiation exposure outside of the x-ray room always result in weekly levels far less than that anticipated by calculation. The total beam-on time is always less than assumed. The average kVp is usually closer to 75 kVp than to 100 kVp. The calculations do not account for the fact that the patient and image receptor always intercept the useful beam. Therefore, although the calculations are intended to result in an MPD (100 mR/wk or 10 mR/wk) outside the x-ray room, rarely will the actual exposure exceed one tenth of the MPD. To confirm this for yourself, keep records for 1 week of kVp, mAs, and beam direction.

RADIATION DETECTION AND MEASUREMENT

Instruments are designed either to detect or measure radiation or to do both. Those designed for detection generally operate in the **pulse** or **rate** mode and are used to indicate the presence of radiation. Those designed to measure the intensity of radiation usually operate in the **integrate** mode; they accumulate the signal and respond with a total exposure or dose. Such an application is called **dosimetry,** and such radiation-measuring devices are called **dosimeters.**

The earliest radiation detection device was the photographic emulsion, and it is still a principal means of radiation detection and measurement. In the intervening years, however, other devices have been developed that have more favorable characteristics than the photographic emulsion for some applications. Table 31-4 lists most of the currently available radiation detection and measurement devices along with some of their principal characteristics and uses.

It is apparent that film has two principal applications in diagnostic radiology: (1) the making of a radiograph and (2) the personnel radiation monitor (film badge). The photographic process was discussed in Chapters 13 and 14. Use of film as a radiation monitor is covered in Chapter 32.

Three other types of radiation detection de-

Table 31-4. Radiation detection and measuring device characteristics and uses

Device	Characteristics and uses
Photographic emulsion	Limited range, sensitive, energy dependent, personnel monitoring, imaging
Ionization chamber	Wide range, accurate, portable survey for fields > 1 mR/hr
Proportional counter	Laboratory instrument, accurate, sensitive, assay of small quantities of radionuclides
Geiger-Müller counter	Limited to <100 mR/hr, portable survey for low fields and contamination
Thermoluminescence dosimetry	Wide range, accurate, sensitive, personnel monitoring, stationary area monitoring
Scintillation detection	Limited range, very sensitive, stationary or portable instruments, photon spectroscopy, imaging

vices are of particular importance in diagnostic radiology. The gas-filled radiation detector is employed widely as a device to measure radiation intensity and to detect radioactive contamination. Thermoluminescence dosimetry (TLD) is used for both patient and personnel radiation monitoring. Scintillation detection is the basis for the gamma camera, an imaging device used in nuclear medicine.

Gas-filled detectors

There are three types of gas-filled radiation detectors: ionization chambers, proportional counters, and Geiger-Müller (G-M) detectors. Although they are different in response characteristics, each is based on the same principle of operation. As radiation passes through gas, it ionizes atoms in its path. This ionization of gas is the basis for these gas-filled radiation detectors.

Consider an ideal gas-filled detector as shown schematically in Fig. 31-4. It consists of a cylindric chamber filled with a gas, which could be air or any of a number of other gases. Xenon under pressure, for instance, is used to measure

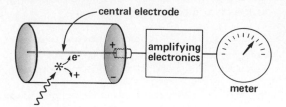

central electrode

amplifying
electronics

meter

Fig. 31-4. Ideal gas-filled detector consists of a cylindric chamber of gas (usually air) and a central collecting electrode. By maintaining a voltage between the central electrode and the wall of the chamber, electrons produced in ionization can be collected and measured.

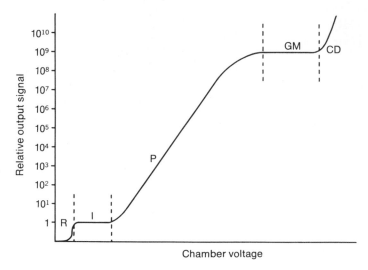

Chamber voltage

Fig. 31-5. Amplitude of the electric signal from a gas-filled detector increases in stages as the voltage across the chamber is increased.

x rays in some CT scanners. Along the central axis of the cylinder is positioned a rigid wire called the **central electrode.** If a voltage difference is impressed between the central electrode and the wall such that the wire is positive and the wall negative, then any electrons liberated in the chamber by ionization will be attracted to the central electrode. These electrons form an electric signal either as a pulse of electrons or a continuous current. This electric signal is then amplified and measured. Its intensity will be proportional to the radiation intensity that caused it.

In general, the larger the chamber, the more gas molecules there are available for ionization and therefore the more sensitive is the instrument. Similarly, if the chamber is pressurized, then more molecules will be available for ionization and a higher sensitivity will result. **A high sensitivity means that an instrument can detect very low radiation intensities.** Sensitivity is not the same as **accuracy.** A high accuracy means that an instrument can detect and **precisely measure** the intensity of a radiation field. Instrument accuracy is controlled by the overall electronic design of the device.

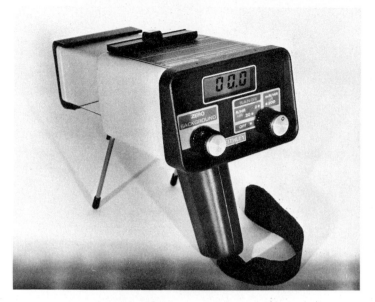

Fig. 31-6. The "cutie pie" portable ion chamber survey instrument is useful for area surveys when exposure levels are in excess of 1 mR/hr. (Courtesy Keithley Instruments, Inc.)

Region of recombination. If the voltage across the chamber of the ideal gas-filled detector is slowly increased from zero to a high level, the resulting electric signal will increase in stages (Fig. 31-5). In the first stage, when the voltage is very low, no electrons will be attracted to the central electrode. The ion pairs produced in the chamber will recombine. This is known as the **region of recombination,** shown as stage R in Fig. 31-5.

Ion chamber region. As the chamber voltage is increased, a level will be reached where every electron released in ionization will be attracted to the central electrode and collected. The voltage at which this occurs varies according to the design of the chamber, but for most conventional instruments it is in the range of 100 to 300 V. This portion of the gas-filled detector performance curve is known as the **ionization region,** indicated by I in Fig. 31-5. Ion chambers are operated in this region.

There are a number of different types of ion chambers used in radiology, the most familiar being the "cutie pie" portable instrument (Fig. 31-6). This instrument is used principally for area surveys. It can measure a wide range of radiation intensities, from 1 mR/hr to several thousand R/hr. It is the instrument of choice for measuring the radiation intensity in areas such as the region of the fluoroscope, around radionuclide generators and syringes, the vicinity of patients containing therapeutic quantities of radioactive materials, and outside protective barriers. There are other, more accurate, ion chambers, which are used for the precise calibration of the output intensity of diagnostic x-ray machines and external beam radiation therapy units (Fig. 31-7). Yet another application of a precision ion chamber is the dose calibrator (Fig. 31-8).

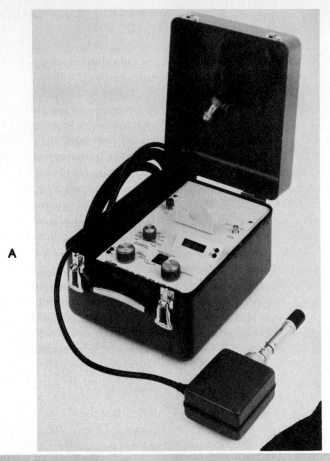

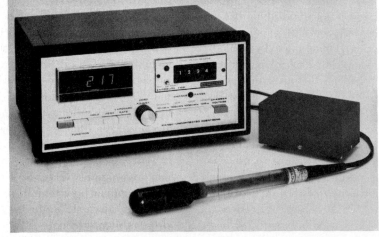

Fig. 31-7. Two representative ion chambers used for accurate measurement. **A,** Used for diagnostic x-ray beams. **B,** Used for therapeutic radiation beams. (**A** courtesy MDH Industries; **B** courtesy Victoreen Instrument Co.)

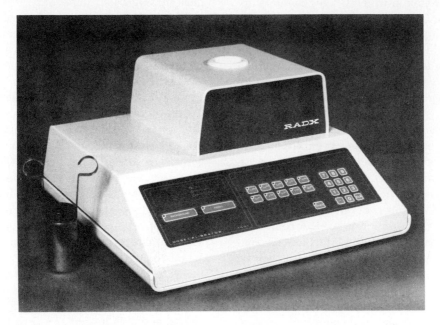

Fig. 31-8. This configuration of an ion chamber is called a dose calibrator. It is used to accurately measure quantities of radioactive material. (Courtesy Radex, Inc.)

These devices find daily use in nuclear medicine laboratories for the assay of quantities of radioactive material.

Proportional region. As the chamber voltage of the ideal gas-filled detector is increased still further above the ionization region, electrons of the filling gas released by primary ionization will be accelerated more rapidly to the central collecting electrode. The faster these electrons travel, the higher the probability that they will cause secondary ionization on their way to the central electrode. These secondary electrons will also be attracted to the central electrode and collected. The total number of electrons collected in this fashion increases with increasing chamber voltage. The result is a rather large electron pulse for each primary ionization. This stage of the voltage response curve is known as the **proportional region.**

Proportional counters are rather sensitive instruments, and they are used principally as stationary laboratory instruments for the assay of small quantities of radioactivity. There are some portable survey instruments that operate in the proportional region, but these are generally used to detect only alpha and beta radiation. One characteristic of proportional counters that makes them particularly useful is their ability to distinguish between alpha and beta radiation. Nevertheless, proportional counters find little application in clinical radiology.

Geiger-Müller region. The fourth region of the voltage response curve for the ideal gas-filled chamber is the **Geiger-Müller (G-M) region.**

This is the region in which Geiger counters operate. In the G-M region the voltage across the ionization chamber is sufficiently high so that when a single ionizing event occurs, a cascade of secondary electrons is produced in a fashion similar to a very brief, yet violent, chain reaction. The effect is that nearly all the molecules of the filling gas are ionized, liberating a large number of electrons; this results in a rather large electron pulse. When ionizing events occur soon after one another, the detector may not be capable of responding to the second event if the filling gas has not been restored to its initial condition. Therefore, a **quenching agent** is added to the filling gas of the Geiger counter to enable the chamber to return to its original condition; subsequent ionizing events can then be detected. The minimum time between ionizations that can be detected is known as the **resolving time.**

Geiger counters are used extensively for contamination control in nuclear medicine laboratories. As a portable survey instrument, it is used to detect the presence of radioactive contamination on work surfaces and laboratory apparatus. It is not particularly useful as a dosimeter because it is difficult to properly calibrate for varying conditions of radiation. It is a sensitive instrument, capable of detecting and indicating single ionizing events. If it is equipped with an audio amplifier and speaker, one can even hear the crackle of individual ionizations. The Geiger counter does not have a very wide range. Most instruments are limited to less than 100 mR/hr (26 μC/kg-hr).

Region of continuous discharge. If the voltage across the ideal gas-filled chamber is increased still further, a condition will be reached whereby a single ionizing event will completely discharge the chamber, as in operation in the Geiger-Müller region. However, because of the high voltage, electrons will continue to be stripped from atoms of the filling gas, producing a continuous current or signal from the chamber. In this condition the instrument is useless for the detection of radiation, and continued operation in this region will result in damage. This region is known as the region of continuous discharge and is indicated as *CD* in Fig. 31-5.

Scintillation detection

Scintillation detection devices are used in several areas of radiologic science. The scintillation detector is the basis for the gamma camera in nuclear medicine and is used in the detector arrays of many computed tomography scanners.

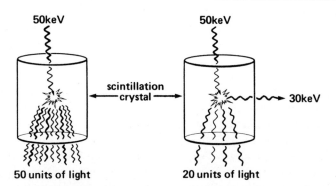

Fig. 31-9. During scintillation, the quantity of light emitted is proportional to the amount of energy absorbed in the crystal.

The scintillation process. Certain types of material will scintillate when irradiated; that is, they emit a flash of light immediately in response to absorption of ionizing radiation. The amount of light emitted is proportional to the amount of energy absorbed by the crystal. Consider for example, the two photon interactions diagrammed in Fig. 31-9. If a 50 keV photon underwent photoelectric absorption in the crystal, all the energy (50 keV) would reappear as light. However, if that same photon underwent a Compton scattering event in which only 20 keV of energy was absorbed, then a proportionately lower quantity of light would be emitted in the scintillation.

Only those materials with a particular crystalline structure will scintillate. At the atomic level the process involves the rearrangement of valence electrons into traps. The return of the electron from the trap to its normal position is immediate in scintillation and delayed in thermoluminescence. This property is considered under an earlier discussion of luminescence (Chapter 14).

Types of scintillation phosphors. Many different types of liquids, gases, and solids can respond to ionizing radiation by scintillation. Scintillation detectors are most often used to indicate individual ionizing events and are incorporated into either fixed or portable radiation detection devices. They can be used to measure radiation either in the rate mode or integrate mode.

Nearly all the noble gases can be made to respond to radiation by scintillation. Such applications are rare, however, because the probability of interaction is small and therefore the detection efficiency is very low.

Liquid scintillation detectors are frequently used in the research laboratory to detect the low-energy beta emissions from carbon-14 (^{14}C) and tritium (^{3}H). ^{14}C and ^{3}H are useful research radionuclides because they present a relatively harmless radiation hazard and are easily incorporated into biologic molecules. These radionuclides emit low-energy beta particles with no associated gamma rays. This makes them hard to detect. With liquid scintillation counting, however, the biologic molecules can be mixed with a liquid scintillation phosphor so that the beta emission interacts directly with the phosphor causing a flash of light to be emitted. Liquid scintillation counters have nearly 100% detection efficiency for beta radiation.

By far the most widely used scintillation phosphors are the inorganic crystals: thallium-activated sodium iodide (NaI:Tl) or thallium-activated cesium iodide (CsI:Tl). The **activator atoms** of thallium are impurities grown into the crystal to control the spectrum of the light emitted and to enhance its intensity. The NaI:Tl crystals are incorporated into gamma cameras. CsI:Tl is the phosphor incorporated into image-intensifier tubes as the input phosphor. Both types of crystals have been incorporated into CT scanner detector arrays.

The scintillation detector assembly. Light produced during scintillation is emitted **isotropically,** that is, with equal intensity in all directions. Consequently, when used as radiation detectors, scintillation crystals are canned in aluminum having a polished inner surface in contact with the crystal. This allows the light flash to be internally reflected and concentrated to the one face of the crystal that is not canned, called the **window.** The aluminum containment is also necessary to hermetically seal the crystal. A **hermetic seal** is one that prevents the crystal from coming into contact with air or moisture. Many scintillation crystals are **hygroscopic;** that is, they will absorb moisture. When moisture is absorbed, the crystals will swell and crack. Cracked crystals are not useful because the crack produces an interface that reflects and attenuates the scintillation.

Fig. 31-10 shows the basic components of a single crystal photomultiplier tube assembly representative of the type employed in a portable survey instrument. The detector portion of the assembly is the NaI:Tl crystal contained in the aluminum hermetic seal. Coupled to the

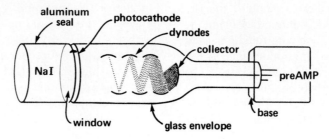

Fig. 31-10. Scintillation detector assembly characteristic of the type used in a portable survey instrument.

window of the crystal is a photomultiplier (PM) tube that converts the light flashes from the scintillator into electrical pulses.

The PM tube is an electron vacuum tube that contains a number of elements. The tube consists of a **glass envelope,** which provides structural support for the internal elements and maintains the vacuum inside the tube. The portion of the glass envelope that is coupled to the scintillation crystal is called the **window of the tube.** The crystal window and the PM tube window are sandwiched together with a silicone grease, which provides **optical coupling** so that the light emitted by the scintillator is transmitted to the interior of the photomultiplier tube with minimum loss.

As the light passes from the crystal into the photomultiplier tube, it is incident on a thin metal coating called a **photocathode,** which consists of a cesium, antimony, and bismuth compound. A photocathode is a device that emits electrons when illuminated. The process is called **photoemission** and is similar to the process of thermionic emission in the filament of an x-ray tube except that the stimulus is light rather than heat.

The flash of light from the scintillation crystal, therefore, is incident on the photocathode, and electrons are boiled off by photoemission. The number of electrons emitted is directly proportional to the intensity of light.

These photoelectrons are accelerated to the first of a series of platelike elements called **dynodes.** Each dynode serves to amplify the electron pulse by **secondary electron emission.** For each electron incident on the dynode, several secondary electrons will be dislodged, emitted, and directed to the next stage. Consequently, there is an electron gain for each dynode in the PM tube. The dynode gain is the ratio of secondary electrons to incident electrons. The number of dynodes and the gain of each dynode determines the overall electron gain of the PM tube. If the dynode gain is g, and n is equal to the number of dynodes, then the overall gain for the PM tube is given by the following:

(31-1)

$$Tube\ gain\ =\ g^n$$

EXAMPLE: An eight-stage PM tube (eight dynodes) has a dynode gain of 3 (three electrons emitted for each incident electron). What is the tube gain?
ANSWER: Tube gain $= 3^8$
$= 6561$

The last platelike element is called the collecting electrode, or **collector.** The collector absorbs the electron pulse from the last dynode and conducts it to the **preamplifier.** The preamplifier provides an initial stage of pulse amplification. It is attached to the **base** of the PM

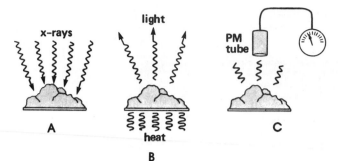

Fig. 31-11. Thermoluminescence dosimetry is a multistep process. **A,** Exposure to ionizing radiation. **B,** Subsequent heating. **C,** Measurement of the intensity of the emitted light.

tube, a structure to provide support for the glass envelope and internal structures. The overall result of scintillation detection is therefore that a single photon interaction produces a burst of light; this in turn produces photoelectron emission, which is then amplified to produce a relatively large electron pulse. **The size of the electron pulse is proportional to the energy absorbed by the crystal from the incident photon.** It is this property of scintillation detection that promotes its use as an energy-sensitive device for **gamma spectrometry** through **pulse height analysis.** Through such application, unknown gamma emitters can be identified, and more sensitive radioisotope imaging can be accomplished by counting only those pulses having energy representing a total photon absorption.

Scintillation detectors are sensitive devices for x and gamma rays. They are capable of measuring radiation intensities as low as single-photon interactions. This property of scintillation detectors results in their use as portable radiation devices in much the same manner as Geiger counters. In fact, a portable scintillation detector is more sensitive than a Geiger counter because it has much higher detection efficiency. For this application, the scintillation detector would be used to monitor the presence of contamination and perhaps low levels of radiation. It is not normally used as a dosimeter because of difficulties involved in calibration.

Thermoluminescence dosimetry

Some materials will glow when heated. This is **thermally stimulated emission of visible light, called thermoluminescence.** In the early 1960s Cameron and co-workers at the University of Wisconsin experimented with some thermoluminescent materials and were able to show that exposure to ionizing radiation caused some materials to glow particularly brightly when subsequently heated. This radiation-induced thermoluminescence has been developed into a sensitive and accurate method of radiation dosimetry for personnel radiation monitoring and for measuring patient dose during diagnostic and therapeutic radiation procedures. Finally, it also enjoys full application in experimental radiation science, especially where small detector size is important and in low-level environmental monitoring. Personnel and patient radiation monitoring are discussed in Chapter 32; however, at this time it is important to know something of the basic principles of thermoluminescence dosimetry. The process of thermoluminescence dosimetry (TLD) is shown schematically in Fig. 31-11.

Following irradiation, the TLD phosphor is placed on a special dish, or planchet, for analysis in an instrument called a TLD analyzer. The temperature of the planchet can be carefully controlled. Directly viewing the planchet is a PM tube. The PM tube is the same type of light-

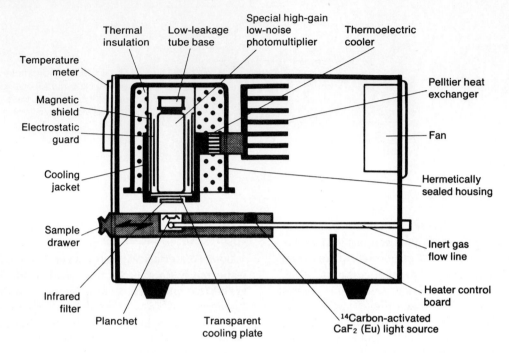

Fig. 31-12. Cutaway schematic of a representative TLD analyzer. (Courtesy Harshaw Chemical Co.)

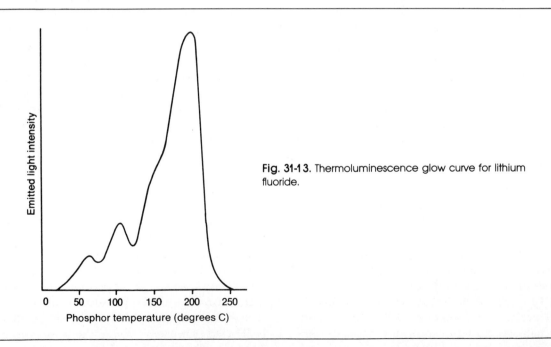

Fig. 31-13. Thermoluminescence glow curve for lithium fluoride.

Table 31-5. Some thermoluminescent phosphors and their characteristics and uses

| | Phosphor | | | |
	Lithium fluoride	Lithium borate	Calcium fluoride	Calcium sulfate
Composition	LiF	$Li_2B_4O_7$:Mn	CaF_2:Mn	$CaSO_4$:Dy
Density $\times 10^3 (kg/m^3)$	2.64	2.4	3.18	2.61
Effective atomic number	8.2	7.4	16.3	15.3
Temperature of main peak (°C)	195	200	260	220
Principal use	Patient and personnel dose	Research	Environmental monitoring	Environmental monitoring

sensitive and light-measuring vacuum tube described previously as a major component of scintillation detectors. The PM tube–planchet assembly encompasses a chamber with a lighttight seal. The output signal from the PM tube is amplified and displayed either on a meter or chart recorder. Fig. 31-12 is a cutaway drawing of a commercially available TLD analyzer.

The glow curve. As the temperature of the planchet is increased, the amount of light emitted by the TLD increases in an irregular manner. Fig. 31-13 shows the light output from lithium fluoride (LiF) with increasing temperature. There are several prominent peaks in this graph, and each occurs because of electron transition in the TL crystal. Such a graph is known as a **glow curve,** and each TL material has a characteristic glow curve. Both the height of the highest temperature peak and the total area under the curve are directly proportional to the energy imparted to the TLD by ionizing radiation. TLD analyzers are electronic instruments designed to measure the height of the glow curve or the area under the curve, and some automatically relate this to exposure or dose through a conversion factor.

Types of TLD material. Many materials, including some body tissues, exhibit the property of radiation-induced thermoluminescence. Materials that are used for TLD, however, are somewhat limited in number and are principally types of inorganic crystals. Lithium fluoride is the most widely used TLD material. It has an effective atomic number of 8.2 and therefore has photon absorption properties similar to that of soft tissue. It is nearly a **tissue equivalent dosimeter.** LiF is relatively sensitive. It can measure doses as low as 10 mrad (0.1 mGy) with modest accuracy, and at doses exceeding 10 rad (100 mGy) accuracy is better than ±5%.

Calcium fluoride that is activated with manganese (CaF_2:Mn) has a higher effective atomic number (Z = 16.3) than LiF, and this makes it considerably more sensitive to ionizing radiation. CaF_2:Mn can measure radiation doses less than 1 mrad (10 μGy) with moderate accuracy. Other types of TLDs are available, and Table 31-5 lists some and their principal characteristics and applications.

Properties of TLD. A particular advantage of TLD is dosimeter size. TLDs can be obtained in several solid crystal shapes and sizes. Rectangular rods measuring 1 × 1 × 6 mm long and flat chips measuring 3 × 3 × 1 mm thick are the most popular sizes. TLDs can also be obtained in powder form, which allows for their irradiation in nearly any configuration. TLDs are also available with the phosphor matrixed with Teflon or plated onto a wire and sealed in glass.

TLDs are reusable. When irradiated, the energy absorbed by the TLD remains stored until released as visible light by heat during analysis. This heating restores the crystal to its original condition and makes it ready for another radiation exposure.

TLDs respond proportionally to dose. If one doubles the dose, the TLD response will also be doubled. TLDs are rugged, and their small size makes them useful for monitoring dose in small areas such as body cavities. TLDs do not respond to individual ionizing events, and therefore they cannot be used in a rate meter type of instrument. TLDs are only suitable for integral dose measurements, but they do not give immediate results.

REVIEW QUESTIONS

1. Define or otherwise identify the following:
   a. TLD
   b. Use factor
   c. Diagnostic protective tube housing
   d. Glow curve
   e. Primary protective barrier
   f. X-ray linearity
   g. Secondary radiation
   h. Occupancy factor
   i. Geiger-Müller region
   j. Resolving time

2. List four conditions that must be considered when computing the thickness of lead required for an x-ray wall.
3. Discuss some of the design features of a fluoroscope intended to control radiation exposure to patient and operator.
4. Diagram the relationship between output signal size and chamber voltage for an ideal gas-filled detector. Identify each region of the curve.
5. A photomultiplier has nine dynodes, each of which has a gain of 2.2. What is the overall tube gain?
6. Discuss the properties of thermoluminescence dosimetry that make it suitable for personnel monitoring.
7. How much filtration is required for a radiographic x-ray tube? A fluoroscopic x-ray tube? Does the tabletop count?
8. What accuracy is required of an SID indicator?
9. A barrier thickness computation results in 0.4 mm Pb. How many pounds per square foot is this? How much gypsum board or glass is equivalent?
10. Given the following conditions of operation:
    20 patients per day
    3.2 films per patient
    80 mAs per view
    Compute the weekly workload.

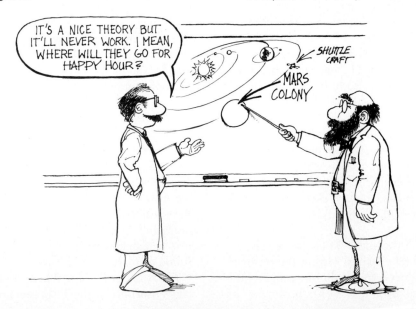

32

Radiation protection procedures

OCCUPATIONAL EXPOSURE

PATIENT DOSE

REDUCTION OF OCCUPATIONAL EXPOSURE

REDUCTION OF UNNECESSARY PATIENT DOSE

All medical health physics activity is directed in some way to minimizing the radiation exposure of radiologic personnel and the radiation dose to patients during x-ray procedures. Radiation exposure of radiologists and radiologic technologists is measured with personnel monitoring devices. Patient dose is usually estimated by conducting simulated x-ray examinations with human phantoms. If radiation control procedures are adopted, occupational exposure and patient dose can be kept acceptably low. Health physicists subscribe to the ALARA program—to keep all radiation exposure as low as reasonably achievable—and radiologic technologists should follow this guide as well.

OCCUPATIONAL EXPOSURE

Radiation dose is measured in units of rad (gray) or millirad. Radiation exposure is mea-

sured in roentgens (coulomb/kg) or milliroentgens. When the exposure is to technologists and radiologists, the proper unit is the rem (sievert) or millirem. The rem is the unit of dose equivalent and is used for radiation protection purposes. Although exposure, dose, and dose equivalent have precise and different meanings, they are used interchangeably in radiology.

When properly employed, exposure (R) refers to radiation intensity in air. Dose (rad) measures the radiation energy absorbed due to a radiation exposure and is used to identify irradiation of patients. Dose equivalent (rem) identifies the radiation energy absorbed by occupationally exposed persons.

Although the maximum permissible dose (MPD) for radiologic personnel is 5000 mrem/ yr (50 mSv/yr), experience has shown that considerably lower exposures than this should be

571

Table 32-1. Average occupational exposure (mrem/yr) of radiologic personnel in four general hospitals in Houston, Texas

	1973-4	1975-6	1977-8	1979-0	1981-2	1983-4	1985-6	Average
Hospital A								
Radiologists	1138	1143	657	384	461	532	252	652
Technologists	207	103	97	112	81	121	88	116
Hospital B								
Radiologists	367	302	282	140	167	336	298	270
Technologists	361	176	427	228	165	223	164	249
Hospital C								
Radiologists	457	829	448	583	331	357	159	452
Technologists	260	266	305	218	207	175	147	225
Hospital D								
Radiologists	616	241	106	187	115	125	94	212
Technologists	241	57	32	92	67	52	45	84

routine. The occupational exposure of radiologic personnel engaged in general x-ray activity should not normally exceed about 500 mrem/yr (5 mSv/yr). Table 32-1 is a summary of the personnel monitoring experience of four large general hospitals in Houston, Texas. Each hospital conducts over 100,000 x-ray examinations per year and has a reasonably proficient radiation control program. Note that there is little difference between the exposure of radiologists and radiologic technologists, although radiologists generally receive slightly higher exposures.

Unquestionably, the highest occupational exposure of diagnostic x-ray personnel occurs during fluoroscopy, portable radiography, and special procedures. During radiographic exposures, the radiologist is rarely present, and the technologist should be positioned behind a protective barrier. When protective barriers are not available, such as during portable examinations, the portable x-ray machine should be equipped with an exposure cord long enough to allow the technologist to leave the immediate examination area. The technologist should wear a protective apron for each such examination.

During fluoroscopy, both radiologist and tech-

nologist are exposed to relatively high levels of radiation. Fig. 31-2 showed this graphically. However, personnel exposure is directly related to the x-ray beam-on time; with care, personnel exposures are acceptably low. Remote fluoroscopy results in low personnel exposures because personnel are usually not in the examination room adjacent to the patient. Some fluoroscopes have the x-ray tube over the table and the image receptor under the table. This geometry offers some advantage to image quality, but personnel exposures are higher because the secondary radiation levels are higher.

Personnel engaged in special procedures often receive higher exposures than do those in general radiologic practice because of the longer fluoroscopic times experienced. The frequent absence of an intensifier tower protective curtain and the extensive use of cineradiography also contribute to higher exposure.

Extremity exposure during fluoroscopy may be significant. Even with protective gloves, exposure of the forearm can approach the applicable MPD (30,000 mrem/yr) if care is not taken. Without protective gloves, hand exposures as high as 75,000 mrem/yr are possible,

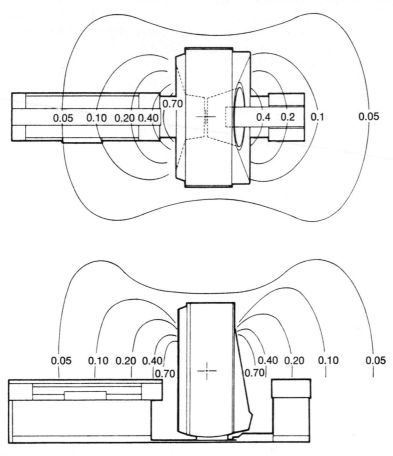

Fig. 32-1. Isoexposure profiles (in mR/scan) in both the horizontal and the vertical planes for a typical CT operation. (Courtesy General Electric Medical Systems.)

and **extremity monitoring must be provided.**

Personnel exposures associated with mammography are low because the low kVp of operation results in reduced scatter radiation. Usually, a long exposure cord and a conventional wall or window wall are sufficient to provide adequate protection. Rarely does a room used strictly for mammography require protective lead shielding. Dedicated mammography x-ray units have personnel protective barriers made

of lead glass, lead acrylic, and even plate glass as an integral component. Such barriers are totally adequate.

Personnel exposures in computed tomography (CT) facilities are exceptionally low. Since the CT x-ray beam is finely collimated and only scatter radiation is present in the scan room, the radiation levels are low compared with those experienced in fluoroscopy. Fig. 32-1 shows the isoexposure profiles for both the horizontal and vertical planes of a typical CT scanner. These data are given as milliroentgen per scan, and they show that personnel can be permitted to remain in the room during scanning. Protective apparel should always be used in such situations.

EXAMPLE: It is necessary for a technologist to remain in the CT room at midtable position during a 20-scan examination. What would be the occupational exposure if no protective apron were worn?

ANSWER: From Fig. 32-1, we may assume an exposure of 0.1 mR/scan.

Occupational exposure =
$$0.1 \text{ mR/scan} \times 20 \text{ scans} = 2 \text{ mR}$$

Nursing personnel and others working in the operating room and in intensive care units are sometimes exposed to x radiation from portable x-ray machines and C-arm fluoroscopes. Although these personnel are often anxious about such exposures, many studies have shown that their occupational exposure is near zero and certainly nothing for concern. The record-keeping requirements of a personnel monitoring program do not warrant providing monitors for these personnel.

Personnel radiation monitors are not necessary during portable radiography except for the radiologic technologist and anyone **routinely** required to restrain or hold patients. Personnel who regularly operate or are in the immediate vicinity of a C-arm fluoroscope should wear a radiation monitor in addition to protective apparel. During C-arm fluoroscopy, the x-ray beam may be on for a relatively long time and the beam can be directed in virtually any position.

It should **never** be necessary for diagnostic x-ray personnel to exceed 5000 mrem/yr. In smaller hospitals, emergency centers, and private clinics, occupational exposures will rarely exceed 500 mrem/yr (50 mSv/yr). Average exposures in most facilities are closer to 100 mrem/yr (1 mSv/yr).

PATIENT DOSE

The exposure of patients to medical x-rays is commanding increased attention in our society for two reasons.

First, the frequency of x-ray examination is increasing among all age groups at a rate of between 6% and 10% per year in the United States. This rate of increase is exceeded in many other countries. This indicates that physicians are relying more and more on x-ray diagnosis to assist them in patient care, even when accounting for the newer imaging modalities.

This is to be expected. X-ray diagnosis is considered much more accurate today than it was in the past because of the more rigorous training programs required of radiologists and radiologic technologists and the improvements in diagnostic x-ray equipment that allow for most difficult, but more substantive, x-ray examination. Efficacy and diagnostic accuracy are much improved.

Second, there is increasing concern among public health officials and radiation scientists regarding the risk associated with medical x-ray exposure. The possible late effects of diagnostic x-ray exposure are of concern not because such exposures are high, but because of unnecessary radiation exposure. If attention is given to good radiation control practices, the same level of diagnostic information can be obtained with lower radiation and therefore with reduced risk.

Estimation of patient dose

Patient dose from diagnostic x-rays is generally reported in one of three ways. The exposure to the entrance surface, or **skin dose**, is most often reported because it is easy to measure. The **gonadal dose** is important because of the suspected genetic responses to medical x-ray exposure. The dose to the gonads is not difficult to measure or estimate. The dose to the **bone marrow** is important because bone marrow is the target organ believed responsible for radiation-induced leukemia.

Table 32-2. Representative radiation quantities from various diagnostic x-ray procedures using a 200-speed image receptor

Examination	Technique (kVp/mAs)	Skin dose (mrad)	Mean marrow dose (mrad)	Gonadal dose (mrad)
Skull	76/100	500	20	<1
Chest	74/5	20	5	<1
Cervical spine	70/80	300	25	<1
Lumbar spine	72/120	600	120	225
Abdomen	74/125	700	60	125
Pelvis	70/100	450	40	150
Pelvimetry (to fetus)	90/120	800	800	800
Extremity	60/50	150	<5	<1
Full-mouth dental	60/3	300	10	<1

Table 32-2 presents some representative values of skin and gonadal dose for various x-ray examinations. The mean marrow dose for each procedure is also presented. Note that these are only approximate values and should not be used to estimate patient dose at any facility. In any given x-ray facility, actual doses delivered may by considerably different. Efficiency of x-ray production and image receptor speed are the most important variables.

These values do provide for relative dose comparisons among various radiographic examinations. Doses during fluoroscopy are too dependent on technique, equipment, and beam-on time to be easily estimated. Usually such doses must be measured.

Skin dose. Exposure to the skin is most often referred to as the patient dose. It is also referred to as entrance exposure, but more accurately described, it is **skin dose**. It is widely used because it is easy to measure and because reasonably accurate estimates can be made in the absence of measurements.

The measurement technique most often employed is thermoluminescence dosimeters (TLD). The size, sensitivity, and accuracy of TLDs make them very satisfactory patient ra-

diation monitors. A small grouping or pack of three to ten TLDs can be easily taped to the patient's skin in the center of the x-ray field. Since the response of the TLD is proportional to dose, they can be used to measure all levels experienced in diagnostic radiology. With proper laboratory technique, the results of such measurements will be accurate to within 5%.

There are two rather straightforward methods for estimating skin dose in the absence of patient measurements. The first requires the use of a nomogram such as that shown in Fig. 32-2. This figure contains a family of curves from which one can estimate the output intensity of a radiographic unit if the tehnique is known or assumed. The output intensity varies widely, so the use of this nomogram method is only good to perhaps ± 50%.

To use this nomogram, one must first know the total filtration in the x-ray beam. This is usually available from the medical physics report, but if not, 3 mm Al is a good estimate. Next, identify the kVp and mAs of the intended examination. Draw a vertical line rising from the value of total filtration until it intersects with the kVp of the examination. From this intersection draw a horizontal line to the left until it intersects the mR/mAs axis. The resulting value of

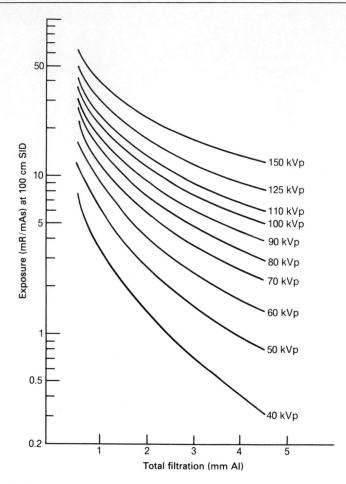

Fig. 32-2. This family of curves is a nomogram for estimating output x-ray intensity from a single-phase radiographic unit. (Courtesy John R. Cameron, University of Wisconsin, Madison.)

mR/mAs is the approximate output intensity of the radiographic unit. Multiply this value times the examination mAs to obtain the approximate patient exposure.

EXAMPLE: With reference to Fig. 32-2, estimate the skin dose from a lateral skull film taken at 66 kVp, 150 mAs with a radiographic unit having 2.5 mm Al total filtration.

ANSWER: Estimate the intersection between a vertical line rising from 2.5 mm Al and a horizontal line through 66 kVp. Extend the horizontal line to the y axis and read 3.8 mR/mAs.

$$3.8 \text{ mR/mAs} \times 150 \text{ mAs} = 570 \text{ mR}$$
$$\approx 570 \text{ mrad}$$

The second method for estimating patient skin dose requires that one know the output intensity for at least one operating condition. During the annual or special radiation control survey and calibration of an x-ray facility, the medical physicist will indicate this output intensity, usually in units of mR/mAs at 80 cm, the approximate source-to-skin distance (SSD), or at 100 cm, the SID. At 70 kVp, radiographic output intensity varies from about 2 to 10 mR/mAs at 80 cm SSD.

With this calibration value available, one would first make adjustment for a different SSD by employing the inverse square law.

EXAMPLE: The output intensity of a radiographic unit is reported as 3.7 mR/mAs (1.0 µC/kg-mAs) at 100 cm SID. What is the intensity at 75 cm SSD?
ANSWER: At 75 cm SSD the intensity will be greater by $(100/75)^2 = (1.32)^2 = 1.78$

$$3.7 \text{ mR/mAs} \times 1.78 = 6.6 \text{ mR/mAs}$$

Having the radiation intensity at the skin, one scales this according to the kVp and mAs of the examination. Output intensity varies according to the square of the kVp.

EXAMPLE: The output intensity at 70 kVp and 75 cm SSD is 6.6 mR/mAs (1.8 µC/kg-mAs). What is the output intensity of 76 kVp?
ANSWER: At higher kVp the output intensity is greater by the square of the kVp or

$$(76/70)^2 = (1.08)^2 = 1.18$$
$$6.6 \text{ mR/mAs} \times 1.18 = 7.8 \text{ mR/mAs}$$

The final step in estimating skin dose in radiography is to multiply the output intensity in mR/mAs by the examination mAs since they are linearly related.

EXAMPLE: If the radiographic technique for an IVP calls for 80 mAs, what is the skin dose when the output intensity is 7.8 mR/mAs (2.1 µC/kg-mAs)?
ANSWER:
7.8 mR/mAs × 80 mAs = 622 mR
                    ≈ 622 mrad

Normally, one would combine each of these steps into a single calculation.

EXAMPLE: The output intensity for a radiographic unit is 4.5 mR/mAs (1.2 µC/kg-mAs) at 70 kVp and 80 cm. If a lateral skull film is taken at 66 kVp, 150 mAs, what will be the skin dose at an 80 cm SSD? What would be the skin dose at a 90 cm SSD?
ANSWER:
At 80 cm SSD:

$$\text{Dose} = (4.5 \text{ mR/mAs}) \left(\frac{66 \text{ kVp}}{70 \text{ kVp}}\right)^2 (150 \text{ mAs})$$

$$= 600 \text{ mR}$$
$$= 600 \text{ mrad}$$

At 90 cm SSD:

$$\text{Dose} = (600 \text{ mrad}) \left(\frac{80}{90}\right)^2$$

$$= 474 \text{ mrad}$$

Skin dose in fluoroscopy is much more difficult to estimate because the radiation field moves and sometimes varies in size. If the field were of one size and stationary, skin dose would be directly related to exposure time. It is usually satisfactory, in the absence of measurements, to estimate fluoroscopic skin dose at 2 rad/mA-min. Stated differently, **for every milliampere of fluoroscopic technique, one can assume a tabletop intensity of 2 rad/min.**

EXAMPLE: A fluoroscopic procedure requires 2.5 minutes at 90 kVp, 2 mA. What is the approximate skin dose?
ANSWER: Skin dose = (2 rad/mA-min)(2.5 min)(2 mA)
                  = 10 rad

Mean marrow dose. The hematologic effects of radiation are rarely, if ever, experienced in diagnostic radiology. However, it is appropriate that we understand the mean marrow dose, one measure of patient dose during diagnostic procedures. The mean marrow dose is that dose of radiation averaged over the entire active bone marrow. For instance, if during a particular examination 50% of the active bone marrow were in the primary beam and received an average dose of 25 mrad (250 µGy), the mean marrow dose would be 12.5 mrad (125 µGy).

Table 32-3. Distribution of active bone marrow
in adults

Anatomic site	Percent of bone marrow
Head	10
Upper limb girdle	8
Sternum	3
Ribs	11
Cervical vertebrae	4
Thoracic vertebrae	13
Lumbar vertebrae	11
Sacrum	11
Lower limb girdle	29
TOTAL	100

Table 32-4. Estimated GSD caused by
diagnostic x-ray examination

Population	Time of study	GSD (mrad)
Australia	1950-1955	159
Sweden	1955	72
Denmark	1956	22
Great Britain	1957-1958	14
Japan	1960	39
New Zealand	1963	12
United States	1964	16
Japan	1969	27
United States	1970	20
Great Britain	1981	12

Table 32-2 includes the approximate mean marrow dose in adults for various types of diagnostic x-ray examinations. In children, these levels would generally be less because the active bone marrow is more uniformly distributed and because the radiographic techniques employed are considerably less. Table 32-3 shows the distribution of active bone marrow in the adult, and this will give some clue as to which diagnostic x-ray procedures involve exposure to large amounts of bone marrow.

In the United States the mean marrow dose from diagnostic x-ray examinations averaged over the entire population is approximately 100 mrad/yr (1 mGy/yr). Such a dose will obviously never elicit the hematologic responses described in Chapter 28. However, it is a dose concept employed by some to estimate, on a population basis, the hazard of one late effect of radiation—leukemia.

Genetically significant dose. Measurements and estimates of gonadal dose are important because of the suspected genetic effects of radiation. Although the gonadal dose from diagnostic x-rays is low for each individual, it may have some significance in terms of population effects. The population gonadal dose of importance is the **genetically significant dose (GSD),** the radiation dose to the population gene pool. **The GSD is defined as the gonadal dose that, if received by every member of the population, would be expected to produce the total genetic effect on the population as the sum of the individual doses actually received.** Thus it is a weighted average gonadal dose. It takes into account those persons who are irradiated and those who are not and averages the results. The GSD can only be estimated through large-scale epidemiologic studies, but with adequate information available it is determined by the equation

(32-1)

$$GSD = \frac{\Sigma D \bar{N} P}{\Sigma N P}$$

Where Σ is the mathematic symbol that means to add or sum values, D is the average gonadal dose per examination, N is the number of persons receiving x-ray examinations, $\underline{N}$ is the total number of persons in the population, and P is the expected future number of children per person.

For computational purposes, therefore, the GSD considers the age, sex, and expected progeny for each person so examined. It also acknowledges the various types of examinations and the gonadal dose per examination type.

Estimates for GSD have been conducted in many different countries. Table 32-4 is a summary of the results of these studies. The most recent authoritative estimate for the United States was reported by the U.S. Public Health Service in 1970 to be 20 mrad (200 μGy). Thus this is a genetic radiation burden over and above the existing average background radiation level of approximately 100 mrad/yr (1 mGy/yr).

Patient dose in special examinations

Dose in mammography. Because of the considerable application of x-rays for examination of the female breasts and the concern for the induction of breast cancer by radiation, it is imperative that we have some understanding of the radiation doses involved in such examinations.

Recall from Chapter 19 that there are three principal methods for mammography, only two of which are generally acceptable. The direct-exposure method is not acceptable because of high patient dose. In direct-exposure mammography the patient skin dose will vary from perhaps 6 to 15 rad/view (60 to 150 mGy/view), and this is unacceptable because the other two methods result in equal if not better images at considerably less patient dose.

When xeromammography was first introduced, it required patient skin doses ranging from 1 to 5 rad/view (10 to 50 mGy/view). More recently these average skin doses have been reduced to the range of 0.5 to 1 rad/view (5 to 10 mGy/view). This reduction in xeromammographic dose has been accomplished principally through changing the recommended technique and some equipment modification. It has been shown that higher tube potential (for example, up to 50 kVp), with the compensating reduction in mAs, is acceptable in xeromammography. Furthermore, increasing the total beam filtration from 0.5 mm Al to as high as 4 mm Al will also result in reduced patient dose with little

sacrifice in image quality. Application of these higher filtration techniques requires alteration of the plate-charging aparatus of the Xerox conditioner and processor.

Screen-film mammography is the lowest-dose procedure. Patient skin doses in the range of 0.3 to 0.8 rad/view (3 to 8 mGy/view) are experienced with screen films. Increasing tube potential much beyond 30 kVp will degrade the image unacceptably in screen-film mammography, and therefore further dose reductions by technique manipulation are unlikely. Faster films and screens, however, may make even lower-dose screen-film mammography possible.

Radiographic grids are now employed in many screen-film mammography examinations. Grid ratios of 3:1 and 4:1 are most popular. The contrast enhancement produced by using such grids is significant but so is the increase in patient dose. Patient dose is increased by 1½ to 2 times with the use of such grids.

The values just cited for patient dose in mammography can be misleading. Because of the low x-ray energies employed in mammography, the dose falls off very rapidly as the beam penetrates the breast. If the skin dose for a craniocaudad view is 1 rad (10 mGy), the dose to the midline of the breast may be only 250 mrad (2.5 mGy) and that at the image receptor perhaps 20 mrad (200 μGy). The biologic effect of such an examination is presumed to be more closely associated with the total energy absorbed by glandular tissue.

It is known that the risk of an adverse biologic response from mammography is vanishingly small; certainly, it is nothing for a patient to be concerned about. However, any possible response is related to the average radiation dose to glandular tissue and not the skin dose. **Glandular dose** varies in a complicated way with variations in x-ray beam quality and quantity. For xeromammography the average glandular dose is approximately 40% of the skin dose. For screen-film mammography it is approximately 15% of the skin dose. Specification of a skin dose

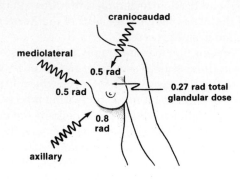

Fig. 32-3. Three-view mammogram results in a total glandular dose that is the sum of the three individual glandular doses.

can also be misleading when one considers a multiview examination. Fig. 32-3 illustrates this dilemma. Consider a three-view screen-film mammogram consisting of craniocaudad, mediolateral and axillary views. The craniocaudad and the mediolateral views produced a skin dose of 0.5 rad (5 mGy) each and the axillary view a dose of 0.8 rad (8 mGy). It would be incorrect to describe this total examination procedure as resulting in a patient dose of 1.8 rad. Skin doses from different projections cannot be added. We must either specify the skin dose for each view or attempt to estimate the total glandular dose.

To estimate the total glandular dose, we can make the approximation that the contribution from each view will be 15% of the skin dose. Consequently, the total glandular dose would be the sum of a 75 mrad (750 μGy) contribution from each of the craniocaudad and mediolateral views and a 120 mrad (1.2 mGy) contribution from the axillary view. The total glandular dose would therefore be 270 mrad (2.7 mGy). **Total glandular dose should never exceed 500 mrad with screen film and 1000 mrad with zeromammography.**

From this discussion, it would seem that patient dose in mammography can be considerably reduced if the number of views is restricted. The axillary view should not be done routinely. For screening programs not more than two views are advisable.

Dose in CT scanning. An important consideration in CT scanning, as with any x-ray procedure, is not only the skin dose but the distribution of dose during the scan.

On the basis of skin dose, CT is comparable with other diagnostic procedures. The skin dose delivered to a patient by a series of contiguous CT scans is somewhat higher than that delivered by a single conventional skull or abdominal radiographic view. However, a typical conventional head or body examination often involves several views. Thus the dose from CT is roughly equivalent to the cumulative dose produced by a series of conventional radiographic views. Furthermore, for most CT examinations considerably less tissue volume is irradiated than in conventional radiography. The CT dose is significantly less than most fluoroscopic procedures.

As was pointed out in Chapter 22, CT differs in many important ways from other radiographic techniques. A regular x-ray film can be likened to a photograph taken with a flash: the patient is "floodlighted" with x-rays to directly expose the image receptor, whether it is film or an image intensifier. CT, on the other hand, scans the patient with a fine collimated beam of x-rays. This difference in delivery also means that the dose distribution from CT is different from conventional radiographic procedures.

Part of the dose efficiency of CT is because of the precise collimation of the x-ray beam. Scat-

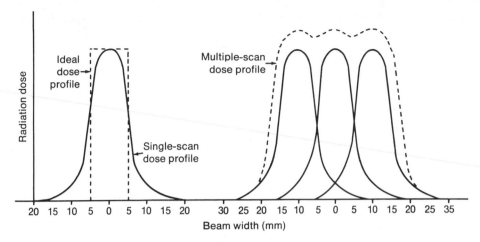

Fig. 32-4. Patient dose distribution in CT is complicated because the profile of the x-ray beam cannot be made sharp.

ter radiation interferes with all types of conventional radiography and increases patient dose while degrading the image. Because CT uses narrow, well-collimated x-ray beams, scatter radiation is significantly reduced. Thus, theoretically, a larger percentage of the x-rays contribute usefully to the image.

The precise collimation used in CT means that only a well-defined volume of tissue is irradiated during each scan. The ideal x-ray beam for CT would have sharp boundaries. There would be no overlap between adjacent scans. Thus, aside from a minimum contribution caused by scatter, the dose delivered to a patient from a series of ideal adjacent CT scans would be the same as from a single scan. Fig. 32-4 illustrates how this ideal situation, however, cannot be attained in practice. The size of the focal spot of the x-ray tube produces some penumbra and blurs the sharp boundaries of the slice. Also, the beam is not precisely parallel, and some spreading occurs as the beam traverses the scan field.

If a series of adjacent scans is performed with an automatically indexing patient couch, the couch movement must be precise. If it moves too much between scans, some tissue will be missed. If it moves too little, some tissue in each scan will be overexposed.

Finally, and perhaps most important, if the prepatient collimators are open too wide, tissues near the interface of each scan may receive twice the dose that they otherwise should. **It is essential that CT collimators be periodically monitored for proper adjustment.** Thus, in practice, a series of adjacent scans delivers a higher dose than a single scan because of the overlap of the beam peripheries.

Dose is more uniformly distributed in CT than in conventional radiography. This uniform dose distribution resembles that experienced in rotational radiotherapy.

Typical skin doses range from 0.5 to 3 rad (5 to 30 mGy) during head scans and 1 to 6 rad (10 to 60 mGy) during body scans. These values are only approximate and vary widely depending on the machine and the radiation technique. Because the CT beam is well collimated, the area of irradiation can be precisely controlled. Thus, radiosensitive areas such as the lenses of the eye can be selectively avoided. Shields as protection from the primary x-ray beam in CT are of little use. Not only does the metal from these shields produce terrible artifacts in the image, but the rotational scheme of the x-ray source greatly reduces their effectiveness as well. The patient, however, can effectively be shielded from the low levels of scatter radiation as long as the direct x-ray beam does not intersect the shield.

As with any radiographic procedure, many factors influence patient dose. For CT the following general proportionality holds true:

$$(32\text{-}2)$$

$$Dose \propto \frac{IE}{\sigma^2 w^3 h}$$

In this proportionality, $\propto$ means "is proportional to," I is beam intensity in mAs, E is average beam energy in keV, σ is system noise, w is pixel size, and h is slice thickness.

Note that, as with conventional radiography, patient dose is proportional to the beam intensity. It is also directly proportional to the average beam energy. The other factors of equation 32-2 are variables that are unique to CT scanning. Sigma (σ) is the noise. This is equivalent to quantum mottle in screen-film radiography and represents random statistical variations in the CT numbers. The w stands for the pixel size, one of the determinants of spatial resolution. The last factor, h, is the slice thickness. **A decrease in either the noise, pixel size, or slice thickness while the other factors remain constant results in increased patient dose.** The relationship shown is a proportionality; the exact constant of proportionality would depend on various machine-dependent parameters such as the rotational mode and the reconstruction algorithm chosen.

All other factors being equal, a scanner that produces a low-noise, high-resolution image does so at the sacrifice of higher patient dose. The challenge in CT, as indeed with all radiographic imaging procedures, is not so much to deliver fantastically good resolution and low noise (since this could be achieved at the cost of very high patient dose) but to use the x-ray beam efficiently, producing the best possible image at a reasonable dose to the patient.

REDUCTION OF OCCUPATIONAL EXPOSURE

The radiologic technologist can do much to minimize the occupational radiation exposure of radiologic personnel. Most do not require sophisticated equipment or especially vigorous training, but simply a conscientious attitude in the performance of assigned duties. Most equipment characteristics, technique changes, and administrative procedures designed to minimize patient dose will also reduce occupational exposure.

In diagnostic radiology at least 95% of the technologist's occupational radiation exposure comes from fluoroscopy, special procedures, and portable radiography. Attention to the cardinal principles of radiation protection (time, distance, and shielding) is the most important aspect of occupational radiation control.

During fluoroscopy, it is intended that the radiologist employ minimum beam-on time. This can be done by careful technique, which includes intermittent activation of the fluoroscopic views rather than one long period of beam-on time. It is appropriate to maintain a log of fluoroscopy time by recording the beam-on time of the 5-minute reset timer.

During fluoroscopy, the technologist should step back from the table when his or her immediate presence and assistance is not required. The technologist should also take maximum advantage of all protective shielding, including apron, curtain, and Bucky slot cover.

Each portable x-ray unit should have a protective apron assigned to it. The technologist should wear an apron during all examinations and maintain maximum distance from the source. **The exposure cord on a portable x-ray unit must be at least 1.8 m long.** the primary beam should never be pointed at the technologist or other nearby personnel.

During conventional radiography, the technologist is positioned behind a control booth barrier. These barriers are usually considered secondary barriers because they only intercept leakage and scatter radiation. Consequently, leaded glass and leaded gypsum board may be unnecessary for such barriers. **The useful beam should never be directed toward the control booth barrier.**

Other work assignments in radiology, such as scheduling, darkroom duties, and filing result in essentially no radiation exposure.

Personnel monitoring

Radiologists and radiologic technologists are routinely exposed to ionizing radiation. The level of exposure is dependent on the type of activity in which they are engaged and how much of it they do. Determining the quantity of radiation they receive requires a program of personnel monitoring. Personnel monitoring refers to procedures instituted to estimate the amount of radiation received by individuals who work around radiation.

Personnel monitoring is required when there is any likelihood that an individual will receive more than one-fourth the maximum permissible dose. Most clinical radiology personnel, therefore, must be monitored; however, it is usually not necessary to monitor radiology secretaries and file clerks. Furthermore, it is usually not necessary to monitor operating room personnel, except perhaps those routinely involved in cystoscopy and C-arm fluoroscopy.

The personnel monitor offers no protection against radiation exposure. It simply measures the quantity of radiation **to which it was exposed,** and therefore is used as an indicator of the exposure of the wearer. There are basically three types of personnel monitors in use in diagnostic radiology: film badges, thermoluminescence dosimeters, and pocket ionization chambers.

Regardless of the type of monitor, it is essential that it be obtained from a certifed laboratory. In-house processing of radiation monitors should not be attempted.

Film badges. Film badges came into general use about the mid-1940s and have been widely employed in diagnostic radiology ever since. Film badges are especially designed devices in which a small piece of film similar to dental radiographic film is sandwiched between metal filters inside a plastic holder. Fig. 32-5 is a view of several typical radiation monitors.

The film incorporated into a film badge is special radiation dosimetry film that is particularly sensitive to ionizing radiation. The density on the exposed and processed film is proportional to the exposure received by the film badge. Carefully controlled calibration, processing, and analyzing conditions are necessary for the film badge to accurately measure occupational exposure. Usually, exposures less than 10 mR (2.6 μC/kg) are not measured by film badge monitors, and the film badge vendor will report only that a minimum exposure (M) was recieved. When higher exposures are received, they can be accurately reported.

The metal filters, along with the window in the plastic film holder, allow estimation of the radiation energy. The usual filters are made of aluminum and copper. If the radiation exposure is a result of penetrating radiation, the image of the filters on the processed film will be faint and there may be no image at all of the window in the plastic holder. If the badge is exposed to soft radiation, the filters will be well imaged and the densities under the filters will allow estimation of the x-ray energy. Often the filters to the front of the badge differ in shape from the filters to the back of the badge. Radiation that had entered through the back of the badge would normally indicate that the person wearing the badge was exposed to considerably higher levels of radiation than indicated, since the radiation would have penetrated through the body before interacting with the film badge. For this reason, **film**

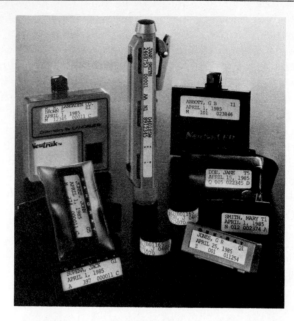

Fig. 32-5. Some representative radiation monitors. Many have metal filters incorporated to help identify the type of radiation and its energy. (Courtesy R. S. Landauer Jr., Inc.)

badges must be worn with their proper side to the front.

Several advantages of film badge personnel monitors continue to make them popular. They are inexpensive, easy to handle, not difficult to process, reasonably accurate, and have been in use for several decades.

Film badge monitors also have disadvantages. Since they incorporate film as the sensing device, they cannot be worn for long periods because of fogging caused by temperature and humidity. Film badge monitors should never be left in an enclosed car or other area where excessive temperatures may occur. The fogging produced by elevated temperature and humidity will result in a falsely high evaluation of exposure. Consequently, film badge monitors should not be worn for longer than 1 month. Film badge monitors do not have the sensitivity of other personnel monitoring devices.

Thermoluminescence dosimeters. Thermoluminescence dosimeters (TLD) are a relatively new type of personnel monitoring device. The sensing material of the TLD monitor is lithium fluoride (LiF) in crystalline form, either as a powder or more often as a small chip approximately 3 mm square and 1 mm thick. When exposed to radiation, the TLD absorbs energy and stores it in the form of excited electrons in the crystalline lattice. When heated, these excited electrons fall back to their normal orbital state with the emission of visible light. The intensity of visible light is measured with a photomultiplier tube and is proportional to the radiation dose received by the crystal. This sequence was described in detail in Chapter 31. A typical TLD monitor is shown in Fig. 32-6.

TLD monitoring devices have several advantages over film. They are more sensitive and more accurate than film badge monitors. Prop-

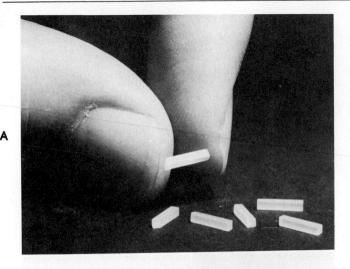

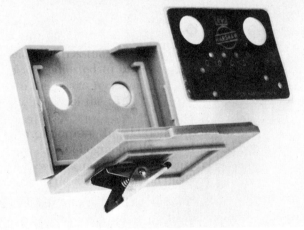

Fig. 32-6. Thermoluminescence dosimeters are used as personnel monitors. **A,** Lithium fluoride chips. **B,** Badge with spring fastener to contain chips. (Courtesy Harshaw Chemical Co.)

erly calibrated TLD monitors can measure exposure as low as 5 mR (1.3 µC/kg). TLD monitors do not suffer from loss of information following exposure to excessive heat or humidity. Consequently, **they can be worn for intervals up to 3 months at a time.** The primary disadvantage of TLD personnel monitoring is cost. The price of a typical TLD monitoring service is perhaps twice that of film badge monitoring.

If the frequency of monitoring is quarterly, however, the price differential becomes less important. TLD has the additional advantage of simplicity. Some departments of radiology process their own TLD personnel monitors, although this is not recommended. This is not so easy with film badges. TLD monitoring is improving constantly and is slowly replacing film badge monitoring.

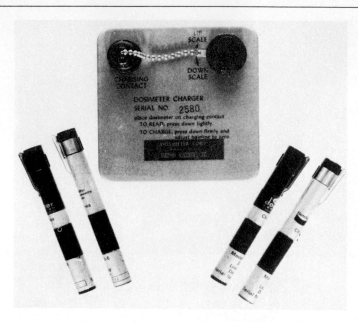

Fig. 32-7. Pocket ionization chambers are occasionally employed in diagnostic radiology.

Pocket ionization chambers. Fig. 32-7 is a photograph of a typical set of pocket ionization chambers with their associated reading instrument. These small devices measure approximately 2 cm in diameter by 10 cm long and are designed to be clipped onto wearing apparel like a writing pen. Pocket ionization chambers are available in several different ranges, but the one usually employed in radiology has a range of 0 to 200 mR (0 to 50 μC/kg). The use of a pocket ionization chamber can be somewhat time consuming. Before it is used, the chamber must be charged to a predetermined voltage so that the scale reading indicates 0. As the chamber is exposed to radiation during the day, the charge is dissipated and neutralized. An additional analysis of the chamber voltage at the end of the day indicates the radiation exposure to which the chamber has been subjected.

Pocket ionization chambers are not employed frequently in diagnostic radiology. Their use re-

quires daily identification of personnel exposures. A manipulation of the charging and reading mechanism is required daily. They are often used for a day or so to monitor nonradiologic personnel such as nurses.

Pocket ionization chambers are reasonably accurate and sensitive, but they do have a limited range. Should exposure to an individual exceed the range of the dosimeter, the precise level of exposure would never be known. Pocket ionization chambers are fairly expensive and can be easily damaged.

Where to wear a personnel monitor. Much discussion and research in health physics have gone into providing precise recommendations about where a radiologic technologist should wear the film badge. The official publications of the National Council on Radiation Protection and Measurements (NCRP) offer little assistance in this regard. They suggest that the technologist "consult a qualified expert." Qualified experts are considered by most to be either certified health physicists (CHP) or certified radiologic physicists (CRP).

Many technologists wear their personnel monitor in front at the waist or chest level because it is convenient to clip the badge over a belt or a shirt pocket. If the technologist is not involved in fluoroscopic procedures, these locations are acceptable.

However, **if the technologist participates in fluoroscopy and wears a protective apron, as recommended, then the personnel monitor should be positioned on the collar above the protective apron.** The maximum permissible dose of 5000 mrem/yr (50 mSv/yr) refers not only to whole-body exposure but also to partial-body exposure of the head, neck, trunk, lens of the eye, gonads, and bone marrow. In other words, the head and neck region are restricted to the same maximum permissible dose as the entire body. It has been shown that during fluoroscopy, when a protective apron is worn, exposure to the collar region is 10 to 20 times greater than that to the trunk of the body beneath the protective lead apron. So, if the personnel monitor is worn beneath the protective apron, it will record a falsely low exposure and will not indicate what could be a hazardous exposure to unprotected body parts.

Nearly all the fifty states' radiation control programs recommend or require that the personnel radiation monitor be worn at collar level.

In some clinical situations it may be advisable to wear more than one personnel monitor. This is not normally necessary for diagnostic radiologic technologists. Two exceptions are monitoring the abdomen during pregnancy and monitoring the extremities during special procedures in which the technologist's hands are in close proximity to the useful beam. Radiologists often should wear extremity monitors during fluoroscopy, as should nuclear medicine technologists when handling radioactive material.

Personnel monitoring report

State and federal regulations require that the results of the personnel monitoring program be recorded in a precise fashion and maintained for review. Monitoring periods and the associated exposure records must not exceed a calendar quarter. Quarterly, monthly, or weekly reports are acceptable, but records reflecting longer periods of time are not.

The personnel radiation monitoring report must contain a number of specific items of information. A representative report is shown in Fig. 32-8 and contains all the information required. The first column is an identification number assigned to the radiation worker and monitor. The second column identifies the type of monitor. The third column lists the employee name and is followed by a column containing the social security number. Additional personal data required include birthdate and sex.

The exposure data that must be included on the form are the current exposure, the cumulative quarterly exposure, the cumulative annual exposure, and the cumulative total exposure. In addition, the cumulative maximum permissible dose and the resulting unused portion of the cumulative maximum permissible dose must be shown on the report. Separate radiation monitors, for example, extremity monitors, would be identified separately from the whole-body monitor. Occasionally, if a personnel exposure involves low-energy radiation, a dose to the skin might occur that is greater than the dose of penetrating radiation. In such case, the skin dose is separately identified. There are areas of the report form for neutron radiation exposure to accommodate nuclear reactor and particle accelerator workers.

The columns associated with cumulative lifetime exposures and the unused portion of the maximum permissible dose require that, when one changes employment, the total radiation exposure history must be transferred to the records of the new employee. Consequently, when one leaves employment, one should automati-

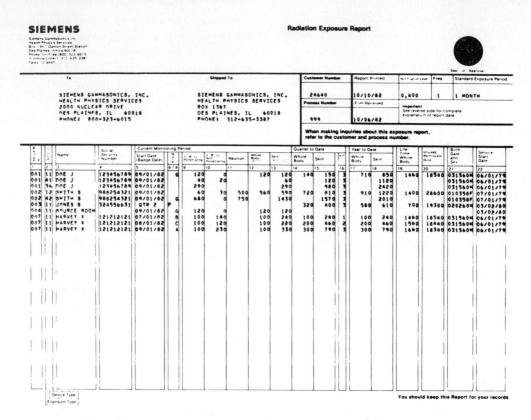

Fig. 32-8. Personnel monitoring report must include the items of information shown here. (Courtesy Siemens Gammasonics, Inc.)

cally receive a report of the previous total radiation exposure history at that facility. Such a report should be given automatically; if it is not, it should be.

When establishing a personnel radiation monitoring program, the supplier of the monitor should be informed of the type of radiation facility involved. That information will influence the method of calibration of the monitors and the control monitors.

The **control monitor** should never be stored in or adjacent to a radiation area. It should be kept in a distant room or office. All monitors should be returned to the supplier together and in a timely fashion so they can be processed together. Lost or inadvertently exposed monitors must be evaluated and an estimate of the true exposure recorded. Unless there are unusual circumstances, the estimate can be made by averaging the previous 6-month exposures.

Protective apparel

The control console is usually positioned behind fixed protective barriers during diagnostic radiographic procedures. It is not normally so positioned during fluoroscopy or portable radiography. **In these instances, protective apparel must be worn.**

Protective gloves and aprons are available in many sizes and shapes. They are usually constructed of lead-impregnate vinyl. Some protective garments are impregnated with tin rather than lead because tin has some advantages over lead as a shielding material in the diagnostic range of x-ray energies. The normal thicknesses for protective apparel are 0.25, 0.5, and 1 mm of lead equivalent. The garments themselves are much thicker than these dimensions, but they provide shielding equivalent to that thickness of pure lead. Table 32-5 summarizes some of the properties of these leaded garments. Of course, maximum exposure reduction is obtained with the 1 mm lead equivalent garment, but an apron of this matierial can weigh as much as 10 kg (22 lb). The wearer could be exhausted by end of the fluoroscopic schedule just from having to carry the protective apron. the x-ray attenuation at 75 kVp for 0.25 mm lead equivalent and 1 mm lead equivalent is 66% and 99%, respectively. Most radiology departments find 0.5 mm lead equivalent protective garments a workable compromise between unnecessary weight and desired protection.

When not in use protective apparel must be stored on properly designed racks. If they are continuously folded or heaped in the corner, cracks may develop. At least once a year aprons and gloves should be fluoroscoped to be sure that no such cracks appear.

Position

During fluoroscopy, all personnel should remain as far from the patient as possible. After loading spot films, the radiologic technologist should take a step or two back from the table when his or her presence is not required. The radiologist should be trained to use the deadman foot switch sparingly. Naturally, when the beam-on time is high, the radiation exposure to patient and personnel will be proportionately high.

Patient holding

Many patients referred for x-ray examination are not physically able to support themselves. Notable examples are infants, the elderly, and

Table 32-5. Some physical characteristics of protective lead aprons

Equivalent thickness (mm Pb)	Weight (lb)	X-ray attenuation (%) by kVp of operation		
		50 kVp	75 kVp	100 kVp
0.25	3-10	97	66	51
0.50	6-15	99.9	88	75
1.00	12-25	99.9	99	94

the incapacitated. **Radiology personnel should never be used to hold these patients.** Mechanical restraining devices should be available. Otherwise, a relative or friend accompanying the patient should be asked to help. As a last resort, other hospital employees such as nurses and orderlies may be used occasionally to hold patients, but **never** radiology employees.

When it is necessary to have another person hold the patient, protective apparel must be provided to that person. An apron and gloves are necessary, and the holder should be carefully positioned and instructed so that he or she is not exposed to the useful beam.

REDUCTION OF UNNECESSARY PATIENT DOSE

There are many sources of unnecessary patient dose over which the technologist has considerable control. Unnecessary patient dose is defined as any radiation dose that is not required for the patient's well-being or proper management and care.

Unnecessary examinations

The technologist has practically no control over what some consider the largest source of unnecessary patient dose, that is, unnecessary x-ray examination. This is almost exclusively the radiologist's responsibility.

Unfortunately, this source of unnecessary patient dose presents a serious dilemma for the radiologist and the clinician. Many x-ray examinations are knowingly requested when the yield of helpful information may be extremely low or nonexistent. When such an examination is performed, the benefit to the patient in no way compensates for the radiation dose. If the examination is not performed, the clinician and radiologist may be severely criticized and then subjected to legal action if the patient's ultimate management results in failure, even though the examination in question would have contributed little, if anything, to effective patient management. In such situations the radiologist is caught between the proverbial "rock and a hard place."

Routine x-ray examinations should not be performed when there is no precise medical indication. substantial evidence shows that such examinations are of little benefit because they are not cost-effective and the disease detection rate is very low. Examples of such cases follow:

1. **Mass screening for tuberculosis.** General screening has not been found effective, and better methods of tuberculosis testing are now available. Some x-ray screening in high-risk groups (for example, medical and paramedical personnel), in service personnel posing a potential community hazard (for example, food handlers or teachers), and in special occupational groups (for example, miners and workers having contact with beryllium, asbestos, glass, or silica) may be appropriate.

2. **Hospital admissions.** Chest x-ray examinations for routine hospital admission when there is no clinical indication of chest disease should not be performed. Among patients who would be candidates for such examinations are those admitted to the pulmonary or surgical service or elderly patients.

3. **Preemployment physicals.** Chest and lower back x-ray examinations are not justified because knowledge gained about previous injury or disease is nil.

4. **Periodic health examinations.** Many physicians now question the utility of the annual executive physical examination. Cer-

tainly, when such an examination is conducted on an asymptomatic patient, it should not include x-ray examination, especially fluoroscopic examination.

Repeat examinations

One area of unnecessary examination that the technologist can influence considerably is that of repeat examinations. The frequency of repeat examinations has been variously estimated to range as high as 10% of all examinations. In the typical busy hospital facility, repeat examinations will not normally exceed 4%. Examinations with the highest retake rates are lumbar spine, thoracic spine, KUB, and abdomen.

Although some repeat examinations are caused by equipment malfunctions, nearly all are caused by technologist error. Studies of causes of repeat examinations have shown that improper positioning and poor radiographic technique resulting in a film too light or too dark are primarily responsible for retakes. Motion and improper collimation are responsible for some retakes. Errors that contribute to repeat examinations but that occur infrequently are dirty screens, use of improperly loaded cassettes, light leaks, chemical fog, artifacts caused by a dirty processor, wrong projection, grid errors, and multiple exposure.

Radiographic technique

In general, the use of high-kVp technique will result in reduced patient dose. Increasing the kVp is always associated with a reduction in mAs to obtain an acceptable film density, and this in turn results in a reduced exposure. This occurs because the patient dose is linearly related to the mAs, but it is related to the kVp by approximately the square.

EXAMPLE: A lateral skull radiograph is obtained at 64 kVp, 80 mAs and results in a skin dose of 400 mrad (4 mGy). If the tube potential is increased to 74 kVp (15% increase) and the mAs reduced by half to 40 mAs, the average radiographic density will remain the same. What will the new skin dose be?

ANSWER: $Dose = (400 \text{ mrad})\left(\dfrac{40 \text{ mAs}}{80 \text{ mAs}}\right)\left(\dfrac{74 \text{ kVp}}{64 \text{ kVp}}\right)^2$

$= (400 \text{ mrad})(0.5)(1.34)$

$= 267 \text{ mrad}$

Of course, the radiologist must be the final judge of radiographic quality. Increasing kVp even slightly may result in images that are too flat for proper interpretation by the radiologist. An area of radiography where very-high-kVp technique is becoming widely accepted is examination of the chest.

Proper collimation is essential to good radiographic technique. New x-ray apparatus is required to be equipped with PBL, but this does not prevent the technologist from reducing the field size still further by collimation. By employing minimum collimation, not only does one reduce the patient dose, but the image quality will be increased as well because scatter radiation will also be reduced.

The image receptor

The image receptor should be selected out of consideration first for the type of examination and second for the radiation dose necessary to provide a quality image. The fastest-speed screen-film combination consistent with the nature of the examination should be employed. It should be kept in mind that the screen speed, in general, controls the patient dose. Rare earth and other fast screens should be used where possible. Routine application of such screens in orthopedic, chest, and magnification radiography is appropriate. In some applications the use of such fast systems may result in bothersome quantum mottle, but this again must be decided by the radiologist. In general, 200 to 400 speed systems are now employed.

Patient positioning

When examining the upper extremities or breast, especially with the patient in a seated position, care should be taken so that the useful beam does not intercept the gonads. Position the patient lateral to the useful beam and provide a protective apron as a shield.

Specific area shielding

X-ray examinations result in a partial-body exposure, although most radiation protection guides and radiation response information are based on whole-body exposure. The partial-body nature of the x-ray examination is controlled by proper beam collimation and the use of specific area shielding.

Use of specific area shielding is indicated when a particularly sensitive tissue or organ is in or near the useful beam. The lens of the eye, breasts, and the gonads are frequently shielded from the primary radiation beam. There are two kinds of specific area shielding devices: the **contact shield** and the **shadow shield**.

Lens shields are always of the contact type. The contact shielding device is positioned directly on the patient. Gonadal shields, on the other hand, can be of either the contact or the shadow type.

Breast shields such as seen in Fig. 32-9 are

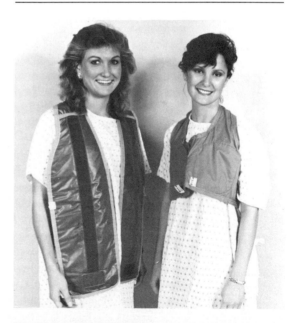

Fig. 32-9. Breast shields are used for juvenile scoliosis examinations. (Courtesy Priscilla Butler, Washington University and Alvin Thomas, Center for Devices and Radiological Health.)

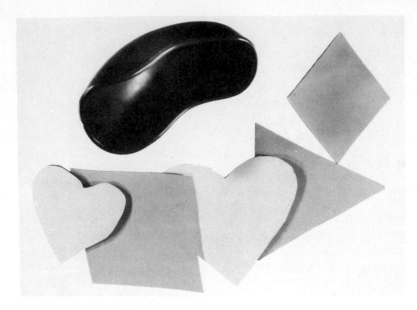

Fig. 32-10. Examples of useful gonadal shields.

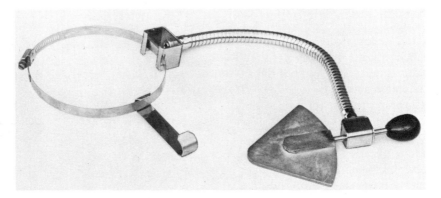

Fig. 32-11. Shadow shield. (Courtesy Nuclear Associates, Inc.)

recommended for use during scoliosis examinations. Such examinations usually employ an AP projection subjecting the juvenile breasts to primary beam x irradiation. However, the PA projection is equally satisfactory since magnification is of little importance. The PA projection results in a breast dose of only about 1% of the AP projection.

Fig. 32-10 shows some examples of contact gonadal shields frequently used for children. When such contact shields are not purchased commercially, a properly cut piece of protective material is perfectly adequate. Shapes such as hearts, diamonds, triangles, and squares have been employed effectively.

An example of the shadow shield is shown in Fig. 32-11. This type of shield is equally as effective as the contact shield and is more acceptable for use with adult patients. Use of such devices however, requires careful attention on the part of the technologist. The shield must shadow the gonads without interfering with adjacent tissue. Improper positioning of the shadow shield can result in a repeat examination and increased patient dose.

The subject of gonadal shielding is sufficiently important to require emphasis. Its use should be governed by the following concepts:

1. Gonadal shielding should be considered for all patients who are potentially reproductive. As an administrative procedure, this would include all patients under the age of 40 and perhaps even older males.
2. Gonadal shielding should be employed when the gonads lie in or near the primary beam.
3. Proper patient positioning and beam collimation should not be relaxed when gonadal shields are in use.
4. Gonadal shielding should only be used when it does not interfere with obtaining the required diagnostic information.

REVIEW QUESTIONS

1. Define or otherwise identify the following:
   a. ALARA
   b. GSD
   c. Image receptor
   d. Shadow shield
   e. Mean marrow dose
   f. The type of radiation present inside a CT room
   g. The units of x-radiation output intensity
   h. Glandular dose
   i. CT noise
   j. Metal filters in a film badge
2. Discuss the three methods for expressing patient dose and their respective applications.
3. What purpose do metallic filters serve in a film badge?
4. Under what circumstances should gonadal shields be employed?
5. What personnel protective measures are usually sufficient for dedicated mammography?
6. What type of examination results in high bone marrow dose?
7. List five factors required to estimate the genetically significant dose.
8. Identify the approximate skin and glandular doses experienced in screen-film mammography and xeromammography.
9. Discuss the use of grids in mammography.
10. The radiographic x-ray intensity at 100 cm SID is 5.8 mR/mAs at 70 kVp. A portable cervical spine examination is conducted at 60 cm SSD, 86 kVp, and 40 mAs. What is the skin exposure?

33

Physical principles of diagnostic ultrasound

NATURE OF ULTRASOUND

ACOUSTIC INTENSITY AND POWER

ACOUSTIC REFLECTION

ACOUSTIC ABSORPTION AND ATTENUATION

The normal range of human hearing is approximately 20 to 20,000 Hz. The **hertz (Hz)** is a unit of frequency; 1 Hz = 1 oscillation per second or 1 cycle per second (cps). In this frequency range, pressure disturbances in the air that are detected by the human ear are called **audible sound. Ultrasound is any sound with higher frequency,** and consequently ultrasound cannot be heard. Subsonic radiation is in the 0 to 20 Hz range, and it also cannot be heard.

There are many examples in nature of species that **transceive** (transmit and receive) ultrasound. Bats and some insects have highly developed ultrasound sensory organs that function up to approximately 120 kHz. No known naturally occurring ultrasound sources exist in the frequency range employed in medical diagnostic or therapeutic ultrasound, which is 1 to 15 MHz.

The first man-made sources of ultrasound appeared in the 1870s. Some credit the Curie brothers, Jacques and Pierre, with first describing the **piezoelectric effect**—the change in elec-

tric charge distribution of certain crystalline materials following a mechanical stress. The Curies, of course, are remembered most for their work with radioactive substances. *Piezo* is a Greek word that means to press, and as used here, it describes the manner in which some substances become electrically polarized when stressed. The piezoelectric effect is the fundamental physical principle for all medical ultrasound.

Another pioneer radiation worker, Roentgen, also participated in early experiments with ultrasound. During the 1880s, Roentgen published a number of papers describing his experiments with high-frequency sound. His efforts in this area were terminated following his discovery of x rays.

Applications of ultrasound, and indeed research of any significance, remained essentially dormant from the turn of the century until near the end of World War I. At this time several engineering groups had the idea of employing ultrasound for the detection of submerged Ger-

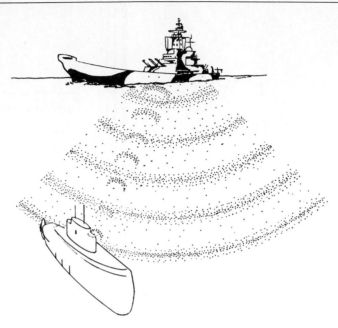

Fig. 33-1. SONAR represents one of the first applications of ultrasound—underwater detection.

man U-boats. The idea was not developed until after World War I. Apparently no practical use was made of ultrasound until World War II, with the development of **SONAR** (**so**und **n**avigation and **r**anging). Fig. 33-1 illustrates the use of SONAR. A beam of ultrasound is transmitted from a surface ship into the depths of the ocean. If it should intersect a submerged object, such as a submarine, a small amount of the ultrasound will be reflected back to the surface and detected. The time required for the ultrasound to travel to the reflecting object and back is directly proportional to the distance from the object. Consequently, SONAR allows the accurate determination of direction and distance. This is the precise basis for diagnostic ultrasound.

During the late 1940s, ultrasound began to find application in industry as a nondestructive testing agent. It was from these applications that its employment in medicine began in the 1950s. Today, diagnostic ultrasound is an essential med-

ical imaging technology, and the future is very bright for its continued improvement and employment.

Medical therapeutic ultrasound is not so widely employed and shows little promise because better modalities are available. Consequently, this chapter is solely concerned with medical **diagnostic ultrasound.** Much of the nomenclature associated with diagnostic ultrasound will be new to the radiologic technologist, and therefore new terms will be defined as used.

NATURE OF ULTRASOUND

Simple harmonic motion and how it can be described by the sinusoidal curve were discussed in Chapter 4. Fig. 4-5 showed three sine curves with their principle parameters—velocity, frequency, and wavelength—identified. As shown, such curves are used to represent characteristics of electromagnetic radiation—x and gamma rays. They are also used to

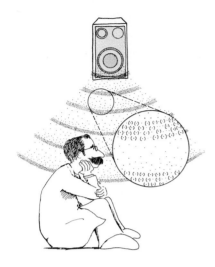

Fig. 33-2. Sound is transmitted through air when molecules are caused to vibrate back and forth along the direction of travel.

represent the physical properties of ultrasound. However, several basic differences exist between electromagnetic radiation and ultrasound.

Electromagnetic radiation is similar to a water wave in that it is **transverse** in nature. When a ripple glides across the surface of a pool, the individual molecules of water remain essentially in the same position. As the ripple passes, these molecules move up and down. The molecules thus move perpendicular, or transverse, to the direction of the wave.

Ultrasound is a **longitudinal wave.** When sound is generated, as in the high-fidelity speaker in Fig. 33-2, the molecules of air are alternately compressed and decompressed (**rarefied**) by the mechanical action of the speaker cone. The sound is transmitted from the speaker to the listener by the air molecules, but the air molecules themselves do not move that distance. The alternate compression and rarefaction created by the motion of the speaker cone produces an alternate to-and-fro motion that is passed from molecule to molecule. This to-and-fro movement of the air molecules is along the

direction of the sound waves, and therefore these waves are called longitudinal.

The use of the terms *transverse* and *longitudinal* as described here are similar to the use applied to magnetic resonance imaging (MRI). The transverse relaxation time, T_2, deals with loss of magnetization in a plane perpendicular to M_0, the net magnetization vector. The longitudinal relaxation time, T_1, is related to growth of M_0 along the same axis as B_0, the main magnetic field.

Unlike electromagnetic radiation, sound waves require a medium for their transmission. X rays can travel in a vacuum. **Matter must be present for sound to travel.**

The two types of ultrasound employed in diagnosis are **continuous wave** and **pulsed wave.** Fig. 33-3 shows the difference between these types of emissions. During continuous-wave emission, the ultrasound generating device, the transducer, vibrates continuously. This type of ultrasound is principally employed in examinations of the fetal heart and of blood flow by the Doppler method. Pulsed ultrasound is employed in most imaging studies, including A-

Continuous wave

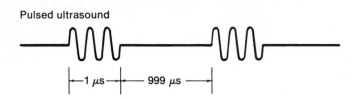

Pulsed ultrasound

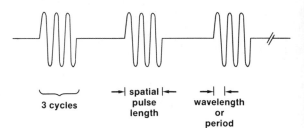

Fig. 33-3. Both continuous-wave and pulsed ultrasound are employed in medical diagnostic ultrasound.

Fig. 33-4. The spatial pulse length is the product of the number of cycles in an ultrasound pulse times the wavelength. If the beam shown here were 1 MHz, the spatial pulse length would be 3 mm.

3 cycles

spatial pulse length

wavelength or period

mode, B-mode, M-mode, and real time. These imaging studies are based on pulse-echo techniques in which a pulse of ultrasound is emitted and the reflected ultrasound wave, or echo, is received by the same transducer after a time delay. In pulse-echo ultrasound the transducer face vibrates rapidly for only a few cycles, usually three to five, and then is at rest for a relatively long time before the next pulse of ultrasound is emitted. Typically, pulses 1 to 5 μs long are separated by 995 to 999 μs periods during which time the transducer receives reflected waves. Such operation results in 1 pulse/1000 μs, or 1 pulse/ms, which is equivalent to 1000 pulses/s. This latter value, 1000 pulses/s, is the **pulse repetition rate (PRR)**.

The time from the beginning of one pulse to the next is called the **pulse repetition period (PRP)**. The pulse repetition rate and the pulse repetition period are reciprocally related as given by:

(33-1)

$$PRP \ (ms) = \frac{1}{PRR \ (kHz)}$$

The **pulse duration (PD)** is the time during which a pulse occurs. It is the product of the number of cycles in a pulse and the period of one cycle. **Period** is the time required for one wavelength or one cycle of ultrasound.

(33-2)

$$PD \ (\mu s) = Number \ of \ cycles \times Period \ (\mu s)$$

In pulse-echo ultrasound, the pulse duration is therefore also equal to the number of cycles in the pulse divided by the frequency.

(33-3)

$$PD \ (\mu s) = Number \ of \ cycles / Frequency \ (MHz)$$

A term derived from these equations, **duty factor (DF),** is important when considering ultrasound intensity during pulse-echo ultrasound. Duty factor is the fraction of time that ultrasound is actually emitted. It can be computed from the following:

(33-4)

$$DF = \frac{PD\ (\mu s)}{PRP\ (ms)\ \times\ 1000}$$

(33-5)

$$DF = \frac{PD\ (\mu s)\ \times\ PRR\ (kHz)}{1000}$$

The factor of 1000 in these equations converts ms and kHz into μs so that the units of the numerator and denominator are equal. When the value of duty factor obtained is multiplied by 100, the result is the duty factor expressed in percent. The duty factor for continuous-wave ultrasound is 1.0 or 100%.

When considering the resolution capabilities of pulse-echo ultrasound, a characteristic of the beam called the **spatial pulse length (SPL)** is employed. This characteristic is illustrated in Fig. 33-4. Spatial pulse length is the length in space over which a pulse occurs. It is determined by the product of the number of cycles in a pulse times the wavelength.

(33-6)

$$SPL\ (mm) = Number\ of\ cycles\ \times\ Wavelength\ (mm)$$

Since spatial pulse length is directly related to wavelength, it is inversely related to frequency.

(33-7)

$$SPL\ (mm) = \frac{Number\ of\ cycles\ \times\ Velocity\ (m/s)}{Frequency\ (MHz)}$$

Wave equation

In Chapter 4 the generalized wave equation was described as follows:

(33-8)

$$Velocity = Frequency \times Wavelength$$

This equation applies to all wave phenomena, transverse and longitudinal. The three characteristics of this wave equation—velocity, frequency, and wavelength—have the same meaning when applied to ultrasound that they have for electromagnetic radiation only their values are different. With electromagnetic radiation, the velocity is constant ($c = 3 \times 10^8$ m/s), and the energy is directly related to the frequency and inversely related to the wavelength. A fourth characteristic—amplitude—does not have direct meaning when describing electromagnetic radiation.

When the wave equation is applied to ultrasound, the velocity is a variable. Frequency and wavelength relate to image resolution and amplitude is the intensity (Fig. 33-5). When dealing with audible sound, frequency is tone or pitch and amplitude is loudness. The velocity of ultrasound depends on the density and compressibility of the medium through which the ultrasound is being transmitted. When standing near a railroad track, one's first indication of an approaching train is the low, rumbling sound transmitted through the rails. The whistle will not be heard for some time because the velocity of sound in air is less than in steel. The velocity is low in gases such as air because of their very large **compressibility** and low density. Generally, **the higher the density, the higher is the velocity of sound.** Table 33-1 shows the velocity of ultrasound in several substances of medical importance. Note that the velocity of ultrasound in bone is twice that in soft tissue and the velocity in soft tissue is five times that in air. **The velocity of ultrasound does not depend on frequency, it is determined by the medium.**

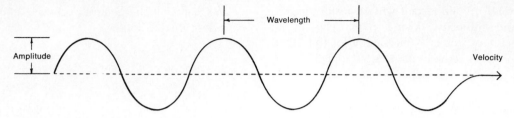

Fig. 33-5. The wavelike representation of ultrasound is similar to that for x rays, except velocity is variable and the amplitude is proportional to the loudness.

Table 33-1. Velocity of ultrasound in several materials of medical interest

Material	Velocity (m/s)
Air	348
Aluminum	2700
Beryllium	12,890
Blood	1570
Bone	3360
Fat	1500
Liver	1550
Muscle	1580
Oil	1500
Polyethylene	920
Soft tissue	1540
Water	1480

Table 33-2. Ultrasound frequency, wavelength, and period in soft tissue

Frequency (MHz)	Wavelength (mm)	Period (μs)
1	1.54	1.00
2.25	0.68	0.44
3.5	0.44	0.29
5	0.31	0.20
7.5	0.21	0.13
10	0.15	0.10
15	0.10	0.07

It is necessary that the velocity of ultrasound be known accurately for proper calibration of ranging and depth localization for a diagnostic instrument.

EXAMPLE: A pulsed ultrasound signal is transmitted through soft tissue to a tissue interface and reflected back. The time required for the complete trip is 60 μs. How deep is the reflecting interface?

ANSWER: $Depth = Velocity \times \frac{1}{2} \, Total \; time$
$= (1540 \text{ m/s}) \, (\frac{1}{2}) \, (60 \times 10^{-6} \text{ s})$
$= 4.62 \times 10^{-2} \text{ m}$
$= 4.6 \text{ cm}$

The other two parameters constituting the wave equation—frequency and wavelength— are inversely proportional. **As ultrasound frequency increases, the wavelength decreases.**

The ability to resolve small objects is directly related to the wavelength of the radiation involved. **High-frequency ultrasound** (short wavelength) results in **better spatial resolution** than low frequency. If this were the only variable, one would employ the highest-frequency ultrasound possible and obtain the best spatial resolution. As frequency is increased, however, the degree of interaction with the conducting medium increases and absorption of the ultrasound beam is increased. **High-frequency ultrasound results in shallow penetration.** For this reason, high-frequency transducers, up to 15 MHz, are employed for ultrasonic examination of small structures such as the eye. Lower-frequency transducers, around 2.5 MHz, are used for abdominal ultrasound examinations.

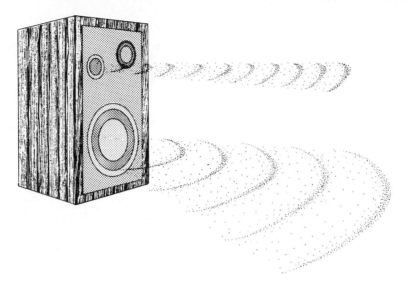

Fig. 33-6. The higher the frequency of sound, the more directional the emission. Bass notes from the woofer will fill the room, but treble notes from the tweeter will be more in the forward direction.

Table 33-2 shows the relationship between frequency, wavelength, and period for ultrasound transmission in soft tissue.

Another frequency-dependent characteristic of ultrasound is its directionality. Unlike sound, medical diagnostic ultrasound is designed to be highly directional and collimated, and this enhances its imaging ability. In general, **as the frequency of sound increases, its dispersion from the source becomes less** and its transmission behaves more like a collimated beam. This characteristic is familiar to high-fidelity enthusiasts. Fig. 33-6 shows a high-fidelity speaker system, which includes a woofer for low frequencies, a midrange speaker, and a tweeter for high-frequency sound. The low-frequency woofer emissions will tend to fill the entire room because sound is emitted from that source nearly **isotropically,** that is, with equal intensity in all directions. On the other hand, the high-frequency sound emitted from the tweeter will be heard most easily when one stands in front of the speaker system. Since this high-frequency sound does not disperse so readily, its perception is low when the listener is positioned to the side. Sound emitted from the midrange speaker shows directional characteristics midway between the woofer and the tweeter.

Diagnostic ultrasound is usually identified by its frequency of operation. In that regard, some summary statements are possible. **As the frequency of ultrasound increases, the following occurs:**

1. The ability to resolve small objects improves.
2. The penetrability of the beam decreases.
3. The beam becomes more collimated and directional.

The final characteristic of the wave equation, amplitude, is also familiar to the audiophile. Amplitude is to the wave equation what intensity, gain, or loudness is to sound. When the amplitude of an ultrasound wave is high, the regions of molecular compression and rarefraction are greater; this results in higher ultrasound intensity and power.

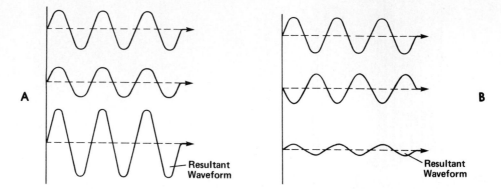

Fig. 33-7. A, Constructive interference occurs when sounds of the same frequency are transmitted in phase. **B,** When sound is transmitted out of phase, destructive interference occurs.

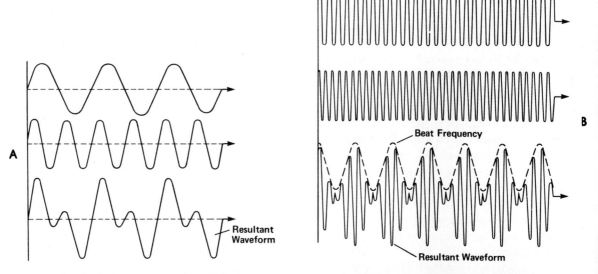

Fig. 33-8. A, When sound of different frequency is transmitted in the same direction, an irregular wave pattern results. **B,** If the frequencies are similar, the resulting interference pattern contains a beat frequency.

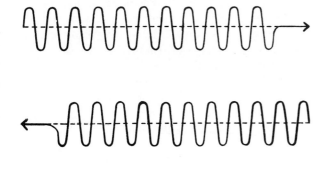

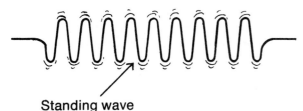

Fig. 33-9. Standing waves are produced when two sound waves travel in opposite directions.

Standing wave

Multiwave relationships

There are many characteristics to wave phenomena that were examined and described more than a century before ultrasonic applications were developed. These early investigations involved visible light, and the wave characteristics described are those of interference, reflection, refraction, diffraction, and scattering. Along with absorption, these are the ways the ultrasound beam is attenuated. A detailed knowledge of these phenomena is unnecessary at this time, but the ultrasonographer should be aware that such relationships exist. Some multiwave relationships are important to acoustic beam shaping, real-time imaging, and acoustic holography.

Wave interference. If multiple waves of equal frequency are transmitted precisely in phase, that is, with peaks and valleys occurring at the same position, the resulting summation wave will have the same frequency but will exhibit increased amplitude (Fig. 33-7, *A*). This phenomenon is called **constructive interference.** If the propagated waves are out of phase so that the maximum molecular compression for one wave occurs at the same point as maximum rarefaction for the second wave, then **destructive interference** occurs (Fig. 33-7, *B*).

When waves of different frequencies are transmitted through the same medium in the same direction, the resulting wave will have an irregular form (Fig. 33-8, *A*). If the frequencies of the associated ultrasound emissions are close to one another (Fig. 33-8, *B*), the resulting interference pattern consists of a low frequency superimposed on a high frequency. The low-frequency sound is called a **beat frequency.**

Standing waves

Standing waves are produced when two waves are traveling in directions opposite to each other. This occurs in diagnostic ultrasound applications with transmitted and reflected waves

(Fig. 33-9). The interference pattern that results is a stationary series of molecular compressions and rarefactions, usually of higher intensity than either the transmitted or reflected wave. Standing waves generated in the body interfere with the diagnostic ultrasound examination and are of no benefit.

Resonance

One type of standing wave is employed to good advantage in diagnostic ultrasound. The active element of the transducer is the **piezoelectric crystal.** It is constructed with parallel acoustic reflecting surfaces so that standing waves will be generated by the to-and-fro motion of the waves being reflected from each surface. If these reflecting surfaces are separated by a distance equal to an integral number of half wavelengths ($n \times \lambda/2$), standing waves will be formed. If the parallel reflecting surfaces are separated by only a half wavelength ($\lambda/2$), the standing waves will **resonate** at a fundamental frequency resulting in maximum intensity of the emitted wave. Ultrasound transducers are designed with this feature in mind so that the active crystal of the tranducer is fabricated to be $\lambda/2$ thick or sometimes $\lambda/4$ thick. This also results in maximum sensitivity for the detection of reflected ultrasound waves.

ACOUSTIC INTENSITY AND POWER

Wave intensity in general is the rate of flow of energy through a unit of area. Acoustic intensity is measured in watts per square centimeter or milliwatts per square centimeter (W/cm^2 or mW/cm^2) and is associated with the amplitude or molecular vibration of the sound wave (Fig. 33-10). Referring to the sine wave model in Fig. 33-5, it is amplitude that is associated with ultrasound intensity.

As the intensity of ultrasound increases, the displacement of an individual molecule in the conducting medium will increase. The total to-and-fro molecular movement will be greater at high intensity. Furthermore, the velocity with

which a molecule moves will be increased. The increased **particle displacement** and **particle velocity** result in increase compression and rarefaction of the conducting medium molecules and therefore increased sound wave pressure—increased intensity.

The intensity of ultrasound, however, is not uniform in space, as illustrated in Fig. 33-11. Its maximum intensity, known as the **spatial peak (SP),** occurs along the central axis of the beam and tapers off to either side. The average intensity across the ultrasound beam is called the **spatial average (SA)** and is considerably less than the spatial peak. Spatial peak and spatial average ultrasound intensities are related by the **beam uniformity ratio (BUR)** as follows:

(33-9)

$$BUR = \frac{SP\ (mW/cm^2)}{SA\ (mW/cm^2)}$$

The value of the beam uniformity ratio is a complex function of transducer design and beam characteristics. It can have values up to 1000:1.

The intensity of pulse-echo ultrasound also varies in time, a **temporal variation.** As with the spatial variation, there are two measures of temporal variation, as shown in Fig. 33-12. The **temporal average (TA)** ultrasound intensity is related to the **temporal peak (TP)** by the duty cycle (DC):

(33-10)

$$DC = \frac{TA\ (mW/cm^2)}{TP\ (mW/cm^2)}$$

If the duty cycle for pulse-echo ultrasound is 0.001, then the temporal peak intensity will be 1000 times greater than the temporal average. The duty cycle for continuous-beam ultrasound is one; therefore the temporal peak intensity and the temporal average intensity are the same.

To identify any ultrasound beam properly, we must refer to both the temporal and spatial char-

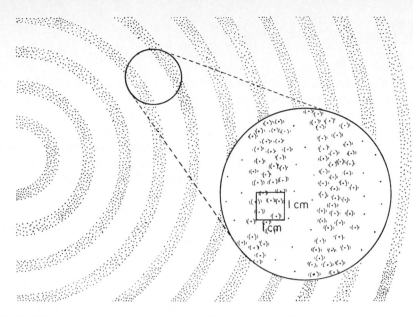

Fig. 33-10. Ultrasound intensity increases when the molecules of the medium are agitated more vigorously. The energy of molecular motion per unit area has units of milliwatts per square centimeter for diagnostic ultrasound.

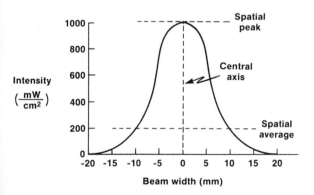

Fig. 33-11. When measuring laterally across the ultrasound beam, the peak intensity occurs along the central axis. The intensity falls off rapidly from the central axis.

Fig. 33-12. Ultrasound intensity varies considerably with time during pulse-echo imaging because the beam is energized intermittently.

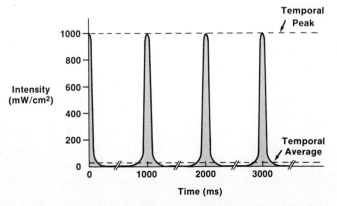

acteristics of the beam. Consequently, four precise intensities are possible: spatial average, temporal average (SATA); spatial peak, temporal average (SPTA); spatial average, temporal peak (SATP); and spatial peak, temporal peak (SPTP).

The defining equations for these intensities follow:

$$(33\text{-}11)$$

$$SATA = \frac{SP \times TP \times DC}{BUR}$$

$$(33\text{-}12)$$

$$SPTA = SA \times TP \times BUR \times DC$$

$$(33\text{-}13)$$

$$SATP = \frac{SP \times TA}{BUR \times DC}$$

$$(33\text{-}14)$$

$$SPTP = \frac{SA \times TA \times BUR}{DC}$$

Average diagnostic ultrasound intensities range from approximately 1 to 10 mW/cm^2. Peak intensities may be in the W/cm^2 range. Industrial applications of ultrasound in numerous nondestructive testing devices employ even higher beam intensities.

Ultrasonic power is the ultrasonic intensity times the cross-sectional beam area and has units of watts or milliwatts. At a given beam intensity, therefore, a broad ultrasound transmission would have higher power than a narrow ultrasound beam, even if individual molecular motion were the same. Power levels are not often cited for ultrasound devices. Suspected biologic effects are presumed to be more related to the energy transmitted through a unit area or absorbed per unit mass than the total power of the system.

The decibel

Only a few laboratories are capable of accurately calibrating ultrasound beam intensity be-

cause of the great technical difficulties involved. The precise beam intensity for medical ultrasound apparatus will vary depending upon the transducer used, the length of the pulse, and the mode of application. Consequently, commercial ultrasound units do not have control or meters indicating beam intensity in mW/cm^2.

The unit employed in describing diagnostic ultrasound intensity is adapted from radio electronics and is the bel or, more frequently, one tenth of a bel, the **decibel (dB).** The decibel is a relative measure and is used to compare the relative intensities of two ultrasound beams, for instance, the transmitted and the reflected beams of diagnostic ultrasound. Usually the comparison is made to the larger of the two beams so that in diagnostic ultrasound the reflected beam intensity is compared with the transmitted beam. When using a decibel, one must remember that **it is (1) relative and (2) logarithmic.** The logarithmic nature allows for expressing very wide ranges with rather small numbers, as described in Chapter 2.

If the intensity of the transmitted beam is identified as I_t and the intensity of the reflected beam as I_r, the intensity of I_r in decibels is given by

$$(33\text{-}15)$$

$$
\begin{aligned}
I_r \ (dB) &= 10 \ (log \ I_r - log \ I_t) \\
&= 10 \ log \ (I_r/I_t)
\end{aligned}
$$

EXAMPLE: If the transmitted ultrasound beam is 100 times as intense as the reflected beam, what is the intensity of the reflected beam?

ANSWER: $I_r = 10 \ log \ 1/100$
$= 10 \ log \ 0.01$
$= 10 \ (-2)$
$= -20 \ dB$

In this example, the reflected beam is said to be 20 dB down or to have lost 20 dB. Decibels are used in high-fidelity specifications to characterize the amplification gain or loudness possible with an amplifier.

Table 33-3. Decibel levels and their relationship to reflected wave intensity and amplification gain

If the intensity of the reflected wave is:	Then its intensity is also:	If the reflected wave is amplified by:	Then the amplification gain will be:
100%	0 dB	×1	0 dB
79%	−1 dB	×2	+3 dB
63%	−2 dB	×3	+4.7 dB
50%	−3 dB	×5	+7 dB
10%	−10 dB	×10	+10 dB
1%	−20 dB	×100	+20 dB
0.1%	−30 dB	×1000	+30 dB

EXAMPLE: A stereo amplifier is described as having a signal amplification of 10,000 to 1. How much gain is this?

ANSWER: $I = 10 \log \left(\dfrac{10,000}{1} \right)$

$\qquad = 10\,(4)$

$\qquad = 40 \text{ dB}$

Amplification gain in decibels is used in ultrasonic apparatus to increase the apparent size of the reflected wave. If a reflected wave is returned with a 20 dB loss, a control on the operating console will allow the ultrasonographer to boost the intensity of the reflected wave +20 dB so that its size will be the same as the transmitted wave. In such a case, a 20 dB gain will have been introduced. Table 33-3 summarizes the relationship between the transmitted intensity and the reflected intensity. Also shown are representative levels of gain applied to the returned wave. In abdominal ultrasound one can expect approximately a 20 dB loss in 10 cm of penetration. Amplifiers employed in diagnostic ultrasound have gains measured as high as 70 dB.

It is interesting to note the extremely wide intensity range possible with the human ear. If the threshold of human hearing is assigned a value of 0 dB, then normal conversation has a value of approximately 70 dB, 10 million times as intense as the threshold level. A factory floor might have a noise level of 80 to 90 dB; current government standards restrict the relative intensity of noise permissible on a factory floor or in any work environment to 90 dB before mandatory ear protective devices are required. During takeoff, a jumbo jet will generate approximately 100 dB of noise, whereas the Concorde supersonic jet was measured as just over 130 dB. The threshold of pain for humans is approximately 140 dB.

ACOUSTIC REFLECTION

Ultrasound is useful as a diagnostic medical tool principally because of reflection at tissue interfaces. The property of ultrasound most responsible for such reflections is called **sonic momentum.** Momentum is the product of mass and velocity. The larger the mass or the higher the velocity, the greater is the momentum. Sonic momentum refers to mass of the conducting molecules and their velocity.

Acoustic impedance. More specifically, the quantity **acoustic impedance (Z)** is used to describe the reflection of sound at an interface. Acoustic impedance is similar to sonic momentum and is determined by similar characteristics. It is a function of the density of the medium and its compressibility, which is measured by the velocity of sound in the medium. In general, **the higher the density, the greater is the acoustic impedance.** Also, **the higher the velocity of**

Table 33-4. Acoustic impedance for several materials of diagnostic importance

Material	Acoustic impedance kg/m² s (10⁻⁶)
Air	0.0004
Aluminum	17
Blood	1.61
Bone	7.80
Brain	1.58
Fat	1.38
Kidney	1.62
Liver	1.65
Muscle	1.70
Oil	1.43
Polyethylene	1.88
Soft tissue	1.63
Water	1.48

Table 33-5. Reflectivity and percentage reflection for various interfaces

Reflecting interface	Reflectivity	Percentage reflection
Fat–muscle	0.01	1.08
Fat–kidney	0.0064	0.64
Muscle–blood	0.007	0.74
Bone–fat	0.476	47.6
Bone–muscle	0.410	41.0
Soft tissue–water	0.0025	0.25
Soft tissue–air	0.999	99.9
Soft tissue–PTZ5 crystal	0.792	79.2
Soft tissue–castor oil	0.0036	0.36

sound in the medium, the greater is the acoustic impedance. The velocity of sound differs from medium to medium because of the freedom of motion of the molecules in the medium, that is, their **stiffness, elasticity,** or **compressibility.** Mathematically, acoustic impedance is described by

(33-16)

$$Z = PV$$

where P is density (kg/m³) and V is velocity (m/s). Acoustic impedance therefore has units of kg/m²s.

EXAMPLE: What is the acoustic impedance of ultrasound in soft tissue?
ANSWER: $Z_{soft\ tissue} = 10^{-3}$ kg/m³) (1.54 × 10³ m/s¹)
$$= 1.54 × 10^6 \text{ kg/m}^2 \text{ s}$$
$$= 1.54 × 10^6 \text{ rayl}$$

Table 33-4 reports the acoustic impedance for several materials of diagnostic importance. Since the acoustic impedance is determined by the velocity of sound in the medium, it is not dependent on the frequency or wavelength of the ultrasound beam. Acoustic impedance is a most important tissue characteristic. The largest re-

flections occur between tissues with great differences in acoustic impedance.

Reflectivity. When an ultrasound wave is incident on a tissue interface, some of the sound will be reflected and some will be transmitted (Fig. 33-13). The transmitted beam will leave the interface at an angle different from that of the incident beam. This deviation of the beam is called **refraction.** In diagnostic ultrasound there is little use for the transmitted beam. Principal interest lies in the reflected beam or actually its intensity relative to the incident beam. This quantity of **intensity ratio** is known as the interface **reflectivity (R)** and is defined as

(33-17)

$$R = \left(\frac{Z_1 - Z_2}{Z_1 + Z_2} \right)^2$$

The percentage of ultrasound reflected at such an interface is

(33-18)

$$Percent\ reflected = \left(\frac{Z_1 - Z_2}{Z_1 + Z_2} \right)^2 × 100$$

EXAMPLE: An ultrasound beam traversing muscle encounters a blood interface. What is the reflectivity at this interface and what percentage of the incident beam will be reflected?

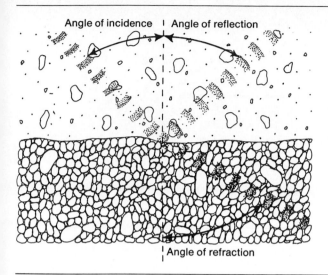

Fig. 33-13. The angle of incidence and the angle of reflection are equal. The angle of refraction depends on the velocity of ultrasound in each medium.

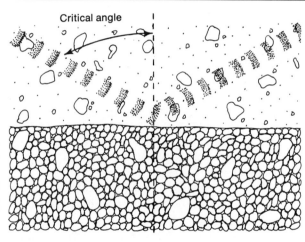

Fig. 33-14. At the critical angle there is total reflection and no refraction.

ANSWER:

$$R = \left(\frac{1.70 \times 10^{10} - 1.61 \times 10^6}{1.70 \times 10^6 + 1.61 + 10^6} \right)^2$$

$$= \left(\frac{0.09 \times 10^6}{3.31 \times 10^6} \right)^2$$

$$= (0.027)^2$$

$$= 0.0074$$

$$Percent\ reflected = 0.74\%$$

Table 33-5 is derived from the previous values reported for acoustic impedance and reports the values of reflectivity at various anatomic interfaces and the percentage of the ultrasound intensity that would be reflected if the beam were incident perpendicular to the interface.

All that was just described assumes perpendicular incidence of the ultrasound beam on the

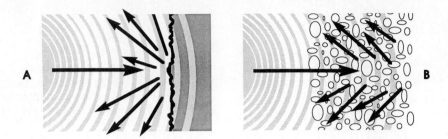

Fig. 33-15. Scattering occurs when diagnostic ultrasound encounters a highly irregular or rough surface **(A)** or heterogeneous tissue such as kidney and liver **(B)**.

reflecting surface. As the angle of incidence increases (Fig. 33-14), the reflected beam is directed farther from the detecting transducer. As the angle increases still farther, total reflection will occur at the interface, but this reflected beam, of course, will not be detected. The angle for total reflection is called the **critical angle,** and it depends on the velocity of sound in each medium.

Scattering. Regardless of the angle of incidence, a large fraction of the transmitted ultrasound beam will be reflected if the dimension or roughness of the tissue interface is large compared to the wavelength of the ultrasound. Such a situation is normal in diagnostic ultrasound and is termed **specular reflection.** The previous discussion of acoustic impedance and reflectivity dealt with specular reflection.

If the dimension or roughness of the tissue interface is small compared to the wavelength of the transmitted ultrasound, then specular reflection will not occur. In such a case, the ultrasound beam becomes diffuse and less intense because of multiple **scattering.** Highly irregular interfaces and heterogeneous tissues result in scattering, as seen in Fig. 33-15. Some of the ultrasound is scattered back to the transducer

and contributes to image formation. This is called **backscattered** ultrasound.

The intensity of specular reflections is very dependent on the angle of incidence of the ultrasound beam. This is not so with the intensity of backscattered ultrasound. Backscattered ultrasound is more a function of the characteristics of the tissue than the angle of incidence. Backscattering allows for imaging of organ interfaces that are not perpendicular to the transducer face. Tissue parenchyma is also imaged with backscattered ultrasound.

Specular reflection and scattering have familiar analogies in visible light. Nearly all incident light is reflected from a mirror as a visible image. Also, nearly all incident light is reflected from frosted glass or a white wall, but there is no image. The mirrored surface is smooth and is analogous to specular reflections. Light is scattered from a white surface because the surface is highly irregular.

ACOUSTIC ABSORPTION AND ATTENUATION

Absorption of ultrasound energy occurs in the conducting medium because of interactions known as **relaxation processes.** Such relaxation is not too unlike that described for MRI. Con-

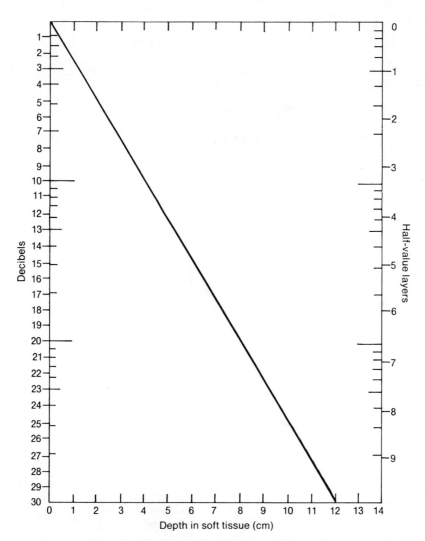

Fig. 33-16. Attenuation of ultrasound in tissue can be measured in decibels or half-value layers. This graph show the attenuation of a 2.5 MHz beam in soft tissue based on an average rate of 1 dB/cm/MHz.

Table 33-6. Half-value layer of ultrasound (− 3 dB) by frequency and absorbing medium

Material (in centimeters)	Frequency				
	1 MHz	2 MHz	5 MHz	10 MHz	20 MHz
Aqueous humor			6	3	1.5
Air	0.25	0.06	0.01		
Blood	17	8.5	3	2	1.00
Bone	0.2	0.1	0.04		
Fat	5	2.5	1	0.5	0.25
Lens of eye			0.3	0.15	0.07
Muscle	1.5	0.75	0.3	0.15	
Polyethylene	0.6	0.3	0.12	0.6	0.03
Soft tissue	3	1.5	0.5	0.3	0.15
Water	1360	340	54	14	3.4

sider the fate of a single molecule displaced by a passing pulse of ultrasound. First, it is pushed forward by the passing compression wave, and then it falls back during the rarefaction phase. The time required for the molecule to fall back following displacement is called its **relaxation time.** For unstructured fluids such as water, the relaxation time is short and beam attenuation is low. Structured fluids such as soft tissue have longer relaxation time and therefore higher attenuation and viscosity.

There are a number of these processes—**thermal relaxation, conductional relaxation,** and **structural relaxation**—but one can best envision such processes collectively as molecular friction. When a sound wave passes through matter and the conducting molecules are agitated to and fro, the transfer of this motion from one molecular layer to the next is not 100% efficient because of relaxation, or friction, among the molecules. Consequently, as ultrasound penetrates through matter, even a homogeneous medium, the ultrasound intensity decreases.

Absorption denotes an all-or-nothing phenomenon, as in the photoelectric absorption of an x ray. In ultrasound the term **attenuation** is more appropriate. In this sense **attenuation refers to the reduction in beam intensity with**

depth in tissue caused by absorption, scattering, and beam divergence. Ultrasound attenuation occurs exponentially in much the same manner as that for x-radiation. The equation describing ultrasound attenuation is also similar:

(33-19)

$$I_x = I_o \, e^{-\mu x}$$

In the equation, I_o is the initial intensity, I_x is the intensity at a depth x, μ is the ultrasound attenuation coefficient measured in dB/cm, and x is depth in tissue. The ultrasonic attenuation coefficient is a function of sonic momentum and frequency and therefore varies with the physical properties of the conducting medium and the ultrasound frequency. **The higher the frequency, the higher is the attenuation coefficient,** and therefore the greater the attenuation. For this reason, the practical upper limit to diagnostic ultrasound is approximately 15 MHz.

Because exponential attenuation does occur, it is convenient and familiar to think in terms of half-value layer (HVL). For an ultrasound beam, **the half-value layer is that thickness of absorbing tissue that will reduce the beam intensity to half its original value.** It is precisely the same definition applied to x-radiation and gamma radiation. Table 33-3 indicated that a 50% reduction in intensity was equivalent to 3 dB loss. Fig. 33-16 takes this relationship still further and shows how attenuation in dB, half-value layer, and depth in soft tissue are related.

As indicated, attenuation is a function of frequency. As a rule of thumb, **ultrasound is attenuated in soft tissue 1 dB/cm/MHz.** In other words, a 3 MHz beam would lose half its intensity in 1 cm and over 90% of its intensity in 10 cm. Table 33-6 lists the thickness of tissue required to attenuate the intensity of an ultrasound beam by 3 dB (one HVL) in several biologic media of interest.

REVIEW QUESTIONS

1. Define or otherwise identify:
   a. Piezoelectric effect
   b. Longitudinal wave
   c. Isotropic
   d. Decibel
   e. Acoustic impedance
   f. Relaxation time
   g. Transceive
   h. Compressibility
   i. Units of acoustic intensity
   j. Ultrasound HVL

2. Discuss the wave equation as it relates to diagnostic ultrasound. What parameters are constant, if any?
3. How deep in soft tissues is an interface when the total time between transmission and reception of an ultrasound pulse is 45 μs?
4. Identify the types of wave interference possible with diagnostic ultrasound.
5. The ratio of the transmitted to the reflected ultrasound beam intensity is 1200 to 1. How many dB of amplification will be required so that the reflected beam is equal to the transmitted beam?
6. The density of a substance is 2.7 x 10^3 kg/m^3, and the velocity of sound in that substance is 2700 m/s^1. What is its acoustic impedance?
7. What is the distance to a destroyer from a submarine if the transmission to reception time is 8.7 s?
8. What is the pulse repetition rate when a 3 μs wide pulse is emitted every 500 μs?
9. What is the wavelength of 2.25 MHz ultrasound in soft tissue?
10. How does the penetrability of an ultrasound beam vary with frequency?

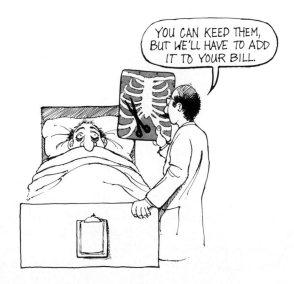

YOU CAN KEEP THEM, BUT WE'LL HAVE TO ADD IT TO YOUR BILL.

34

Diagnostic ultrasound instrumentation and operation

ULTRASOUND TRANSDUCER
ULTRASONIC BEAM
OPERATIONAL MODES
BIOLOGIC EFFECTS

Diagnostic ultrasound has developed into a widely used medical imaging modality in just a few short years. In addition to radiologists, a number of other physician specialists employ it. A principal reason for its wide application is its ease of use and the relatively low cost of the instrumentation. The heart of diagnostic ultrasound is the transducer.

ULTRASOUND TRANSDUCER

A **transducer** is any device that converts energy from one form into another. An ultrasound transducer converts electric energy into ultrasound energy and ultrasound energy back into electric energy. Similar audible sound transducers exist, and they are called loudspeakers and microphones. Ultrasound transducers have no such special names. Operation of an ultrasound transducer is based on the **piezoelectric effect**.

The piezoelectric effect is demonstrated graphically in Fig. 34-1. When a suitable crystalline material is stimulated electrically, the crystal will expand along its short axis. If the polarity of the electric signal is reversed, the crystal will contract. If the electric signal oscillates at a high frequency, then the crystal will alternately expand and contract at the same frequency. In such a situation, the crystal face behaves in the same manner as a high-fidelity speaker cone, and this mechanical motion produces ultrasound at the same frequency as the applied electric signal. More precisely, therefore, an ultrasound transducer converts an electric signal into mechanical motion and the mechanical motion into ultrasound.

The reverse is also possible. Ultrasound incident on a suitable crystalline material will transfer the energy of compression and rarefaction into contraction and expansion of the crystal. This in turn will cause an oscillating electric signal. This process is also the piezoelectric effect.

There are several components to the trans-

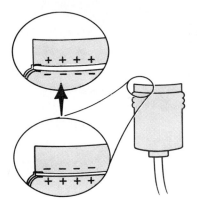

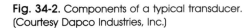

Fig. 34-1. Piezoelectric effect is the distortion of crystal shape by an electric stimulus and the generation of an electric signal by mechanical distortion of the crystal.

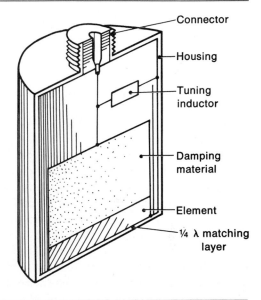

Connector

Housing

Tuning inductor

Damping material

Element

¼ λ matching layer

Fig. 34-2. Components of a typical transducer. (Courtesy Dapco Industries, Inc.)

ducer (Fig. 34-2). The **case** provides structural support for the internal filling and mechanical support so the device can be manipulated by hand rather ruggedly. The **face** of the transducer assembly is a protective acoustic window designed to match the active crystal and transmit the ultrasound beam through acoustic coupling to the patient. A **matching layer** with acoustic impedance between that of the face and tissue may be attached to improve ultrasound transmission into tissue by reducing surface reflectivity.

The active element of the transducer is the **piezoelectric crystal.** The material most frequently used is lead zirconate titanate (**PZT**). Quartz, barium lead zirconate, barium lead titanate, and lithium sulfate have also been used. The manufacturing process for crystal growth

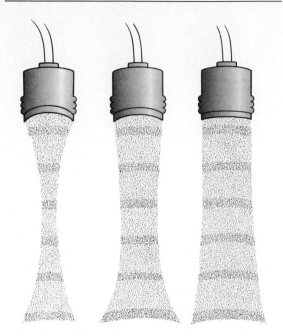

Fig. 34-3. Beam focusing can be accomplished by shaping the face of the transducer.

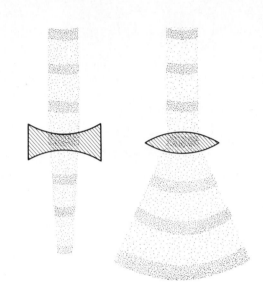

Fig. 34-4. Sometimes acoustic lenses are employed to focus ultrasound beams.

and shaping is precise and highly critical. To optimize the efficiency of ultrasound transmission and reception, the thickness of the crystal must be a half or a quarter wavelength. For a 2.5 MHz transducer, crystal thickness is 0.31 mm or 0.15 mm. At 10 MHz the crystal thickness is only 70 μm or 35 μm. The diameter of the crystal face is likewise critical. Crystal diameter controls the profile of the ultrasound beam. One way of focusing the ultrasound beam is accomplished by shaping the crystal and face.

In pulse-echo ultrasound, it is important that the source of ultrasound not be allowed to **reverberate** or **ring**. Consequently, the piezoelectric crystal is backed by material designed to damp or cushion the movement of the crystal so that, when the electric stimulus is removed, the crystal will cease motion immediately. This **backing material** is similar to one's hand placed on the rim of a ringing bell to soften the sound. Backing material is often absent in transducers designed for continuous-beam ultrasound. The piezoelectric crystal and backing material are surrounded by acoustic insulation to further confine the ultrasound beam. Electric signals are transmitted through a **connector** on the back of the transducer to each face of the piezoelectric crystal. The crystal faces are coated with electrically conducting material.

Beam focusing

The crystal shape controls the focus of the ultrasound beam. As shown in Fig. 34-3, flat-faced transducers show relatively broad beam transmission. As the transducer face is made more concave, the beam becomes more focused.

In addition to shaping the transducer face, beams can be focused with acoustic lenses (Fig.

34-4). These lenses can be placed at any point in the ultrasound beam but are normally built into the transducer. Acoustic lenses take advantage of the property of refraction of sound to change the direction of the sound wave. Such lenses can be made of polystyrene, nylon, other plastic materials, and aluminum. Most transducers manufactured for medical imaging are focused. The manufacturer will identify the focal length of such transducers.

ULTRASONIC BEAM

To this point we have described ultrasound as a sinusoidally varying wave. Doppler systems usually employ continuous waves of ultrasound, although some Doppler systems employ relatively long pulses of ultrasound. Pulse-echo systems (A-mode, B-mode, and M-mode) employ the very short pulses of ultrasound. For instance, a 2.5 MHz ultrasound transducer used for pulse-echo technique would typically have a pulse 1-microsecond long followed by a 999-microsecond dead time. The pulse repetition rate is thus 1 kHz. Pulse repetition rates of 500 and 5000 Hz are encountered. At 2.5 MHz for 1 microsecond, each pulse would contain two and a half cycles of ultrasound.

The more cycles present in an ultrasound pulse, the purer will be the frequency of the beam. Continuous-wave ultrasound has essentially one frequency, the resonant frequency of operation.

Pulse-echo ultrasound, however, may contain many frequencies in each pulse because of the difficulty in starting and stopping a pulse. In general, the fewer the cycles in a pulse, the more frequencies it will contain.

Bandwidth is an electrical engineering term used to express the range of frequencies in an ultrasound pulse. Another borrowed electrical engineering term is **quality factor (QF)**, which describes the purity or homogeneity of the ultrasound pulse. Quality factor is determined by dividing the resonant frequency by the bandwidth:

(34-1)

$$QF = \frac{Resonant\ frequency\ (MHz)}{Bandwidth\ (MHz)}$$

The narrower the bandwidth, the greater is the quality factor.

The wave front

Consider the three audio speakers in Fig. 34-5. In general, as the source of sound becomes smaller, the emission of sound becomes more isotropic. If the smallest speaker in Fig. 34-5 had a cone diameter of one-half wavelength ($\lambda/2$), the emitted sound pattern would appear as in Fig. 34-6, *A*.

This figure actually represents an ultrasound transducer having diameter of $\lambda/2$. If it were replaced by a line of several similar transducers, each emitting sound isotropically, the phenomenon of constructive and destructive interference would result in alternate regions of enhancement and reduction of the sound wave as it emerges from these multiple sources. Such a multiple-source generator of sound creates a sound **wave front** (Fig. 34-6, *B*), and it is the wave front that is employed in diagnostic ultrasound. The transducer behaves as though it were many individual small sources of sound, each contributing to the wave front.

Near field and far field

A transducer whose crystal diameter is an integral multiple of the primary wavelength (for example, thirty times) will emit an ultrasound beam characterized by a strong **plane wave front.** This plane wave front has two distinct regions, each with differing physical characteristics.

The region nearest the transducer face is called the **near field,** or **Fresnel zone,** and it is characterized by a highly collimated beam with great variation in ultrasound intensity from wave front to wave front.

The zone farthest from the transducer face is

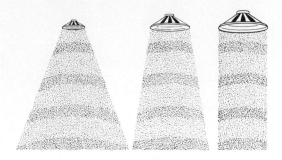

Fig. 34-5. For any given frequency, the larger the sound source, the more directional will be the sound.

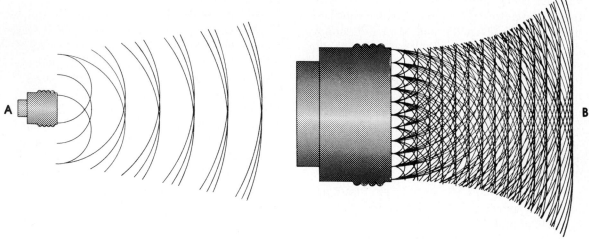

Fig. 34-6. A, Spheric sound waves are emitted from a transducer that has a diameter of one half wavelength. **B,** Plane wave fronts are emitted from larger transducers.

Fig. 34-7. There are two distinct regions to the ultrasound beam, the near field and the far field.

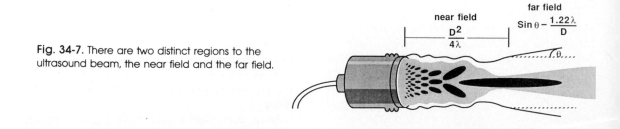

Table 34-1. Near-field lengths and far-field divergence of commercially available transducers

Transducer diameter (mm)	Frequency (MHz)	Near-field length (cm)	Far-field divergence
8	10	10.4	1°21'
8	5	5.2	4°25'
12	2.5	1.1	1°48'
12	5.0	11.7	1°48'
15	1.0	9.1	2°52'
20	1.0	6.5	5°23'

called the **far field,** or **Fraunhofer zone.** The far field is characterized by a divergence of the ultrasound beam and a more uniform ultrasound intensity. These features of the ultrasound beam are shown schematically in Fig. 34-7. **Best image resolution occurs at the near-field, far-field transition.**

The diameter and length of the near field and the divergence of the far field are determined by the transducer diameter and the ultrasound frequency. The equations governing these relationships are given in Fig. 34-7. In general, the following relationships exist:

1. As the transducer diameter is increased, the near field is lengthened and the far-field divergence is decreased.
2. As frequency is increased, the near field is lengthened and the far-field divergence is decreased.

Table 34-1 shows some representative field properties of commercially available transducers.

Resolution

When internal structures are scanned with an ultrasound beam to produce a two-dimensional image, the quality of the image will be directly related to the spatial resolution of the system. Spatial resolution in diagnostic ultrasound is the ability of the system to identify closely separated tissue interfaces. Ultrasound imaging involves axial and lateral resolution.

Axial resolution, sometimes called longitudi-

nal resolution, is a measure of the ability of the ultrasound system to identify closely separated interfaces that lie on the **axis** of the ultrasound beam (Fig. 34-8). If the interfaces are widely separated, they will be easily identified. As the interfaces become close together, however, the returning echoes from each interface may not be distinguishable from each other so that separately returning echoes appear as one.

Axial resolution depends on the length of the ultrasound pulse. Therefore a pulse of ultrasound containing ten complete wavelengths will have worse axial resolution than one containing three wavelengths. In practice, most ultrasound pulse-echo systems emit beams of two to five wavelengths in duration. Normally, the ultrasonographer cannot alter this condition. As ultrasound frequency increases, however, the wavelength decreases, and therefore the length of the ultrasound pulse decreases. Consequently, at higher frequencies better axial resolution is obtained. Table 34-2 presents typical values of axial resolution as a function of frequency. **For optimum axial resolution, one should apply the highest frequency, which will also provide the necessary tissue penetration.** Furthermore, at high frequency, the near field is longer and the far field more collimated. This contributes to improved axial and lateral resolution.

Lateral resolution, sometimes called **azimuthal resolution,** refers to the resolution of objects in a plane perpendicular to the axis of the beam.

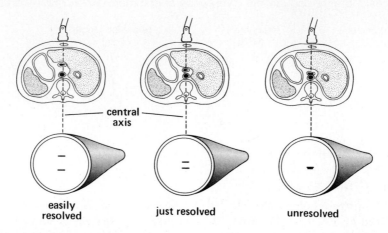

Fig. 34-8. Axial resolution is the ability to resolve closely separated objects or interfaces on the axis of the ultrasound beam.

Table 34-2. Axial resolution determined by the frequency of operation

Frequency (MHz)	Wavelength in soft tissue (mm)	Axial resolution (mm)
1	1.54	4.6
2.25	0.68	2.0
3.5	0.44	1.3
5	0.31	0.8
7.5	0.21	0.6
10	0.15	0.5
15	0.1	0.3

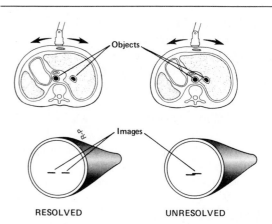

Fig. 34-9. Lateral resolution measures the ability of the ultrasound system to detect closely separated objects lying in a plane perpendicular to the beam axis.

Fig. 34-9 demonstrates the concept of lateral resolution. When one scans laterally across objects, echoes will be returned to the transducer during the entire period that it is positioned over the objects. If the objects were only points, they would appear as a line whose length was equal to the effective width of the ultrasonic beam. If one now scans two point objects separated by a distance greater than the effective beam width, two straight lines will appear. As the point objects are moved close together, the image lines will likewise move closer together until they merge into one line. **The minimum object separation distance at which the two lines can still be distinguished is the lateral resolution.** This lateral resolution is approximately equal to the effective beam width, and consequently it depends on transducer size and somewhat on frequency. **The larger the size of the transducer, the worse is the lateral resolution. The higher the frequency, the better is the lateral resolution.**

Lateral resolution is considerably more important to image quality than axial resolution because it is the parameter that limits image quality. A typical abdomen scan at 2.5 MHz will have axial resolution of approximately 2 mm, but lateral resolution of only 1 to 2 cm. At 10 MHz, lateral resolution as small as 2 mm is obtainable.

OPERATIONAL MODES

At present a number of operational modes are available to the ultrasonographer. Two are static imaging modes, A-mode and B-mode; two are dynamic imaging modes, M-mode and real time; and one, Doppler mode, is a ranging mode. All find application in diagnostic ultrasound, and each has its own area for special application. A-mode is particularly useful for measuring midline shifts of the brain. B-mode is perhaps the one most widely employed, and it is used primarily for abdominal imaging. M-mode finds its principal application in dynamic imaging of internal structures. Real-time ultrasound allows

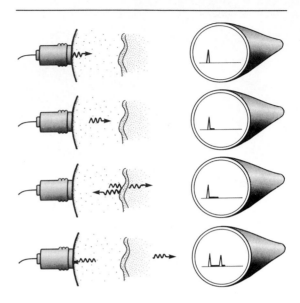

Fig. 34-10. In pulse-echo ultrasound a short pulse transverses tissue until it is reflected at an interface. The time required for the reflected pulse to return to the transducer determines the position of the blip on the CRT screen.

for observation of structures in motion. Doppler ultrasound is used for depth and flow measurements and investigations of moving surfaces. It finds principal application in fetal heart monitoring and peripheral blood flow measurements.

All but Doppler ultrasound employ **pulse-echo technique.** The basis for this technique is simple. Fig. 34-10 shows the emission of a single pulse and reflection from interfaces. The first reflection occurs at the transducer-patient interface, and it is the most intense. Each succeeding tissue interface results in a reflection, the intensity of which is reduced by depth into the patient. The time required for the pulse to be reflected and returned to the transducer determines the indicated position of the interface by a blip on the CRT screen.

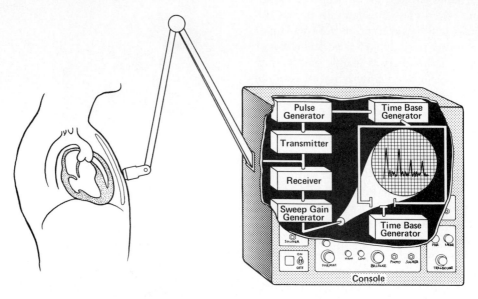

Fig. 34-11. Basic components of A-mode ultrasound and the image display format.

A-mode display

Some of the earliest work with diagnostic ultrasound employed **A-mode (amplitude mode)** display. In this mode ultrasound is emitted in pulses by the transducer, which then also receives echoes or reflections from tissue interfaces. This type of ultrasound emission is called **pulse-echo** technique. The returning echoes are displayed on a CRT as a series of blips. The distance between blips is proportional to the distance between interfaces, and the height of each blip is proportional to the intensity of the reflected beam. Therefore distal reflections produce smaller blips than do proximal reflections. The basic components and display mode for this type of ultrasonography are shown in Fig. 34-11.

A-mode ultrasound employs either one or two transducers. In a two-transducer application, one transducer is used to transmit and the other to receive. For observations in the brain, the transmitting transducer is placed on one side of the head and the receiving transducer on the other. In the one-device mode, the same transducer is used to transmit and receive.

The main purpose for employing A-mode is to measure the depth of interfaces and to detect their separation accurately. This type of operation relies on axial resolution, which was shown to depend on the pulse length and the frequency of operation.

A-mode instruments are relatively inexpensive, rugged, and easy to use. Since depth and separation are the critical measurements, A-mode instruments do require frequent, if not daily, calibration. A 2.5 cm thick lucite or polystyrene block is approximately equivalent to 2 cm of tissue and can be employed as a quick calibration tool on a regular basis. A-mode ultrasound was the first to be used, but today it is rarely employed.

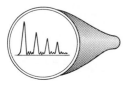

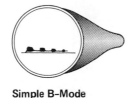

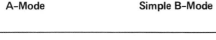

A-Mode   **Simple B-Mode**

Fig. 34-12. Relationship between A-mode display and a simple B-mode display.

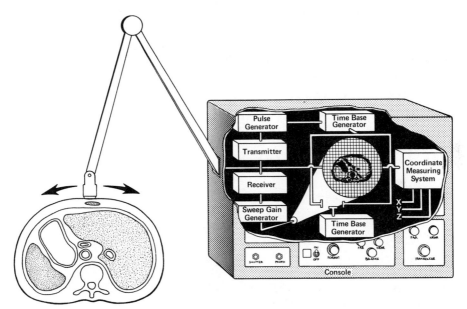

Fig. 34-13. Basic components of a B-scanner and the image format.

B-mode display

In the A-mode display, the height of the blip is proportional to the intensity of the reflected wave. If that blip is now squeezed down to a dot on the CRT display, its brightness will be proportional to the intensity of the reflected wave (Fig. 34-12). This type of display is **B-mode (brightness mode).**

B-mode by itself has little application in diagnostic ultrasound. However, if the spatial po-

sition and direction of the ultrasound beam are mechanically coupled to the CRT display and the B-mode pulses individually stored while the transducer is moved about the body, an image will appear that is the summation of many individual B-mode lines. Such an imaging system is called **compound B-mode** (Fig. 34-13). Although this type of scan is correctly identified as compound B-mode, use of the general term **B-scan** is universally employed.

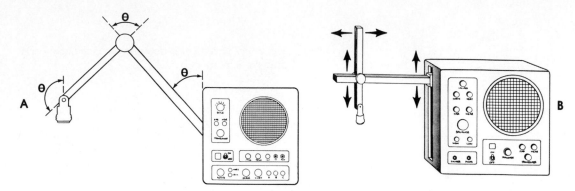

Fig. 34-14. **A,** Sine and cosine potentiometers measure angles. **B,** Linear potentiometers measure distance.

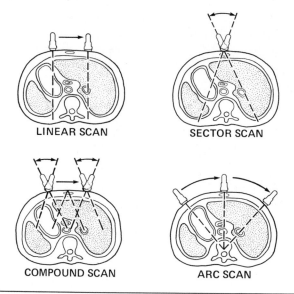

LINEAR SCAN   SECTOR SCAN

COMPOUND SCAN   ARC SCAN

Fig. 34-15. Types of transducer motions used in ultrasound scanning.

Critical to the B-scan image is the proper mechanical alignment and indication for position and direction. This alignment is accomplished with electric potentiometers, or **pots.** The electrical resistance of the potentiometer changes with its position, which allows for easy indication of transducer position. Linear and sine-cosine potentiometers are employed. Most B-scanners have a transducer attached to a swinging, crane-type arm (Fig. 34-14, A). This type of apparatus would employ sine-cosine potentiometers. Al-ternatively, the transducer can be fixed on a rigid frame (Fig. 34-14, B), so that linear potentiometers are required.

The ultrasonographer has multiple options for the manner in which the B-mode transducer is manipulated. The transducer can be moved linearly over the patient to provide a rectangular field of view, it can be angulated to provide a sector field of view, or a combination of both can be employed (Fig. 34-15).

The spatial resolution of a B-scanner is deter-

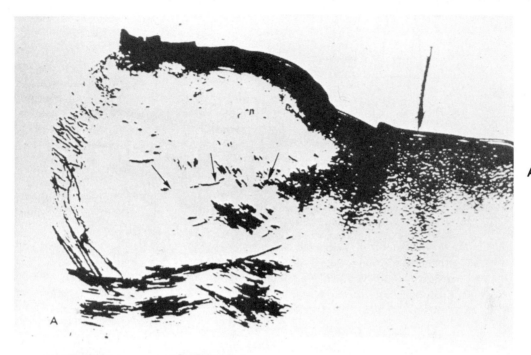

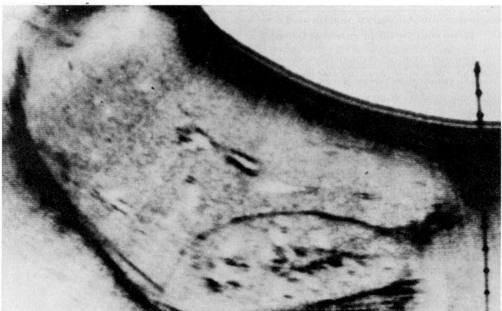

Fig. 34-16. Abdominal images formed by ultrasound. **A,** Bistable ultrasound. **B,** Gray-scale ultrasound. (Courtesy P. Athey, Baylor College of Medicine, Houston, Tex.)

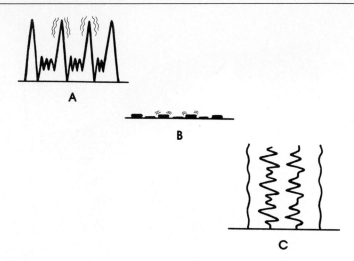

Fig. 34-17. If the A-mode image contains moving interfaces and is converted to a B-mode display so that the vertical axis is time driven, M-mode display results. **A,** A-mode. **B,** B-mode. **C,** M-mode.

mined not only by the transducer characteristics, but also by the mechanical-electrical linkage that determines the position and direction of the transducer. Resolution in B-scanning is described for both axial and lateral objects.

Early B-scanners incorporated a **bistable** display mode. This type of display shows very high contrast—only bright spots or blank screen with no intermediate intensities on the face of the CRT. **Gray-scale display** subsequently has been developed, and it provides a range of intermediate display intensities. Gray scale is possible by using a small, dedicated computer and a special type of CRT tube—a **scan converter.** Fig. 34-16 demonstrates the difference between bistable and gray-scale ultrasound.

Analog and digital scan convertors are used in diagnostic ultrasound, but the trend is definitely to digital scan convertors. Currently, nearly all diagnostic ultrasound units incorporate digital scan convertors and microprocessors. With a digital scan convertor, data are stored in digital form and displayed as an image

matrix similar to computed tomography (CT) and magnetic resonance imaging (MRI). This allows **digital ultrasound** images to be post-processed for more flexible image analysis and interpretation.

M-mode display

If a pulse-echo transducer is positioned over the heart and operated in the A-mode, the image will contain a number of blips, some of them stationary and some vibrating back and forth. The stationary blips indicate motionless interfaces, and their amplitude is proportional to the intensity of the echo. The vibrating blips represent interfaces that are in motion relative to the transducer. The magnitude of the vibration of each blip represents the degree of movement of the tissue interface. Such an image is shown schematically in Fig. 34-17, *A.*

If this A-scan display is now converted to a single B-scan, the image would contain a series of dots, some fixed and some moving (Fig. 34-17, *B*). The moving dots, of course, are related

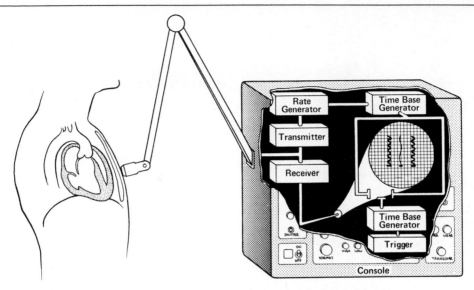

Fig. 34-18. M-mode produces a strip chart for tracing moving tissue interfaces.

to the moving tissue interfaces. If the y axis of the display is now driven as though it were the paper in a strip-chart recorder, a tracing of the dots will result. The stationary dots will trace a regular pattern according to the motion of the associated tissue interface (Fig. 34-17, *C*).

This type of ultrasound display is called **M-mode (motion mode)** (Fig. 34-18). It is also sometimes referred to as TM-mode (time-motion mode), PM-mode (position-motion mode), and UCH (ultrasonic cardiography), since its principal application is to monitor the heart. From the M-mode display the x axis is a depth axis; the y axis is a time axis that can be used to measure the time between successive heartbeats. An advanced feature of M-mode display allows it to be synchronized with an electrocardiogram tracing for even better evaluation of cardiac function.

Doppler ultrasound

Another method of ultrasonically monitoring the movement of tissue interfaces is based on the **Doppler effect.** Christian Johann Doppler noted in 1842 that the wavelength of light varied according to the relative motion of the source of light and the observer. If the source or observer or both are moving toward each other, the light received will have a shorter wavelength (higher frequency) than that emitted. On the other hand, if the source and observer are moving apart, the received light will have a lower frequency than that emitted.

Application of this effect in astronomy allows observers to determine the expansion and contraction of various parts of the universe. Stars moving away from the earth produce light that appears shifted to the red, or longer, wavelength region of the spectrum. Stars moving toward the earth appear more blue.

This effect is illustrated for sound in Fig. 34-19. A familiar example of the Doppler effect is that of the passing train. The sound from the whistle of the train appears very high pitched (high frequency, short wavelength) as it approaches an observer. When the train passes,

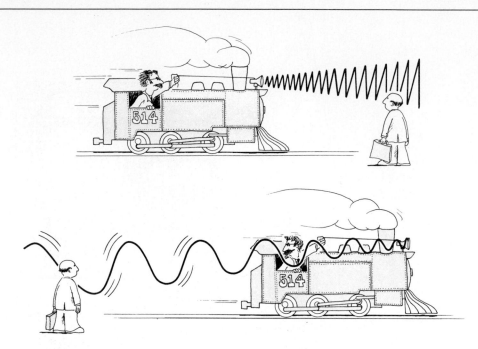

Fig. 34-19. Doppler effect describes the apparent change in frequency of emitted sound when either the source or the receiver is in motion. As a train passes, the pitch of its whistle changes from high to low.

however, the pitch makes an abrupt change to a lower note or lower frequency.

A continuous ultrasound beam is emitted in Doppler applications. When the reflected beam is received by the transducer, the change in frequency caused by the Doppler effect is electronically determined.

The mathematics associated with Doppler ultrasound to measure this frequency shift are rather simple. The frequency shift, F_D, is called the **Doppler shift frequency.** If F_T is the transmitted frequency and F_R the frequency of sound reflected from the moving tissue interface, then

(34-2)

$$F_D = F_T - F_R$$

However, if one knows the velocity of sound in the medium (V) and the velocity of the in-

terface (u), then the Doppler shift frequency becomes

(34-3)

$$F_D = F_T \frac{2u}{V}$$

EXAMPLE: Consider an ultrasound device designed to monitor fetal heartbeat by the Doppler method. If the transmitting frequency (F_T) is 2 MHz, the velocity of sound is 1540 m/s, and the velocity of the interface is 20 cm/s, what is the Doppler shift frequency?

ANSWER: $F_D = F_T \dfrac{2u}{V}$

$$= (2 \text{ MHz}) \left(\frac{2 \times 20 \text{ cm/s}}{1540 \text{ m/s}} \right)$$

$$= (2 \times 10^6/\text{s}) \left(\frac{0.4 \text{ m/s}}{1540 \text{ m/s}} \right)$$

$$= 519/\text{s}$$

$$= 519 \text{ Hz}$$

This illustrates one of the properties of Doppler ultrasound that makes it particularly effective for monitoring the fetal heart. The Doppler shift frequency is in the audible range, and therefore an audioamplifier and speaker are all that is necessary to listen to the fetal heart. It is sometimes called an **ultrasound stethoscope.**

The transducer used in Doppler ultrasound incorporates two crystals, one to transmit and one to receive. Because of this simplicity, the cost of a Doppler ultrasound unit is less than 10% of that of a compound B-scanner.

Real-time imaging

Real-time ultrasound is dynamic imaging. It is to compound B-mode what fluoroscopy is to radiography. Real-time ultrasound is finding increasing application in abdominal and obstetric imaging. It has several distinct advantages over B-mode imaging:

1. The cost of equipment can be considerably less.
2. The image obtained is not nearly so dependent on operator skill.
3. The time required for real-time examination is generally less because of the ease with which the equipment can be handled.
4. Several commercial versions are available, including mobile systems (Fig. 34-20).

The real-time transducer assembly is larger than a B-mode transducer; therefore, the ultrasonographer must make certain that the patient being examined is well oiled for proper acoustic coupling. The transducer probe is then moved over the surface of the patient in any direction and angle until the anatomic region of interest is found. The dynamic (moving) image may then be stored on videotape for subsequent viewing, or stop-action frame photographs may be obtained.

Real-time ultrasound does have disadvantages. The real-time image results from the ultrasound beam interacting with the tissue interface from only one direction, whereas with B-mode, one can move the transducer while storing the image from many directions for ul-

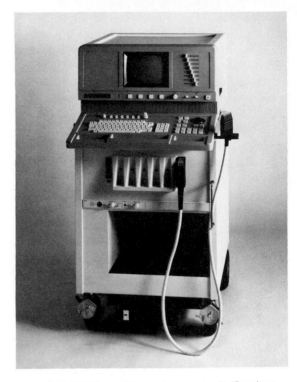

Fig. 34-20. Mobile real-time ultrasound unit. (Courtesy Acuson.)

timate composition. Consequently, the **lateral resolution is better with B-mode than with real time.**

The three types of real-time ultrasound devices are the mechanical device, the linear array, and the phased array.

Mechanical scanners. Mechanical assemblies were the first type of real-time scanners to be developed. Almost no mechanical scanners are manufactured now. These units employ a single or multiple transducers. Some employ a water bath for better acoustic coupling.

The transducer assembly is motorized so that the ultrasound beam is mechanically swept across the desired field of view in an oscillating fashion. Each sweep results in one **image frame,** and frame rates up to fifteen frames per second are possible. The mechanical arrangement allows the transducer to be moved in a linear fashion for a rectangular field of view or in an angular fashion for a sector field of view.

There were significant problems with early mechanical real-time ultrasound scanners. The frame rate was limited, the field of view was restricted, and distortion was commonplace. In addition, there were difficulties with the mechanical design, resulting in vibration and instability of the system. Consequently, mechanical real-time scanners, although available commercially, have not been popular.

Linear array scanning. Consider the line of thirty-two transducers contained in a single case, as illustrated in Fig. 34-21. Such a transducer assembly is called a **linear array.** If each transducer is small, for example, 2 mm, then the overall length of the active array will be 6.4 cm. This defines the field of view as a 6.4 cm field.

To accomplish real-time monitoring, each transducer is fired in sequence from number 1 to number 32, and this results in thirty-two **image scan lines.** These thirty-two scan lines then constitute one **frame** of information. The frame rate is sometimes selectable, but generally, for multiple-transducer real time, imaging is set at thirty frames per second.

When individual transducers are energized sequentially, they must remain active long enough to receive the reflected ultrasound wave. Such a system is identified as a **sequential linear array.** A **segmental linear array** is shown in Fig. 34-22. In a segmental linear array, four

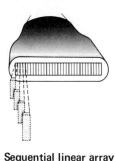

Fig. 34-21. Linear transducer array employing multiple transducers activated sequentially.

Sequential linear array

Fig. 34-22. Linear transducer array can be activated segmentally for enhanced image quality.

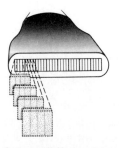

Segmental linear array

or five contiguous transducers are energized simultaneously so that each pulse of ultrasound results in four or five scan lines. In a typical system, transducers numbers 1 to 5 will be energized for one pulse and produce five scan lines. The second ultrasound pulse will be emitted by transducers 2 to 6, which again will produce five scan lines of information. Next, transducers 3 to 7 are energized to produce an additional five scan lines of information. The advantage of the segmental linear array is that it provides for increased image line density over the sequential array and consequently results in better image quality.

The linear array results in a rectangular image format, the lateral dimensions of which are determined by the physical size of the transducer assembly; the depth of penetration is a function of ultrasound frequency.

The lateral resolution is limited by the center-to-center distance of each transducer element and the frequency of operation. Since it is necessary to pack a number of transducers along a short distance, the far-field ultrasound pattern becomes very poor because of the small size of each transducer. This contributes to the poor lateral resolution. Acoustic focusing can be employed to improve this lateral resolution.

Phased array scanners. The phased array transducer assembly is very similar to the linear array. The phased array device incorporates **segmental excitation** of the transducer elements, but the electronic control of emission and reception results in a sector scan. The sector scan is accomplished not only by segmental sequencing of the transducer elements, but also by electronic circuitry incorporating **delay** to precisely time the excitation and reception of ultrasound by each transducer element.

If the thirty-two transducer elements of a linear array are excited simultaneously, the result is similar to the pulsing of a single transducer having a diameter equal to the length of the transducer array. A plane wave front is emitted (Fig. 34-23, *A*). If the linear array is excited in

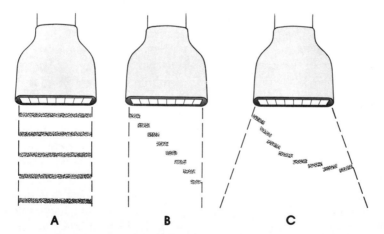

Fig. 34-23. **A,** Linear transducer array will emit a plane wave front if transducers are excited simultaneously. **B,** It will emit a series of parallel wave fronts if transducers are excited segmentally. **C,** With phased electronic circuitry control, each segmental plane wave can be directed.

segmental fashion, a series of wave fronts will be emitted, all parallel to one another and all traveling in the forward direction (Fig. 34-23, B). If the excitation of each transducer in each segment is delayed somewhat from its neighbor, it is possible to direct the plane wave front at an angle from the transducer face rather than directly forward (Fig. 34-23, C). The delaying of excitation of each transducer element is known as phasing, and such an assembly is called a **phased array.**

Phased array imaging produces a sector scan having a maximum sector angle of 90 degrees. The sector is produced by steering the ultrasound wave front through phased segmental excitation of the transducer elements. The scan line rate, frame rate, and depth of scan are interdependent and are often operator selectable. Electronic delay lines on the receiver circuitry allow some depth of focusing by synchronizing the returning reflected pulses.

To accommodate the sector-scanning nature of the phased array, the total transducer size is smaller than that for the linear array—generally 1 to 3 cm in length. The individual transducers are so small that they begin to radiate isotropically as a point source, and this increases the noise of the system and degrades the image somewhat. The axial resolution with the phased array system approaches that which is possible with a single-element transducer of comparable size. The lateral resolution is poor, as with the linear array, but can be improved somewhat with the use of acoustic focusing.

The scan line rate is determined by the size of the transducer and the rate at which it is pulsed. The frame rate is a function of overall transducer size and pulse rate. The depth of scan is a function of transducer frequency and electronic delay line circuitry that allows depth focusing by synchronizing returning pulses.

Experience has shown that the minimum acceptable scan line concentration is one line per millimeter for rectangular scans and one line per degree for sector scans.

The **annular phased array** is an extension of the linear phased array in which transducers are arranged in concentric rings. The electronics are more difficult, but multiple-plane images are possible.

Currently, phased array real-time ultrasound is the principal ultrasonic imaging technique. A promising extension of this technique is the **duplex scanner,** which incorporates a multielement transducer for real-time phased array imaging with Doppler detection of motion. Such systems are finding great application in blood flow imaging. Blood vessel wall, plaque, and lumen are presented as B-scan images and blood flow is detected by Doppler frequency shifts, all in real time. With color imaging, even the direction of blood flow is shown. Red indicates the blood is flowing away, and blue indicates it is flowing toward the transducer. The relative velocity of flow is indicated by the intensity of the color.

BIOLOGIC EFFECTS

Diagnostic ultrasound was introduced into obstetric practice in 1966 and is now a routinely employed clinical tool. Because such examinations occur at a time of particular sensitivity of the fetus to all environmental influences, it is absolutely essential that we understand the effects of ultrasound and the doses required to cause those effects. **We know that no manifest injury or late effect has ever occurred in humans exposed to diagnostic levels of medical ultrasound.** We also know that much higher levels can produce measurable effects. Additional research is in process in many laboratories to define the effects, if any, of diagnostic levels of ultrasound.

Because of past experience with ionizing radiation and the many years required to precisely identify the nature and degree of its hazard, physicians are somewhat timid in their application of diagnostic ultrasound. Since the available evidence indicates no effect at these levels, a diagnostic ultrasound examination should never be refused out of fear of radiation effects.

Mechanisms of action

An expression used by radiobiologists to describe the manner in which radiation produces a biologic effect is **the mechanism of action.** For ionizing radiation, the mechanism of action is ionization and excitation. For ultrasound, the mechanism of action is temperature elevation, cavitation, and various viscous stresses.

Thermal effects

Ultrasound irradiation can elevate the temperature of tissue through molecular agitation and the relaxation processes previously described. Extremely intense levels are required to produce a measurable temperature elevation in tissue. The hazard from temperature elevation is, of course, not specific to ultrasound. At the local tissue level, temperature elevation can result in structural changes in macromolecules and membranes and changes in the rates of biochemical reactions.

Cavitation

Even in the absence of elevated temperature, ultrasound-induced structural and functional changes in macromolecules and cells can occur. Such changes are often associated with the phenomenon of **cavitation.** When an aqueous suspension such as tissue is irradiated with ultrasound, if the relaxation forces are sufficiently violent, tiny bubbles of gas, or cavities, will form. As cavitation increases, more energy is absorbed from the incident ultrasound beam. Cavitation can result in the disruption of molecular bonds and the production of the free radicals H* and OH* produced by the dissociation of H_2O vapor.

Viscous stresses

When a tissue interface is present, the viscosity of tissue on each side of the interface will probably not be equal. As ultrasound interacts along this interface, the differences in the viscosity result in a force known as a **viscous stress** exerted on the boundary. In cellular layers near the boundary, small-scale fluid motions called **microstreaming** are produced as a viscous stress. Such stresses can disrupt membranes and cells in the region of the interface.

Effects on living tissue

If the ultrasound intensity is sufficiently high, many of the effects earlier described as resulting from ionizing radiation exposure can be produced. Chemical bonds can be disrupted, macromolecules can be degraded, chromosome aberrations can be produced, and cells can be killed. To observe such effects, ultrasound intensities in excess of 10 W/cm² delivered over considerable periods of time are necessary.

At the whole-body level the only effects of any significance that can be measured are those associated with irradiation in utero. All the information available in this regard has been obtained from experimental animal irradiation using ultrasound intensity orders of magnitude higher than those employed in diagnostic ultrasound. Irradiation early in pregnancy, through the period of major organogenesis, results in an elevated level of prenatal and neonatal death. Irradiation during organogenesis can result in gross congenital abnormalities. No such human effects have been observed. No evidence for ultrasound-induced latent malignant disease exists.

Dose-response relationships

None of the results just cited as either whole-body effects or molecular and cellular effects has been observed following diagnostic levels of ultrasound. Diagnostic ultrasound is emitted in the intensity range of 1 to 10 mW/cm².

The absolute minimum dose level reported for observable effects in experimental specimens is 100 mW/cm² and then only following many hours of continuous radiation. Fig. 34-24 is a summary of the results of many experiments de-

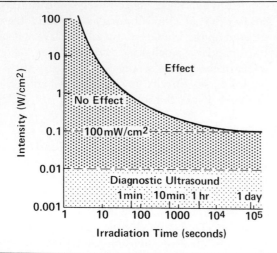

Fig. 34-24. Minimum ultrasound intensity levels reported to produce measurable biologic effects and the associated irradiation time.

signed to identify the lowest intensity level necessary to produce an effect. This composite evaluation shows the effects of ultrasound to be a function of both intensity and time of exposure. The higher the intensity, the shorter is the exposure necessary to produce an effect. At intensities in the diagnostic ultrasound range, however, no duration of exposure has been shown to produce an effect. Consequently, we presume that ultrasound-induced bioeffects are threshold in nature.

The American Institute of Ultrasound in Medicine (AIUM) recently issued the following statement on the clinical safety of diagnostic ultrasound:

Diagnostic ultrasound has been in use for over 25 years. Given its known benefits and recognized efficacy for medical diagnosis, including use during human pregnancy, the American Institute of Ultrasound in Medicine herein addresses the clinical safety of such use: 'No confirmed biological effects on patients or instrument operators caused by exposures at intensities of present diagnostic instruments have ever been reported. Although the possibility exists that such biological effects may be identified in the future, current data indicate that the benefits to patients of the prudent use of diagnostic ultrasound outweigh the risks, if any, that may be present.'

REVIEW QUESTIONS

1. Define or otherwise identify:
   a. Reverberation
   b. Doppler effect
   c. Wave front
   d. M-mode
   e. Scan convertor
   f. Axial resolution
   g. Phased array
   h. Cavitation
   i. Near field
2. Diagram an ultrasound transducer and identify the function of each part.
3. Describe how the near field and the far field vary with transducer size and frequency of operation.
4. What limits lateral resolution?
5. Using a 2.25 MHz transducer in the Doppler mode, a reflected beam has frequency of 2.12 MHz. What is the Doppler frequency?
6. What is the Doppler frequency from question 5 if the beam is reflected from an interface whose velocity is 8 cm/s?
7. Describe the characteristics of A-mode, B-mode, M-mode, and Doppler ultrasound.
8. What is the difference between sequential arrays and segmental arrays?
9. Discuss the advantages and disadvantages to linear arrays.
10. What is the shape of the dose-response relationship for ultrasound?

Sources for supplementary teaching materials

American Association of Physicists in Medicine
335 East 45th Street
New York, New York 10017

American College of Medical Physics
Medical University of South Carolina
171 Ashley Avenue
Charleston, South Carolina 29425

American College of Radiology
1891 Preston White Drive
Reston, Virginia 22091

American Society of Radiologic Technologists
15000 Central Avenue S.E.
Albuquerque, New Mexico 87123

Center for Devices and Radiological Health
5600 Fishers Lane
Rockville, Maryland 20857

Continuing Professional Education Center, Inc.
127 Wall Street
Princeton, New Jersey 08540

Eastman Kodak Company
Radiography Markets Division
343 State Street
Rochester, New York 14650

E.I. du Pont de Nemours & Co., Inc.
Photo Products Department
Wilmington, Delaware 19898

General Electric Medical Systems
4855 N. Electric
Milwaukee, Wisconsin 53201

Liebel-Flarsheim Company
2111 East Galbraith Road
Cincinnati, Ohio 45208

The Machlett Laboratories, Inc.
1063 Hope Street
Stamford, Connecticut 06909

Mallinckrodt Inc.
675 McDonnell Boulevard
St. Louis, Missouri 63127

National Council on Radiation Protection and
    Measurements
7910 Woodmont Avenue
Bethesda, Maryland 20814

Phillips Medical Systems, Inc.
710 Bridgeport Avenue
Shelton, Connecticut 06484

Picker International
595 Miner Road
Highland Heights, Ohio 44143

Radiological Society of North America, Inc.
1415 West 22nd Street
Oak Brook, Illinois 60521

Siemens Medical Systems, Inc.
186 Wood Avenue South
Iselin, New Jersey 08830

U.S. Nuclear Regulatory Commission
Office of Information
Washington, D.C. 20555

Victoreen, Inc.
10101 Woodland Avenue
Cleveland, Ohio 44104

APPENDIX B

Universal constants

Table B-1. Universal constants

Constant	Unit
Avogadro's number	$N_a = 6.02 \times 10^{23}$ atoms/g atomic weight
Planck's constant	$h = 6.62 \times 10^{-27}$ erg-s
	$= 6.62 \times 10^{-34}$ J-s
	$= 4.15 \times 10^{-15}$ eV-s
Velocity of light	$c = 3 \times 10^{8}$ m/s
	$= 3 \times 10^{10}$ cm/s
Base of natural logarithms	$e = 2.7183$
Pi	$\pi = 3.1416$
Electronic charge	$e = 1.6 \times 10^{-19}$ C
	$= 4.8 \times 10^{-10}$ esu
	$= 1.6 \times 10^{-20}$ emu

Useful units in radiology

Table C-1. SI prefixes

Factor	Prefix	Symbol
10^{18}	Exa	E
10^{15}	Peta	P
10^{12}	Tera	T
10^{9}	Giga	G
10^{6}	Mega	M
10^{3}	Kilo	k
10^{2}	Hecto	h
10^{1}	Deca	da
10^{-1}	Deci	d
10^{-2}	Centi	c
10^{-3}	Milli	m
10^{-6}	Micro	μ
10^{-9}	Nano	n
10^{-12}	Pico	p
10^{-15}	Femto	f
10^{-18}	Atto	a

Table C-2. SI base units

Quantity	Name	Symbol
Length	Meter	m
Mass	Kilogram	kg
Time	Second	s
Electric current	Ampere	A

Table C-3. SI derived units expressed in terms of base units

Quantity	SI unit Name	SI unit Symbol
Area	Square meter	m^2
Volume	Cubic meter	m^3
Speed, velocity	Meter per second	m/s
Acceleration	Meter per second squared	m/s^2
Density, mass density	Kilogram per cubic meter	kg/m^3
Current density	Ampere per square meter	A/m^2
Concentration (of amount of substance)	Mole per cubic meter	$mole/m^3$
Specific volume	Cubic meter per kilogram	m^3/kg

Table C-4. SI derived units with special names

Quantity	SI unit			
	Name	Symbol	Expression in terms of other units	Expression in terms of SI base units
Frequency	Hertz	Hz		$1/s$
Force	Newton	N		$m\ kg/s^2$
Pressure, stress	Pascal	Pa	N/m^2	kg/ms^2
Energy, work, quantity of heat	Joule	J	N m	$m^2\ kg/s^2$
Power	Watt	W	J/s	$m^2\ kg/s^3$
Electric charge	Coulomb	C		s A
Electric potential	Volt	V	W/A	$m^2\ kg/As^3$
Capacitance	Farad	F	C/V	$sA^2/m^2\ kg$
Electric resistance	Ohm	Ω	V/A	$m^2\ kgA^2/s^3$
Conductance	Siemens	S	A/V	$s^3A^2/m^2\ kg$
Magnetic flux	Weber	Wb	V s	$m^2\ kg/s^2A$
Magnetic field (B)	Tesla	T	Wb/m^2	kg/s^2A
Luminous flux	Lumen	lm		cd sr

Table C-5. Summary of new and old radiologic units

Quantity	Name	Symbol	Expression	
			Other units	SI base units
Activity	Bequerel (curie)	Bq (Ci)	3.7×10^{10} Bq	$1/s$
Absorbed dose	Gray (rad)	Gy (rad)	J/kg (10^{-2} Gy)	m^2/s^2
Dose equivalent	Sievert (rem)	Sv (rem)	J/kg (10^{-2} Sv)	m^2/s^2
Exposure	Coulomb per kilogram (roentgen)	R	C/kg (2.58×10^{-4} C/kg)	sA/kg

APPENDIX D

Conversion tables

Table D-1. Length

Unit	Equivalent in meters
1 centimeter (cm)	10^{-2} meter (m)
1 micron (μm)	10^{-6} meter
1 nanometer (nm)	10^{-9} meter
1 angstrom (Å)	10^{-10} meter
1 mile (mi)	1609 meters

Table D-2. Mass-energy*

Electron volts	Joules	Grams	Atomic mass units
1.0	1.60×10^{-19}	1.78×10^{-33}	1.07×10^{-9}
6.24×10^{18}	1.0	1.11×10^{-14}	6.69×10^{9}
5.61×10^{32}	8.99×10^{13}	1.0	6.02×10^{23}
9.32×10^{8}	1.49×10^{-10}	1.66×10^{-24}	1.0

*(1 J = 10^{7} ergs; 4.19 J = 1 calorie; 1 BTU = 1.06×10^{10} ergs.)

Table D-3. Time

Years	Days	Hours	Minutes	Seconds
1	365	8.75×10^{3}	5.26×10^{5}	3.15×10^{7}
	1	24	1.44×10^{3}	8.64×10^{4}
		1	60	3.6×10^{3}
			1	60

Review of basic physics

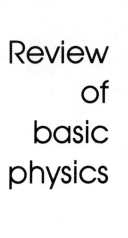

ELECTROSTATICS

1. The addition or removal of electrons is called electrification.
2. Like charges repel; unlike charges attract.
3. Coulomb's law of electrostatic force:

$$F = c \frac{Q_A Q_B}{d^2}$$

4. Only negative charges can move in solids.
5. Electrostatic charge is distributed on outer surface.
6. The concentration of charge is greater when the radius of curvature is greater.

ELECTRODYNAMICS

Ohm's law: $V = IR$
A series circuit:

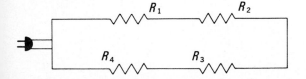

1. $V_T = V_1 + V_2 + V_3 + V_4$
2. I is the same through all elements.
3. $R_T = R_1 + R_2 + R_3 + R_4$

A parallel circuit:

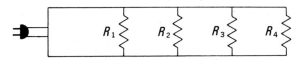

1. V is the same across each circuit element.
2. $I_T = I_1 + I_2 + I_3 + I_4$
3. $\dfrac{1}{R_T} = \dfrac{1}{R_1} + \dfrac{1}{R_2} + \dfrac{1}{R_3} + \dfrac{1}{R_4}$

Electric power: $P = IV = I^2R$ [(A) (V) = W]
Work: $Work = QV$ [(C) (V) = erg]
Potential: $V = Q/x$ [C/cm = V]
Capacitance: $C = Q/V$ [C/V = F]

MAGNETISM

1. Every magnet has a north pole and a south pole.
2. Like poles repel; unlike poles attract.
3. Gauss's law:

$$F = k \frac{M_1 M_2}{d^2}$$

ELECTROMAGNETISM

1. A magnetic field is always present around a conductor in which a current is flowing.
2. Changing magnetic fields can produce an electric potential.
3. Transformer law:

$$\frac{V_p}{V_s} = \frac{N_p}{N_s}$$

CLASSICAL PHYSICS

Linear force: $F = ma$ [(kg)(m/s^2) = N]
Momentum: $p = mv$ [(kg)(m/s)]
Mechanical work (or energy): $Work$ (or E) = Fs
   [(N)(m) = J]
Kinetic energy: $E = \frac{1}{2}mv^2$ [(kg)(m^2/s^2) = J]
Mechanical power: $P = Fs/t$ [(N)(m)/s = J/s]

Conservation of momentum between A and B*:

$$m_A v_A + m_B v_B = m_A v_A' + m_B v_B'$$

Conservation of kinetic energy between A and B*:

$$\tfrac{1}{2}m_A(v_A)^2 + \tfrac{1}{2}m_B(v_B)^2 = \tfrac{1}{2}m_A(v_A')^2 + (\tfrac{1}{2}m_B')^2$$

---

*v, Initial velocity; v', final velocity.

Answers
to
numeric
questions

CHAPTER 1

3. 86,000 V; 0.2 A
4. 36,000 eV
5. 0.015 R

CHAPTER 2

4. a. $^{33}/_{32}$
   b. $^{13}/_{24}$
   c. 18
5. a. 0.7
   b. 0.081
   c. 0.467
6. a. 1.48×10^{6}
   b. 4×10^{-3}
   c. 7.11×10^{5}
7. a. 8×10^{10}
   b. 4×10^{10}
   c. $x = 1$
   d. $x = 2\frac{1}{7}$
8. 118 N; 19.6 N
9. 8045 J
10. 68 kg, 13.9 m/s^{2}

CHAPTER 3

2. a. 17 orders of magnitude
   b. 0.0000000001 m and 10,000,000 m

3.
Atom	Protons	Neutrons	Electrons	Nucleons
$^{17}_{8}O$	8	9	8	17
$^{27}_{13}Al$	13	14	13	27
$^{60}_{27}Co$	27	33	27	60
$^{226}_{88}Ra$	88	138	88	226

4. 100.03463 amu; 1.66×10^{-22} g
6. 200 electrons
7. (a) 57.4 keV, (b) 66.7 keV, (c) 69.5 keV
9. (a) 5 Ci, (b) 3.8 Ci, (c) 277 mCi

CHAPTER 4

3. 400 m/s; 2400 m, or about 1½ miles
4. 3×10^{12} Hz
5. 2.88 m
6. 9.6×10^{18} Hz
7. 2.6×10^{19} Hz; 1.13×10^{-11} m
8. 1.76×10^{-14} J; 1.18×10^{-4} amu
9. 0.75 mR/mAs; 0.93 mR/mAs
10. 7.1 mR/mAs

CHAPTER 5

2. The electrostatic force will be reduced to one fourth its original value.
3. The magnetic force will be reduced to one fourth its original value.
4. 1.56×10^{20} electrons; 0.14 μg
5. (a) 50 Ω, (b) 2.4 Ω
6. (a) 2.2 A, (b) 45.8 A
7. (a) 70 V, (b) 16.8 V
8. (a) 242 W, (b) 5042 W

CHAPTER 6

4. 242 kV
5. 27
6. 6.6 kW; yes
7. 1000 to 1
8. 100 A
9. 120; 60; 1; 6; 1
10. 100%; 100%; 13%; 4%

CHAPTER 7

3. The rotating target will have 94 times more area than the stationary target.
4. 302.5 V
5. 71.7 V peak
6. 5 V
7. 6 A
8. 30 dashes
9. 104.5 kV

CHAPTER 8

2. a. 66.7 keV; 0.0186 nm
   b. 12.02 keV; 0.103 nm
4. 0.59
7. 0.014 nm
8. 12.15 cm²; 886 mR/s

CHAPTER 9

3. 23.962 keV
4. Approximately 96
8. 38.9 keV; 9.28 keV; 11.505 keV; 12.023 keV; 12.1 keV
10. 653; 1

CHAPTER 10

1. d. 15%
3. 667 mR
4. 1083 mR
5. 1.32 times
6. 100 mAs
7. (a) 48 mR, (b) 39 mR
8. 2.6 mm Al; 4.4 mm Al
9. 3.2 mm Al
10. a. 196 mR
    b. 148 mR
    c. 127 mR

CHAPTER 11

3. 0.75×0.92 inch

CHAPTER 12

3. a. 13%; 8%; 4%
   b. 87%; 92%; 96%
4. a. 0.33
   b. 1.10
   c. 1.13
5. 8:1
6. 85 lines/in
7. 8%
8. a. 369 μm
   b. 8.7:1
   c. 5.6%
9. 1.8
10. 5×12 inches

CHAPTER 15

6. 20

CHAPTER 16

4. 3; black
5. 2.5
6. A is faster. A, 67; B, 22
7. 11.1 cm
8. 0.07 mm

CHAPTER 17

4. 80 mAs
5. 1200 mA
6. 10 ms

CHAPTER 18
5. 4212
8. 3.75 cm
10. 24 mm

CHAPTER 19
5. 20; 19.5; 17.4; 2.6; 2.1; 0.5 keV
7. 2.8 times as high

CHAPTER 20
8. 4.096×10^9 bits
9. a. 11
   b. 1101
   c. 1001000
   d. 10010011
   e. 1110010101110
10. a. 11
   b. 17
   c. 49
   d. 114
   e. 171

CHAPTER 21
8. 102,400
9. 0.2 mm
10. 256 gray levels

CHAPTER 22
2. 22.5 degrees
4. 60
5. $0.2 \ mm^3$
6. 0.63 mm
7. 0.4 mm

CHAPTER 23
3. 86 MHz
4. 11 MHz, 65 MHz
6. 20 MHz

CHAPTER 24
3. 2 T

CHAPTER 25
3. Seven x-ray rooms
4. One x-ray room
5. Two x-ray rooms
6. Yes initially, but 5742 square feet would be needed after 5 years of growth.

CHAPTER 26
7. 0.85
8. 2.7

CHAPTER 27
3. $HOH^+ + e^-$; $H^+ + OH^*$; $OH^- + H^*$
4. 5%
5. 4.5

CHAPTER 28
3. 300 rad; 500 rad

CHAPTER 29
3. 1.2
4. 15 cases/10^6 persons/rad/yr
5. 4.5

CHAPTER 30
2. 252 mR
3. 4.32 R
4. 933 mrad
8. 12.5 mR/hr
9. 281 mR
10. 0.26 mR

CHAPTER 31
5. 1207
10. 427 mA min/wk

CHAPTER 32
10. 973 mR

CHAPTER 33
3. 3.5 cm
5. 30.8 dB
6. $7.29 \times 10^6 \ kg/m^2 \ s^1$
7. 6.4 km
8. 2000 pulses/s
9. 0.68 mm

CHAPTER 34
5. 130 kHz
6. 233 Hz

Index